Basic
pharmacology
for nurses

Basic pharmacology for nurses

JESSIE E. SQUIRE, R.N., B.A., M.Ed.

Professor Emeritus, De Anza College School of Nursing,
Cupertino, California, Foothill Junior College District;
formerly Instructor, Foothill College School of Vocational Nursing,
Los Altos Hills, California, Foothill Junior College District;
formerly Instructor, Hayward-Fairmont School of Vocational Nursing,
Hayward Adult and Technical School, Hayward Unified School District,
Hayward, California

BRUCE D. CLAYTON, B.S., Pharm.D.

Associate Professor and Vice-Chairman, Department of Pharmacy Practice,
College of Pharmacy, University of Nebraska Medical Center,
Omaha, Nebraska

SEVENTH EDITION

Illustrated

The C. V. Mosby Company

ST. LOUIS • TORONTO • LONDON   1981

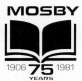

MOSBY

1906 **75** 1981
YEARS

A TRADITION OF PUBLISHING EXCELLENCE

SEVENTH EDITION

Previous editions copyrighted 1957, 1961, 1965, 1969, 1973,
1977

Printed in the United States of America

The C. V. Mosby Company
11830 Westline Industrial Drive, St. Louis, Missouri 63141

Library of Congress Cataloging in Publication Data

Squire, Jessie E
  Basic pharmacology for nurses.

  Bibliography: p.
  Includes index.
  1. Pharmacology. 2. Nursing. I. Clayton,
Bruce D., 1947-   joint author. II. Title.
[DNLM: 1. Pharmacology—Nursing texts. QV 4
S777b]
RM300.S67   1981   615'.1   80-26574
ISBN 0-8016-4743-6

AC/VH/VH 9 8 7 6 5 4   03/C/314

Preface

The original purpose of this book remains intact: to motivate the learner to administer medications with concern for safety, precision, and attention to important physiologic factors. The responsibility for teaching the patient has added a dimension to the nursing role that must be developed at the basic level. This text can assist in that dimension, as a self-help tool in the basic program and as a quick review for the graduate nurse.

This text presents basic information related to drug administration, source, purpose, effect, side effects, contraindications, route, and dosage. It provides important considerations in accurate dosage, apothecary and metric measurements, conversion techniques, calibrated instruments for measure and administration, multiple and unit dosage concepts, the use of various syringes, and opportunities for practice in the preparation and administration of medicines.

Many of the procedures and practice lessons have been designed not only for class study and participation but also for self-teaching. These have proved a definite aid to students for home study after class presentation of the subject and to many graduates as a means of independent study. The student should be urged to form a habit of using a medical dictionary and the detailed and helpful glossary at the end of the text for unfamiliar terms.

The time planned for presentation of the text depends on the individual using the text. The self-learner will set a pace necessary to achieve preset goals. The instructor may wish to allow 50 to 60 hours as a course presentation.

We have prepared the chapters on drugs affecting body systems to fulfill two purposes simultaneously:

1. These chapters can be used as a separate unit for review of basic factual knowledge of effects and dosage of drugs. Drugs affecting a particular body system may be discussed in conjunction with clinical experience involving the particular body system and the course in body structure itself.
2. The chapters can be integrated with fundamental courses and clinical conferences pertaining to the care of patient for valuable associative learning in the total care of the patient.

These purposes complement each other, and the repetition is of great value in the learning process. If extensive arithmetic review is needed, our suggestion is that 24 to 30 hours be devoted to this review in a separate course or as a preentrance course that makes use of a basic elementary school arithmetic text.

For this seventh edition we have again reviewed the suggestions offered by our readers and have revised the text to incorporate these suggestions wherever feasible. We offer our gratitude and sincere appreciation for this assistance.

The following revisions have been made in the seventh edition:

1. Many new drugs and their main effects, dosages, side effects, and interactions have been added.
2. Certain chapters with similar information have been combined to permit greater continuity.
3. All chapters have been reviewed to eliminate drugs seldom or no longer used.
4. Greater emphasis has been placed on drug action, side effects, and drug interactions to help the student anticipate adverse effects before they become severe.
5. Additional illustrations and tables have been placed in various chapters to aid in the learning process.
6. New information has been added on intravenous therapy, physiologic concepts, administration techniques, and nursing responsibilities.
7. All end-of-chapter assignments have been rewritten and include questions on additional drugs. Questions are presented to follow the order of the chapter material. Many assignments end with questions on drug dosage as a review of basic arithmetic and dosage.

As in the sixth edition, the student can complete the test questions in the assignments at the end of each chapter that cover the material presented thus far by the instructor, hand in answers to the test questions at the beginning of the next class hour, ask for any explanations needed, and thus use the tests for preparation for class examinations.

v

Our thanks and sincere appreciation are extended to the many student nurses and graduate nurses and reviewers of our text for their most helpful suggestions and criticisms. A special note of thanks must go to Francine E. Clayton for her encouragement and support of this edition.

Jessie E. Squire
Bruce D. Clayton

Contents

CHAPTER 1

Pharmacology, therapeutic methods, and drugs

PHARMACOLOGY

1. Pharmacology (Greek: *pharmakon,* drugs; *logos,* science) deals with the study of drugs and their actions.
2. Emphasis is placed on the interactions of chemical compounds and living systems.

THERAPEUTIC METHODS

1. The different ways diseases can be treated are called therapeutic methods.
2. Examples of therapeutic methods are:
   a. Drug therapy—treatment with drugs.
   b. Hormonal therapy—treatment with preparations from endocrine glands of animals, such as:
      (1) Insulin from the pancreas of cattle, sheep, pigs, and fish
      (2) Thyroid extracts from the thyroid glands of any food animal
   c. Diet therapy—treatment with diet, for example:
      (1) Reducing diets to cause loss of weight
      (2) Sugar-free diets for diabetes
      (3) Low-salt diets for kidney disease
   d. Serum therapy—treatment with serums to lessen the effects of allergic disorders.
   e. Physiotherapy—treatment with natural physical forces, such as:
      (1) Water
      (2) Light
      (3) Heat

DRUGS

1. Drugs (Dutch: *droog,* dry) are chemical substances used as medicines.
2. Long ago, dried plants probably were the greatest source of medicines, thus the word *drug* was applied to them.

Nineteenth-century drug therapy

Our modern approaches to drug therapy are rooted in the primitive origins of mankind and require more time and space than one text can cover. Some important contributions of the nineteenth century were:

1. Chemistry gradually became known as a highly specialized science, with biochemistry and pharmaceutical chemistry as important subdivisions.
2. Famous pharmaceutical discoveries of this period included:
   a. Discovery of the alkaloid morphine, obtained from opium, by a German apothecary, Sertürner, 1815.
   b. Discovery of quinine, strychnine, and veratrine by Pelletier and Caventou.
   c. Discovery of emetine by Pelletier and Magendie.
   d. Discovery of atropine by Brandes.
   e. Discovery of codeine by Robiquet.
   f. Discovery and use of ether as a general anesthetic by Dr. Crawford W. Long of Georgia, 1842.
   g. Use of chloroform as a general anesthetic by Dr. J. T. Simpson (Sir J. T. Simpson), 1847.
   h. The first of the coal-tar products, synthetic organic compounds, appeared about 1856.
      (1) Trying to discover a synthetic quinine, Perkin instead discovered the first coal-tar dye, called "Perkin's purple" or mauve.
      (2) This led to the preparation in the laboratory of a large family of medicinal agents, such as salicylic and benzoic acids, which duplicated products previously obtained from natural sources. Others were new to science, such as antipyrine and acetanilid, forerunners to today's analgesics, aspirin, and acetaminophen.
3. These discoveries and the invention of many new and convenient dosage forms led to the establishment of large-scale manufacturing plants, which made it possible to administer drugs in attractive and palatable forms for accurate dosage.
4. The first of the important national pharmacopeias appeared.
   a. The French *Codex* (1818) was first to be produced.

1

b. The first *Pharmacopeia of the United States of America* appeared in 1820.

c. The national standard for Great Britain was printed in 1864 and replaced those used in London, Edinburgh, and Dublin.

d. The pharmacopeia for Germany appeared in 1872, replacing numerous local volumes.

5. Philosophically, drug therapy began to replace empiricism.

a. Fewer drugs were prescribed, and those prescriptions given were accompanied with greater knowledge of their action.

b. Purging and bloodletting declined in popular use.

c. Harmful patent medicine and nostrums were exposed, and legal action to protect the patient's safety began to be taken.

Twentieth-century drug therapy

1. In the twentieth century, an era of great progress in medicine and pharmacy, pharmacology was emphasized.

a. The strengthening and improving of the work of the professional organizations, such as the American Pharmaceutical Association and the American Society of Hospital Pharmacists.

b. The promotion of legislation controlling the experimentation, manufacture, and sale of food, drugs, and cosmetics. The most important acts to achieve positive legislation controlling the manufacture and sale of drugs were the U.S. Food and Drug Acts of 1906, 1938, and 1962, the Harrison Narcotic Act of 1914, and the Controlled Substances Act of 1970.

2. More progress in pharmacology has probably been made in the past 50 years than in all the years before this period. Such changes occurred probably because of the changing concepts concerning the causes of disease. The development of many biologic preparations, such as the vaccines, antitoxins, serums, and antibiotics, and the synthetic production of drugs in the laboratory helped make this period a time of great progress.

3. A few key discoveries in this century that benefited mankind included:

a. 1908—Synthesis of sulfanilamide, an antibacterial agent, by Gelmo, a German organic chemist.

b. 1912—Phenobarbital, a sedative-hypnotic and anticonvulsant, was introduced.

c. 1918—The effects of quinidine in atrial fibrillation were reported by Frey.

d. 1922—Discovery of insulin by Banting and Best in their laboratory in Toronto, Canada.

e. 1930s—Development of many sulfonamide derivatives as antiinfective agents. A few (sulfamethoxazole, sulfisoxazole, and sulfasalazine) are still in common use.

f. 1938—Phenytoin was introduced for the symptomatic treatment of epilepsy by Merritt and Putnam.

g. 1941—The first patient was treated with penicillin.

h. 1948—The first of the adrenocorticosteroids, cortisone, was used in medicine.

i. 1952—Chlorpromazine, first of many phenothiazine derivatives, was used in psychiatric patients.

j. 1954—Meprobamate, first of the "minor tranquilizers," was introduced to medical therapy.

k. 1957—Chlordiazepoxide, first of the benzodiazepine derivatives, was released.

l. 1958—Haloperidol, a major antipsychotic agent, became available.

m. 1966-70—Levodopa was studied and then released, opening a new era in the treatment of parkinsonism.

The 1960s and 1970s have shown major advances in the refinement of chemical agents for the control of infection and the treatment of hypertension, psychiatric disorders, ulcer disease, and various forms of cancer. The twentieth century has often been called the golden age in pharmacy and medicine, but many new drugs and treatments in the field of medicine yet remain to be discovered. What will the future bring?

ASSIGNMENT

1. Define pharmacology. On what is the emphasis in pharmacology placed?

2. Explain the meaning of therapeutic methods. Outline the examples of therapeutic methods and their examples.

3. What is the origin of the word *drugs?* What is the meaning of the word drugs? Long ago, what were the greatest source of medicines?

4. Outline some important contributions of the nineteenth century to drug therapy, as discussed under #2 of important contributions, a through h.

5. What led to the establishment of large-scale manufacturing plants for drugs? What caused the administration of drugs in attractive and palatable forms for accurate dosage?

6. List the first of the important national pharmacopeias and tell when it appeared.

7. Philosophically, drug therapy began to replace empiricism. What does empiricism mean? What changes occurred because of this?

8. In twentieth-century drug therapy, what changes occurred?

9. Name the three most important acts to achieve positive legislation during the twentieth century and give their dates. You will read about and hear about these acts fre-

quently throughout your pharmacology course and during your life as a nurse. Be familiar with them.

10. Outline the key drug discoveries that benefited mankind in this century. Be familiar with this list and the dates of these discoveries. Can you see how difficult it would be to decide which ones were the most important discoveries?

11. What have been major advances in drug therapy during the 1960s and 1970s?

12. Which century has been called the golden age in pharmacy and medicine? Do you think it will always remain so?

CHAPTER 2

Sources, names, information sources, and standards

FOUR MAJOR SOURCES (ORIGINS) OF DRUGS
Animal sources

1. An example of a drug from an animal source is thyroid.
   a. Thyroid is obtained from the thyroid gland in the neck of pigs and cattle.
   b. The thyroid glands are dried and the fat is removed. The dried glandular substance is then made into tablets. This substance may be further purified until only the important active substances remain. These pure compounds are thyroxine and triiodothyronine.
   c. Thyroid medicine is used to treat hypothyroidism, a condition caused by deficiency of thyroid hormone. In this condition, there is too little secretion of thyroxin from the thyroid gland.
2. Another example of a drug from an animal source is insulin.
   a. Insulin is obtained from the pancreas ("sweetbread") of animals such as sheep, hogs, and cattle. The pancreas is an organ found behind the stomach in many of the lower animals and in human beings.
   b. Insulin is used to treat and control diabetes mellitus. One of the numerous symptoms of this disease is sugar in the urine.

Vegetable or plant sources

1. Drugs from vegetable sources are obtained by drying the roots, bark, sap, leaves, flowers, and seeds of medicinal plants. They are then prepared for medicinal use by chemists in pharmaceutical companies.
2. An example of a drug from a vegetable or plant source is digitalis.
   a. Digitalis is obtained from a wild flower called purple foxglove. The dried leaves of the plant are called digitalis.
   b. The plant is cultivated in England, Germany, and North America for the drug markets. It grows wild in Australia, Europe, and the United States.

c. The purple foxglove leaves contain a number of active glycoside principles. Important active principles are digitoxin and digoxin.
d. Digitalis is given for arrhythmias or congestive heart failure (see Chapter 16).

Active principles of plants

Parts of the plant that are processed for medicinal use, such as leaves, roots, or seeds, are known as the crude drug.

Alkaloids (al′kah-loidz)

Alkaloids are one group of basic substances found in plants.
1. They are alkaline (basic) in reaction, thus the name.
2. They are bitter in taste.
3. They may be powerful in physiologic activity.
4. EXAMPLES
   a. Atropine and scopolamine (belladonna alkaloids found in the nightshade plant, *Atropa belladonna*)
   b. Morphine, cocaine, quinine, nicotine, and caffeine

Glycoside (gli′ko-sid)

Glycoside is a compound found in plants that contains a carbohydrate molecule. One example is the cardiac glycoside digitalis, which has a characteristic action on the heart (see Chapter 16).

Resin (rez′in)

Resin is a naturally occurring solid, brittle, amorphous substance from plants and trees that is soluble in alcohol. An example is the colonic irritant found in the laxative cascara.

Gums

Gums are mucilaginous excretions of various plants.
1. Some absorb water and are used in bulk-type laxatives.

2. Tragacanth is a gum used in certain skin preparations for its emulsifying effect.

Oils

Oils include two types:
1. Fixed oils do not evaporate on mild warming and occur as solids, semisolids, or liquids. Example: oleum ricini—castor oil.
2. Volatile oils are extracted from aromatic plants and readily evaporate. EXAMPLE: methyl salicylate—oil of wintergreen.

Mineral sources

1. Drugs may be extracted from metallic and nonmetallic mineral sources. They are usually in the form of acids, bases, and salts found in food.
2. An example of a drug from a mineral source is dilute hydrochloric acid, given to control or prevent indigestion caused by too little secretion of hydrochloric acid from the stomach glands.
3. Calcium, another mineral, is found in green vegetables and also is given therapeutically.
4. Potassium chloride 10% is an important drug given to assist in electrolyte balance, especially in diuretic therapy.

Synthetic sources

1. Most drugs in use today are synthetically produced. Synthesis is the process of making a compound by alteration of other compounds or elements. Chemists know the elements in a medicine and can make most medicines synthetically by chemical formulation in the laboratory.
2. Some examples of synthetic medicines are:
   a. Steroids, used in treatment of arthritis and other diseases.
   b. Sulfonamides or chemotherapeutic agents, used to kill microorganisms or to slow their growth.
   c. Meperidine hydrochloride (Demerol), a narcotic analgesic.

DRUG NAMES

Many drugs have a variety of names. This may cause confusion to the patient, physician, and nurse, so care must be taken in obtaining the exact name and spelling for a particular drug name.

Chemical name

1. This name usually is meaningful chiefly to the chemist.
2. By means of the chemical name, the chemist understands an exact description of the chemical constitution of the drug and the exact placing of the atoms or atomic groupings.

Generic name (nonproprietary name)

1. Before a drug becomes official, it is given a generic name or common name.
2. A generic name is simpler than the chemical name and may be used in all countries by any manufacturer.
3. Generic names are provided by the United States Adopted Names (USAN) Council, an organization sponsored by the United States Pharmacopeial Convention, the American Pharmaceutical Association, and the American Medical Association.
4. The generic name is not capitalized.
5. Occasionally, it is less expensive to order by generic rather than by brand name. Medicare recommends that physicians prescribe by generic name.

Official name

1. The official name is the name under which the drug is listed by the Food and Drug Administration. The FDA is empowered by federal law to name drugs for human use in the United States.
2. It is now customary that the FDA accepts the generic name given by the USAN Council as the "official name."

Trademark or brand name (proprietary name)

1. A trademark or brand name has the symbol ® at the upper right of the name. This indicates the name is registered and its use restricted to the manufacturer of the drug who is the legal owner of the name.
2. Some drug companies place their official drugs on the market under trade or proprietary names instead of official names. The trade names are deliberately made easier to pronounce, spell, and remember.
3. The first letter of the trade name is capitalized.

Example of nomenclature:
Chemical name: 4-dimethylamino-1, 4, 4a, 5, 5a, 6, 11, 12a-octahydro-3,6,10,12,12a-pentahydroxy-6-methyl-1,11,dioxo-2-naphthacenecarboxamide
Generic name: tetracycline
Official name: Tetracycline, USP
Brand names: Achromycin®, Panmycin®, Tetracyn®

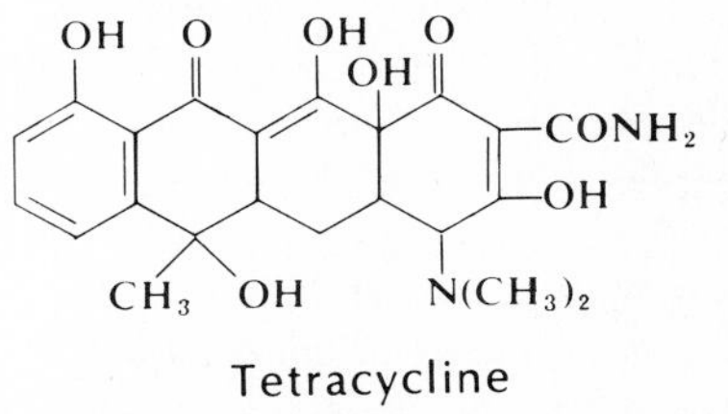

Tetracycline

Fig. 2-1. Tetracycline, an antibiotic.

DRUG STANDARDS

Standardization is needed to ensure uniformity of purity and potency of drug products. Before 1820, many drugs were found in different parts of the United States in varying degrees of purity. This problem was solved by the establishment of an authoritative book that set forth required standards of purity for drugs as well as methods of assay to determine purity. It is called the *Pharmacopeia of the United States of America*.

The United States Pharmacopeia (USP), 20th revision, and The National Formulary (NF), 15th revision

1. The USP and NF are published by the United States Pharmacopeial Convention, a nonprofit, nongovernmental corporation. The latest edition, published in 1980, represents the first time these two established reference books have been combined into one volume.
2. The primary purpose of this volume is to provide standards for identity, quality, strength, and purity of substances used in the practice of health care.
3. The standards set forth in the USP and NF have been adopted by the Food and Drug Administration as ''official'' standards for the manufacture and quality control of medicines produced in the United States.
4. This book is revised every 5 years. Supplements are published more frequently to keep it up to date.

USAN and the USP Dictionary of Drug Names

1. This reference text is a dictionary of nonproprietary names, brand names, code designations, and Chemical Abstracts Service registry numbers for drugs.
2. USAN (United States Adopted Names) represents a program sponsored by the United States Pharmacopeial Convention, the American Pharmaceutical Association, and the American Medical Association. The USAN program is responsible for producing simple and useful nonproprietary (generic) names for drugs.
3. Manufacturers or individuals submit a proposal for a name to the USAN Council announcing that a certain chemical compound has therapeutic potential and that they plan to run investigations on its use in human beings. The Council studies the chemical name, applies a series of nomenclature guidelines, and then selects the USAN. It is now customary that the Food and Drug Administration accepts the adopted generic name as the FDA ''official name'' for a chemical compound.
4. This dictionary is a compilation of over 11,000 drug names. Each monograph contains the USAN, a pronunciation guide, the molecular and graphic formula, chemical and brand name, manufacturer, and therapeutic category.

DRUG INFORMATION SOURCES
American Drug Index

1. The *American Drug Index* is edited annually by Norman F. Billups, Ph.D., and is published by J. B. Lippincott Co. of Philadelphia.
2. Drugs are listed alphabetically by generic name and brand name.
   a. Generic name monographs contain recognition of the drug to the *United States Pharmacopeia, National Formulary,* or *United States Adopted Names,* the chemical name, use, and cross-references to brand names.
   b. Each brand name monograph lists the manufacturer, composition and strength, pharmaceutical forms available, package size, dosage, and use.
3. Other features of this reference book include a list of common medical abbreviations; tables of weights, measures, and conversion factors; a glossary to aid in interpretation of the monographs; a labeler code index to identify drug products; and a list of manufacturers' addresses.

American Hospital Formulary Service

1. This two-volume set is published by the American Society of Hospital Pharmacists, Washington, D.C. It is updated with five supplements yearly.
2. This reference work contains monographs on virtually every single-drug entity available in the United States. The monographs emphasize rational therapeutic procedures. Each monograph is subdivided into sections on chemistry, absorption, distribution, metabolism and excretion, mechanism of action, uses, cautions, and dosage. The index is cross-referenced by both generic and brand names.
3. The *American Hospital Formulary Service* has been adopted as an official source by the Public Health Service and the Veteran's Administration. It has also been approved for use by the American Hospital Association, the Catholic Hospital Association, and the American Pharmaceutical Association.

Drugs of Choice

1. *Drugs of Choice* is edited by Walter Modell and published by The C. V. Mosby Co., St. Louis.
2. It is revised every 2 years.
3. It contains contributions from more than 40 outstanding specialists who give their opinions of the drugs in current use in their own fields of specialization.
4. The book provides clear, concise, and practical answers to questions of drugs of choice for actual therapeutic problems.
5. Included is an alphabetic index of drugs in common use.

Drug Interactions

1. This book is edited by Philip Hansten, Pharm. D. and published by Lea & Febiger of Philadelphia.
2. Part I of the book provides a description of drug-drug and drug-food interactions. Part II discusses drug effects on clinical laboratory tests.
3. Each individual monograph on interactions lists the drugs and laboratory tests involved, the mechanism by which the interaction occurs, the clinical significance of each interaction, and the management of the interaction should it occur.
4. The book is well indexed and extensively referenced to provide additional data should the reader require further information on a particular interaction.

Evaluations of Drug Interactions

1. This book is prepared and published by the American Pharmaceutical Association of Washington, D.C.
2. It is divided into three sections:
   a. The first and largest section contains alphabetically listed monographs of drug-drug interactions. Each monograph contains an abstract of the monograph, other related drugs that might cause the same reaction, the mechanism of action of the interaction, a well-referenced review of the clinical literature that has reported the interaction, and recommendations on the management of the interaction.
   b. The second section provides a review of the basic principles of drug interactions.
   c. The third section discusses the pharmacologic aspects of drug interactions by therapeutic classes rather than by individual drugs as described in the first section.

Handbook of Non-Prescription Drugs

1. This book is prepared and published by the American Pharmaceutical Association, Washington, D.C.
2. It is the most comprehensive text available on medications that may be purchased over-the-counter in the United States.
3. Chapters are divided by therapeutic activity, such as antacid products, cold and allergy products, nutritional supplements, mineral and vitamin products, and feminine hygiene products.
4. Each chapter provides a brief review of anatomy and physiology, evaluation of the symptoms being treated, suggested treatments with appropriate dosages, and a listing of medications with their ingredients.
5. Three particular advantages of this book for the health professional are:
   a. A list of questions to be asked of the patient to determine whether treatment should be recommended.
   b. Product selection guidelines for determining the most appropriate products.
   c. Counseling to be conveyed to the patient on how to properly use the product recommended.

Martindale—the Extra Pharmacopoeia

1. This 2,000-page volume is edited by Ainley Wade and published by The Pharmaceutical Press in London.
2. It is one of the most comprehensive texts available for information on drugs in current use throughout the world. In addition to extensive, referenced monographs (part 1) on the pharmacologic activity and side effects of 3,130 medicinal agents, there are short monographs (part 2) on another 1,000 agents that are either considered obsolete or too new for inclusion in part 1. Part 3 gives the composition and manufacturers of more than 1,450 over-the-counter pharmaceutical products.
3. The index contains more than 43,000 entries. Medicinal agents are indexed by official names, chemical names, synonyms, and proprietary names.

Medical Letter

1. The *Medical Letter,* published by Drug and Therapeutic Information, Inc., New York, is a semimonthly periodical.
2. It contains brief, independent comments on newly released drug products and related topics by a board of competent authorities who use the knowledge of specialists in various fields.
3. The letters contain data on drug action and comparative clinical efficacy.
4. The *Medical Letter* has the advantage of presenting timely and critical summations of new drugs during the early period of promotion of the drug. Such appraisals must, necessarily, be tentative.

Package brochures

1. Before a new drug is marketed, the manufacturer develops a comprehensive but concise description of the drug, indications and precautions in clinical use, suggestions for dosage, known adverse actions, contraindications, and other pharmacologic information relating to the drug.
2. Federal law requires that a brochure accompany each package of the product.
3. The brochure must be approved by the Food and Drug Administration before the product is released for marketing.

Physicians' Desk Reference (PDR)

1. The PDR is published annually by Medical Economics, Inc., Oradell, N.J.
2. It contains a listing of almost 2,500 therapeutic agents arranged in seven sections. Each section uses a different page color for easy access.
   a. Section 1 (white), Manufacturers' Index—an alphabetic listing of each manufacturer, their addresses, emergency phone numbers, and a partial list of available products.
   b. Section 2 (pink), Product Name Index—a comprehensive alphabetic listing of brand name products discussed in the Product Information section of the book.
   c. Section 3 (blue), Product Classification Index—products are subdivided by therapeutic classes, such as analgesics, laxatives, oxytocics, and antibiotics.
   d. Section 4 (yellow), Generic and Chemical Name Index—products are listed by their generic or chemical names, with references to the Product Information section.
   e. Section 5, Product Identification Section—each manufacturer has provided color pictures of the actual sizes of their tablets and capsules. This section is an invaluable aid in product identification.
   f. Section 6 (white), Product Information Section—This section lists the major products of manufacturers, with information on action, uses, administration, dosages, contraindications, composition, and how each drug is supplied.
   g. Section 7 (green), Diagnostic Product Information—an alphabetic listing by manufacturer of many diagnostic tests used in hospital and office practice.
3. This reference text also provides a list of poison control centers and their telephone numbers.

DRUG LEGISLATION

Drug legislation protects the consumer and patient. The need for such protection is great because of the zeal of manufacturers and advertising agents and the many methods by which the public can be informed today, such as radio, television, newspapers, and magazines. The public is increasingly aware of new drugs but lacks a knowledge of the effect and dangers of many drugs.

Federal Food, Drug, and Cosmetic Act, June 25, 1938 (amended 1952, 1962)

The Food and Drug Administration of the Department of Health and Welfare has the responsibility for enforcing this law. Important contents of the law include habit-forming drugs, which must be listed quantitatively on the label, with the label containing a warning that the drug is habit forming. Dangerous drugs are to be used only by or on the prescription of a physician, dentist, or veterinarian. Warning statements must appear on the label of certain drugs; for example, cathartics must bear a statement that such drugs should not be taken in the presence of abdominal pain or cramps and that they may be habit forming. Nose drops, such as ephedrine and Neo-Synephrine, are to be labeled with a statement that continued use may cause nervousness and inability to sleep and that people with high blood pressure, heart disease, thyroid trouble, or diabetes should not take such preparations except on competent advice.

The 1938 act authorized the federal Food and Drug Administration to determine the safety of drugs before marketing. One of the main causes of this provision was the more than 100 deaths in 1937 resulting from ingestion of a diethylene glycol solution of sulfanilamide. This sulfanilamide preparation had been marketed as an "elixir of sulfanilamide" without benefit of investigation of the toxicity of the solvent. The only charge that could be made against the drug was that it was misbranded an "elixir," because it did not meet the definition of elixir. Thus, a provision of the 1938 act was made to prevent premature marketing of new drugs not properly tested for safety. Manufacturers are required to submit new drug applications to the government for review of safety studies before products can be sold.

The Durham-Humphrey Law in 1952 amended the 1938 act in regard to drugs. It tightened control by restricting the refilling of prescriptions.

The Kefauver-Harris Drug Amendment in 1962 was brought about by the thalidomide tragedy in which many infants were born malformed. This amendment provides for greater control and surveillance over the distribution and clinical testing of investigational drugs. It provides the authority to require that drugs be efficacious as well as safe. The intent is to protect the public and the clinical investigator by ensuring that adequate preclinical studies are done on the drug before the investigator is asked to do human studies.

The intent of the 1962 drug law, to protect the public and the clinical investigator, is made more effective by the following provisions:

1. Manufacture of all drugs under adequate control and good manufacturing practices.
2. Government certification of both the safety and effectiveness of all drugs for human use.
3. Substantial evidence of the effectiveness of new drugs before marketing.
4. Prompt reporting by manufacturers to the government of adverse reactions attributed to new drugs and antibiotics.

5. Truthful statements in prescription drug advertisement concerning the effectiveness, side effects, and contraindications of the advertised drugs.
6. Annual registration with the Food and Drug Administration of all persons and firms engaged in the manufacturing, reporting, and labeling of drug products.
7. Inspection of every registered establishment at least once every 2 years.

The new law further authorizes the Food and Drug Administration to do the following:

1. Withdraw approval of drugs when substantial doubt arises as to their safety or in the absence of substantial evidence of effectiveness.
2. Establish official names for drugs in the interest of usefulness and simplicity.
3. Exercise greater controls over shipments of investigational drugs for testing in humans.
4. Have access during inspection of prescription drug manufacturing establishments to all matters that have a bearing on possible violations of the law with respect to such drugs, including records, files, papers, processes, controls, and facilities.

Regulations pertaining to labeling

Labels on containers, circulars, pamphlets, and brochures must comply with the following points:

1. No false or misleading statement.
2. Dosages and frequency must be clearly stated and must not be dangerous to health when used as recommended on the label.
3. Name, business address, and lot number of the manufacturer.
4. An accurate statement of the contents.
5. A warning if the drug is habit forming.
6. Quantity, kind, and proportion of specific ingredients.
7. Directions for use and contraindications, with adequate warnings for:
   a. Children
   b. Persons with pathologic (disease) conditions
8. When the drug is unsafe for self-medication, the label must state Caution: Federal Law Prohibits Dispensing Without A Prescription.
9. The label must designate presence of official drugs by their official names, and if nonofficial, must bear generic name of the drug.

Harrison Narcotic Act, 1914 (amended several times)

The Harrison Narcotic Act regulated the importation, manufacture, sale, and use of opium, cocaine, and all their compounds and derivatives. Its purpose was to limit

and prevent the indiscriminate use of such drugs and to prevent the spread of the drug habit. The law has been repealed and replaced by the Controlled Substances Act of 1970.

Controlled Substances Act, 1970

The Comprehensive Drug Abuse Prevention and Control Act was passed by Congress in the fall of 1970. This new statute, commonly referred to as the "Controlled Substances Act," repeals almost 50 other laws written since 1914 that relate to the control of drugs. The new composite law is designed to improve the administration and regulation of manufacturing, distributing, and dispensing of drugs found necessary to control.

The Drug Enforcement Administration (DEA) was organized to enforce the Controlled Substances Act, to gather intelligence, and to train and conduct research in the area of dangerous drugs and drug abuse. The DEA is a bureau of the Department of Justice. The director of the DEA is responsible to the Attorney General of the United States.

The basic structure of the Controlled Substances Act consists of five classifications or "schedules" of controlled substances. The degree of control, the conditions of record keeping, the particular order forms required, and other regulations depend on these classifications. Following are the five schedules, their criteria, and examples of drugs within each schedule.

Schedule I (C-I) drugs have:
1. A high potential for abuse
2. No currently accepted medical use in the United States
3. A lack of accepted safety for use under medical supervision
EXAMPLES: LSD, marijuana, peyote, STP, heroin, hashish

Schedule II (C-II) drugs have:
1. A high potential for abuse
2. A currently accepted medical use in the United States
3. An abuse potential that may lead to severe psychologic or physical dependence
EXAMPLES: secobarbital, pentobarbital, amphetamines, morphine, meperidine, methadone, methaqualone, Percodan

Schedule III (C-III) drugs have:
1. A high potential for abuse, but less than drugs in schedules I and II
2. A currently accepted medical use in the United States
3. An abuse potential that may lead to moderate or low physical dependence or high psychologic dependence
EXAMPLES: Empirin with codeine, Doriden, Fiorinal, paregoric, Noludar, Tylenol with codeine

Schedule IV (C-IV) drugs have:
1. A low potential for abuse, relative to those in schedule III
2. A currently accepted medical use in the United States
3. An abuse potential that may lead to limited physical or psychologic dependence, relative to drugs in schedule III

EXAMPLES: phenobarbital, Equanil, chloral hydrate, paraldehyde, Librium, Valium, Dalmane, Tranxene

Schedule V (CV) drugs have:
1. A low potential for abuse, relative to those in schedule IV
2. A currently accepted medical use in the United States
3. An abuse potential of limited physical or psychologic dependence liability, relative to drugs in schedule IV

EXAMPLES: terpin hydrate with codeine, Lomotil, Robitussin A-C

The Attorney General, after public hearings, has authority to reschedule a drug, bring an unscheduled drug under control, or remove controls on scheduled drugs.

Every manufacturer, physician, dentist, pharmacy, and hospital that manufacturers, prescribes, or dispenses any of the drugs listed in the five schedules must register annually with the Drug Enforcement Administration.

A physician's prescription for substances named in this law must contain the physician's name, address, DEA registration number and signature, the patient's name and address, and the date of issue. The pharmacist cannot refill such prescriptions without the approval of the physician.

All controlled substances for ward stock must be ordered on special hospital forms that are used to help maintain inventory and dispersion control records of the schedule drugs. When a nurse administers a schedule II drug, under a physician's order, the following information must be entered on the controlled substances record: name of the patient, date of administration, drug administered, and drug dosage.

Possession of controlled substances

Federal and state laws make the possession of controlled substances a crime, except in specifically exempted cases. The law makes no distinction between professional and practical nurses in regard to possession of controlled drugs. Nurses may give controlled substances only under the direction of a physician or dentist who has been licensed to prescribe or dispense these agents. Nurses may not have controlled substances in their possession unless they are giving them to a patient under a doctor's order, or the nurse is a patient for whom a doctor has prescribed schedule drugs, or the nurse is the official custodian of a limited supply of controlled substances on a ward or department of the hospital. Controlled substances ordered but not used for patients must be returned to the source from which they were obtained (the doctor or the pharmacy). Violation or failure to comply with the Controlled Substances Act is punishable by fine, imprisonment, or both.

Effectiveness of legislation of drugs

Effectiveness of legislation depends on the interest and determination used to enforce these laws, the appro-

priation of adequate funds for this enforcement, the vigor used by proper authorities in their enforcement, the interest and cooperation of professional people and the public, and the education of the public concerning the dangers of unwise and indiscriminate use of drugs in general, vitamins, drugs for obesity, glandular preparations, and cancer "cures." Many organizations help in this education, including the American Medical Association, American Dental Association, American Heart Association, American Society for the Control of Cancer, and local, state, and county health departments.

Food and Drug Administration

The Food and Drug Administration (FDA) is charged with the enforcement of the federal Food, Drug, and Cosmetic Act. Methods used to enforce this act include, among others, seizure of offending goods and criminal prosecution of responsible persons or firms in federal courts. The Kefauver-Harris Amendment requires, in addition, that pharmaceutical firms report at regular intervals to the FDA all adverse effects associated with their new drugs. The FDA also has an adverse-reaction reporting program, with about 450 cooperating reporting sources helping to discover reactions not revealed by previous clinical or pharmaceutic studies.

Public Health Service

The Public Health Service is a part of the U.S. Department of Health and Welfare. It has many functions, such as regulating biologic products. This refers to "any virus, therapeutic serum, antitoxin, or analogous product applicable to the prevention, treatment, or cure of diseases or injuries of man." The Public Health Service maintains control over these products by inspecting and licensing the establishments that manufacture them and by examining and licensing the products themselves.

Federal Trade Commission

The Federal Trade Commission is an agency of the federal government directly responsible to the president. It has the power to suppress false or misleading drug advertising to the general public.

ASSIGNMENT

Review previous lessons and questions according to the direction of your instructor.

1. List the four major sources (origins) of drugs. Give an example of each source and tell the main use of each example.
2. What is the most common source of most drugs in use today? Give two examples of drugs from synthetic sources.
3. Explain the following and give an example of each. You need not use the detailed chemical name.

a. Drug name

b. Generic name (nonproprietary name)

c. Official name

d. Trademark or brand name (proprietary name)

4. Give the generic, official, and brand name of tetracycline and its chemical name to familiarize yourself with the meaning of chemical name. (It is not necessary to memorize it.)

5. Explain what is meant by drug standards. Why is it important to have drug standards? How was the problem of purity and potency of drug products solved? What is the name of the authoritative book that requires adherence to the standards of purity and potency of drug products?

6. What are the names of the two official books published by the United States Pharmacopeial Convention? What are their abbreviations? When was the latest edition published? When were these two reference books combined into one volume? What is the primary purpose of this volume? What agency has adopted the standards set forth in it? How often is it revised? How is it kept up to date?

7. Explain the meaning and purpose of the USAN and the USP *Dictionary of Drug Names.*

8. How often is the *American Drug Index* edited and how are the drugs listed? What other features are included in this reference book?

9. Name the publisher of the *American Hospital Formulary Service* and tell how often it is updated. Name the services, administrations, and associations that have adopted the *American Hospital Formulary Service* as an official source.

10. Who edits and publishes *Drugs of Choice?* How often is it revised? Explain the format of the book. Become familiar with this book; it is one of several books you will use often during this course and as a graduate nurse.

11. Explain the purpose and importance of *Drug Interactions.* Describe the arrangement of this book.

12. Explain the purpose and importance of *Evaluation of Drug Interactions.* Who prepares and publishes this book? Describe the arrangement in sections of this book.

13. Who prepares and publishes the *Handbook of Non-Prescription Drugs?* It is the most comprehensive text available on what type of medications? How are its chapters divided? Name three particular advantages of this book for the health professional.

14. Name the publisher of the *Martindale—The Extra Pharmacopoeia.* This text is one of the most comprehensive books available for information on drugs in current use throughout the _____. List the contents on Part 1, Part 2, and Part 3 to show how the book is divided. How are medicinal agents indexed?

15. Name the publisher of *Medical Letter* and tell how often it is published. What does it contain? What advantage does the *Medical Letter* have? Why should appraisals of some of the newer drugs be tentative?

16. Explain package brochures. What does federal law require of them? What agency must approve the brochure before the product is released for marketing?

17. Who publishes *Physicians' Desk Reference* (PDR) and how often? Describe the contents of each section of the PDR. What else does the PDR provide as vital information? Become familiar with the arrangement of the contents of this book; you will use it often both as a student and a graduate nurse. Obtain a copy of the PDR from your nursing school library or your instructor and look up the trade and generic name, purposes, route of administration, contraindications, symptoms of untoward side effects, and usual dosage of the following drugs to familiarize yourself with the use of this book.

a. Coumadin

b. Digoxin

c. Demerol

d. Hydrodiuril

18. What is the purpose of drug legislation?

19. What are some important contents of the federal Food, Drug, and Cosmetic Act? What did the 1938 amendment to this act do? What was the cause of this amendment? What did the Durham-Humphrey Law in 1952 do in amending the 1938 act? What did the Kefauver-Harris Drug Amendment in 1962 do and why? What is the intent of the 1962 drug law? Drugs first marketed between 1938 and 1962 may meet claims made for them, or they may not. Which is correct?

20. List the provisions of the 1962 drug law of the Federal Food, Drug, and Cosmetic Act. Name four additional authorizations of this law.

21. List the regulations pertaining to labeling.

22. Go to your drugstore and record the information from the labels of the following. Do they meet the legal requirements?

a. Anacin

b. Contac

c. Infrarub

d. Nyquil

e. Pepto-Bismol

f. Preparation H

23. Explain the Harrison Narcotic Act, 1914. Has this law been repealed? What act replaced it?

24. When was the Comprehensive Drug Abuse Prevention and Control Act passed (Controlled Substances Act)? What is its purpose? Why was the Drug Enforcement Administration (DEA) organized? The DEA is a bureau of what department? The director of the DEA is responsible to whom? What is the basic structure of the Controlled Substances Act? List the five schedules of this act and give three examples of drugs under each schedule.

25. After public hearings, what authority can the Attorney General exercise in regard to drugs that fall under any of the five schedules of the Controlled Substances Act of 1970?

26. What rule must be followed by every manufacturer, physician, dentist, pharmacy, and hospital that manufacturers, prescribes, or dispenses any of the drugs listed in the five schedules of the Controlled Substances Act of 1970?

27. What must a physician's prescription contain for substances regulated by the Controlled Substances Act?

28. How must controlled substances for ward stock be ordered for the hospital under the Controlled Substances Act?

29. When a nurse administers a schedule II drug under a physi-

cian's order, what information must be entered on the Controlled Substances record?

30. Federal and state laws make the possession of controlled substances a crime, except in specifically exempted cases. Describe the specifically exempt cases in which a nurse may have or give such drugs. Can a nurse have controlled substances in her possession without these exemptions? Study the law in this regard and its exemptions and know it well. What is done with controlled substances ordered for patients but not used? What is the punishment for violation or failure to comply with the Controlled Substances Act?

31. On what does effectiveness of legislation of drugs depend? What organizations help to educate the public in increasing the effectiveness of drug legislation?

32. Explain the methods used to enforce the Food and Drug and Cosmetic Act.

33. Name some of the functions of the Public Health Service. It is a part of what department? How does the Public Health Service maintain its control?

34. To whom is the Federal Trade Commission responsible? What is its purpose?

CHAPTER 3

Solid and liquid dosage forms

SOLID DOSAGE FORMS

Capsules

1. Capsules are small, cylindric gelatin containers that hold a dry powder or liquid medicinal agent.
2. Capsules are a convenient way of administering drugs with an unpleasant odor or taste. They are available in various sizes (Fig. 3-1).
3. Capsules can also be used as a delayed-action dosage form. The granules inside the capsule are prepared so some will dissolve almost at once and other granules, which are coated with a substance to delay disintegration, will dissolve later. EXAMPLE: Contac cold capsules.
4. A trade name indicating that the drug is a delayed-action dosage form is Spansule.

Creams

1. Creams are solid emulsions containing medicinal agents for external application.
2. EXAMPLE: hydrocortisone cream—a corticosteroid applied to rashes caused by an allergic reaction.

Extracts

1. Extracts are concentrated, solid preparations of drugs obtained by dissolving the crude drug in alcohol or water. The solution is then allowed to evaporate.
2. The remaining sediment is the extract. It is usually four to five times as strong as the crude drug itself and is incorporated into tablets or capsules.
3. EXAMPLE: cascara sagrada, used as a laxative.

Lozenges

1. Lozenges are flat disks containing a medicinal agent in a suitably flavored base. The base may be a hard sugar candy or the combination of sugar with sufficient mucilage to give it form.
2. Lozenges are placed in the mouth to slowly dissolve, liberating the antiseptic or astringent ingredient.
3. EXAMPLE: cough lozenges—given to stop irritation or a dry, tickling cough.

Ointments

1. Ointments are semisolid preparations of medicinal substances in an oily base such as lanolin or petrolatum. They are intended for external application to the skin or mucous membranes.
2. EXAMPLE: triamcinolone ointment—used for treatment of contact dermatitis.

Pills

1. A pill is an obsolete dosage form. It was made by rolling the drug and binder into a sphere. It is now used, however, as a common term for both tablets and capsules.

Powders

1. Powders are drugs ground into a fine powder and stored or used in this form.
2. EXAMPLE: douche powders are completely soluble and are intended to be dissolved in water prior to use as antiseptics or cleansing agents for a body cavity.

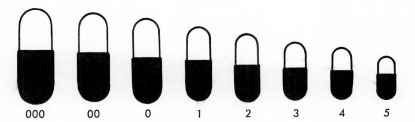

Fig. 3-1. Various sizes and numbers of gelatin capsules, actual size. (From Bergersen, B. S.: Pharmacology in nursing, ed. 14, St. Louis, 1979, The C. V. Mosby Co.)

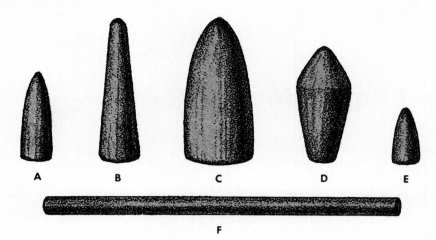

Fig. 3-2. Various forms of suppositories. **A, B,** and **E,** Rectal. **C** and **D,** Vaginal. **F,** Urethral. (From Bergersen, B. S.: Pharmacology in nursing, ed. 14, St. Louis, 1979, The C. V. Mosby Co.)

Suppositories

1. Suppositories are mixtures of drugs with a firm base such as cocoa butter. They are molded into a shape suitable for insertion into a body opening such as the rectum or the vagina.
2. The suppositories melt at body temperature. This allows the drug to come in contact with the mucous membranes of, for example, the rectum or vagina. The drug then produces a local or systemic effect (Fig. 3-2).
3. EXAMPLES: glycerin and Dulcolax—drugs to move the bowels.

Tablets

1. Tablets are dried, powdered drugs that have been compressed into small disks. Many are easily dissolved. EXAMPLE: aspirin.
2. Tablets may also have special coatings that allow the tablet to dissolve slowly, releasing the medicinal agent over a prolonged time. Trade names of slow-release tablets are Extentabs and Dospan.

LIQUID DOSAGE FORMS
Ampules and vials

1. Ampules and vials are glass containers (Fig. 3-3) containing powdered or liquid drugs.
2. Ampules are sealed glass containers and usually contain one dose of the drug. Vials are glass containers with rubber stoppers and usually contain a number of doses of the drug.
3. Vials and ampules are used for drugs given by injection. The powdered drugs are redissolved with the proper diluent before being drawn up into a syringe for injection.

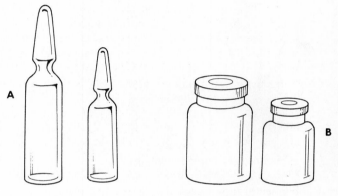

Fig. 3-3. A, Single-dose ampules. **B,** Multi-dose ampules. (From Bergersen, B. S.: Pharmacology in nursing, ed. 14, St. Louis, 1979, The C. V. Mosby Co.)

4. EXAMPLE: ampicillin—an antibiotic that, because of instability, must be redissolved, using proper aseptic technique, prior to use.

Elixirs

1. Elixirs are palatable preparations of drugs made up with alcohol, sugar, and some aromatic or pleasant-smelling substance.
2. EXAMPLES:
   a. Elixir of terpin hydrate—a cough medicine.
   b. Elixir of phenobarbital—a sedative and anticonvulsant.

Emulsions

1. Emulsions are suspensions of oils or fats in water. The suspension is maintained by emulsifying agents such as sodium lauryl sulfate.
2. EXAMPLE: Intralipid—a 10% solution of essential fatty acids used for intravenous nutrition.

Fluidextracts

1. Fluidextracts are concentrated fluid preparations of drugs made by dissolving the crude plant drug in the fluid that dissolves it most readily, for example, water or alcohol.
2. EXAMPLE: fluidextract of cascara—a laxative.

Gels

1. Gels are aqueous suspensions of insoluble drugs in hydrated form; particles are smaller than in the magma suspensions.
2. EXAMPLE: aluminum hydroxide gel (Amphojel)—an antacid.

Liniments

1. Liniments are mixtures of drugs with soap, oil, water, or alcohol to be used for external application only. Usually applied by rubbing, liniments relieve pain and produce heat to the skin by increasing blood circulation.
2. EXAMPLE: liniment of camphor—a counterirritant.

Lotions

1. Lotions are usually aqueous preparations that contain suspended matter. They are commonly used as soothing applications to protect the skin and relieve rashes and itching.
2. Some lotions have a cleansing action, while others have an astringent, or drawing, action.
3. To prevent increased circulation and itching, lotions should generally be patted on the skin instead of rubbed on.
4. All lotions should be shaken before using.
5. EXAMPLE: calamine lotion.

Magma

1. Magma are bulky suspensions, in water, of drugs or preparations that are insoluble. They look like milk or cream.
2. EXAMPLE: milk of magnesia—a laxative.

Prefilled syringes

These contain a prepared dosage ready for immediate use.

Spirits

1. Spirits are preparations of volatile (evaporating into vapor) substances dissolved in alcohol.
2. EXAMPLE: spirit of peppermint—given by drops, in a small amount of water, as a flavoring agent.

Suspensions

1. Suspensions are solid, insoluble particles dispensed in a liquid.
2. All bottles of suspensions must be shaken well before use.
3. EXAMPLE: Dilantin Suspension—an anticonvulsant.

Syrups

1. Syrups contain medicinal agents dissolved in a sugar and water solution. They are particularly effective for masking the taste of a drug.
2. EXAMPLE: cherry syrup.

Tinctures

1. Tinctures are diluted alcoholic extracts of drugs. They vary in strength from 10% to 20%.
2. EXAMPLE: tincture of belladonna.

The physician prescribes the medicine and treatment.
The nurse carries out the physician's orders.
Self-medication is dangerous. Consult your physician first.
There is in every medicine a possible danger.
When in doubt—ASK!

ASSIGNMENT

Review previous lessons and questions according to the directions of your instructor.

1. Capsules are (one choice is correct)
   a. Dried, powdered drugs compressed into small disks
   b. Drugs shaped into small balls or spheres
   c. Drugs contained in small, cylindric gelatin containers
   d. Sealed glass containers

2. Capsules (more than one choice is correct)
   a. Are available in one size only
   b. Are simply another way of giving an oral medicine
   c. Can be considered a convenient way of administering drugs with an unpleasant odor or taste
   d. Can also be used as a delayed-action dosage form
   e. In delayed-action dosage form have all their granules dissolve later to avoid indigestion
3. Define creams and give an example.

4. Extracts are (more than one choice is correct)
   a. Dried, powdered drugs compressed into small disks
   b. Concentrated solid preparations of drugs obtained by dissolving the drug in alcohol or water; the solution is then allowed to evaporate, leaving the sediment extract
   c. Crude or other drugs ground into a powder
   d. Drugs always contained in a small gelatin cylinder
   e. The sediment remaining after evaporation, which is usually four to five times as strong as the crude drug itself and is incorporated into tablets or capsules
5. Lozenges are (more than one choice is correct)
   a. Dried, powdered drugs compressed into small disks
   b. Flat disks containing a medicinal agent in a suitably flavored base
   c. Drugs shaped into small balls or spheres
   d. Placed in the mouth to slowly dissolve, releasing the medicine
   e. Given to stop irritation or a dry, tickling cough
6. Define ointments and give their purpose.
7. Are pills commonly used today? How were they made? The term pill is now used as a common term for which two medicinal forms?
8. Define powders and give an example.
9. Suppositories are (more than one choice is correct)
   a. Mixtures of drugs with a firm base such as cocoa butter and shaped into balls or triangles
   b. Mixtures of drugs with a firm base such as cocoa butter and molded into a shape suitable for insertion into a body opening such as the rectum or the vagina
   c. Glass capsules
   d. Mixtures that melt at body temperature to allow the drug to come in contact with the mucous membranes of, for example, the rectum or vagina; the drug then produces a local or systemic effect
10. Tablets (more than one choice is correct)
    a. Are dried, powdered drugs that have been compressed into small disks, many of which are easily dissolved
    b. Are drugs shaped into small spheres or balls
    c. May also have special coatings that allow the drug to dissolve slowly, releasing the medicinal agent over a prolonged time
    d. Include Extentabs, a trade name for a slow-release medicinal agent
11. Ampules and vials (more than one choice is correct)
    a. Are gelatin containers
    b. Are glass containers containing powdered or liquid drugs
    c. Are usually used for more accurate oral medication dosage
    d. Are used for drugs given by injection

e. Ampules are sealed glass containers and usually contain one dose of the drug
   f. Vials are glass containers with rubber stoppers and usually contain a number of doses of the drug
   g. The powdered drugs are redissolved with the proper diluent before being drawn up into a syringe for injection
12. Define elixirs and give two examples.
13. Define emulsions and give an example.
14. Define fluidextracts and give an example.
15. Define gels and give an example.
16. What are liniments? What is the method of administration? How do liniments relieve pain and produce heat to the skin?
17. Define lotions. Tell their common use, effect, and action. Explain the correct application of lotions. Give an example of a lotion. Should a lotion be shaken or not shaken before use?
18. Define magma and give an example.
19. What is meant by the term "prefilled syringes"?
20. Spirits are (one choice is correct)
    a. Made with sugar and water
    b. Preparations of volatile (evaporating into vapor) substances dissolved in alcohol
    c. Preparations that do not stay mixed
    d. Preparations that are four or five times the strength once the sediment is ready for use
21. Define suspensions and give an example. Should the bottle be shaken before use?
22. Syrups are made (one choice is correct)
    a. Without sugar
    b. In a sugar and water solution
    c. With alcohol alone
    d. With a base that emphasizes alcohol to mask the taste of the drug
23. Tinctures are (one best choice)
    a. Diluted alcoholic extracts of drugs that vary in strength from 10% to 20%
    b. Drugs made with sugar and water
    c. Fluid mixtures that stay together for short periods
    d. Drugs made with alcohol, sugar, and water

Questions to discuss with your instructor.

1. Should a drug prepared for one route of administration be used for another?
2. What should a nurse do if the physician orders a drug given by injection and the drug is only available in an oral form?
3. Should a nurse give drugs that have been prepackaged by the clinical pharmacist? Who is responsible in this situation for a medication error?

CHAPTER 4

Some concepts of drug action

Bioavailability is a consideration of the highest importance in drug effectiveness and safety, according to the American Pharmaceutical Association. The bioavailability of a drug depends on (1) the relative amounts of an administered drug that reach the general circulation or the site of action and (2) the rate at which this occurs.

Often, the amount of drug that reaches the general circulation does not produce the effect expected from the amount of the drug taken. This may be attributed to the condition of the patient, the formula of the drug, or the process by which it is manufactured. In drug therapy, the physician and the clinical pharmacist need to consider the following:

1. The dosage required for desirable effects and the dosage at which the drug begins to produce untoward effects.
2. The method and rate of biotransformation (metabolism). This information is contained in the literature that accompanies the drug and must be carefully scrutinized by both professionals before a drug is prescribed and administered to any individual.

A drug is given with a definite goal, either to reach the general circulation and affect the entire body, or to limit its action to a target site or location and bring about a desirable therapeutic response at its site of action.

For a drug to reach its site of action it must transport itself across various body membranes by a process of diffusion or active transport. Some membranes, the mucosa of the intestines, or the skin may be many cell layers thick, but this alone does not influence the distribution of drugs. The cell membrane itself determines permeability since it contains a lipoidal barrier and pores that permit the passage of lipid-soluble substances. Once a drug reaches the plasma, it must cross the capillary wall to reach its final site of action. Lipid-soluble substances diffuse through the entire capillary membrane; lipid-insoluble substances may pass through the pores.

ABSORPTION

Absorption is the process by which a drug is made available to the body fluids for distribution. The rate at which this occurs depends on the physical properties of the drug, such as solubility and route of administration.

A drug molecule usually consists of two charged parts with some negative and some positive portions. In solution, some of these particles separate and drift; this is termed "ionization." Substances that do not ionize pass readily through the lipoidal layer of the gastrointestinal tract and are distributed more rapidly.

Routes of administration

1. Oral—lipid membrane is more permeable to lipid-soluble forms of drugs that remain unionized (see acid-base balance).
   a. Solutions absorb rapidly.
   b. Drugs that are weak acids (aspirin, sulfonamides, barbiturates) tend to remain unioinized in gastric contents and are readily absorbed.
   c. Drugs that are weak bases (ephedrine, erythromycin) are not absorbed from the stomach but are absorbed from the alkaline (base) medium of the small intestine.

   Acid-base balance *(acidity-alkalinity of a solution)*
   1. pH = 7: solution is neutral
   2. pH greater than 7: solution is basic (alkaline)
   3. pH less than 7: solution is acidic
      Stomach pH = 1.3
      Small intestine pH = 5.7
      Large intestine pH = 7.8
      Blood pH = 7.4

The process of converting the drug to a soluble form can be controlled by pharmaceutical action and is an important consideration in the drug form used (for example, solution, suspension, capsule, and tablets with various coatings). Before a solid drug taken orally can enter the bloodstream, it must dissolve in the gastrointestinal fluids and be transported across the lipoidal membrane (Fig. 4-1).

The rate of drug absorption depends on (1) the solubility of the drug preparation (aqueous preparations are more rapidly absorbed than are suspensions or colloidal preparations; for example, regular insulin vs. protamine insulin) and (2) blood flow through the tissue (absorption from a subcutaneous site), which is slow if peripheral circulation is impaired.

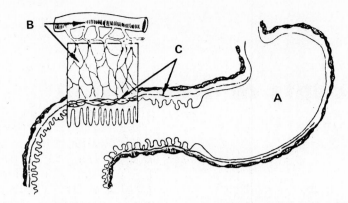

Fig. 4-1. Oral route for absorption. **A,** Lumen of gastrointestinal tract. **B,** Blood vessel. **C,** Lipoidal layer.

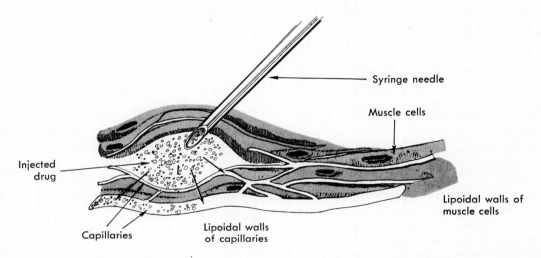

Fig. 4-2. Route of absorption of intramuscular medication. (Arrows indicate lipoidal barriers.)

2. Parenteral
   a. Subcutaneous: slowest absorption rate, especially if peripheral circulation is impaired.
   b. Intramuscular: more rapid rate because of greater blood flow per unit weight of muscle (Fig. 4-2). Cooling an area of injection will slow the rate of absorption and may be used to combat undesirable effects. Heat or massage will speed up the rate of absorption.
   c. Intravenous: the drug is disseminated through the body, the effects are rapid, and attempts to halt or slow the effect require use of drugs that neutralize or deactivate the drug given; thus, extreme care is essential in utilizing this route.

OTHER FACTORS INFLUENCING DRUG ACTION

1. *Pregnancy.* Precautions against administration of drugs that pass the placental barrier are necessary because of the deficiency of enzyme systems in the fetus. Drugs that have teratogenic effects are identified in the accompanying literature and should not be used. Certain drugs may also be secreted in breast milk.
2. *Age.* The volume of distribution of a drug is a function of body mass; thus, the body weight and surface area are the parameters for determining drug dosage. This suggests smaller dosages for children and elderly persons.
3. *Idiosyncrasy.* If the reaction is not usual and the cause is not clearly understood, it may be because of genetic deficiencies in certain enzymes.
4. *Drug allergy.* An immunologic mechanism from a previous sensitizing exposure may result in an acute hypersensitivity reaction.
5. *Cumulation.* The body does not eliminate one dose before another dosage is given. Digoxin is a drug notable for its cumulative side effects and should be

given at proper intervals, with attention to manifestation of toxic symptoms indicative of cumulation.

6. *Tolerance.* This is the need for increasing amounts of a drug to obtain the same effect. Tachyphylaxis is the term used to described a rapidly developing tolerance, which accounts for the drug user's need to increase dosages of "uppers."

7. *Drug antagonism.* One drug may negate the effect of another. It is very important that the physician be aware of "over-the-counter" drugs the patient may be self-administering when prescribing drugs that may be antagonistic.

8. *Potentiation.* Drugs given together may have a greater effect than when either is used alone. This may be desirable (Demerol and Phenergan) or undesirable (alcohol and tranquilizers).

DRUG ACTION DEFINITIONS

1. *Depressant.* Slows down activity of body systems or organs (produces drowsiness). EXAMPLES: phenobarbital, flurazepam.

2. *Stimulant.* Speeds up activity of body systems or organs (increases and strengthens pulse and respirations). EXAMPLES: caffeine, amphetamine.

3. *Irritant.* Local stimulation of cells or organs (certain laxatives stimulate the bowel musculature to produce peristalsis, leading to a bowel movement). EXAMPLE: bisacodyl.

4. *Demulcent.* Protects the surface of the skin or mucous membrane from irritation. EXAMPLE: antidiarrheals, such as bismuth, calcium carbonate, and pectin.

5. *Side effect.* A "by-product" reaction or one other than the main effect desired, such as a skin rash resulting from taking a drug designed to combat infection.

DURATION CHARACTERISTICS OF DRUGS AND THEIR ACTIONS

1. *Cumulative effect.* When drugs are not eliminated from the body as rapidly as they are absorbed, there is a "storing up" effect that may produce a toxic condition.

2. *Additive effect.* To increase effectiveness, one drug may be combined with one or more additional drugs.

3. *Selective action.* This is the power to act on a certain part of the body. A drug such as isoproterenol stimulates the heart to beat more rapidly.

4. *Tolerance.* A decreased response occurs with some drugs when dosages have been repeated over a period of time.

5. *Addictive effect.* This is the physical or psychic dependence on certain drugs, such as narcotics.

Termination of drug action occurs (1) when the drug is eliminated by the lungs, kidneys, intestines, skin, or saliva, (2) when the drug is redistributed, or (3) when a drug tolerance develops. The physician responds by adjusting the dosages and intervals to prolong the action of the drug or by discontinuing its administration.

It is a nursing responsibility to determine that a patient who self-administers his own drugs understands the purpose, effects, dosage, method of administration, and possible adverse effects. The nurse should develop a precise, current drug history, an understanding of the patient's unique problems, and a method of instruction for the patient and the patient's family that will encourage the patient, when appropriate, to assume responsibility for a personal care plan. The nurse must emphasize the importance of informing the physician of all over-the-counter medication taken.

ASSIGNMENT

1. Explain how the following determine the effect of drugs.
   a. Bioavailability
   b. pH
   c. Solubility
   d. Ionization
   e. Rate of absorption
   f. Lipoidal barrier
   g. Route of administration
   h. Rate of excretion

2. List the routes of administration from most rapid to slowest rate of absorption. Explain your reason for this placement.

3. The rate of absorption for subcutaneous and intramuscular injections depends on
   a. _____
   b. _____
   You may increase this rate by _____
   You may decrease this rate by _____

4. List the points the drug history of a patient should include.

5. Give an example of a drug that might produce each type of action listed.
   a. Depressant
   b. Stimulant
   c. Irritant
   d. Cumulative
   e. Demulcent
   f. Additive
   g. Selective
   h. Tolerance
   i. Side effect

6. You are requested to give your patient digoxin 0.25 mg orally. Fill in the following.
   a. Generic and proprietary name
   b. Purpose
   c. Usual dosage
   d. Routes of administration
   e. Nursing implications
   f. Points in patient teaching
   g. Manifestation of toxic effect
   h. Laboratory and ECG procedures
   i. Side effects expected
   j. Conditions for which this drug is used

See Index as well as this chapter to help you answer questions 7 to 17.

7. Oxygen, coffee, tea, and chocolate have a _____ effect on the body.

8. Alcohol, aspirin, and codeine have a _____ effect on the body.

9. What effect do the digitalis glycosides have on the heart rate? _____
The term for this action is a _____.

10. Oral contraceptives might be said to _____ (*depress* or *stimulate*) a body activity.

11. Atropine is given to the cardiac patient to _____ (*stimulate* or *depress*) output.

12. Atropine is given to the surgical patient to _____ (*stimulate* or *depress*) salivary excretion.

13. Aspirin, codeine, and Demerol would _____ (*enhance* or *suppress*) pain; this would affect the vital signs usually by _____ (*elevating* or *lowering*) them.

14. Explain the relationship of drug tolerance to initial dosages of analgesics in terminal cancer patients.

15. Explain the rationale for the following order of a preoperative medication: Demerol 100 mg, scopolamine 0.4 mg, and Vistaril 10 mg IM 1 hour before surgery.

16. What physical manifestation of a drug idiosyncrasy to Demerol might be observed following an initial dosage administered postoperatively?

17. What are some symptoms that lead patients to report drug allergies to their physician?

18. Do all persons respond correctly to the question: Do you have any allergies? What can the nurse do to elicit an accurate response?

CHAPTER 5

A review of arithmetic

Although many hospitals are using the "unit dosage" system in dispensing drugs, it is still the responsibility of the nurse to ascertain that the medication administered is exactly as prescribed by the physician. To give an accurate dosage, the nurse must have a working knowledge of basic mathematics. This review is offered so that you may individually determine areas in which you may need improvement.

ROMAN NUMERALS

Toward the end of the sixteenth century two systems of numbers emerged, Roman and Arabic. They are the basis for our communications in mathematics today, are used interchangeably, and are used by the physician in prescribing drugs.

Roman numerals 1 through 100 are used frequently in medicine; key symbols are as follows:

$$X = 10 \quad L = 50 \quad C = 100 \quad D = 500 \quad M \ 1000$$

To add, place the Roman numeral after the key symbol. To subtract, place the Roman numeral before the key symbol.

EXAMPLE: 109 = CIX   99 = XCIX

Express in Roman numerals:

3 _____	20 _____	101 _____
9 _____	18 _____	499 _____
10 _____	49 _____	1979 _____

Express in Arabic numerals:

IV _____	XXXIX _____	MCMLXX _____
VI _____	LIV _____	CXIX _____
XVIII _____	XCIV _____	LIX _____

FRACTIONS

Fractions are one or more of the separable parts of a substance, or less than a whole number or amount.

EXAMPLE: $1 - \dfrac{1}{2} = \dfrac{1}{2}$.

Common fraction

A common fraction is part of a whole number. The numerator (dividend) is the number above the line. The denominator (divisor) is the number below the line. The line separating the numerator from the denominator tells us to divide.

EXAMPLE: $\dfrac{1}{2} =$ the 1 is divided by the 2

Types of common fractions

1. *Simple:* contains *one* numerator and *one* denominator: $^1/_4$, $^1/_{20}$, $^1/_{60}$, $^1/_{100}$
2. *Complex:* may have a simple fraction in the numerator or denominator:

$$^1/_2 \text{ over } 4 = \frac{^1/_2}{4}, \ ^1/_2 \text{ over } ^1/_4 = \frac{^1/_2}{^1/_4}$$

3. *Proper:* numerator is smaller than denominator: $^1/_8$, $^2/_5$, $^1/_{100}$
4. *Improper:* numerator is larger than denominator: $^4/_3$, $^6/_4$, $^{100}/_{10}$
5. *Mixed number:* a whole number and a fraction: $4^5/_8$, $6^2/_3$, $1^5/_{100}$
6. *Decimal:* fractions written on the basis of a multiple of ten: $0.5 = {}^5/_{10}$, $0.05 = {}^5/_{100}$, $0.005 = {}^5/_{1000}$
7. *Equivalent:* fractions that have the same value: $^1/_3$ and $^2/_6$

Working with fractions

1. *Reducing to lowest terms.* Divide both the numerator and the denominator by a number that will divide into both (a common denominator).

EXAMPLE: $\dfrac{25}{125} \div \dfrac{25}{25} = \dfrac{1}{5}$

Reduce the following:

$$\frac{5}{100} \qquad \frac{3}{21} \qquad \frac{6}{36} \qquad \frac{12}{244} \qquad \frac{2}{4}$$

2. *Adding common fractions.* When denominators are the same figure, add the numerators.

EXAMPLE: $\dfrac{1}{4} + \dfrac{2}{4} + \dfrac{3}{4} = \dfrac{6}{4} = 1\dfrac{1}{2}$

Add the following:

$$\frac{2}{6} + \frac{3}{6} + \frac{4}{6} \qquad \frac{1}{100} + \frac{3}{100} + \frac{5}{100}$$

When the denominators are unlike, change the fractions to equivalent fractions by finding the lowest common denominator.

EXAMPLE: $\frac{2}{5} + \frac{3}{10} + \frac{1}{2} = 1\frac{1}{5}$

(use 10 as common denominator)

Divide 5 into 10 and multiply by 2 $= \frac{4}{10}$

Divide 10 into 10 and multiply by 3 $= \frac{3}{10}$

Divide 2 into 10 and multiply by 1 $= \frac{5}{10}$

Add $\frac{4}{10} + \frac{3}{10} + \frac{5}{10} = \frac{12}{10} = 1\frac{1}{5}$

Add the following:

$$\frac{2}{8} + \frac{4}{64} + \frac{5}{16} \qquad \frac{3}{7} + \frac{9}{14} + \frac{1}{28}$$

3. *Adding mixed numbers.* Add the fractions first; then add the whole numbers.

EXAMPLE: $2\frac{3}{4} + 2\frac{1}{2} + 3\frac{3}{8}$

a. Determine common denominator of fractions:

$$\frac{3}{4} = \frac{6}{8}, \quad \frac{1}{2} = \frac{4}{8}, \quad \frac{3}{8} = \frac{3}{8}$$

b. Add the fractions:

$$\frac{6}{8} + \frac{4}{8} + \frac{3}{8} = \frac{13}{8} = 1\frac{5}{8}$$

c. Add whole numbers:

$$2 + 2 + 3 = 7$$

d. Add b and c:

$$1\frac{5}{8} + 7 = 8\frac{5}{8} \text{ answer}$$

Add the following:

$$\frac{1}{4} + \frac{3}{4} \qquad \frac{1}{2} + \frac{1}{3} + \frac{1}{6} \qquad 15\frac{3}{5} + \frac{4}{50}$$

$$\frac{1}{3} + \frac{4}{9} + \frac{3}{19} \qquad \frac{1}{5} + \frac{14}{25} + \frac{11}{50}$$

$$3\frac{3}{10} + 4\frac{2}{5} + 5\frac{3}{15}$$

4. *Subtracting.* To find the least common denominator, subtract the smaller numerator from the larger. Reduce the remainder to its lowest terms.

EXAMPLE: $\frac{1}{4} - \frac{3}{16} = \frac{4}{16} - \frac{3}{16} = \frac{1}{16}$

5. *Subtracting mixed numbers.* When the numerator of the fraction in the top number is smaller than the numerator of the bottom number, it is necessary to borrow from the whole number, in the top number.

EXAMPLE: $4\frac{1}{4} - 1\frac{3}{4}$ (Note: you cannot subtract $\frac{3}{4}$ from $\frac{1}{4}$)

$$3\frac{5}{4} - 1\frac{3}{4} = 2\frac{2}{4} = 2\frac{1}{2}$$

Subtract the following:

$$\frac{7}{8} - \frac{3}{6} \qquad \frac{6}{12} - \frac{2}{24} \qquad \frac{1}{3} - \frac{1}{4}$$

$$6\frac{7}{8} - 3\frac{1}{16} \qquad 12\frac{1}{9} - 5\frac{7}{36}$$

Decimals as fractions

Now let us think of $1.00. The decimal point is after the "1," so this is read "one dollar." A decimal point in front of a number, in regard to the dollar, would make the amount less than a dollar. For example, 75 cents expressed as a fraction of a dollar would be $^{75}/_{100}$. Seventy-five cents expressed as a decimal part of a dollar would be $.75. Twenty-five cents expressed as a fraction of a dollar would be $^{25}/_{100}$; expressed as a decimal part of a dollar, it would be $.25. (Decimal points will be discussed later in the chapter.)

The fraction $^{25}/_{100}$ is twenty-five hundredths of one hundred or, in this case, of the whole dollar. The fraction $^{75}/_{100}$ is seventy-five hundredths of the hundred, or dollar. Notice the spelling of hundredths. This indicates less than the whole amount and shows that it is different from hundred, or less than one hundred. Be careful to spell hundredths correctly. The same is true of "tenths," "thousandths," and "ten-thousandths." They all indicate less than the whole amount. Notice the spelling of these words.

MULTIPLICATION
Multiplying a whole number by a fraction

1. Multiply the whole number by the numerator (top number).
2. Write the answer (product) over the denominator (bottom number).
3. Change the improper fraction to a mixed number.

EXAMPLE: $3 \times \frac{5}{8} = \frac{15}{8} = 1\frac{7}{8}$

Multiply the following:

$$2 \times \frac{3}{4} \qquad 15 \times \frac{3}{5} \qquad 9 \times \frac{3}{33} \qquad 4 \times \frac{9}{28} \qquad 6 \times \frac{5}{100}$$

Multiplying two fractions

1. Multiply the numerators (top numbers) together.
2. Multiple the denominators (bottom numbers) together.
3. Reduce your answer to its lowest terms.

EXAMPLES: $\dfrac{1}{4} \times \dfrac{2}{3} = \dfrac{2}{12}$ or reduced $\dfrac{1}{6}$

$\dfrac{5}{6} \times \dfrac{9}{10} = \dfrac{45}{60}$ or reduced $\dfrac{3}{4}$

Using cancellation to speed your work

1. Divide both the numerator and the denominator by the same number.
2. Then multiply both numerators and both denominators for the final answer.

EXAMPLE: $\dfrac{5}{6} \times \dfrac{9}{10}$

$$\dfrac{\overset{1}{\cancel{5}}}{\underset{2}{\cancel{6}}} \times \dfrac{\overset{3}{\cancel{9}}}{\underset{2}{\cancel{10}}} = \dfrac{3}{4}$$

Multiplying mixed numbers

To multiply mixed numbers change the mixed numbers to improper fractions.

EXAMPLES: $3\dfrac{1}{2} \times 2\dfrac{1}{5} = \dfrac{7}{2} \times \dfrac{11}{5} = \dfrac{77}{10} = 7\dfrac{7}{10}$

$16 \times 2\dfrac{1}{4} = \dfrac{16}{1} \times \dfrac{9}{4} = \dfrac{144}{4} = 36$

Multiply the following:

$1\dfrac{2}{3} \times \dfrac{3}{6} \qquad 1\dfrac{7}{8} \times 1\dfrac{1}{4}$

Multiplying whole numbers and decimals

1. Point off as many places in the answer, from the right, as there are places in the decimal involved in the multiplication.
2. The multiplier is the bottom number with the × or multiplication sign before it.
3. The multiplicand is the top number.

EXAMPLES:

500	1000	1000
× .02	× .04	× .009
10.00 (10)	40.00 (40)	9.000 (9)

7.25	500
× 4	× .009
29.00 (29)	4.500 (or 5)

Note in the last example that the first number after the decimal point in the answer is 5. Instead of the answer remaining 4.5 it becomes the next whole number, 5. This would be true if the answer were 4.5, 4.6, 4.7, 4.8, or 4.9. In each case the answer would become 5. If the answer were 4.1, 4.2, 4.3, or 4.4 the answer would remain 4.

When the first number after the decimal point is 5 or above, the answer becomes the next whole number. When the first number after the decimal point is less than 5, the answer becomes the whole number in the answer.

Multiply the following:

1,200	575	515	510
× .009	× .02	× .02	× .04

Multiplying a decimal by a decimal

1. Multiply the problem as if the numbers were both whole numbers.
2. Point off in the answer, from the right, as many decimal places as there are in both of the numbers that were to be multiplied.

EXAMPLE:

3.75
× .5
1.875 = 2

There are two decimal places in 3.75 and one decimal place in .5, making three decimal places. Point off three decimal places from the right. Round off the answer to 2.

Multiplying numbers with zero

EXAMPLES:

1. Multiply 223 by 40.
   a. Multiply 223 by 0. Write the answer, 0, in the unit column of the answer.
   b. Then multiply 223 by 4. Write this answer in front of the 0 in the product.

223
× 40
8920

2. Multiply 124 by 304.
   a. First multiply 124 by 4. The answer is 496.
   b. Now multiply 124 by 0. Write this answer, 0, under the 9 in 496.
   c. Multiply 124 by 3. Write this answer in front of the 0 in the product.

124
× 304
496
3720
37696

DIVISION

Dividing fractions

1. Change the division sign to a multiplication sign.
2. Invert the divisor (number by which you divide).

EXAMPLES: $4 \div \dfrac{1}{2} = \dfrac{4}{1} \times \dfrac{2}{1} = \dfrac{8}{1}$ or 8

$\dfrac{1}{8} \div \dfrac{1}{4} = \dfrac{1}{8} \times \dfrac{4}{1} = \dfrac{4}{8}$ or $\dfrac{1}{2}$

Divide the following:

$$2 \div \frac{3}{8} \qquad \frac{5}{8} \div \frac{7}{10} \qquad \frac{1}{8} \div \frac{1}{6}$$

If the divisor is a whole number, remember that the denominator of a whole number is always 1. Thus, a divisor of 4 becomes $\frac{1}{4}$ when inverted.

EXAMPLE: $\frac{1}{8} \div 4 = \frac{1}{8} \times \frac{1}{4} = \frac{1}{32}$

Divide the following:

$$3\frac{1}{8} \div 2\frac{1}{16}$$

Dividing with a mixed number

1. Change the mixed number to an improper fraction.
2. Change the division sign to a multiplication sign.
3. Invert the divisor.

EXAMPLES: $4\frac{1}{2} \div \frac{3}{4} = \frac{9}{2} \div \frac{3}{4} = \frac{\overset{3}{\cancel{9}}}{\cancel{2}} \times \frac{\overset{2}{\cancel{4}}}{\cancel{3}} = \frac{6}{1}$ or 6

$6\frac{1}{4} \div 1\frac{1}{4} = \frac{25}{4} \div \frac{5}{4} = \frac{\overset{5}{\cancel{25}}}{\cancel{4}} \times \frac{\overset{1}{\cancel{4}}}{\cancel{5}} = \frac{5}{1}$ or 5

Dividing decimals

1. If the divisor (number by which you divide) is a decimal, make it a whole number by moving the decimal point to the right of the last figure.
2. Move the decimal point in the dividend (the number divided) as many places to the right as you moved the decimal point in the divisor.
3. Place the decimal point for the quotient (answer) directly above the new decimal point of the dividend.

EXAMPLES (*Can you work the ones without answers?*):

$.25 \overline{)\ .10} = 25 \overline{)\ 10.00}^{.40} \qquad .03 \overline{)\ 9.93} = 3 \overline{)\ 993}^{331}$

$.4 \overline{)\ 1.68} = 4 \overline{)\ 16.8}^{4.2}$

DECIMAL FRACTIONS

When fractions are written in decimal form, the denominators are not written. The word *decimal* means "10." The first place to the right of the decimal point means tenths, the second place means hundredths, the third place means thousandths, the fourth place means ten-thousandths, and so on.

EXAMPLES: .3   is read three tenths
.05   is read five hundredths
.465 is read four hundred sixty-five thousandths

.0007 is read seven ten-thousandths
2.25   is read two and twenty-five hundredths

On prescriptions another way of expressing the decimal is by using a slanted line.

EXAMPLES:
1	mg = 0.001	g = 0/001	g
0.1	mg = 0.0001	g = 0/0001	g
30	mg = 0.030	g = 0/030	g
100	mg = 0.100	g = 0/100	g
1000	mg = 1.000	g = 1/0	g
250	mg = 0.250	g = 0/250	g

Changing decimals to common fractions

1. Remove the decimal point.
2. Place the appropriate denominator under the number.
3. Reduce to lowest terms.

EXAMPLES: $.2 = \frac{2}{10} = \frac{1}{5} \qquad .20 = \frac{20}{100} = \frac{1}{5}$

Change the following:

.3 _____   .25 _____
.4 _____   .50 _____
.5 _____   .75 _____
.05 _____   .002 _____

Changing common fractions to decimal fractions

Divide the numerator of the fraction by the denominator.

EXAMPLE: $\frac{1}{4}$ means $1 \div 4$ or $4 \overline{)\ 1.00}^{.25}$

Change the following:

$\frac{1}{2}$ means _____ $\frac{3}{4}$ means _____

$\frac{1}{6}$ means _____ $\frac{1}{50}$ means _____

$\frac{2}{3}$ means _____

PERCENTS
Determining percent one number is of another

1. Divide the smaller number by the larger number.
2. Multiply the quotient by 100 and add the percent sign.

EXAMPLE: A certain 1000 parts solution is 10 parts drug. What percent of the solution is drug?

$1000 \overline{)\ 10.00}^{.01} \quad .01 \times 100 = 1.$ or 1%

Changing percents to fractions

1. Omit the percent sign to form the numerator.
2. Use 100 for the denominator.

3. Reduce the fraction.

EXAMPLES: $5\% = \dfrac{5}{100} = \dfrac{1}{20}$ $75\% = \dfrac{75}{100} = \dfrac{3}{4}$

Change the following:

$25\% = \dfrac{25}{100} =$ $2\% = \dfrac{2}{100} =$

$15\% = \dfrac{15}{100} =$ $12\frac{1}{2}\% = \dfrac{12.5}{100} =$

$10\% = \dfrac{10}{100} =$ $\frac{1}{4}\% = \dfrac{\frac{1}{4}}{100} =$

$20\% = \dfrac{20}{100} =$ $150\% = \dfrac{150}{100} =$

$50\% = \dfrac{50}{100} =$ $4\% = \dfrac{4}{100} =$

Changing percents to decimal fractions

1. Omit the percent signs.
2. Insert a decimal point *two places to the left* of the last number, or express as hundredths, decimally.

EXAMPLES: $5\% = .05$ $15\% = .15$

Change the following:

$4\% =$ $25\% =$

$1\% =$ $50\% =$

$2\% =$ $10\% =$

Note in these examples that those numbers that were already hundredths, such as 10%, 15%, 25%, 50%, merely need to have the decimal point placed in front of the first number, since they are already expressed in hundredths: where 1%, 2%, 4%, 5% needed to have a zero placed in front of the number to express them as hundredths.

Change these percents to decimal fractions:

$12\frac{1}{2}\% =$ $\frac{1}{4}\% =$

If the percent is a mixed number, it should have the fraction expressed as a decimal. Then change the percent to a decimal by moving the decimal point two places to the left.

EXAMPLES: $12\frac{1}{2}\% = 12.5\%$ or $.125$
$\frac{1}{4}\% = 0.25\%$ or $.0025$

Changing common fractions to percents

1. Divide the numerator by the denominator.
2. Multiply the quotient by 100 and add the percent sign.

EXAMPLE: $\dfrac{1}{50} = 50\overset{.02}{\overline{\smash{)}1.00}} = .02 \times 100 = 2\%$

Change the following:

$\dfrac{1}{400} =$

$\dfrac{1}{8} =$

Changing decimal fractions to percents

1. Move the decimal point two places to the right.
2. Omit the decimal point if a whole number results.
3. Add the percent signs. (This is the same as multiplying the decimal fraction by 100 and adding the percent sign.)

EXAMPLE: $.01 = 1.00 = 1\%$ (or $\dfrac{1}{100}$)

Change the following:

.05 =
.25 =
.15 =
.125 =
.0025 =

Points to remember in reading decimals

1. 1. is the whole number 1. When it is written 1.0 it is still one or 1.
2. The whole number is usually written like this: 1 or 2 or 3 or 4, and so on.
3. The whole number also can be written with the decimal point after the number: 1.0, 2.0, 3.0, 4.0
4. Can you read this one? 0.1. This is one-tenth. There is one number after the decimal point.
5. Can you read this one? .1. This is also one-tenth. The zero in front of the decimal point does not change its value. One-tenth can be written, then, in two ways: 0.1 and .1.
6. Remember that in writing the number 1. or 1.00, the decimal point is after the number. This makes the number a whole number. It is read the whole number 1.

RATIOS

A ratio expresses the relationship that one quantity bears to another.

EXAMPLES: 1:5 means 1 part of a drug to 5 parts of a solution.
1:100 means 1 part of a drug to 1000 parts of a solution.
1:500 means 1 part of a drug to 500 parts of a solution.

A common fraction can be expressed as a ratio.

EXAMPLE: $\dfrac{1}{5}$ is the same as 1:5

The ratio of one amount to an amount expressed in

terms of the same unit is the number of units in the first divided by the number of units in the second. The ratio of 2 ounces of a disinfectant to 10 ounces of water is 2 to 10 or 1 to 5 or $^1/_5$. This ratio may be written $^1/_5$ or 1:5.

The two numbers compared are called the terms of a ratio. The first term of a true ratio is always one, or 1. This is the simplest form of a ratio.

Changing ratio to percent

1. Make the first term of the ratio the numerator of the fraction whose denominator is the second term of the ratio.
2. Divide the numerator by the denominator.
3. Multiply by 100 and add the percent sign.

EXAMPLE: $5:1 = \dfrac{5}{1} \times 100 = 500\%$

Change the following:

$1:5 =$

Changing percent to ratio

1. Change the percent to a fraction and reduce fraction to lowest terms.
2. The numerator of the fraction is the first term of the ratio, and the denominator is the second term of the ratio.

EXAMPLE: $^1/_2\% = \dfrac{^1/_2}{100} = \dfrac{1}{200} = 1:200$

Change the following:

$2\% =$
$50\% =$
$75\% =$

Simplifying ratios

Ratios can be simplified as ratios or as fractions.

EXAMPLE: $25:100 = 1:4$ or $\dfrac{25}{100} = \dfrac{1}{4}$

Simplify the following:

$4:12 =$
$5:10 =$
$10:5 =$
$75:100 =$
$^1/_4:100 =$
$15:20 =$
$3:9 =$

PROPORTIONS

A proportion shows how two *equal* ratios are related. This method is good because it is possible to prove that your answer is correct, and it is especially useful in solutions.

1. Three factors are known. The fourth *unknown* (what you are looking for) is represented by x.
2. The first and fourth terms of a proportion are called extremes. The second and third are the means. The product of the means equals the product of the extremes, or multiplying the first and fourth equals the second and third.

EXAMPLE:
$$\overset{extreme}{1} \times \overset{mean}{2} = \overset{mean}{2} \times \overset{extreme}{4}$$

Proof: $1 \times 4 = 4$ and $2 \times 2 = 4$

If you did not know one number you could solve for it as follows:

EXAMPLE:
$$1:2 = 2:x$$
$$1x = 4$$
$$x = 4 \div 1 = 4$$
$$x = 4$$

Proof: $1 \times 4 = 4$ and $2 \times 2 = 4$

Solve the following:

$6:12 = 24:x$

ASSIGNMENT

Review previous lessons and questions according to the direction of your instructor. Attempt to solve the following problems without referring to the review. Check your mistakes to find the type of problem you need to review.

1. Express in Roman numerals.
   a. 17 _____   e. 75 _____
   b. 65 _____   f. 45 _____
   c. 99 _____   g. 38 _____
   d. 100 _____   h. 59 _____
2. Express in Arabic numerals.
   a. CX _____   e. XLVIII _____
   b. LX _____   f. IV _____
   c. XLV _____   g. XXV _____
   d. XXX _____   h. XC _____
3. Change to whole or mixed numbers.
   a. $^{12}/_6$ _____   e. $^{64}/_8$ _____
   b. $^{19}/_3$ _____   f. $^{38}/_7$ _____
   c. $^{25}/_{25}$ _____   g. $^{89}/_8$ _____
   d. $^{48}/_5$ _____   h. $^{125}/_5$ _____
4. Add the following fractions.
   a. $^1/_4$ b. $2^3/_5$ c. $^1/_{10}$ d. $^7/_9$
       $^3/_8$ $1^1/_3$ $^3/_5$ $^9/_{10}$
       $^1/_3$ $4^1/_2$ $^5/_8$ $^2/_{15}$
5. Add the following decimal fractions.
   a. 0.65   b. 0.375   c. 0.6
      0.019   0.5   0.4758
      0.010   0.69   0.352
6. Add the following.
   a. 256.789   b. 3.542   c. 85.65
      83.45   89.650   910.86
      6.500   33.3   1100.78

7. Subtract the following fractions and mixed numbers.

   a. $3/5$ b. $2^1/4$ c. $1^6/10$ d. $8^1/2$
   $-1/10$ $-3/8$ $-3/5$ $-6/8$

8. Subtract the following decimal fractions.

   a. 15.650 b. 265.39 c. 34.5 d. 189
   $-$ 8.35 -100.13 -26.5 $-$ 5.29

9. Multiply the following.

   a. $2/3 \times 3/16$ b. $15 \times 1^4/5$ c. $3^1/5 \times 10$ d. $6^1/2 \times 2$

10. Multiply the following.

    a. 675.5×0.78 c. 910.24×0.8
    b. 150×0.34 d. 88.40×0.30

11. Divide the following.

    a. $5/8$ by $7/10$ b. 2 by $3/4$ c. $2/5$ by $2^1/2$

12. Divide the following.

    a. 86 by 23.5 b. 15.75 by 2.5 c. 156.9 by 4.5

13. Which is the larger fraction?

    a. $1/2$ or $2/5$ _____ c. $1/150$ or $1/200$ _____
    b. $3/4$ or $5/8$ _____ d. $1/50$ or $1/75$ _____

14. Change the following to decimal fractions.

    a. $3/4$ _____ c. $1^5/10$ _____
    b. $9/10$ _____ d. $4^1/4$ _____

15. Change the following to percents.

    a. $1/2$ _____ c. 0.0009 _____
    b. 0.07 _____ d. $1/3$ _____

16. Solve the following.

    a. 2% of 80 _____ c. 0.08% of 800 _____
    b. 0.5% of 2000 _____ d. 5% of 100 _____

17. Read the following. Tell what the answer is *in words*, showing you know how to read these first decimal points you were taught. You will have many more in different strengths to learn in the next few chapters. Review *Points to remember in reading decimals* in this chapter.

    a. 1. _____
    b. 0.1 _____
    c. .1 _____
    d. 1.00 _____
    e. 5 _____

18. Express the following as ratios.

    a. $1/8$ _____ c. $1/250$ _____
    b. $1/50$ _____ d. $1/125$ _____

19. Solve the following.

    a. $9 : x : : 5 : 300$ _____
    b. $x : 60 : : 4 : 120$ _____
    c. $5 : 3000 : : 15 : x$ _____
    d. $0.7 : 70 : : : x : 1000$ _____
    e. $1/400 : : x : : 2 : 1600$ _____
    f. $0.2 : 8 : : x : 20$ _____
    g. $100,000 : 3 : : 1,000,000 : x$ _____
    h. $1/4 : x : : 20 : 400$ _____

    NOTE: x is the unknown factor. It may be a mean or an extreme in either of the four positions in any problem.

20. Develop ten problems from each of the 19 types presented in this assignment. Bring the problems to the next class for discussion.

CHAPTER 6

Systems of weights and measures

Two systems of weighing and measuring drugs are the *apothecary* and the *metric*. In the United States we are changing to the latter; until change is complete, nurses will need to know commonly used values in each.

APOTHECARY SYSTEM

Apothecary is an ancient word meaning pharmacist or druggist, with the units of measurement under this system ancient as well.

Apothecary weight

For weighing solids the units are, in increasing order of magnitude (smallest to largest), as follows:

grain (smallest)	ounce
scruple	pound (largest)
dram	

The grain was originally derived from the average weight of a grain of wheat. The symbol for grain is "gr." The dram (originally, drachma or drachm) was a Greek silver coin. The symbol for dram is "ʒ." The ounce, whose symbol is "℥," is $^1/_{12}$ of a troy pound. The pound is of Roman origin and signifies a balance. The symbol "lb" is the abbreviation for the Latin word *libra,* which means pound.

In apothecary weight 12 ounces equal 1 pound (same weight as those of troy weight). In avoirdupois weight 16 ounces equal 1 pound. Avoirdupois weight is used in weighing all articles except drugs, gold, silver, and precious stones.

$$20 \text{ grains (gr)} = 1 \text{ scruple}$$
$$3 \text{ scruples or } 60 \text{ grains} = 1 \text{ dram (ʒ)}$$
$$(1 \text{ dram} = 4 \text{ ml or } 4 \text{ cc})$$
$$8 \text{ drams or } 480 \text{ grains} = 1 \text{ ounce (℥)}$$
$$12 \text{ ounces} = 1 \text{ pound (lb)}$$

Apothecary volume

For measuring fluids the units are, from smallest to largest, as follows:

minim (smallest)	pint
fluidram	quart
fluidounce	gallon (largest)

The unit of fluid measure is a minim (see Fig. 6-1). This is approximately the quantity of water that would weigh a grain. The symbol for minim is "♏." The symbol "O" is the abbreviation for the Latin word *octarius.* It means an eighth of a gallon and is the same as a pint. The symbol "C" is taken from the Latin word *congius.* It means a vessel or container that holds a gallon.

$$60 \text{ minims (♏)} = 1 \text{ fluidram (fʒ)}$$
$$8 \text{ fluidrams or } 480 \text{ minims} = 1 \text{ fluidounce (f℥)}$$
$$16 \text{ fluidounces} = 1 \text{ pint (pt or O)}$$
$$2 \text{ pints} = 1 \text{ quart (qt)}$$
$$4 \text{ quarts} = 1 \text{ gallon (C)}$$

It might be of aid to visualize a dram as approximately equal to one teaspoonful in household measure.

Symbols and abbreviations

When symbols are used, the quantity is usually expressed in Roman numerals. These Roman numerals are placed after the symbols. For example, 2 grains is written gr ii; 2 drams, ʒ ii; and 2 ounces, ℥ ii. Sometimes drams and ounces are written ʒ 2 and ℥ 2. Fractions are expressed in Arabic numerals, gr $^1/_4$, gr $^1/_8$, gr $^1/_2$, gr $^1/_{150}$.

The symbol "ss" may be used for one-half: $1^1/_2$ grains is written gr iss. The symbol "ss" comes from the Latin *semi, semisis,* meaning half.

The minim (♏) is the approximate equivalent of the drop, but it is not identical to the drop. To help you realize that it is an approximate equivalent to the drop, note the following:

1. A minim of water is approximately equal to 1 drop.
2. A minim of an alcoholic solution, such as tincture of belladonna, equals 2 drops.
3. A minim of ether is about 3 drops.
4. A minim of a gummy substance is less than 1 drop.

Minims should always be measured when the doctor orders a drug in minims. A minim glass should be used for accuracy. When the doctor orders drops, they may be measured with a medicine dropper. The abbreviation for drops is "gtt," from the Latin *gutta,* meaning drops.

The abbreviation for grain in the apothecary system should always be written "gr." This prevents confusing it with the abbreviation "g" for gram in the metric sys-

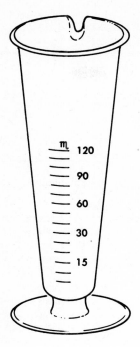 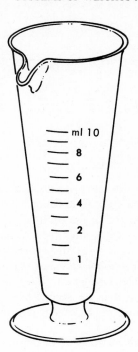

Fig. 6-1. Fluid measures.

tem. Since 1 gram equals 15 grains, a serious error could result.

Write the following correctly:

3 grains _____		10 drops _____
1¹/₂ grains _____		15 minims _____
4 drams _____		¹/₄ grain _____
2 ounces _____		1 dram _____
¹/₂ grain _____		1 ounce _____

METRIC SYSTEM

The metric system was invented by the French in the late eighteenth century. A committee of the Academy of Sciences, working under government authority, recommended a standard unit of linear measure. For a basis of measurement they chose a fourth of the earth's circumference measured across the poles. One ten-millionth of this distance was accepted as the standard unit of linear measure.

The committee calculated the distance from the equator to the North Pole from surveys that had been made along the meridian that passes through Paris. The distance divided by 10,000,00 was chosen as the unit of length, or the meter.

Metric standards were adopted in France in 1799. The International Metric Convention met in Paris in 1875, and as a result of this meeting the International Bureau of Weights and Measures was formed. The first task of the International Bureau of Weights and Measures was the preparation of an international standard meter bar and an international standard kilogram weight. Duplicates of these were made for all participating countries to the convention.

A measurement line was selected on the international standard meter bar. The distance between the two lines of measurement on the bar is the official unit of the metric system. The standards given to the United States are preserved in the U.S. Bureau of Standards, Washington, D.C. There are 25 millimeters in 1 inch (2.5 centimeters).

Metric weight

The unit of weight is the gram. This is the weight of 1 cubic centimeter of water at 4° centigrade. The symbol for gram is "g." A milligram is one-thousandth (0.001) of a gram. Its symbol is "mg." One kilogram is equivalent to 2.2 pounds.

Metric volume

The unit of volume is the liter. A liter is equal to 1000 ml (milliliters) or 1000 cc (cubic centimeters) or 1 quart. One milliliter weighs 1 gram.

Divisions of the gram and the milligram

In the division of the gram the amounts are usually written and read as decimal fractions of the gram. The same is true of the milligram.

Can you read the following decimal fractions?

0.1 g	.05 g
1.0 g	1.25 mg
.25 mg	

Table 6-1. Prefixes in metric system

Prefixes	Meaning	Written as	Units
milli—one-thousandth	1/1000	.001	"meter" for length
centi—one-hundredth	1/100	.01	"gram" for weight
deci—one-tenth	1/10	.1	"liter" for capacity
unit—one	1	1.0	
deka—ten	10/1	10.	
hecto—one hundred	100/1	100.	
kilo—one thousand	1000/1	1000.	

Remember: one number after the decimal point is read as tenths; two numbers after the decimal point as hundredths; three numbers after the decimal point as thousandths; and four numbers after the decimal point as ten-thousandths. In such cases the values are all fractions, or less than the whole—in the examples here, less than a gram or less than a milligram. If the decimal point is after the number, such as the second problem (1.0 g), it indicates that the number is a whole number and is read 1 gram.

The prefixes in the metric system that indicate multiples of the unit are of Greek derivation; those that indicate subdivisions are of Latin origin. (See Table 6-1). In the divisions of the gram the amounts are usually written and read as decimal fractions of the gram. For example, a dosage is never written as a decigram; it is expressed as 0.1 g. The use of the milligram is becoming more common, for example, nicotinic acid, vitamin B_6, 100 mg (same as 0.1 g).

A milligram is one-thousandth of a gram. It is less than a gram. A microgram is one-thousandth of a milligram. The use of decimals always suggests that the quantity is metric.

If the drug is a solid, the unit will be g, such as sulfisoxazole 1.0 (Sulfisoxazole, a sulfa drug, is a chemotherapeutic agent—a drug that kills certain microorganisms.) If the drug is a liquid, the unit will be ml, for example, elixir phenobarbital, 4 ml (1 dram or 1 teaspoon). Elixir phenobarbital is a drug given to quiet the patient or overcome nervousness.

EXAMPLES 1.0 g = one gram
          1 ml = one milliliter

Write the following dosages:

0.5 g	_____	1.0 mg	_____
0.05 g	_____	4.0 mg	_____
0.3 g	_____	18.3 mg	_____
0.4 g	_____	25.0 mg	_____
0.6 g	_____	0.0006 g	_____
0.4 mg	_____	4.0 ml	_____
0.625 mg	_____		

Table 6-2. Handy equivalents*

Apothecary	Metric
15 minims	= 1 ml (cc)
30 minims ($1/2$ dram)	= 2 ml (cc)
60 minims (1 dram)	= 4-5 ml (cc)
1 grain	= 0.065 g
5 grains	= 0.3 g (or $1/3$ g)
10 grains	= 0.6 g
15 grains	= 1.0 g
$7^1/2$ grains	= 0.5 g ($1/2$ g)

*Review the equivalents. All of these must be memorized and reviewed often. You will use them in pouring medicines.

CONVERSION OF METRIC AND APOTHECARY UNITS
Converting grams to grains (or milliliters to minims)

Multiply the number of grams (or milliliters) by 15.

EXAMPLES:
1. Change 30 grams to grains.

$$30 \times 15 = 450 \text{ gr}$$

2. Change 1 gram to grains.

$$1g \times 15gr/g = 15gr$$

Use ratio and proportion.

$$\frac{g}{1} : \frac{gr}{1} : : \frac{g}{15} : \frac{gr}{x}$$
$$x = 15$$
$$1 \text{ g} = \text{gr } 15$$

Converting grains to grams

Divide the number of grains by 15 (or multiply by 0.065).

EXAMPLES:
1. Change 30 grains to grams.

$$30 \div 15 = 2 \text{ g}$$

2. Change 5 grains to grams.

$$0.065 \text{ g/gr} \times 5 \text{ gr} = 0.325 \text{ g}$$

Converting grams to milligrams

Multiply by 1000 and move the decimal point of the grams three places to the right.

EXAMPLE: The physician orders the patient to have 0.250 g of a drug. The label on the bottle of medicine says 250 mg, meaning that each capsule contains 250 mg of the drug.

To change the gram dose into milligrams multiply 0.250 by 1000 and move the decimal point three places to the right (a milligram is one-thousandth of a gram); 0.250 g = 250 mg, so you would give one tablet of this drug.

TRY THIS ONE: The physician orders the patient to have 0.1 g of a drug. The label on the bottle states the strength of the drug is 100 mg.

To change the gram dose into milligrams, move the decimal point three places to the right: 0.1 g = 100 mg, exactly what the bottle label strength states.

Convert the following grams (g) to milligrams (mg):

0.2 g = _____ mg
.250 g = _____ mg
.125 g = _____ mg
.0006 g = _____ mg
0.004 g = _____ mg

Converting milligrams to grams

Divide by 1000 and move the decimal point of the milligrams three places to the left.

EXAMPLES: 200 mg = 0.2 g
0.6 mg = .0006 g

Convert the following milligrams to grams:

0.4 mg = _____ g
0.12 mg = _____ g
0.2 mg = _____ g
0.1 mg = _____ g
500 mg = _____ g
125 mg = _____ g
100 mg = _____ g
200 mg = _____ g
50 mg = _____ g
400 mg = _____ g

Can you take the gram dosages in these answers and convert them to milligrams?

Converting ounces to pints

Divide the number of ounces by 16 (16 ounces in 1 pint).

EXAMPLE: Convert 320 ounces to pints.

320 ÷ 16 = 20 pt

Converting pints to quarts

Divide the number of pints by 2 (2 pints in 1 quart).

EXAMPLE: Convert 10 pints to quarts.

10 ÷ 2 = 5 qt

Converting quarts to gallons

Divide the number of quarts by 4 (4 quarts in 1 gallon).

EXAMPLE: Convert 4 quarts into gallons.

4 ÷ 4 = 1 C

Solid dosage for oral administration

If the dosage *on hand* and the dosage ordered are both in the same system, the problem is to give the patient the *correct* dosage ordered from what you have.

EXAMPLE: Physician orders patient to have 1.0 g of a medicine. The medicine bottle states that each capsule in the bottle contains 0.5 g.

PROBLEM: You do not have the 1.0 g as ordered; instead, you have a bottle of 0.5-g capsules. How many capsules will you give?

SOLUTION: You may use two methods:

1. $\dfrac{\text{Dosage desired}}{\text{Dosage on hand}} = \dfrac{1.0 \text{ g}}{0.5 \text{ g}} = 2$ You will give two 0.5-g capsules to give the 1.0 g ordered.

2. $\dfrac{\text{g}}{0.5} : \dfrac{\text{Capsule}}{1} :: \dfrac{\text{g}}{1.0} : \dfrac{\text{Capsule}}{x}$ $\begin{array}{l} 0.5x = 1.0 \\ x = 2 \end{array}$

Proof: 0.5 × 2 = 1.0
1.0 × 1 = 1.0

EXAMPLE: Physician orders patient to have 1000 mg of ampicillin. You have on hand a bottle of tablets labeled 0.25 g per tablet. (0.25 g = 250 mg)

SOLUTION:

1. $\dfrac{\text{Dosage desired}}{\text{Dosage on hand}} = \dfrac{1000 \text{ mg}}{250 \text{ mg}} = 4$ Give four 0.25-g tablets.

2. $\dfrac{\text{mg}}{250} : \dfrac{\text{tablet}}{1} :: \dfrac{\text{mg}}{1000} : \dfrac{\text{tablet}}{x}$ $\begin{array}{l} 250x = 1000 \\ x = \dfrac{1000}{250} = \end{array}$

4 tablets

Proof: 250 × 4 = 1000
1000 × 1 = 1000

Solve the following yourself using both rules (desired:on hand) and proportion:

1. Physician orders aspirin 600 mg. You have aspirin gr v per tablet.
2. Physician orders Gantrisin 0.25 g. You have Gantrisin 500 mg per tablet.
3. Physician orders pentobarbital 200 mg. You have pentobarbital $1^1/_2$-gr capsules.

Table 6-3. Metric doses and apothecary equivalents*

Liquid measure		Weight	
Metric	**Approximate apothecary equivalents**	**Metric**	**Approximate apothecary equivalents**
1000 ml†	1 quart	30 g	1 ounce
750 ml	1½ pints	15 g	4 drams
500 ml	1 pint	100 g	2½ drams
250 ml	8 fluidounces	7.5 g	2 drams
200 ml	7 fluidounces	6 g	90 grains
100 ml	3½ fluidounces	5 g	75 grains
50 ml	1⅓ fluidounces	3 g	45 grains
30 ml	1 fluidounce	2 g	30 grains (½ dram)
15 ml	4 fluidrams	1.5 g	22 grains
10 ml	2½ fluidrams	1 g	15 grains
8 ml	2 fluidrams	0.75 g	12 grains
5 ml	1¼ fluidrams	0.6 g	10 grains
4 ml	1 fluidram	0.5 g	7½ grains
3 ml	45 minims	0.4 g	6 grains
2 ml	30 minims	0.3 g	5 grains
1 ml	15 minims	0.25 g	4 grains
0.75 ml	12 minims	0.2 g	3 grains
0.6 ml	10 minims	0.15 g	2½ grains
0.5 ml	8 minims	0.12 g	2 grains
0.3 ml	5 minims	0.1 g	1½ grains
0.25 ml	4 minims	75 mg	1¼ grains
0.2 ml	3 minims	60 mg	1 grain
0.1 ml	1½ minims	50 mg	¾ grain
0.06 ml	1 minim	40 mg	⅔ grain
0.05 ml	¾ minim	30 mg	½ grain
0.03 ml	½ minim	25 mg	⅜ grain
		20 mg	⅓ grain
		15 mg	¼ grain
		12 mg	⅕ grain
		10 mg	⅙ grain
		8 mg	⅛ grain
		6 mg	1/10 grain
		5 mg	1/12 grain
		4 mg	1/15 grain
		3 mg	1/20 grain
		2 mg	1/30 grain
		1.5 mg	1/40 grain
		1.2 mg	1/50 grain
		1 mg	1/60 grain
		0.8 mg	1/80 grain
		0.6 mg	1/100 grain
		0.5 mg	1/120 grain
		0.4 mg	1/150 grain
		0.3 mg	1/200 grain
		0.25 mg	1/250 grain
		0.2 mg	1/300 grain
		0.15 mg	1/400 grain
		0.12 mg	1/500 grain
		0.1 mg	1/600 grain

*From United States Pharmacopeia XX.
†A milliliter (ml) is the approximate equivalent of a cubic centimeter (cc).

EXAMPLES: Physician orders 3 g. You have grains.
PROBLEM: How can you give 3 g from grains? To convert grams to grains, multiply the number of grams by 15.
SOLUTION: 3g × 15 = 45 grains
or   15 : 1 : : x : 3 = gr 45

Prepare 45 grains to give the 3.0 g ordered.
Solve the following:

$$6.0 \text{ g} = \underline{\hspace{2cm}} \text{ gr}$$
$$500 \text{ mg} = \underline{\hspace{2cm}} \text{ gr}$$
$$60 \text{ mg} = \underline{\hspace{2cm}} \text{ gr}$$
$$.1 \text{ g} = \underline{\hspace{2cm}} \text{ gr}$$

EXAMPLE: Physician orders aspirin gr 45. You have aspirin in grams.
PROBLEM: How can you give aspirin gr 45 from the grams you have on hand? To convert grains to grams, divide the number of grains by 15.
SOLUTION: 45 ÷ 15 = 3 g in gr 45
or   0.06 : 1 : : x : 45 = 3 g

Prepare 3 g to give the gr 45.
Solve the following:

$$\text{gr x} = \underline{\hspace{2cm}} \text{ g}$$
$$\text{gr 3} = \underline{\hspace{2cm}} \text{ mg}$$
$$\text{gr xv} = \underline{\hspace{2cm}} \text{ g}$$

Conversion problems

Some students understand problems in tablet dosage for oral administration if presented with their fractional equivalents as follows.

1. Physician orders patient to receive 2 g of a drug in oral tablet form. The medicine bottle label states the strength on hand is 0.5 g. This means each tablet in the bottle is the strength 0.5 g.
   How many tablets would you give the patient—1, $1^1/_2$, 2 $2^1/_2$, 3, 4, or 5? Answer: 4
   What strength are you asked to give ? 2 g
   What strength is on the bottle label? 0.5 g
   What is the fractional equivalent of 0.5 g? $^1/_2$ g
   How many $^1/_2$ (0.5-g) tablets would equal 2 g?

   $$2 \div {}^1/_2 = {}^2/_1 = {}^2/_1 = 4 \text{ tablets}$$

2. Physician orders patient to receive 0.2 mg of a drug in oral tablet form. The medicine bottle label states the strength on hand is 0.1 mg. This means each tablet in the bottle is the strength 0.1 mg.
   How many tablets would you give the patient—$^1/_2$, 1, $1^1/_2$, 2, 3, or 4? Answer: 2
   What strength are you asked to give? 0.2 mg
   What is the fractional equivalent of 0.2 mg? $^2/_{10}$
   What strength is on the bottle label (on hand)? 0.1 mg
   What is the fractional equivalent of 0.1 mg? $^1/_{10}$
   How many $^1/_{10}$-mg (0.1-mg) tablets would equal $^2/_{10}$ mg (0.2 mg)? 2

$$\begin{array}{r} 0.1 \text{ mg} = 1 \text{ tablet} \\ 0.1 \text{ mg} = 1 \text{ tablet} \\ \hline 0.2 \text{ mg} = 2 \text{ tablets} \end{array}$$

or $^2/_{10} \div {}^1/_{10} = {}^2/_{10} \times {}^{10}/_1 = 2$ tablets

3. Physician orders patient to receive 0.5 mg of a drug in oral tablet form. The medicine bottle label states the strength on hand is 0.25 mg. This means each tablet in the bottle is the strength 0.25 mg.
   How many tablets would you give the patient—$^1/_2$, 1, $1^1/_2$, 2, $2^1/_2$, 3, 4, or 5? Answer: 2
   What strength are you asked to give? 0.5 mg
   What fractional equivalent equals 0.5 mg? $^1/_2$ mg
   What strength is on the bottle label? 0.25 mg
   What fractional equivalent equals the strength on hand? $^1/_4$ mg
   How many $^1/_4$-mg (0.25-mg) tablets would equal $^1/_2$ mg (0.5 mg)? 2

$$\begin{array}{l} 0.25 \text{ mg} = {}^1/_4 \text{ mg or 1 tablet} \\ 0.25 \text{ mg} = {}^1/_4 \text{ mg or 1 tablet} \\ \hline 0.50 \text{ mg} = {}^1/_2 \text{ mg or 2 tablets} \end{array}$$

or $^1/_2 \div {}^1/_4 = {}^1/_2 \times {}^4/_1 = 2$ tablets

You must realize in this problem that the answer 0.50 mg is the same as 0.5 mg, which is the strength ordered.

4. Physician orders patient to receive 0.25 mg of a drug in oral tablet form. The medicine bottle label states the strength on hand is 0.5 mg. This means that every tablet in the bottle is the strength 0.5 mg.
   How many tablets would you give? $^1/_2$, 1, $1^1/_2$, 2, $2^1/_2$, 3, 4, or 5? Answer: $^1/_2$
   What strength did the physician order? 0.25 mg
   What is the fractional equivalent of the strength the doctor ordered? $^1/_4$ mg
   What strength is on the bottle label? 0.5 mg
   What is the fractional equivalent of the strength on the bottle label (on hand)? $^1/_2$ mg
   Which is less: 0.5 mg ($^1/_2$ mg) or 0.25 mg ($^1/_4$ mg)? 0.25 mg ($^1/_4$ mg)
   Was the amount ordered less than the strength on hand or more? Less

   0.5 mg = $^1/_2$ mg or 1 tablet.
   0.25 mg = $^1/_4$ mg or half as much or $^1/_2$ tablet
   or $^1/_4 \div {}^1/_2 = {}^1/_4 \times {}^2/_1 = {}^1/_2$ tablet

All this problem asked was: if you have 0.5-mg or $^1/_2$-mg tablets on hand, how many tablets would you need to give 0.25 mg ($^1/_4$ mg)? Realize that $^1/_4$ is half of $^1/_2$.

Liquid dosage for oral administration

1. Physician orders 60 ml of a liquid medication. How many ounces will you give?

60 ml ÷ 30 (30 ml = 1 oz) = 2 oz

Give 2 oz to get 60 ml.

2. Physician orders 45 ml. How many ounces will you give?

$$45 ÷ 30 = 1\frac{1}{2}\ oz$$

3. Physician orders 6 drams. How many milliliters (cubic centimeters) will you give?

4 ml = 1 dram
4 × 6 = 24 ml (cc)

Converting weight to kilograms

Many physicians request that this metric measure be used to record the body weight of their patients; since the scales used in many hospitals are still calibrated in pounds, the conversion from pounds to kilograms is required.

1. To convert weight in kilograms to pounds, multiply the kilogram weight by 2.2.

EXAMPLE: 25 kg × 2.2 lb = 55 lb

Convert the following:

35 kg = _____ lb
16 kg = _____ lb
65 kg = _____ lb

2. To convert weight in pounds to kilograms, divide the weight in pounds by 2.2.

EXAMPLE: 140 lb ÷ 2.2 kg = 63.5 kg

Convert the following:

125 lb = _____ lb
9 lb = _____ lb
180 lb = _____ lb

The weight of a liter of water at 40° C is 1 pound.

FAHRENHEIT AND CENTIGRADE (CELSIUS) TEMPERATURES

In some hospitals the centigrade thermometer is used to test the temperature of solutions and the Fahrenheit clinical thermometer is used to take the patient's temperature. The nurse should be familiar with both the centigrade and the Fahrenheit scale. Here are some of the main points about centigrade and Fahrenheit thermometers (Fig. 6-2).

1. Centigrade and Fahrenheit thermometers look alike.
2. Both are made of the same-sized tube containing mercury.
3. The column of mercury in each thermometer rises to the same height when placed in a beaker of freezing water and to the same height in boiling water.
4. The centigrade and Fahrenheit thermometers dif-

fer from each other in the way they are graduated.
5. On the centigrade thermometer the point at which water freezes is marked "0."
6. On the Fahrenheit thermometer the point at which water freezes is marked "32."
7. The boiling point in centigrade is 100°.
8. The boiling point in Fahrenheit is 212°.
9. The space between the 0° point and the 100° point on the centigrade scale is divided into equal spaces or degrees.
10. The value of graduations (degrees) on the centigrade thermometer differs from the value of degrees on the Fahrenheit thermometer.
11. There are 180 spaces between the freezing and boiling points on the Fahrenheit thermometer.
12. In order to change readings on the centigrade thermometer to the Fahrenheit scale, the centigrade reading is multiplied by 180/100 or 9/5 and then added to 32.
13. To change Fahrenheit reading to centigrade scale, subtract 32 from the Fahrenheit reading and multiply by 5/9.

To understand why thermometer readings are interpreted in the way explained in point 12 and to understand your conversion formula better, read points 4 to 12 again several times.

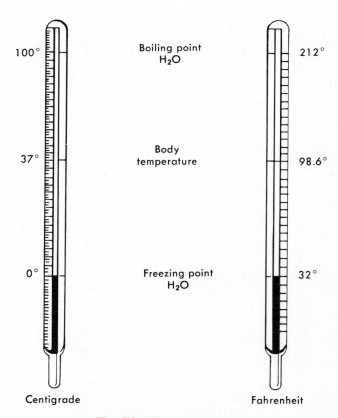

Fig. 6-2. Clinical thermometers.

Formula for converting Fahrenheit temperature to centigrade temperature

$$(\text{Fahrenheit} - 32) \times \frac{5}{9} = \text{centigrade}$$

$$(F - 32) \times \frac{5}{9} = C$$

EXAMPLE: Change 212° F to C.

$$(F - 32) \times \frac{5}{9} = C$$

$$212 - 32 = 180$$

$$180 \times \frac{5}{9} = \frac{900}{9} = 100° \text{ C}$$

Convert the following Fahrenheit temperatures to centigrade:

98.6° F = _____ C
102.4° F = _____ C
95.2° F = _____ C

Formula for converting centigrade temperature to Fahrenheit temperature

$$(\text{Centigrade} \times \frac{9}{5}) + 32 = \text{Fahrenheit}$$

$$(C \times \frac{9}{5}) + 32 = F$$

EXAMPLE: Change 100° C to F.

$$(C \times \frac{9}{5}) + 32 = F$$

$$100 \times \frac{9}{5} = \frac{900}{5} = 180$$

$$180 + 32 = 212° \text{ F}$$

Convert the following centigrade temperatures to Fahrenheit:

37° C = _____ F
35° C = _____ F
41° C = _____ F

Try these problems in converting centigrade to Fahrenheit and Fahrenheit to centigrade.

1. The nurse takes the following temperatures with Fahrenheit clinical thermometers: patient A, 104° F; patient B, 99° F; patient C, 101° F. The physician asks what the centigrade temperature is for each patient. Work your problems to convert Fahrenheit temperatures to centigrade. Check your answers. (Answers: patient A, 40° C; patient B, 37.2° C; and patient C, 38.3° C.)

2. The nurse takes the following temperatures with centigrade clinical thermometers: patient D, 37° C; patient E, 37.8° C; patient F, 38° C. The physician asks what the Fahrenheit temperature is for each patient. Work your problems to convert centigrade to Fahrenheit. Check your answers. (Answers: patient D, 98.6° F; patient E, 100° F; and patient F, 100.4° F.)

Many hospitals today have conversion tables available on the wards. This saves time and possibility of error in doing problems. The nurse simply refers to the particular temperature on one scale and finds the conversion listed in a column beside it. However, try to remember the formula for each conversion.

ASSIGNMENT

Review previous lessons and questions according to the direction of your instructor.

1. Name the two systems of weighing and measuring drugs.
2. What is the meaning of the word *apothecary*?
3. Which is the smallest unit of weight in the apothecary system—the pound, dram, grain, or scruple?
4. What is the original derivation of the grain? Give the symbol for grain.
5. What is the origin of dram? What is its symbol?
6. Give the symbol for ounce. The ounce is what proportion of a troy pound?
7. Give the abbreviation for pound and the Latin word from which it originates.
8. In apothecary weight 12 ounces equal what part of a pound?
9. In avoirdupois weight how many ounces equal 1 pound? What are the uses for avoirdupois weight?
10. Eight drams equal how many grains and how many ounces?
11. In the measurement of fluids (apothecary volume) which is the smallest unit—the fluidram, minim, fluidounce, or pint?
12. What is the unit of fluid measure? What is its symbol? Tell the meaning of the symbol "O" and its word origin. Tell the origin of the symbol "C" and its meaning.
13. Sixty minims equal how many fluidrams? Give the symbol also.
14. Eight fluidrams equal how many fluidounces? Give the symbol also.
15. A fluidram is *approximately* the same as what household measure?
16. Sixteen fluidounces equal how many pints? Give the symbol for pint.
17. Two pints equal how many quarts?
18. Four quarts equal how many gallons?
19. Write the following correctly, as they would appear on medicine orders.
    a. ½ grain
    b. 1 grain
    c. 1 ounce
    d. 1½ grains
    e. 5 grains
    f. 2 grains
    g. 2 ounces
    h. 1 dram
20. What does the symbol "ss" mean?
21. What is the approximate equivalent of a minim? Explain

the examples given to emphasize this approximation. What is the symbol for minim? If the doctor orders a dosage in drops for his patient, the drug should be measured with what? If the physician orders a dose in minims for his patient, the dose should be measured with what?

22. Give the abbreviation for drops and tell the origin of this abbreviation.

23. What is the abbreviation for grain? Why is it important to write and read carefully "grain" (apothecary) and "gram" (metric) and their symbols?

24. What is the unit of weight in the metric system? What is the symbol for gram? A milligram is what part of a gram? What is its symbol? What is the equivalent in pounds of one kilogram?

25. What is the unit of volume in the metric system? A liter equals how many milliliters, how many cubic centimeters, and how many quarts?

26. One cc weighs how much? One ml weighs how much?

27. Give the abbreviation for gram. Be sure to write or print it plainly so it will not be confused with the grain of the apothecary system.

28. How is one number after a decimal point read—as tenths, hundredths, or thousandths? How are two numbers after a decimal point read—as tenths, hundredths, thousandths, or ten-thousandths? How are three numbers after a decimal point read—as tenths, hundredths, thousandths, or ten-thousandths? How are four numbers after a decimal point read—as tenths, hundredths, thousandths, or ten-thousandths?

29. Express the following amounts in *words* to show that you can read decimal numbers correctly.
   a. 0.1 gram
   b. 0.05 gram
   c. 0.25 milligram
   d. .250 milligram
   e. .0006 gram
   f. 1.0 gram
   g. .1 gram
   h. 1.25 milligram

30. Are amounts with decimal points in front of the number the same as or less than the whole amount?

31. A milligram is what part of a gram? Is it less than or more than a gram? A microgram is one-thousandth of a milligram—true or false?

32. Are the terms tenths, hundredths, thousandths, and ten-thousandths more or less than tens, hundreds, thousands, and ten thousands? You can see that you must *spell* and *pronounce* the terms correctly to assure accuracy.

33. The use of decimals always means that the quantity is in which system, apothecary or metric?

34. If the drug is a solid, how will it usually be expressed—in ml, teaspoonfuls, or g?

35. If the drug is a liquid, will it usually be expressed in ml (or cc) or g?

36. Write in *words* to show you can read the decimals and symbols for the following dosages *(spell correctly amounts and symbols)*.
   a . 0.4 mg _____
   b. 0.05 g _____
   c. 0.5 g _____
   d. 1.0 mg _____
   e. 0.625 mg _____
   f. 4.0 mg _____
   g. 0.0006 g _____
   h. 25.2 mg _____
   i. .1 mg _____
   j. .250 mg _____
   k. .25 mg _____
   l. 0.1 mg _____
   m. .0002 mg _____
   n. 0.25 mg _____
   o. 5 g _____

37. Change the following grams (metric) to grains (apothecary).
   a. 15 g
   b. 30 g
   c. 1 g

38. Change grains (apothecary) to grams (metric).
   a. 1 grain
   b. 5 grains
   c. 10 grains
   d. 15 grains

39. Using Table 6-3 on apothecary and metric equivalents, fill in the following.
   a. 15 minims = _____ ml (cc)
   b. 60 minims = _____ ml (cc)
   c. 7½ grains = _____ g

40. Give the rule for converting grams to milligrams, and work the two examples given for this rule in this chapter. Convert the following grams (g) to milligrams (mg).
   a. .250 g
   b. .125 g
   c. .0006 g
   d. .5 g

41. Give the rule for converting milligrams to grams. Convert the following milligrams to grams.
   a. 500 mg
   b. 100 mg
   c. 0.1 mg
   d. 50 mg
   e. 200 mg
   f. 0.6 mg

42. Convert all the answers from problem 41 from grams to milligrams for further practice.

43. Give the rule for converting ounces to pints. Convert the following ounces to pints.
   a. 16 ounces
   b. 32 ounces
   c. 320 ounces

44. Give the rule for converting pints to quarts. Convert the following pints to quarts.
   a. 20 pints
   b. 6 pints
   c. 8 pints

45. Give the rule for converting quarts to gallons. Convert the following quarts to gallons.
   a. 8 quarts
   b. 12 quarts
   c. 4 quarts

46. Study these measurements and know them well before taking any test. Review them constantly. You will use them often. (See Table 6-3 on metric and apothecary equivalents.)

    a. 4-5 ml   = _____ dram
    b. 15 ml   = _____ drams
    c. 30 ml   = _____ ounces
    d. 250 ml   = _____ fluidounces
    e. 1000 ml = _____ quart
    f. 8 ml   = _____ fluidrams
    g. 5 ml   = _____ fluidrams
    h. 1 ml   = _____ minims
    i. 2 ml   = _____ minims
    j. 500 ml   = _____
    k. 1 g   = _____ grains
    l. 0.6 g   = _____ grains
    m. 0.5 g   = _____ grains
    n. 0.3 g   = _____ grains
    o. 0.1 g   = _____ grains
    p. 60 mg   = _____ grain

    q. 30 mg   = _____ grain
    r. 15 mg   = _____ grain
    s. 10 mg   = _____ grain
    t. 8 mg   = _____ grain
    u. 1 mg   = _____ grain
    v. 0.1 mg   = _____ grain

47. Work all of the problems on the three pages following Table 6-3, including the ones using fractional equivalents. The review of fractions is worthwhile, and many students understand what the problem asks when they use fractional equivalents.

48. Work the problems converting kilograms (kg) to pounds, and the problems converting weight in pounds to kilograms.

49. List the main points about centigrade and Fahrenheit thermometers. Learn these well since they will help you to remember conversion of Fahrenheit to centigrade and centigrade to Fahrenheit. Write the formula down for each problem and work the ones given in the discussion of this conversion.

CHAPTER 7

Administration and dosage of medicines

MEDICINE ORDERS

The physician either writes the order for a medication on the patient's chart or gives it to the nurse by telephone, later confirming the order by signature.

If the nurse or pharmacist questions an order, it is that person's responsibility to check with the physician for clarification before administering or dispensing the drug.

The order *must* include date, time, drug, dosage, route, frequency, and duration. Some drugs have a time limit, and the order for renewal must be rewritten before the nurse can continue to administer the medication (for example, antibiotics, narcotics, and hypnotics). Orders for narcotics must be rewritten every 72 hours in most hospitals. Today, protection for the patient is enhanced by the unit dosage system used in many hospitals. The drugs are prepared by the pharmacist, who has transcribed these orders from a carbon copy of the physician's order sheet; this does not replace standard nursing precautions but provides an additional safety check beneficial to the physician, pharmacist, nurse, and patient.

PRESCRIPTIONS

Prescription writing is simpler today than it was many years ago. Modern drug companies prepare medicines in such a practical and attractive form that much less work is made for today's pharmacist in preparing and compounding drugs.

A prescription is a written formula that is given by a physician to a pharmacist for the preparation of a medicine. A prescription has four parts:

1. Superscription includes name of patient, date, and symbol ℞, meaning "take thou"
2. Inscription includes names and amounts of ingredients to be used
3. Subscription includes directions to the pharmacist
4. Signature includes directions to be written on the label

The quantities of drug to be given are written in either the metric or the apothecary system. The language commonly used is English.

EXAMPLE:
For Mr. Obedy Zedia

℞	Date _____
Ammonium chloride	10 g
Syrup citric acid	48 ml
Syrup glycyrrhiza, to make	120 ml

Mix and label: 1 teaspoonful every 4 hours

Dr. E. T. Yedlow
240 E. 16th St.

THE MEDICINE GLASS

The medicine glass has the following graduations or measurements:

teaspoons (tsp)	ounces (oz)
tablespoons (tbs)	milliliters (ml)
dessertspoons (dssp)	

Some medicine glasses are measured in cubic centimeters (cc). Milliliters and cubic centimeters are the same. Measurements of teaspoons, tablespoons, and dessertspoons are in the household measuring system. Measurements in ounces are in the apothecary system, and measurements in milliliters or cubic centimeters are in the metric system.

Many nurses have difficulty with the problem of approximate equivalents. The subject seems confusing to them, since they are so impressed with the necessity of accuracy in measuring medications. For example, how many minims in an ounce? One possible answer is 480 minims (8 drams × 60 minims). Another possible answer is 450 minims (30 ml × 15 minims).

The explanation of approximate equivalents lies in this important point: in handling medications, an error that is 10% or less is considered legitimate and negligible by pharmacists in approximating equivalents from one system to the other. Notice that the difference in answers falls below this permissible margin of error in the example given.

The nurse should realize that this margin of error is recognized as safe and has been already provided for. The nurse must not exceed this margin of error by making a mistake in dosage; the dosage must be accurate and exact.

Table 7-1. Some measurements and equivalents* for pouring medicines (to be memorized)

4 ml (4-5 ml)	=	1 teaspoon	or	1 dram	or	60 drops (gtt)
1 ml	=	$^1/_4$ teaspoon	or	$^1/_4$ dram	or	15 to 16 drops (gtt)
2 ml	=	$^1/_2$ teaspoon	or	$^1/_2$ dram	or	30 to 32 drops (gtt)
15 ml	=	3 teaspoons	or	4 drams	or	$^1/_2$ ounce (oz)
30 ml	=	6 teaspoons	or	8 drams	or	1 ounce (oz)
1 *table*spoon	=	3 teaspoons	or	15 ml	or	$^1/_2$ ounce (oz)
2 *table*spoons	=	6 teaspoons	or	30 ml	or	1 ounce (oz)
6 fluidounces	=	1 teacupful	or	150 to 180 ml		
8 fluidounces	=	1 glassful	or	240 to 250 ml		
1 pint				480 ml	or	$^1/_2$ liter
2 pints	=	1 quart	or	1000 ml	or	1 liter
4 quarts	=	1 gallon	or	4000 ml	or	4 liters

*These equivalents are approximate only. In practice, the cubic centimeter and the milliliter are equal. In reality, the cubic centimeter is less than the milliliter by 0.000028 cc.

Table 7-2. Further handy equivalents*

1 dram (weight) = 4 grams
1 ounce = 30 grams (or ml)
4 drams or 3 teaspoons = $^1/_2$ ounce or 15 ml or 240 minims
8 drams or 6 teaspoons = 1 ounce or 30 ml or 480 minims
2 drams or 1.5 teaspoons = $^1/_4$ ounce or $7^1/_2$ ml or 120 minims
2.5 drams or 2 teaspoons = $^1/_3$ ounce or 10 ml or 150 minims
60 drops = 1 teaspoon or 1 dram or 4 ml

*These equivalents are approximate only. Remember: 5 ml equals 1 teaspoon or 1 dram (4 to 5 ml).

The meniscus

When aqueous (watery) or alcoholic solutions are poured into medicine glasses, surface tension causes the portion of the fluid that is in contact with the glass to be drawn upward, and the surface of the fluid becomes concave. Concave means hollow and rounded, or incurved, as in the interior or inside of a sphere or ball.

The reading of the dose of liquid medicine must always be made at the lowest point of the meniscus when the glass is held level with the eyes.

Procedure: reading the medicine glass

Materials needed

Medicine glasses, one for each student and one for instructor.
Pitcher of water for instructor to use; water may be colored with harmless dye to simulate liquid medicine.

Introduction

It is of vital importance to the nurse to learn how to read the medicine glass correctly, accurately, and quickly. This will prevent error in dosage and harm to the patient. The measurements we discuss now are commonly used in measuring doses of medicines. It is therefore necessary that the nurse memorize both measurements and understand their meanings.

It is necessary to remember these measurements in pouring 4 ml. One dram is the same as 1 teaspoon (4 to 5 ml). Medicine glasses are marked for one measurement "ml." This means milliliters. The measurement ml is the same as cc. If you are asked to pour 4 cc of a medicine, look for "ml" on the medicine glass. You will not find "cc."

Instructions

1. Hold medicine glass at eye level and straight. Medicine cannot be measured accurately if the glass is slanted. Most beginners do not hold the medicine glass straight and level. Watch this.
2. Turn glass around in hand until "ml" is found.
3. Place thumbnail on the line marked 5 at bottom of glass; 5 ml is the approximate equivalent of 4 cc or 1 3 or 1 teaspoon.
4. Turn glass to your left slowly until "tea" (spoon) is found at top of glass.
5. Place thumbnail on the 1-teaspoon line.
6. Turn glass to your right until 5 ml is reached. Note that 5 ml is the same as 1 teaspoon. Most texts use the approximate equivalent, 4 ml being the same as 1 teaspoon.
7. Turn glass to your left again until "tea" is found.
8. Place thumbnail on the 2-teaspoon line.
9. Turn glass to right until "ml" is reached.
10. Note that the milliliter equivalent is slightly under 10 ml.
11. Note that 2 teaspoons are the same as 8 ml.
12. Repeat steps 1 to 11 several times, finding 1 teaspoon, 2 teaspoons, and 4 to 5 ml and noting the equivalents, to ensure familiarity and understanding.
13. Turn medicine glass until the ounce (oz) measurement is found.
14. Place thumbnail on the $^1/_2$-ounce line.
15. Turn glass slightly to your left until "ml" is found.
16. Note that $^1/_2$ ounce is the same as 15 ml.
17. Turn glass slightly to your left until "oz" is found.
18. Place thumbnail on the 1-ounce (1-oz) mark.
19. Turn glass slightly to your right until "ml" is found.
20. Note that 30 ml is the same as 1 ounce (1 oz).
21. Find the following measurements: 10 ml, 20 ml, 25 ml, and 30 ml.
22. Find the following measurements: $^1/_4$ oz, $^1/_2$ oz, $^3/_4$ oz, and 1 oz.

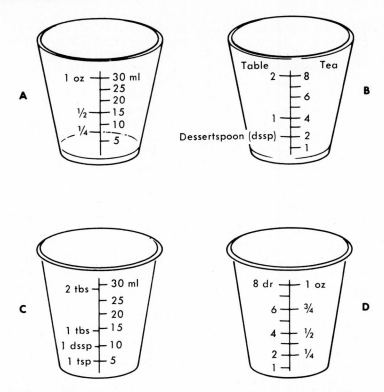

Fig. 7-1. A, Medicine glass graduated in apothecary (ounces) and metric (milliliters or cubic centimeters) measures. **B,** Medicine glass graduated in household measures; teaspoons and tablespoons are those most commonly used. **C** and **D,** Disposable medicine cups.

23. Find the "table" (spoon) measurement.
24. Place thumbnail on the 2-tablespoon mark.
25. Turn glass slightly to your left until "tea" is found. How many teaspoons make 2 tablespoons? How many teaspoons make 1 tablespoon?
26. Repeat steps 13 to 25 several times until measurements are understood.
27. After instructor pours 2 teaspoons of water into your glass, hold medicine glass at eye level and straight to find meniscus. The reading of the dose of medicine must always be made at the lowest point of the meniscus when the glass is held level with the eyes. Note that the surface of the fluid becomes concave, or hollow, or rounded, or incurved. This is the lowest point for reading the meniscus.

Many hospitals are now using disposable cardboard or plastic medicine glasses. There are several types in use. Notice the differences in two types shown in the drawings of such glasses (Fig. 7-1). The differences lie chiefly in the arrangement of measurement units. One type of disposable medicine glass, as shown in Fig. 7-1, *C,* for example, arranges the measurements of tablespoon and milliliter next to each other. Another type of medicine glass arranges the measurements of ounce and milliliter next to each other. Your instructor will show you examples of these medicine glasses if your hospital uses them.

Some hospitals use tiny soufflé cups as containers for tablets and capsules and medicine glasses of the cardboard disposable type for liquid medicines.

Review

1. Take a medicine glass home for study.
2. Remember that in unit dosage system, each drug comes prepared in its own container, from which it is administered.
3. Compare each measurement by practicing the steps in dosage discussed under Procedure. Practice several times until you understand the dose.
4. Memorize the medicine glass measurements from Fig. 7-1. Understand each measurement—this makes memorizing easier. Memorizing must be done, and it must be done with understanding.

Medicine-ticket abbreviations

For some common abbreviations you must know to read medicine tickets, refer to the tables on the inside back cover of the text. Your instructor will show you medicine orders used in your hospital.

You must understand clearly the difference between s.o.s. and p.r.n.; s.o.s. refers to *one dose only*—more than one dose should not be given. p.r.n. means when required, or *as often as necessary;* nurses may use their own judgment about repeating the dose. Consult your team leader, instructor, head nurse, or supervisor if it becomes necessary to repeat a dose under a p.r.n. order. *You must memorize the abbreviations, and you must memorize them with understanding.*

Student nurses tend to confuse abbreviations for the number of times per day and the number of hours apart for administration of drugs. These are summarized here as an aid in learning them.

q.h. = every hour
q.2h. = every two hours
q.3h. = every three hours
q.4h. = every four hours
b.i.d. = twice a day
t.i.d. = three times a day
q.i.d. = four times a day

(Note that the "h" in q.2h., q.3h., q.4h., means *hour*, and the "d" in b.i.d., t.i.d., q.i.d., means *day*.)

Procedure: measuring and giving liquid medicines

NOTE: This lesson may be used by instructor for demonstration. Medicine tickets are made up by instructor (or can be made by students in class practice, with adequate supervision). Instructor can then select any medicines desired for class practice, fitting them to the procedure.

Materials needed

Units for each student, usually 8 units, or as many as the instructor thinks can be observed. The pharmacist will make up these units for the instructor, using appropriate colors and labeling each medication "placebo" or "classroom practice."

8 medicine bottles, 4 to 6 oz, elixir terpin hydrate
8 medicine bottles, 4 to 6 oz, elixir phenobarbital
8 medicine bottles, 4 to 6 oz, milk of magnesia, for $^1/_2$ and 1 oz practice
8 medicine tickets for elixir terpin hydrate, 4-ml dose
8 medicine tickets for elixir phenobarbital, 4-ml dose
8 medicine tickets for elixir phenobarbital, 8-ml dose
8 medicine tickets for milk of magnesia, $^1/_2$-oz dose
8 medicine tickets for milk of magnesia, 1-oz dose
10 medicine glasses for each student (these can be obtained from affiliating hospitals, can be of the disposable cardboard type, or can be ordered by instructor for classroom use)
Drinking straws, several (to familiarize students with these)
8 small cloths for wiping the necks of bottles
3 or four pitchers of water on table for use by students in diluting drugs
Long table (to accommodate three or four students on each side)
Oilcloth or plastic covering for table to prevent spillage discoloration.

Introduction

Measuring and giving medicines are important responsibilities of the nurse. There is an element of danger in practically every medicine prescribed if it is not given correctly. Carelessness on the part of the nurse can cause injury or even death to the patient. Errors can be prevented by always following the safety rules in pouring.

1. Read the label three times: (1) before pouring, (2) after pouring, and (3) as you check the label on the bottle with the medicine ticket and return the bottle to the shelf.
2. Concentrate. Think of pouring medicine—nothing else.
3. Shake medicines before pouring, if labeled "to be shaken."
4. *Never* use an unlabeled bottle. There is *NO* exception to this rule.
5. Hold medicine glass straight and at eye level while pouring.
6. Always check the medicine ticket order with the physician's order from the patient's chart.

Instructions

1. Wash your hands.
2. Look for the medicine ticket labeled "Elixir Terpin Hydrate."
3. Look at the patient's name on the medicine ticket.
4. Look for the expiration date, or "stop date." If ticket has expired, take it to supervisor for renewal or to be discontinued. Supervisor or head nurse obtains orders from the physician for this.
5. Notice the exact dose of the medicine on the medicine ticket.
6. Remove bottle from shelf or table, checking label.
7. Compare bottle label and dose with medicine ticket.
8. Shake bottle well.
9. Remove cap.
10. Place cap top side down on table.
11. Read label on bottle again.
12. Read medicine ticket again.
13. Hold medicine glass straight and at level with your eyes.
14. Hold medicine bottle with label in the palm of your hand. This prevents pouring medicine over the label and smearing it.
15. Place thumbnail on medicine glass on exact dosage mark.
16. Check name of medicine and dosage on your medicine ticket.
17. Pour dose of medicine. (Instructor will pass down the group, checking quickly the dose of each student with the student's ticket and medicine glass.)
18. Read the label again as the bottle is returned to the shelf or table. Compare the name and dose of medicine on the medicine ticket with the name and strength of the medicine on the bottle label and with the amount of medicine in the medicine glass.
19. Wipe off neck of bottle with cloth and replace cap.
20. Add water to medicine for dilution, pouring up to the $^1/_2$-oz mark. This does not mean adding $^1/_2$ oz of water—enough water is added until the $^1/_2$-oz mark is reached. This is sufficient dilution.
21. Take medicine to patient. If you were actually on a ward you would follow these rules:
    a. Check patient's name before giving medicine; look at bed tag at foot of bed and patient's identification wrist bracelet. Ask patient his name if he is able to give it. If he is unable and you have any doubt about the patient's identification, consult your team leader, head nurse, supervisor, or instructor.
    b. Give patient the medicine with a drinking tube if necessary to add to his comfort.

c. *Never* leave medicine at a patient's bedside.
d. Patient may have half to one glass of water following medication if he wishes, except with cough medicines.
e. Do not dilute cough medicines. Instruct patient not to drink fluids or eat for 15 to 30 minutes after taking cough medicines to obtain best effects of the drug.
f. Give iron medications and acid medicines through a drinking tube, since they destroy or discolor the enamel on the teeth if administered over a prolonged period in a medicine glass.

22. Find the next medicine ticket according to the directions of your instructor. The previous steps are then repeated over and over, giving you a chance to pour a few doses of liquid medicine in 4 and 8 ml doses, and a few in $1/2$ and 1 oz. Pour in as close to unison as possible, with instructor supervision. Eight students can be given this practice in 30 minutes, or sixteen students per hour.

(NOTE: If any time remains at conclusion of the class practice, students may practice pouring 4- or 5-ml dosages, 8- to 10-ml dosages, and any other dosages that seem to present difficulty; 4- to 5-ml dosages seem to cause the most difficulty.)

PATIENT DRUG PROFILE OR MEDICINE TICKET

The unit dosage method is intended as a safety measure to provide the nurse with a premeasured dosage in the proper container. This method requires the same precautionary measures as those in using stock supplies.

Each drug given requires that certain information be available to the nurse to use at the patient's bedside. Both the ticket and profile forms achieve this purpose. Both contain the same information, room and bed numbers, name, drug, dosage, route, frequency, start date, stop date, and identification of person transcribing the drug orders.

In addition, the patient profile contains the diagnosis, age, allergies, and other pertinent information. It is used to chart and make drug charges and becomes a permanent part of the patient's chart.

The pharmacist shares responsibility in translating and dispensing drugs the physician has ordered, thus affording the nurse an additional safeguard. (NOTE: The nurse and the pharmacist share responsibility for the safe and accurate administration of all medication given to patients.)

Medicine trays

The card system medications are placed on a tray in which the medication for each individual is separate and identified with a medicine ticket for each drug. Paper soufflé cups are used for solid drugs, and plastic disposable medicine glasses are used for liquid preparations (Fig. 7-2).

Medicine carts (procedure commonly used)

The unit dosage system employs carts that contain individual compartments for each patient's 24-hour supply of drugs. Each patient's drug profile is kept in a rack on top of the cart.

The cart is wheeled into the patient's room, the drug to be administered is removed from the patient's individual compartment, checked against the drug profile, given, charted, and charged to the patient. The cart is sent to the pharmacy to be checked and replenished once daily. (Fig. 7-3).

Underlying principles in giving medicines

General rules and regulations have been developed to administer medications safely and efficiently; good judgment requires deviation from these as circumstance dictates, but you must carefully evaluate the situation beforehand and seek advice if uncertain.

1. Give your entire attention to preparing and giving medications.
2. Check the labels, container, syringe, or vial for name of drug dosage and route of administration.
3. Do not give medicine from a container that is not properly labeled.
4. Do not give medicines prepared by another person (exception: the clinical pharmacist).
5. Check fractional dosages and medicines such as insulin, anticoagulants, digitalis preparations (injectable), and IV additives with another licensed nurse.
6. Use a properly calibrated instrument to measure the dose desired.
7. Do not return an unused dose of medicine to a stock bottle.
8. Do not break a tablet unless it has been scored by the pharmaceutical company.
9. Do not save an opened vial that does not have a rubber stopper.
10. Verify the patient's identity:
    a. Check name, room number, physician, and hospital number on wristband.
    b. Ask patient to tell you his name.
    c. Check with family or staff members who can positively identify the patient.
11. Check patients for medications upon hospital admission, determine the physician's intent, and either remove or leave the medications at the patient's bedside, depending on hospital policy. (This requires the nurse to monitor the patient's self-administration of drugs.)
12. On his discharge, determine that the patient has the proper medication and understands how to take it correctly.

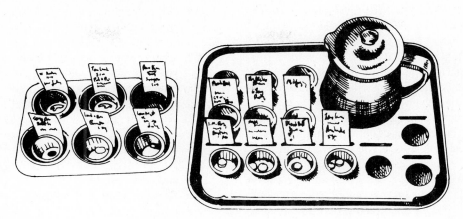

Fig. 7-2. Tray for medication card system.

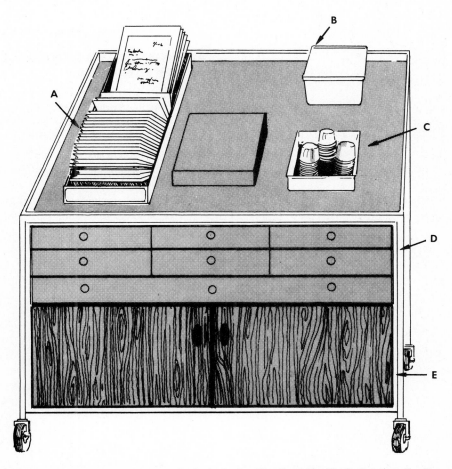

Fig. 7-3. Cart for unit dosage system method. **A,** Patient Rand profile. **B,** Syringe needle disposer. **C,** Container with medicine glasses. **D,** Drawers with compartments for individual patient medications. **E,** Cupboard for injectable equipment and stock medications.

13. Do not leave the tray or cart of medicines unattended.
14. Do not record a medication until after it has been given.
15. Remain with the patient until you have determined that he has taken the medication.
16. Answer questions posed by the patient appropriately after determining what information the physician has given to him.
17. Indicate, in the case of p.r.n. or one-time medications, the patient's reaction to a drug as well as the problem that caused you to give the medication.
18. Record when a drug is not given and the reason why it was not given.
19. Question when in doubt and report any medication error immediately to the proper authority.
20. Develop careful, safe habits by utilizing the technique appropriate to the situation at hand. Determine hospital and agency policies and function within the framework of these regulations.

Some additional points:
1. Hold medicine glass at eye level when pouring liquids.
2. Place thumbnail on meniscus.
3. Shake liquids (if label indicates).
4. Pour from back of the bottle to keep label clean.
5. Measure drops with a dropper.
6. Measure minims with an instrument calibrated in minims.
7. Dilute medicines according to directions.

8. Know purpose, dosage, and effect before administering any drug.
9. Relate medication to patient's disease and treatment; know why this patient is receiving this particular medication.
10. Check expiration date; know hospital rules for renewal order.
11. Know usual dosage and route of administration; question pharmacist or physician if in doubt.
12. Narcotics are kept under double lock. Neither leave the key unattended nor surrender the key to an unauthorized person.
13. Keep external and internal substances separate and clearly marked.
14. Remember the five rights of medication administration. Give
    a. The right medicine
    b. To the right patient
    c. At the right time
    d. In the right manner
    e. In the right amount

ADMINISTRATION OF MEDICATIONS BY OTHER ROUTES

Prior to administering any medication, you should wash your hands thoroughly with soap and water.

Administration of ear drops

1. Allow drops to warm to body temperature by having the patient hold the bottle in his hand for a few minutes.
2. Look into the external ear canal to determine whether

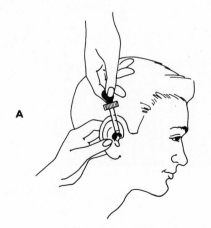
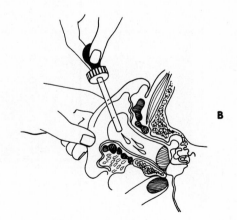

Fig. 7-4. Ear drops. **A,** Ask patient to turn his head to the side so that the ear being treated faces upward. Manipulate the external ear gently to expose the external canal. **B,** Direct medication toward the internal wall of the canal. (From Dison, N.: Clinical nursing techniques, ed. 4, St. Louis, 1979, The C. V. Mosby Co.)

significant ear wax has accumulated. If the canal appears to be impacted, the canal should be cleaned before drops are instilled. If the eardrum is intact and if the physician approves, irrigate the ear canal with 3% saline (2 tablespoons of salt per quart of warm water), using an ear syringe.

3. Have the patient lie on his side with the ear to be treated upward.
4. Shake the medicine if required and draw up into the dropper.
5. To allow the drops to run in (Fig. 7-4):
    a. Adults—pull the pinna (earlobe) back and up and allow the drops to fall in the external canal.
    b. Children—pull the pinna (earlobe) back and down and allow the drops to fall in the external canal.
6. Do not insert the dropper into the ear and do not allow the dropper to come into contact with any portion of the ear.
7. Have the patient remain on his side for a few minutes to allow the medication to reach the eardrum.
8. Insert a soft cotton plug if ordered. Never pack the plug tightly into the ear.

Administration of eye drops

See Chapter 22 on Drugs affecting the eye.

Administration of nose drops

1. Instruct the patient to gently blow his nose.
2. Draw the medicine into the dropper (Fig. 7-5). To properly regulate dosage, draw only what should be instilled.
3. Have the patient lie down and tilt his head backward over the edge of the bed.
4. Insert the dropper $1/3$ to $1/2$ inch into the nasal passage and instill the medicine.
5. Have the patient remain in this position for several minutes to allow the medication to be absorbed.
6. Instruct the patient not to blow his nose unless absolutely necessary.
7. Each patient should have his own bottles of nasal solutions to prevent cross-contamination of patients.

Insertion of rectal suppositories

1. When possible, have the bowel evacuated before insertion of the suppository.
2. If suppositories are soft and unmanageable, hold the foil-wrapped suppository under cold water to harden prior to insertion.
3. Put on a disposable glove or a finger cot to protect the finger used for insertion (index finger for adults, fourth finger for infants).
4. Ask the patient to lie on his side and draw his upper leg up toward his waist (Fig. 7-6).
5. Unwrap the suppository.

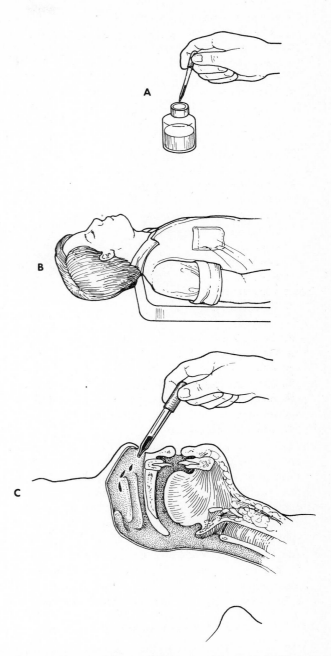

Fig. 7-5. Nose drops. **A,** Draw proper dose into dropper. **B,** Tilt patient's head backward. **C,** Cross section showing instillation of drops.

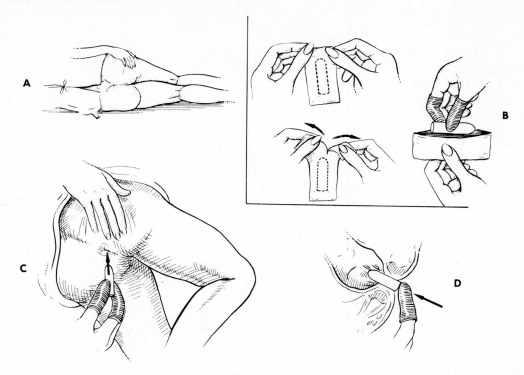

Fig. 7-6. Rectal suppositories. **A,** Position of patient. **B,** Open wrapper and remove suppository. **C,** Insert suppository. **D,** Cross section showing insertion of suppository. Advance suppository beyond anal sphincter. (From Dison, N.: Clinical nursing techniques, ed. 4, St. Louis, 1979, The C. V. Mosby Co.)

6. Lubricate the suppository with a water-soluble lubricant such as K-Y jelly (do not use mineral oil or Vaseline). If a lubricant is not available, wet the rectal orifice with tap water.
7. Place the tip of the suppository at the rectal entrance and ask the patient to take a deep breath and exhale through his mouth (many patients will have an involuntary rectal gripping when the suppository is pressed against the rectum). Gently insert the suppository about an inch beyond the orifice past the internal sphincter.
8. Ask the patient to remain lying on his side for 15 to 20 minutes to allow melting and absorption of the medication.
9. Discard used materials and wash hands thoroughly.

Administration of rectal retention enemas

1. For maximum absorption, the bowel should be evacuated prior to the enema.
2. Collect all of the apparatus and mix the solution prior to preparing the patient.
3. Ask the patient to lie on his side and draw his upper leg up toward his waist (Fig. 7-7).
4. Remove the protective cap and lubricate the catheter tip with tap water.

5. Place the tip of the catheter at the rectal entrance and ask the patient to take a deep breath and exhale through his mouth. This maneuver will help relax the rectal sphincter.
6. Gently insert the catheter tip past the internal sphincter and administer the enema slowly, using no more than 120 ml of solution, to prevent peristaltic activity from expelling the solution.
7. After instillation, remove the catheter and ask the patient to lie flat for 30 minutes.
8. Discard used materials and wash hands thoroughly.

Administration of parenteral medications

See Chapter 8 on Syringes, dosages, and injection sites.

DRUGS AND THE AGING INDIVIDUAL

Physiologic changes that alter drug actions:
1. Gastrointestinal
   a. Changes in quality and quantity of digestive enzymes (slow the rate of transfer from the gastrointestinal tract to the bloodstream).
   b. Reduction in absorbing cells, gastrointestinal motility, and intestinal blood flow.
2. Decrease in efficiency of circulation alters distri-

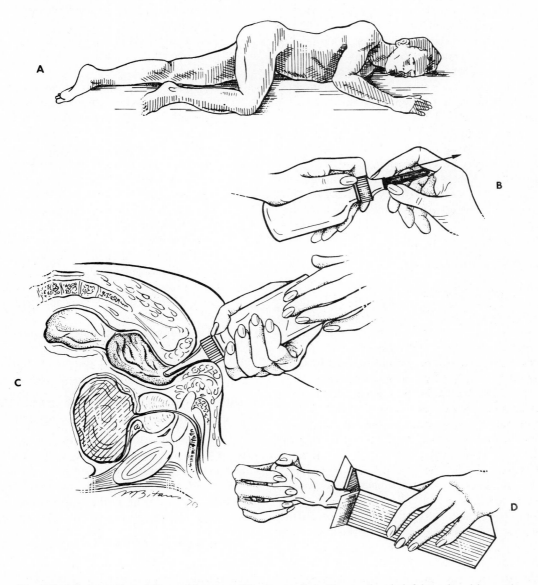

Fig. 7-7. Administration of disposable enema (Fleet enema). **A,** Place patient in left lateral position, unless knee-chest position has been specified. **B,** Remove protective covering from rectal tube and lubricate tube with lubricant contained in this cover. **C,** Insert lubricated rectal tube into rectum and insert solution by compressing plastic container. **D,** Replace used container in its original container for disposal. (Courtesy C. B. Fleet Co., Lynchburg, Va. From Dison, N.: Clinical nursing techniques, ed. 4, St. Louis, 1979, The C. V. Mosby Co.)

bution of drugs to target tissues and reduces the amount of blood entering the liver and kidneys; this influences the rate of metabolism and excretion of drugs.

Lowering of body temperature will reduce the rate at which drugs are absorbed at the site of administration and metabolized. (The oral suspension form is preferable to the suppository from the standpoint of absorption.)

A decrease in the amount of cellular and intracellular fluids suggests a higher concentrated form of the active drug in the elderly which makes adequate hydration essential to dilute the drug concentration and reduce the possibility of drug intoxication.

3. A decreasing metabolic rate and efficiency, indicating that some drug dosages should be less for the elderly than the young adult.
4. The ability of the kidneys to eliminate drugs decreases. A decreasing efficiency in tubular function means drugs may be reabsorbed into the blood more easily, thus enhancing the likelihood of cumulative effect.

Drug reaction in the elderly

A cardinal sign of drug reaction in the elderly is a behavioral change in the level of mental function, usually termed confusion. By treating such symptoms with psychotropic drugs it is possible to bring about a form of drug-induced senility. When the term *confusion* is used, the specific change in behavior should be described, and the drug therapy being utilized should be reviewed as the possible causative factor. It is a nursing function to be aware of possible side effects and to intervene by withholding the drug until after consulting the physician.

Measures to prevent undesirable drug reactions in the elderly

1. Careful monitoring of the numbers and dosages of drugs prescribed.
2. Use of active, current drug history of all medicinal substances consumed, including over-the-counter drugs.
3. Frequent review of the patient's drug program, establishment of goals, and evaluation to determine that the drugs being given are meeting these goals.
4. Health teaching programs directed toward involving the patient and his family in safe, effective medication practice. Develop a pattern with the patient and his family of reviewing and discussing over-the-counter drugs used with the physician so that the physician is aware of the patient's total drug regimen and can consider this when prescribing drugs.
5. Appropriate laboratory testing, including blood sugar determination, digitalis blood levels, and prothrombin time.

Helpful suggestions in giving medication to the elderly

1. Facilitate swallowing by moving the patient to a sitting position.
2. Have fluid, water, or juice poured beforehand.
3. Inform the patient in simple terms what you are going to do.
4. If several tablets or capsules are to be given, offer them one at a time and allow the patient a moment to rest between each.
5. Ascertain that the patient has swallowed the medication by encouraging him to talk or by inspecting the inside of the mouth while applying gentle pressure to the lower jaw to open the mouth.
6. Remember that semisolids such as applesauce and Jell-O are sometimes easier to swallow than liquids and are good vehicles for the medication.
7. Give liquids slowly after determining that the swallowing reflex is intact by gently rotating the index finger over the Adam's apple.
8. Administer the most important medication first.
9. Do not leave medications at the bedside (unless physician has ordered).
10. Do not increase the level of anxiety by attempting to hurry the patient; avoid a negative reaction if possible.
11. Give additional fluids unless the fluid intake is restricted.
12. Use every opportunity to teach the patient and his family about the drug he is receiving.

MEDICATING INFANTS AND CHILDREN
Factors influencing dosage prescribed

The physician orders the dosage of medication to be given to an individual child based on one of two parameters: (1) weight or (2) body surface area. Body size and weight are important considerations for dosage, since the distribution of a drug in the body depends on the relationship of the drug to tissue mass.

Calculation of dosages

The physician prescribes the dosage. The nurse or pharmacist must accurately prepare the dosage and be prepared to question a dose that seems out of the safe dosage range.

Common dosage problems in pediatrics

1. Fractional dosage.

EXAMPLE: The physician orders Polycillin 35 mg. Drug available is Polycillin 50 mg in 5 ml.

$$\frac{mg}{50} : \frac{ml}{5} :: \frac{mg}{35} : \frac{ml}{x}$$

$$50x = 175$$
$$x = 3.5 \text{ ml}$$

Administer 3.5 ml.

2. Conversion of administration units.

EXAMPLE: Drug available is Neomycin 150 mg/tsp. How many milligrams are there in each ml?

$$1 \text{ tsp} = 5 \text{ ml}$$

$$\frac{mg}{150} : \frac{ml}{5} :: \frac{mg}{x} : \frac{ml}{1}$$

$$5x = 150$$
$$x = 30 \text{ mg}$$

3. Conversion of apothecary units.

EXAMPLE: Drug available is acetaminophen gr v/tsp. Convert to mg/tsp.

$$\text{gr i} = 60 \text{ mg}$$

$$\frac{gr}{5} : \frac{tsp}{1} :: \frac{gr}{1} : \frac{mg}{60}$$

$$t \text{ tsp} = 300 \text{ mg}$$

Table 7-3. Determination of children's doses from adult doses on the basis of body surface area*

Age	Weight†		Surface area† (m²)	Fraction of adult dose‡
	kg	lb		
	2.0	4.4	0.15	0.09
Birth	3.4	7.4	0.21	0.12
3 weeks	4.0	8.8	0.25	0.14
3 months	5.7	12.5	0.29	0.17
6 months	7.4	16	0.36	0.21
9 months	9.1	20	0.44	0.25
1 year	10	22	0.46	0.27
1½ years	11	25	0.50	0.29
2 years	12	27	0.54	0.31
3 years	14	31	0.60	0.35
4 years	16	36	0.68	0.39
5 years	19	41	0.73	0.42
6 years	21	47	0.82	0.47
7 years	24	53	0.90	0.52
8 years	27	59	0.97	0.56
9 years	29	65	1.05	0.61
10 years	32	71	1.12	0.65
11 years	36	78	1.20	0.70
12 years	39	86	1.28	0.74

*From Done, A. K.: Drugs for children. In Modell, W., editor: Drugs of choice 1972-1973, St. Louis, 1972, The C. V. Mosby Co., p. 55.
†Approximate average for age.
‡Based on adult surface area of 1.73 m².

4. Combination conversions.

EXAMPLE: Drug available is Demerol 1 gr/ml. drug ordered is Demerol 15 mg. What volume must be administered?

$$\frac{\text{Desired dose (15 mg)}}{\text{Available dose (1 gr)}} = \frac{\text{Desired volume } (x)}{\text{Available volume (ml)}}$$
$$(1 \text{ gr} = 60 \text{ mg})$$

$$\frac{15}{60} = \frac{x}{1} \text{ ml}$$

$$\frac{1}{4} = \frac{x}{1} \text{ ml}$$

$$4x = 1 \text{ ml}$$
$$x = .25 \text{ ml}$$

Administer 0.25 ml of Demerol.

5. Reconstituting a powdered medication.

EXAMPLE: Drug available is penicillin G 1,000,00 units per vial. Instructions from drug company are to add 10 ml of sterile water for 100,000 units per milliliter. The order is for 750,000 units in an IV solution. Prepare this solution. Add 10 ml of sterile water to the 1,000,000 units. How many ml of reconstituted penicillin G are then added to the IV solution?

$$\frac{\text{units}}{1,000,000} : \frac{ml}{10} :: \frac{\text{units}}{750,000} : \frac{ml}{x}$$

$$1,000,000x = 7,500,000$$
$$x = 7.5 \text{ ml}$$

Add 7.5 ml to the IV solution.

6. Intravenous solution drip rates.

EXAMPLE: Pediatric drip sets (1 ml = 60 gtt) for this problem. Order 80 ml to run in 8 hours. How many drops per minute?
   a. Change 80 ml to drops. 80 × 60 = 4,800 gtt
   b. Change 8 hours to minutes. 8 × 60 = 480 minutes
   c. Divide 480 minutes into 4,800 drops. 10 gtt per minute

Suggestions for giving medicines to children

1. Utilize the information that the parent gives you regarding previous experiences with medicines; encourage the parent to assist.
2. Give honest, simple explanations and answers to questions.
3. Approach in a firm but kindly manner with the attitude that the nurse expects cooperation.
4. Disguise the taste of unpleasant medications with substances permitted in the child's diet.
5. Prevent aspiration by giving the medication slowly and in small amounts.
6. Plastic containers, medicine cup, eyedropper, or syringe (without needle) may be used; purse the child's lips to keep the medicine from running out of the mouth.

7. Realize that the quadriceps muscle is the best site for intramusclar injections and that the site should be changed frequently.
8. Give injections as rapidly as possible to avoid a fear-provoking experience.
9. If restraints are required, help the child understand that your purpose is to protect and not to punish. Permit the cooperative child to take his own medication.
10. After a rectal suppository is inserted, hold it in by holding the buttocks together for 5 or 10 minutes.
11. Suppositories should be divided by the pharmacist, who can ensure as accurate a dosage as possible.
12. Note reactions to a drug that would indicate intolerance or allergy.
13. Reward the child who has been cooperative with praise.
14. Use every opportunity to teach the parents and the child the appropriate information regarding the drug therapy.
15. Pass along successful methods to the other nursing personnel via the plan of care card.
16. Utilize the five rights and the proper techniques used in adult dosages.
17. Question when in doubt and report any error immediately.

ASSIGNMENT

Review previous lessons and questions according to the directions of your instructor.

1. Who orders a medication for the patient? How may this be done? If nurses or pharmacists question an order, what is their responsibility? What must an order for medication include? Give examples of drugs that have a time limit and must be reordered. What is the time limit for narcotics?
2. List the four parts of a prescription and what they include.
3. Give the following equivalents and memorize them well.
   a. 30 ml   = _____ teaspoons
                   or _____ drams
   b. 2 ml   = _____ teaspoons
                   or _____ drams
   c. 4 ml (4-5 ml) = _____ teaspoons
                   or _____ drams
   d. 15 ml   = _____ teaspoon
                   or _____ drams
   e. 1 tablespoon = _____ teaspoons
                   or _____ ml
   f. 2 tablespoons = _____ ml
                   or _____ ounces
   g. 8 fluidounces = _____ glassful
                   or _____ ml
   h. 1 pint   = _____ cc
                   or _____ liter
   i. 2 pints   = _____ quart
                   or _____ ml

   j. 4 quarts   = _____ gallons
                   or _____ ml
   k. 30 ml   = _____ cc
                   or _____ ounces
   l. 15 ml   = _____ cc
                   or _____ ounces
   m. 6 fluidounces = _____ teacupful
                   o or _____ ml
   n. 1 ml   = _____ teaspoon
4. In practice, the cubic centimeter and the _____ are equal. Why is it necessary in using a medicine glass to know this?
5. Define and describe the meniscus.
6. With a medicine glass in your hand follow the introduction and instructions of the Procedure: reading the medicine glass. Read these 27 steps through and follow the instructions four times. Know the equivalents emphasized in this procedure.
7. List the information that must be on the medicine ticket.
8. Know the common abbreviations of the following.
   a. of each _____
   b. before meals _____
   c. freely as desired _____
   d. water _____
   e. two times a day _____
   f. bedtime _____
   g. with _____
   h. discontinue _____
   i. gram _____
   j. grain _____
   k. drop _____
   l. hypodermic _____
   m. hour _____
   n. hour of sleep _____
   o. night _____
   p. nothing by mouth _____
   q. every day _____
   r. after meals _____
   s. by mouth _____
   t. when required _____
   u. every hour _____
   v. every two hours _____
   w. every three hours _____
   x. every four hours _____
   y. four times a day _____
   z. without _____
   aa. if necessary _____
   bb. a half _____
   cc. three times a day _____
   dd. immediately _____
9. Tell the times that the label is read during the pouring of medicines.
10. List four safety rules in pouring medicines.
11. Explain the patient drug profile or medicine ticket.
12. From the underlying principles in giving medicines select ten that seem to you to be the most important.
13. List the five rights of medication administration.
14. Explain each procedure for the following administration: ear drops, eye drops, and nose drops. What is the proce-

dure for insertion of rectal suppositories and rectal retention enemas? Give a brief account of administration of parenteral medications.

15. Give two keynotes to success in administering medicines to elderly patients who have difficulty in swallowing. If several tablets or capsules must be administered to aged patients, should they be given all at once or one at a time? If the aged patient is unable to place tablets or capsules in his mouth, what should the nurse do? List the helpful suggestions in administering medication to the elderly.

16. What two factors does the physician consider in determining the dosage for infants and children?
17. Can medicine be left at the bedside of children, aged patients, or any patient?
18. Work each one of the problems discussed under Common dosage problems in pediatrics.
19. Outline the suggestions for administering medicines to children. Be prepared to discuss these in class.

CHAPTER 8

Syringes, dosages, and injection sites

THE 3-CC SYRINGE

You will find the reading of the 3-cc syringe simple. Remember that 1 cc equals 15 to 16 ♏ and 3 cc equals 45 to 48 ♏. The 3-cc syringe is used commonly for intramuscular injections and is graduated in units of 0.1 cc. It is also used for subcutaneous injections.

To give you an idea of the amount of a minim, remember that a minim is approximately equal to a drop. Minims and drops are not identical, however.

Procedure: reading a 3-cc syringe

Materials needed

3-cc syringes, 1 for each student
Large blackboard drawing showing cubic centimeter measurement; no needles are necessary

Introduction

This procedure will be valuable for home study. Follow the directions, using the 3-cc syringe or pictures of a 3-cc syringe.

Instructions

1. There are three parts to a syringe (Fig. 8-1): (a) The barrel, which has the measurements printed on it. It also contains the drug. (b) The plunger, which is made of clouded glass or plastic. It has a head—the rounded, button-like part. Always hold the plunger by the head. Never touch the clouded glass part, since this comes in contact with the drug. (c) The hub, to which the needle fits. Sometimes the hub is made of glass and sometimes of metal.
2. Hold the plunger by the head. Use your right hand, unless you are left-handed. Do not touch the end that fits into the barrel.
3. With your left hand hold the barrel with the hub pointed straight down.
4. With your right hand place the plunger gently into the open

barrel. Do not allow the plunger to touch the outside of the barrel. This would contaminate it, since you handled the outside of the barrel with your fingers.
5. Ease the plunger into the barrel as far down as it will go. Do not force a plunger into position. That might jam the plunger and make it difficult to remove, or it might break the syringe.
6. Hold the syringe in your left hand in a horizontal position.
7. With your right hand hold the head of the plunger. Do not touch the hub of the syringe with your hand or fingers. This would contaminate it.
8. Roll the syringe gently around with your right hand until "cc" measurements are seen. The 3-cc mark will be found on the upper part of the barrel. Each time the plunger is drawn back and the dose determined, expel the air by pushing forward on the head of the plunger. This prepares you for the next dose practice.
9. Draw the plunger slowly back with your right hand until the lowest edge of the plunger rests on the line ¹/₂. This is ¹/₂ cc or one half of a cubic centimeter.
10. Draw the plunger slowly back until it rests on the line marked 1. This is 1 cc.
11. Draw the plunger slowly back until it rests on the line 1¹/₂. This is 1¹/₂ cc.
12. Draw the plunger slowly back until it rests on the line 2 cc. This is 2 cc.
13. Draw the plunger slowly back until it rests on the line 2¹/₂ cc. This is 2¹/₂ cc. Then draw it back to 3 cc. This is 3 cc.
14. Push the plunger forward toward the hub as far as it will go.
15. Notice the lines marking the divisions of ¹/₂ cc, ¹/₂ to 1 cc, 1 to 1¹/₂ cc, 1¹/₂ to 2 cc, 2 to 2¹/₂ cc, and 2¹/₂ to 3 cc.
16. Notice that there are 5 lines between zero and ¹/₂ cc, between ¹/₂ cc and 1 cc, and so on. Each line represents ¹/₅ of the *particular* measurement, or 0.1 of the whole cubic centimeter.

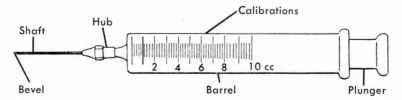

Fig. 8-1. Parts of a syringe.

17. Draw the plunger back slightly until it rests on the *first* line. This is $^1/_5$ of the $^1/_2$ cc.
18. Draw the plunger back slightly until it rests on the *second* line. This is $^2/_5$ of the $^1/_2$ cc.
19. The next line is $^3/_5$ of the $^1/_2$ cc. The next line is $^4/_5$ of the $^1/_2$ cc, and the next line is $^5/_5$ of the $^1/_2$ cc, or $^1/_2$ cc.
20. Draw the plunger back until it rests on the line after $^1/_2$ cc. This would be $^6/_{10}$ of 1 cc.
21. The next line is $^7/_{10}$ of 1 cc. The next line is $^8/_{10}$ of 1 cc. The next line is $^9/_{10}$ of 1 cc, and the next line is $^{10}/_{10}$ of 1 cc, or 1 cc.
22. The remainder is read in the same manner.
23. Note that the syringe holds *no more than* 3 cc.
24. Roll the syringe slightly away from you until the minim measurement side is exposed.
25. Notice that the syringe holds a total of 48 ♏.
26. Each line represents 1 ♏.
27. Draw the plunger slightly back until it rests on the *first* line. This is 1 ♏.
28. Draw the plunger back to the next line. This is 2 ♏.
29. Draw the plunger back to the next line. This is 3 ♏.
30. Draw the plunger back to the next line. This is 4 ♏.
31. Draw the plunger back to the next line. Notice that it is a longer line than the others. This is 5 ♏. It is not marked 5, but is halfway between zero and 10.
32. The next line is 6 ♏, the next line is 7 ♏, the next is 8 ♏, the next is 9 ♏, and the next longer line is 10 ♏.
33. Now draw the plunger back to 11 ♏, 12 ♏, 13 ♏, 14 ♏, and the longer line at 15 ♏; 15 ♏ is not marked 15, but is halfway between 10 and 20 and is represented by a longer line.

34. Draw the plunger back to 16 ♏.
35. Roll the syringe toward you until "cc" can be read. Note that 1 cc is the same as 16 ♏. Remember there are 15 to 16 ♏ in 1 cc.
36. Roll the syringe slightly away from you until minims can be read.
37. Draw the plunger back to 20 ♏.
38. Draw the plunger back to 22 ♏, 25 ♏, 27 ♏, 28 ♏, 30 ♏, and 32 ♏. Notice there are two lines beyond the 30 ♏ mark. This is 32 ♏.
39. Roll syringe slightly toward you until "cc" can be read. Notice that there are 32 ♏ in 2 cc and 48 ♏ in 3 cc.

THE I-CC OR TUBERCULIN SYRINGE

This syringe is calibrated to measure dosages of 1.0 cc (ml) or less. It is commonly used to measure pediatric dosages, immunizing agents, or for skin testing for allergenic reactions (see Fig. 8-2).

Procedure: reading a tuberculin syringe

Materials needed
1 syringe for each member of the class or 1 syringe for every two students

Introduction
Obtain a tuberculin syringe from your instructor. The tuberculin syringe is graduated in 0.01 cc or $^1/_{100}$ of a cubic centimeter. It has a double scale: minim measurement on one side of the syringe and 0.01 cc, or $^1/_{100}$ of a cubic centimeter, on the other side. The total amount of the syringe in cubic centimeters is 1 cc. In minims it is 16 ♏.

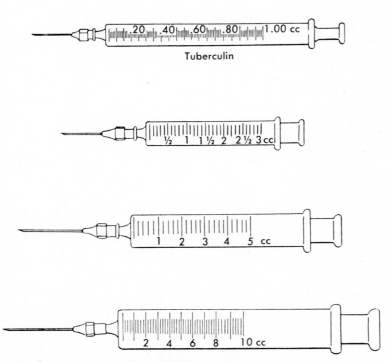

Fig. 8-2. Commonly used syringes.

Instructions

1. Place the plunger in the barrel of the syringe. (Follow the instructions given for a 3-cc syringe.)
2. Hold the syringe in a horizontal position in your left hand.
3. Hold the head of the plunger with your right hand.
4. Turn the syringe slowly until the cc measurements can be read. (The 1-cc measurement can be found on the upper part of the barrel.)
5. Realize that each line means 0.01 cc, or $1/100$ of 1 cc.
6. Notice that every five lines there is a longer line. The first longer line represents $5/100$, the second longer line $10/100$, the third longer line $15/100$, and the fourth longer line $20/100$ of a cubic centimeter. Note that $20/100$ is marked with a "20" but that $5/100$, $10/100$, and $15/100$ are not labeled.
7. Draw the plunger back to the first short line. (This is $1/100$ of a cubic centimeter—0.01 cc.)
8. Draw the plunger back to the second short line. (This is $2/100$ of a cubic centimeter—0.02 cc.)
9. Draw the plunger back to the third short line. (This is $3/100$ of a cubic centimeter or 0.03 cc.)
10. Draw the plunger back to the fifth line. Notice that this line is the first longer line. (This is $5/100$ of a cubic centimeter or 0.05 cc.)
11. Draw the plunger back to $6/100$, $7/100$, $8/100$, $9/100$, and the next line, which is longer, or $10/100$ of a cubic centimeter. (Realize that $10/100$ is the same as $1/10$ of a cubic centimeter. The fraction is reduced to lowest terms. Expressed as a decimal, it is 0.1 cc.)
12. Draw the plunger back to $16/100$, $17/100$, $18/100$, $19/100$, and the next line, which is longer, or $20/100$ of a cubic centimeter. (Note that the number 20 is printed above the line. Realize that all of these divisions are fractions of the whole amount, which is 1 cc. They are less than 1 cc.)
13. Draw the plunger back to $40/100$ and $50/100$ of a cubic centimeter. (Realize that $50/100$ can be reduced to the fraction $1/2$; $50/100$ is, then, $50/100$ cc, or $1/2$ cc.)
14. Draw the plunger back to $95/100$, then to $100/100$, or the entire amount of 1 cc.
15. Roll the syringe around until the minim measurement can be read.
16. Notice that the total number of minims is 16.
17. Notice that the first long line represents 4 ℳ.
18. Notice that there are eight lines between zero and 4 ℳ, 4 ℳ and 8 ℳ, 8 ℳ and 12 ℳ, and so on.
19. The first short line between zero and 4 ℳ represents $1/8$ of 4 ℳ, the second short line is $2/8$ (or $1/4$) of 4 ℳ, the third short line is $3/8$ of 4 ℳ, and the fourth short line is $4/8$ (or $1/2$) of 4 ℳ, or 2 ℳ. Realize that $2/8$ of 4 ℳ is 1 ℳ.
20. Draw the plunger back to $5/8$ of 4 ℳ, $6/8$, $7/8$, and $8/8$, or 4 ℳ.
21. Realize that each line on the minim measurement marks a unit equal to $1/8$ of the particular measurement. Show, for example, $1/8$ of 4 ℳ, $2/8$ of 8 ℳ, and $5/8$ of 12 ℳ.
22. *On the tuberculin syringe, each line on the minim measurement side does not represent 1 ℳ. This should be understood.*

THE TUBEX AND PREFILLED DISPOSABLE SYRINGES

1. A prefilled, premeasured sterile cartridge needle unit and syringe is available and requires the same safety measures regarding dosage and technique as other injectables (Fig. 8-3).
2. The use of prefilled disposable syringes is becoming widespread. The routes are subcutaneous, intramuscular, and intravenous, depending on the medication to be administered.
3. Some advantages are:
   a. Time saved in calculating and preparation.
   b. Accuracy of dosage.
   c. Diminished potential for transmission of organisms between patients, since the cartridge and needle are destroyed after one use.
   d. Less hazard to the person administering the drug from allergenic sensitization and hypersensitive reaction, since this person does not come in contact with the medication.
   e. Space saved in storage.

DOSAGES

For parenteral subq, IM, and intradermal medications, the amount of medication ordered and the amount available frequently are the same; the main caution then is to be absolutely certain that they are the same, especially if the apothecary value is used for one and the metric for the other.

Many times the physician will order a fraction of the amount on hand, or two different drugs may be ordered, both in fractional quantities. This is frequently the case for the patient who is going to surgery.

There are two methods used to calculate fractional dosages. Learn to use the one most comfortable for you.

1. Use the formula: dose ordered divided by dose available multiplied by the total strength of drug in cc (ml) or minim.

   EXAMPLES:
   a. Physician orders codeine phosphate 15 mg.
      (1) You have codeine phosphate 30 mg/cc (ml).
      (2) 15 mg ÷ 30 mg = $1/2 \times 1/1 = 1/2$
      (3) $1/2 \times 1$ cc (ml) = $1/2$ cc. Give 0.5 cc of the codeine phosphate 30 mg/ml to give 15 mg ordered.
   b. Physician orders Demerol 25 mg. You have available 100 mg/cc (ml).

   $$\frac{25 \text{ mg}}{100 \text{ mg}} \times 1 \text{ cc (ml)} = 1/4 \times 1 =$$

   $$1/4 \text{ ml or } .25 \text{ ml}$$

2. Use ratio and proportion:

   $$\frac{mg}{30} : \frac{ml}{1} :: \frac{mg}{15} : \frac{ml}{x}$$

   $$30x = 15$$

   $$x = 15 \div 30 = \frac{15}{30} = 1/2 \text{ ml or } 0.5 \text{ ml}$$

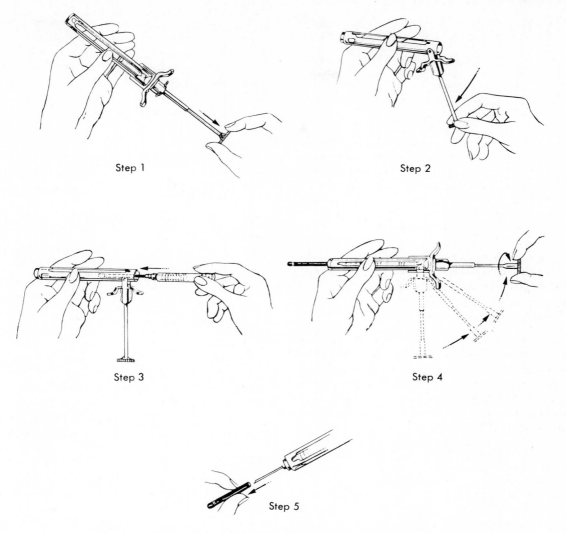

Step 1

Step 2

Step 3

Step 4

Step 5

Fig. 8-3. Placing a prefilled cartridge of medication in a Tubex.

EXAMPLES:

a. The physician wants the patient to have 75 mg of the drug. The label on the bottle states there are 100 mg to each cc (ml). See the simple formula.
   What does the physician want administered?
   What strength is on hand?
   $$\frac{75}{100} = \frac{3}{4}$$

   $$\frac{3}{4} \times 1 \text{ cc} = 0.75 \text{ cc (ml)}$$

or

   $$\frac{mg}{100} : \frac{cc}{1} : : \frac{mg}{75} : \frac{cc}{x}$$
   $$100x = 75$$
   $$^{75}/_{100} = {}^{3}/_{4} \text{ of 1 cc}$$
   $$x = 0.75$$

b. The physician orders the patient to receive 25 mg of a drug. The medicine bottle reads 100 mg to 1 ml.

   $$\frac{25}{100} = {}^{1}/_{4} \text{ of 1 ml}$$

   $$\frac{mg}{100} : \frac{cc}{1} : : \frac{mg}{25} : \frac{cc}{x}$$
   $$100x = 25$$
   $$x = {}^{25}/_{100} =$$
   $${}^{1}/_{4} \text{ of 1 ml or 0.25 ml (cc)}$$

c. The physician orders the patient to receive 20 mg of a drug. The medicine bottle reads 100 mg to 1 ml.

   $$\frac{mg}{100} : \frac{cc}{1} : : \frac{mg}{20} : \frac{cc}{x}$$
   $$100x = 20$$
   $$x = {}^{20}/_{100} = {}^{1}/_{5} \text{ of 1 ml or 0.2 ml (cc)}$$

d. The physician orders the patient to receive 75 mg of a drug. The label on the bottle states there are 100 mg to 2 ml.

$$\frac{mg}{100} : \frac{cc}{2} :: \frac{mg}{75} : \frac{cc}{x}$$

$$100x = 150$$
$$x = {}^{150}/_{100} = 1.5 \text{ ml (cc)}$$

e. The physician orders the patient to have 10 mg of a drug. The medicine bottle reads 50 mg to 1 ml.

$$\frac{mg}{50} : \frac{cc}{1} :: \frac{mg}{10} : \frac{cc}{x}$$

$$50x = 10$$
$$x = {}^{10}/_{50} = {}^{1}/_{5} \text{ of 1 ml or 0.2 ml (cc)}$$

Proof: $^{1}/_{5} \times 50 = 10$
$1 \times 10 = 10$

CALCULATION OF PREOPERATIVE HYPODERMIC MEDICATION FOR FRACTIONAL DOSAGE

Mrs. H. is going to surgery for an appendectomy (removal of the appendix) at 9 AM. The physician orders 50 mg of Nembutal Sodium, 20 mg of Demerol, and 0.4 mg of atropine to be administered to her by hypodermic injection at 8 AM. These are intramuscular injections. You find that you have on hand the following strengths: Nembutal Sodium ampule, 100 mg per 2 ml; Demerol, 50 mg per 1 ml; and atropine, 0.6 mg per 1 ml.

You will draw the Nembutal in a separate syringe (see Fig. 8-4) and give it in a separate injection, since Nembutal cannot be mixed with other drugs.

You will draw the proper doses of Demerol and atropine in one syringe and administer in one injection, thus making a total of two separate injections: Nembutal as one injection, Demerol and atropine as the second injection.

Nembutal:
Remember the formula:

$$\frac{\text{Dose ordered}}{\text{Dose available}} \times \text{Total strength of the drug in ml}$$

What does the physician want? Nembutal Sodium, 50 mg
What strength is on hand? Nembutal Sodium, 100 mg per 2 ml

$$\frac{50}{100} \text{ mg} = \frac{1}{2}$$

$$\frac{1}{2} \times 2 \text{ ml} = 1 \text{ ml (cc)}$$

Administer 1 ml or 50 mg ($^{1}/_{2}$ of 100 mg). Draw this dose into one syringe and place on hypodermic tray, following usual hypodermic syringe technique.

Demerol:
What does the physician want? Demerol, 20 mg
What strength is on hand? Demerol, 50 mg per 1 cc (1 ml)

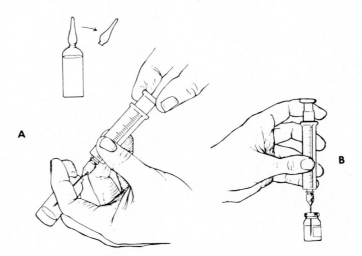

Fig. 8-4. Techniques for withdrawing parenteral medications from an ampule and a multiple dose vial. **A,** Withdrawing medication from an ampule. An ampule may be made like the one in the lower left portion of this illustration—it will break easily when pressure is exerted at the constricted portion—or the ampule may be made so that a metal file must be used at the neck to secure a clean break. **B,** Inserting hypodermic needle into a stoppered vial. When a hypodermic needle is inserted into a vial of this type, it is important that air be injected first to facilitate withdrawal of the liquid medication. Note that the plunger has been withdrawn and is supported by the index finger. After the plunger has been pushed down to the end of the barrel, the vial can be turned and held much like the ampule in **A.** The desired amount is then drawn into the syringe.

$$\frac{20}{50} = \frac{2}{5}$$

$$\frac{2}{5} \times 1 \text{ ml (50 mg)} = 0.4 \text{ ml (cc)}$$

Administer 0.4 ml (²/₅ of total strength 50 mg per 1 ml).

Atropine:

What does the physician want? Atropine, 0.4 mg
What strength is on hand? Atropine, 0.6 mg per 1 ml

$$\frac{0.4}{0.6} = \frac{2}{3}$$

$$\frac{2}{3} \times 1 \text{ ml (0.6 mg)} = 0.66 \text{ cc or } 0.6 \text{ ml (cc)}$$

Administer 0.66 ml (²/₃ of the total strength, 0.6 mg per 1 ml).

Draw the 0.4 ml of Demerol into a second syringe, using the usual syringe technique. Draw the 0.66 ml of atropine into the same syringe.

You, now have a reading on the syringe of 1.06 ml, of which 0.4 ml is Demerol and 0.66 ml is atropine.

Remember: Once you have drawn a drug into a syringe and are about to draw a second drug into the same syringe, wedge the narrow neck of the plunger of the syringe against the barrel of the syringe with your little finger. Do not push forward with the plunger when injecting the needle of the syringe into the second bottle. This prevents pushing the first drug into the second bottle.

INJECTION SITES

It is necessary that the medication ordered be given into the tissue that has been prescribed, otherwise the

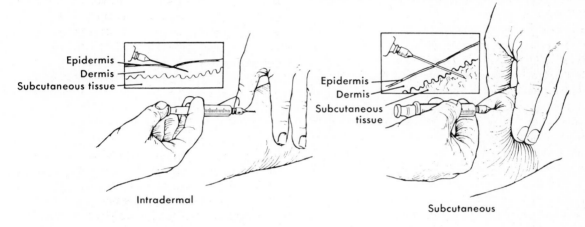

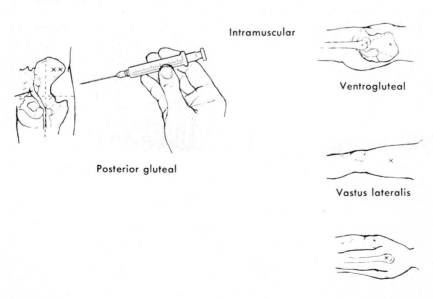

Fig. 8-5. Injection sites.

effects may be harmful to the patient. These sites and method of injection follow:

1. Intradermal (intracutaneous) injections are given by means of a tuberculin syringe with ⅝-inch, 26-gauge needle. A minute amount of solution is injected just under the outer layers of skin. The trajectory of the needle is parallel to the outer skin surface, between the epidermis and the dermis and avoiding subcutaneous tissue (Fig. 8-5).
2. Subcutaneous (subq; sc; hypodermic) injections are given by means of a 3-cc or tuberculin (1-cc) syringe with a ⅝-inch 25-gauge, needle. Trajectory of the needle is at a 45° angle to the outer skin surface (Fig. 8-5). (Note: A tuberculin syringe has a total volume of 1 cc and is calibrated in 0.01 ml.)

Subcutaneous injections

1. Needle should be inserted through the skin with a quick, even movement.
2. Plunger of syringe should be withdrawn slightly to determine and prevent penetration into a blood vessel.
3. Outer surface of upper arm, anterior surface of thigh, and lower abdomen are common sites.
4. Injection is made slowly and steadily.
5. Volume is limited to 0.5 to 2 ml. Larger amounts of fluids (250 to 500 cc) may be given into tissues by a process called hypodermoclysis, using the areas of loose connective tissue found:
   a. Under the breasts
   b. Upper surfaces of the thighs
   c. Subscapular region of the back
6. Chart the injection site, for example, sc—rt. arm, left thigh.
7. Massage skin after injection if indicated in drug literature.

Intramuscular injections

1. Tuberculin (1-cc) or 3-cc syringe.
2. Needles from 1 to 3 inches and 19 to 22 gauge, depending on the site of injection.
3. Trajectory of needle is at a 90° angle.
4. Usual sites are the buttocks:
   a. Posterior gluteal. Divide buttocks into four quadrants and insert needle at 90° angle into upper, outer quadrant.
   b. Ventrogluteal. Using your left hand, place the index finger on right iliac spine of the patient and the middle finger stretched back and slipped to a point just below the crest of the ilium, with your palm resting on the patient's hip. The injection site is the apex of the triangle between the index and middle finger. Insert needle at a 90° angle.
   c. Vastus lateralis. Spot injection site a handsbreadth

above the knee and an equal distance below the greater trochanter. Insert needle at a 90° angle.
   d. Deltoid. Cover the head of the humerus. Insert below the acromion and lateral to the axilla.

Parenteral solutions

Medications given by injection must be in a solution available to the circulating blood.

Reconstituting a powdered medication

Some drugs are unstable in a liquid form and must be stored in a crystal or powder form until ready for use. Once they are mixed, they must be used within the time span the pharmaceutical company has indicated on the label. These companies are required to present instructions for reconstituting the drug, and such instructions should be followed meticulously.

EXAMPLE:
   Drug available: ampicillin 125 mg in a 1-cc vial.
   Instructions: End quantity of solution equals the volume of sterile water added to the vial.
   Physician orders 50 mg ampicillin (IM).
   1. Add 1 ml (cc) sterile water to the 125 mg ampicillin = 125 mg/1 ml.
   2. 125 mg : 1 ml : : 50 mg : x = 0.4 ml.
   Administer 0.4 ml from the 1-cc vial.

Work these problems:
   1. Desired: glucagon 0.5 mg IM.
      Instructions: Dilute 1 mg of glucagon powder with 1 ml of its own diluting solution.
      How many milliliters will you give?
   2. Desired: Librium 25 mg IM.
      Available: 100 mg in a 5-ml dry amber ampule, and a 2-ml vial of special diluent.
      Instructions: Add the 2 ml of diluent to the ampule containing the Librium powder.
      How many milliliters will you administer?
   3. Desired: Staphcillin 75 mg IM.
      Available: Staphcillin 1 g IM.
      Instructions: Add 1.5 ml *sterile* water for a total volume of 2 ml.
      How many milliliters will you administer?

INTRAVENOUS THERAPY

The L.P.N. is responsible for knowing state regulations and hospital policy. Do not attempt venipuncture if you are unqualified.

Nursing responsibilities

1. The same principles apply to IV solutions as to all other medications, with a special caution to *check the physician's order sheet* before starting an infusion or superimposing on to one that is already infusing.
2. Inspect the IV bottle.

a. Check the label for correct solution and concentration information.

b. Check for cloudiness or foreign matter.

c. Check for chips or cracks in the bottle.

d. Determine that the closure is intact.

e. Check vacuum bubbles in solution after inversion. Absence of a hissing sound when administration set is opened indicates contamination or a break in technique. Do not use!

3. IV additives: in many hospitals today the clinical pharmacist prepares these solutions; however, many hospitals still place this responsibility with the nurse.

a. Do not initiate (unless an emergency) a solution prepared by another nurse.

b. Use the principles of sterile technique.

c. Perform compatibility checks for each solution.

(1) Refer to the compatibility charts available from pharmaceutical companies that usually are posted in each hospital.

(2) Use a solution's own diluent or the exact diluent recommended by the manufacturer.

(3) Read the bold-print cautions in the package insert on how to mix the solution.

(4) Nothing should be mixed with blood or blood products.

(5) Try not to mix more than one antibiotic in the same IV solution.

(6) If you do not know the compatibility of drugs to be mixed and you cannot find out, do not mix them.

Usual causes of medication errors

1. Dilutions miscalculated. Check your figures with another nurse, a pharmacist, or a physician.

2. Mislabeling or absence of labeling. Check for correct information.

a. Patient's name and room number.

b. Times to start, to stop, and to monitor the rate of infusion.

c. Number of bottle (for example, No. 1 or No. 2) to facilitate accounting for total intake.

d. Additives: drug name and dosage—preferably a colored form to stand out.

e. Report and record the exact amount of solution absorbed on your shift and the amount remaining to be carried forward to the next shift.

Regulation of rate of parenteral infusions

Drugs may be added to intravenous fluid and given over a prescribed number of minutes or hours. The flow must be constant. A fast rate followed by a slow rate, simply to extend the time, does not accomplish the purpose of administration. To regulate the flow over a definite period, you must know how many drops are given

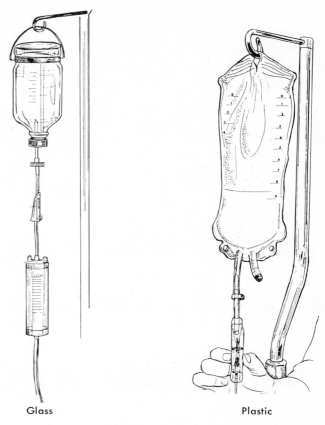

Glass   Plastic

Fig. 8-6. Intravenous fluid and container sets.

over a definite number of minutes. Certain sets deliver 15 drops of an aqueous solution per milliliter. Check each set for the number of drops per milliliter it will deliver. (See Fig. 8-6.)

EXAMPLES:
Administer 1 liter (L) over a period of 5 hours. 1 L = about 15,000 drops; 5 hours = 300 minutes.

$$\frac{50 \text{ drops per minute}}{300 \overline{)\ 15,000}} \textit{ or } 15{,}000 \text{ drops :}$$
$$300 \text{ min : : } x \text{ drops : 1 min}$$

1. A 20-ml ampule of aminophylline contains 25 mg/ml or 500 mg. This may be diluted to 200 ml with sodium chloride injection and administered at a rate of 25 mg per minute to relieve bronchiolar spasm.

$$500 \text{ mg : } 200 \text{ ml : : } 25 \text{ mg : } x = 10 \text{ ml}$$

Ten milliliters of the dilution is to be administered per minute. Approximately how many drops per minute are given? Answer: 150

$$\frac{20 \text{ minutes}}{150 \overline{)\ 3{,}000}}$$

A faster rate may cause some patients to feel the excessive stimulating effect of the drug and may cause circulatory collapse.

2. How many drops per minute are given for (assume 15 drops per milliliter):
   a. 25 ml per hour   *Answer:*   6 gtt per minute
   b. 1 L in 6 hours   *Answer:*   41 gtt per minute
   c. 500 cc in 5 hours   *Answer:*   25 gtt per minute

VENIPUNCTURE

1. Venipuncture is performed to:
   a. Withdraw a blood sample.
   b. Instill IV fluids or medications or both.
2. Before administering any drug IV:
   a. Determine that the preparation is intended for IV administration.
   b. Ascertain that the drug(s) are compatible with the IV solution, or with each other.
   c. Do not use substances with an oil base or unsterile substances.
   d. Do not prepare solutions for the next shift or leave partially used, opened vials.
   e. Observe for air bubbles or solution leaking from tubing. A rubber inset in the tubing that does not reseal itself can result in an air embolus.
3. The steps in performing a venipuncture for the recorded purpose include (Fig. 8-7):
   a. Check physician's order, type of fluid, medications to be added, and rate of infusion.
   b. Based on this information, assemble equipment—IV solution, administration set, tourniquet or sphygmomanometer, antiseptic solution, needle (steel or plastic), sterile 2 by 2 inch gauge, and tape.
   c. Prepare IV solution and tubing, clearing line of air, and have handy to connect to needle hub.
   d. Select the site. For long-term therapy choose a vein that is naturally splinted by such long bones as the ulna or radius.
   e. Apply pressure per tourniquet or sphygmomanometer above site.
   f. Palpate vein to determine depth and direction.
   g. Cleanse site with Betadine or 70% alcohol.
   h. Place left thumb on the skin about 2 inches distal to injection site; this exerts tension on the superficial skin to prevent it from retracting or curling away from needle point.
   i. Insert needle through skin (see Figs. 8-3 to 8-5 for technique in steel and plastic needle).
   j. When venous blood flow is established:
      (1) For blood sample, withdraw amount needed per syringe, release tourniquet, remove needle, and apply pressure with sterile compress until bleeding ceases. Label specimen and send with request slip to the laboratory.
      (2) For infusion, connect tubing to needle, release tourniquet, and anchor needle and tubing to arm or hand with tape. Some hospitals

apply a dressing with antibiotic ointments at the needle site.
   k. Determine the rate of flow of solution:

$$\frac{\text{ml of solution} \times \text{number of drops/ml}}{\text{hours of administration} \times 60 \text{ min}} = \text{gtt/min}$$

Regulate the flow by counting the drops from 15 seconds, multiplying by 4, and adjusting clamp on tubing.
   l. Mark IV bottle with patient's name, medications added, start time, stop time, hourly intervals between, and number of bottle; for example, #1, #2, #3.
   m. Chart time, fluid, medication, needle used, site, number, and rate of flow.
   n. Keep an accurate record of fluid intake during your shift and residual to credit to the oncoming personnel.

Monitoring the IV infusion

1. Check mechanical difficulties for obstruction of tubing or filter and either irrigate or change.
2. If the bevel of the needle is occluded by a wall of the vein, then rotate needle.
3. Check outflow of blood from needle by lowering IV bottle below IV site and observing for blood return from hub of needle into the tubing. This method of lowering the bottle to check for blood return prevents contamination of the IV.
4. Use glass syringe to aspirate blood clot from needle. Do *not* attempt to clear needle by flushing with fluid because this will dislodge the clot and may cause thrombophlebitis.
5. Check site frequently for infiltration, redness, tenderness, or swelling.
6. Check vital signs and objective complaints offered by the patient.

Adding additional fluids

1. Check additional fluids against physician's order sheet. Frequently, an initial order is changed.
2. Supply the exact preparation ordered.
3. Ascertain that tubing is free of air and filled with solution.
4. Use careful aseptic technique.
5. Regulate flow rate and label bottle correctly.
6. Chart time, solution, amount, and number of bottle.

Changing IV tubing

1. It is recommended that IV tubing be changed every 24 hours. Check with your hospital policy.
2. Tubing must be changed if the filter becomes clogged or the tubing contaminated.
3. Steps in changing IV tubing:
   a. Remove old tubing from bottle, add new tubing to

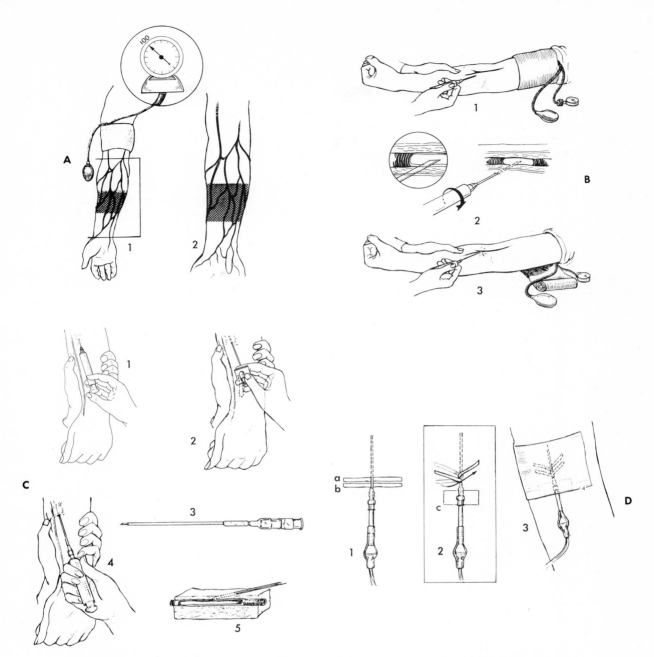

Fig. 8-7. Venipuncture. **A,** Preparation for venipuncture. *1,* A sphygmomanometer or tourniquet is applied to the upper arm and inflated to distend the veins. *2,* An average pattern of superficial veins. The preferred area for fluid therapy is shaded. **B,** Venipuncture with steel needle. *1,* Tension of the thumb, distal to the site of venipuncture, stretches the skin and stabilizes the vein. The needle, attached to a syringe, is inserted through the skin adjacent to the vein. *2,* The needle is held at little less than a 45° angle for penetration of the skin. When the needle enters the vein, the bevel is rotated to prevent puncture of the posterior wall of the vessel. *3,* The needle and syringe are lowered nearly parallel to the skin for advancement into the vein. **C,** Venipuncture with plastic needle. *1,* Formation of skin wheal with local anesthetic agent. *2,* A pathway for the plastic needle is formed by puncturing the skin with large-bore steel needle. *3,* Plastic needle, Jelco IV catheter placement unit. *4,* The plastic needle is attached to syringe for introduction through the preformed channel. *5,* Cross section showing needle being introduced through the channel. **D,** Securing plastic needle. *1,* Approximate placement of narrow strips of tape. The first tape, *a,* is anchored before the second one, *b,* is placed. The tape must adhere to the distal end of the plastic needle. *2,* Method of fastening tape to needle and skin. Tape beneath hub is placed with its adhesive side up, *c.* Its adherence to overlying tape prevents movement of the needle, which may contribute to separation and loss of the plastic tube. *3,* A large piece of tape completes stabilization of the needle. It is labeled to show the date of insertion and that plastic needle is in place.

bottle, and run solution through the tubing to fill it with solution and clear air bubbles.

   b. Disengage old tubing from needle and place the adaptor of the new tubing into the needle. Do this quickly and aseptically by keeping the adaptor sterile until insertion.

4. Changing of IV tubing in the case of a new veni-puncture site is recommended to prevent infection.

5. The specific procedure required for a venipuncture site is established by the physician or the hospital.

Discontinuing an infusion

1. Check physician's order sheet.
2. Bring sterile alcohol sponge and bandage to the bedside.
3. Remove tape, holding needle firmly to prevent a rotation that might traumatize the vein.
4. Hold alcohol sponge over site of insertion with fingers of one hand. Gently and slowly remove the needle with the other hand, keeping the needle parallel with the skin to assure its removal intact.
5. Apply pressure to wound as soon as needle is removed and place a bandage over the puncture site.
6. Chart time, amount of fluid infused, and appearance of site.
7. Warm, moist compresses may be applied to an infiltrated area or irritated puncture site; these must be applied with care to avoid burns to the skin.
8. Report any error immediately; the physician will need to institute corrective measures as soon as possible to prevent irreversible consequences to the patient.

ASSIGNMENT

Review previous lessons and questions according to directions of your instructor.

1. Identify the parts of a syringe.
2. Name the parts of the syringe to avoid contamination and explain why.
3. Measure the following quantities of colored fluid in the appropriate syringe.
     a. 2.5 ml
     b. 1.20 ml
     c. 36 minims
     d. 0.02 minims
     e. 0.30 ml
     f. 0.8 ml
     g. $^3/_{10}$ of 1 ml
     h. 2 minims
     i. 4.5 ml
     j. 0.09 ml
     k. 3.2 ml
     l. $^5/_5$ of $^1/_2$ ml
     m. 15 minims
     n. 52 minims
     o. 1.5 ml

4. Measure the following doses on a tuberculin syringe.
     a. 0.01 cc ($^1/_{100}$ of 1 cc)
     b. 0.02 cc ($^2/_{100}$ of 1 cc)
     c. 0.10 cc ($^{10}/_{100}$ of 1 cc)
     d. 0.15 cc ($^{15}/_{100}$ of 1 cc)
     e. 0.05 cc ($^5/_{100}$ of 1 cc)
     f. 0.49 cc ($^{49}/_{100}$ of 1 cc)
     g. 0.50 cc ($^{50}/_{100}$ of 1 cc)
     h. 1.00 cc ($^{100}/_{100}$ of, or entire cc)

5. On the minim side of the tuberculin syringe what does the first short line between 0 and 4 ♏ represent? Find the fourth short line on the minim side of the tuberculin syringe. What does it represent? Each line on the minim measurement side *does not* represent 1 ♏, or *does* represent 1 ♏. Which is correct?

6. Would a prefilled syringe have some special advantage on the emergency drug tray?

7. Examine the emergency drugs on your hospital unit and bring to class a list of those drugs found in prefilled syringes.

8. What are some advantages of prefilled syringes? Can you think of any dangers?

9. How would you respond to a patient's question: "What is this shot that you are giving me?"

10. What will you do if your patient protests an injection or intravenous infusion?

11. Why must you record the injection site?

12. You are requested by the RN in charge to administer an IV solution of 5% DW/0.2% normal saline 1000 ml. What will be your response?

13. Assume you accept the responsibility for question 12; outline the steps in
      a. Venipuncture
      b. Initiating infusion
      c. Monitoring infusion
      d. Care of site
      e. Changing tubing
      f. Discontinuing
      g. Charting

14. Solve the following problems:
      a. Desired: Adrenalin 0.2 ml of 1:1000 solution subq. Available: 1 ml/1:1000 solution.
      b. Desired: old tuberculin 0.01/ml intradermally. Available: as ordered.
      c. Desired: 0.5 ml influenza virus vaccine subq. Available: 1 ml/ampule.
      d. Desired: 0.1 ml influenza virus vaccine.
      e. Desired: Pitocin 0.5 ml IM. Available: 1 ml/ampule.
      f. Desired: Pitocin 1 ml/1000 ml 5% D/W intravenous to run at 100 ml/hour. Available: Pitocin 0.5 ml/ampule and D5/W 500-cc bottle.
      g. Desired: posterior pituitary injection 0.3 ml subq. Available: 1 ml/ampule.
      h. Desired: 40 mg Vasoxyl in 250 ml D5/W IV to be infused at the rate of 5 mg/min. Available: 20 mg Vasoxyl/1-ml ampules.
      i. Desired: lidocaine IV 1 mg/kg body weight. Patient weighs 150 pounds. How many milligrams will you administer?

j. Desired: sodium bicarbonate 89.2 mEq IV push. Available: 44.6 mEq/50 cc. How many cubic centimeters (milliliters) will you administer?

k. Desired: Nalline 0.2 mg injected into umbilical vein. Available: 0.2 mg/ml.

l. Desired: Lasix 120 mg IV over 2 minutes. Available: 20 mg/2 ml.

m. Desired: Hykinone 2.5 mg IV. Available: 10 mg/ml.

n. Desired: 1.0 g erythromycin in 80 cc D5/W IV. Rate infuse in 30 minutes. Available: 1 g/20 ml sterile water.

o. Desired: digoxin 1.0 mg IV push. Available: digoxin 0.5 mg/2 ml.

p. Desired: penicillin G 3,000,000 U/1000 cc D5/W to run in 4 hours. Available: 5,000,000/10 ml.

q. Desired: 500 mg ampicillin/1000 cc D5W/0.45% sodium chloride solution. Rate 30 gtt/min. Reconstruction directions say dilute each 500 mg ampicillin powder with 5 ml of sterile water.

15. The physician wants the patient to have 50 mg of a drug. The label on the bottle states there are 100 mg to each cc (ml). Did you have an answer in minims? This could have been worked in cubic centimeters (or milliliters). Try it.

16. The physician wants the patient to have 40 mg of a drug. The label on the bottle states there are 50 mg to each cc (ml). Is your answer in minims?

17. The physician wants the patient to have 20 mg of a drug. The label on the bottle states there are 100 mg to 1 ml. Is your answer in minims?

18. The physician wants the patient to have 75 mg of a drug. The label on the bottle states there are 100 mg to 2 ml. What is the strength on the label? 100 mg to how many ml? Is your answer in cubic centimeters (milliliters)?

19. The physician wants the patient to have 25 mg of a drug. The label on the bottle states there are 100 mg to 2 ml. What is the strength on the label? 100 mg to how many ml?

20. The physician wants the patient to have 20 mg of a drug. The label on the bottle states there are 100 mg to 1 ml. What is the strength on the label? 100 mg to how many ml?

21. The physician wants the patient to receive gr $1/200$ of a drug. The bottle label states gr $1/100$ per 1 ml. Notice that

these doses are expressed in *grains*. How do you divide a fraction by a fraction?

22. Draw up the following in your syringe:
    a. 1 ml
    b. $1/2$ ml
    c. $1^1/2$ ml
    d. 2 ml
    e. 1 ℳ
    f. 3 ℳ
    g. 5 ℳ
    h. 12 ℳ
    i. 15 ℳ
    j. 16 ℳ
    k. 24 ℳ
    l. 30 ℳ
    m. 32 ℳ
    n. There are how many minims in 1 cc (1 ml)?
    o. There are how many minims in 2 cc (2 ml)?

23. The physician wants the patient to have 75 mg of a liquid drug by hypodermic injection. The label on the bottle states there are 100 mg per 1 cc (1 ml). How much will you administer?

24. Work the following problems so that your answer is in minims. How many minims equal 1 cc (1 ml)?
    a. The physician wants the patient to have 20 mg of a liquid drug by hypodermic injection. The label on the bottle states there are 100 mg per 1 cc (1 ml). How much will you administer?
    b. The physician wants the patient to have 25 mg of a liquid drug by hypodermic injection. The label on the bottle states there are 100 mg per 1 cc (1 ml). How much will you administer?
    c. The physician wants the patient to have 50 mg of a liquid drug by hypodermic injection. The label on the bottle states there are 100 mg per 1 cc (1 ml). How much will you administer? Give your answer in both minims and cc (ml).
    d. The physician wants the patient to have 10 mg of a liquid drug by hypodermic injection. The label on the bottle states there are 100 mg per 1 cc (1 ml). How much will you administer?

CHAPTER 9

Diabetes and insulin

The part of the body most involved in diabetes is the organ called the pancreas. This is a gland that lies just behind and below the stomach. In recent years studies have shown that other glands may contribute to the condition of diabetes.

In the innermost substance of the pancreas there are cells arranged in small groups or clusters. These cells, called islands of Langerhans, supply the substance known as insulin.

Insulin is necessary to help the body use and store sugar. The process of changing sugar into a form the body can use takes place in the liver. The sugar is stored in the liver and released to other parts of the body when it is needed.

DIABETES

In diabetes the supply of insulin is inadequate. The result of this inadequate supply of insulin is that sugar cannot be stored or used by the body. It is then excreted into the urine. Diabetes is treated by diet, by injection of insulin, or by oral medications.

Diabetic diet

A diabetic diet contains the kinds and amounts of foods required for the particular patient. The diet is prescribed especially for that patient and is helpful to him alone in the treatment of his condition.

The diet contains low-carbohydrate fruits and vegetables and is usually sugar-free. Each serving is weighed carefully or measured by tablespoon or cup. The physician prescribes the diet, and the dietitian and nurses see that the orders are carried out.

A patient taking insulin should eat all the food prescribed in the diet, or a sugar-insulin imbalance may occur with reactions. This is because too little food was eaten for the insulin dose given, or the patient may have vomited. Such problems should be reported at once to the team leader, head nurse, supervisor, or physician.

Insulin

Insulin was discovered by Sir Frederick Banting, Charles Best, and John Macleod of Toronto, Canada and was made available to the public in 1922.

Extra insulin is required when there is not enough body insulin available from the pancreas to take care of the required diet. This insulin is obtained from a preparation of animal insulin and is sold in bottles. It acts as body insulin does to help lower the level of sugar in the blood.

Insulin is administered by injection and must be given in exact dosage (Fig. 9-1). The physician determines the dose necessary for the particular patient, since insulin can cause severe reactions. It is a good idea for the nurse to know these reactions and how the physician treats them.

Many attempts have been made to obtain a preparation of insulin that is active after oral administration. No attempt has been successful. In the last few years, however, a few drugs have been found that do have blood sugar–lowering action when given by mouth. These are the sulfonylureas. They were discovered after it was observed that some of the antibacterial sulfonamides had hypoglycemic or blood sugar–lowering effects. It is thought that the sulfonylureas act by increasing the ability of the pancreas to secrete insulin. These drugs are not oral insulin, and it is incorrect to call them such. They are oral hypoglycemic agents.

Oral hypoglycemic agents

There are some oral substitutes for insulin that are effective for certain patients, such as tolbutamide (Orinase). It is indicated in uncomplicated diabetes mellitus of a stable type, with onset in maturity, that cannot be controlled by diet alone. Orinase lowers blood sugar and controls glycosuria, polyuria, and polydipsia. It cannot be used in juvenile diabetes mellitus or in complicated diabetes mellitus. It is available in 0.5-g tablets for oral administration. The dose is carefully regulated by the physician and depends on the patient's blood sugar level and sugar in the urine. Patients should be converted from injection type of insulin to tolbutamide gradually so that aggravation of the diabetes will not occur.

Another antidiabetic agent in tablet form is chlorpropamide (Diabinese). It is said to have more potency than tolbutamide in both acute and chronic administration and to show excellent response in maturity-onset diabetes. It is available in 100- and 250-mg tablets. Other oral anti-

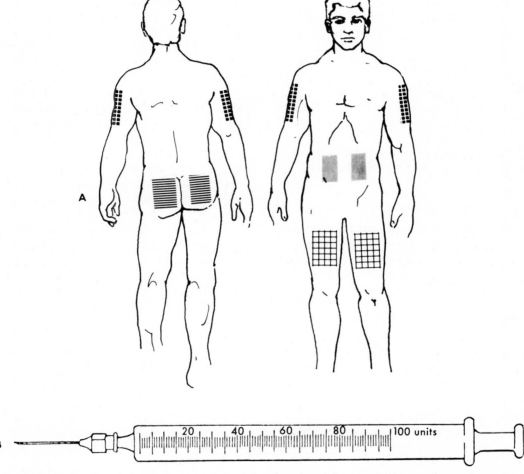

Fig. 9-1. A, Sites for subcutaneous injections of insulin for the diabetic patient (record site used and rotate for each injection). **B,** Insulin syringe calibrated in units (100 U/1 cc).

Table 9-1. Oral hypoglycemic agents available in the United States*

Type	Drug	Half-life (hours) peak†	Duration (hours)†
Sulfonyl-urea	Acetohexamide Dymelor (Lilly)	6-8 (includes metabolites)	12-24
	Chlorpropamide Diabinese (Pfizer)	30-36	60
	Tolazamide Tolinase (Upjohn)	7	10-14
	Tolbutamide Orinase (Upjohn)	4-6	6-12

*Adapted from Ryan, S. A., and Clayton, B. D.: Handbook of practical pharmacology, ed. 2, St. Louis, 1980, The C. V. Mosby Co.
†The times listed are averages based on a newly diagnosed diabetic patient. Factors modifying these times include patient variation, site and route of administration, and dosage.

diabetic agents similar to the other two are acetohexamide (Dymelor) and tolazamide (Tolinase) (see Table 9-1).

Some possible causes of diabetes mellitus

Some possible causes of diabetes mellitus are (1) heredity (if both parents are diabetic, all the children can possibly be diabetic, although this is not certain); (2) obesity (overweight); (3) indulgence in sweets for long periods; and (4) too little exercise.

Some common symptoms of diabetes

Some common symptoms of diabetes are (1) increased urination (polyuria), which is caused by glucose acting as an osmotic diuretic (a diuretic is a drug or food that increases urine output); (2) increased appetite (polyphagia), resulting from the loss of nourishment because glucose (sugar) is lost in the blood and urine; (3) increased thirst (polydipsia), caused by the great loss of body fluids through the urine; and (4) increase in blood sugar, since the body cannot use the glucose because of lack of insulin. This unused sugar accumulates in the blood. At a certain point, which is about 170 mg/100 ml, sugar will spill into the urine. Normal blood contains about 80 to 120 mg of glucose in every 100 ml (cc) of blood. Diabetic blood shows a glucose content of greater than 140 mg for every 100 ml (cc) of blood.

At the present time no diabetic patient is cured, but symptoms are brought under control with the aid of diabetic diets, drugs, and exercise.

Some complications of diabetes

Complications that may occur are (1) acidosis (this will be discussed in more detail); (2) arteriosclerosis (hardening of the arteries); (3) hypoglycemia (too little sugar in the blood); and (4) infections, especially of the feet (feet and toes may become gangrenous and amputation may be necessary; care of feet and toenails is most important in prevention of infections).

Acidosis. Acidosis occurs in untreated cases of diabetes. Glucose (sugar) cannot be oxidized without insulin, so the patient must burn excessive amounts of fat. When the oxidation of fats is incomplete, some of the products of incomplete combustion appear in the urine. These products of incomplete combustion are diacetic acid, acetone, and beta-hydroxybutyric acid. They are known collectively as ketones. Acidosis caused by ketones is called ketoacidosis. If this condition is not corrected, the patient will go into a coma (state of unconsciousness).

Symptoms. Symptoms of acidosis include (1) headache, nausea, and vomiting; (2) pains in abdomen; (3) feeling of exhaustion, dizzy sensations, and drowsiness; (4) fruity odor to the breath (from acetone); (5) rapid, shallow breathing; (6) rapid pulse; and (7) coma (if symptoms are not brought under control).

Treatment. Treatment means constant effort, testing, and observation of the patient for hours, sometimes days, by both physician and nurse.

1. Physician orders insulin in large doses (sometimes 40 to 50 units or more, depending on the severity, for first dose).
2. Twenty units or more of insulin may be given every 15, 30, or 60 minutes thereafter, depending on the results of urine and blood sugar tests.
3. If the patient is unconscious or unable to void, the physician may order catheterization to obtain urine specimens for tests. Urine is examined for sugar, the amount of sugar present, and the presence of ketones.
4. When symptoms are brought under control, the physician reduces the dose of insulin.
5. The nurse must keep the patient warm and his circulation good and therefore should change the patient's position often.
6. The nurse must pay particular attention to patient mouth care to prevent sordes.
7. Fluids are administered by mouth if the patient is conscious. The physician may order additional fluids to be administered by intravenous injection to overcome dehydration.

It is obvious that diabetes mellitus is a serious disease if untreated and that insulin is a valuable drug used in the control of diabetes mellitus. The more the nurse can learn about insulin—the different kinds of insulin, insulin dosage, and insulin reactions—the safer the patient will be.

Table 9-2. Commercially available forms of insulin*

Type of insulin	Onset† (hours)	Peak† (hours)	Duration† (hours)	Appearance	Shape of bottle	Glycosuria‡	Hypoglycemia‡
Fast-acting							
Insulin injection USP (regular insulin)	1/2-1	3-6	5-8	Clear	Round	Early AM[1]	Before lunch[3]
Prompt insulin zinc suspension USP (Semilente)	1/2-1	4-6	12-16	Opaque	Hexagonal	Early AM[1]	Before lunch[3]
Intermediate-acting							
Globin zinc insulin injection USP	1-4	6-8	16-18	Clear	Round	Before breakfast and lunch[2]	3 to supper[3]
Insulin zinc suspension USP (Lente)	1-2	8-12	24-28	Opaque	Hexagonal	Before lunch[2]	3 to supper[3]
Isophane insulin suspension USP (NPH)	1-2	8-12	24-28	Opaque	Square	Before lunch[2]	3 to supper[3]
Long-acting							
Extended insulin zinc suspension USP (Ultralente)	4-8	16-18	36+	Opaque	Hexagonal	Before lunch and bedtime[2]	2 AM to breakfast[3]
Protamine zinc insulin (PZI) suspension USP	1-8	16-24	36+	Opaque	Round	—	2 AM to breakfast[3]

*Adapted from Ryan, S. A., and Clayton, B. D.: Handbook of practical pharmacology, ed. 2, St. Louis, 1980, The C. V. Mosby Co.
†The times listed are averages based on a newly diagnosed diabetic patient. Factors modifying these times include patient variation, site and route of administration, and dosage.
‡Most frequently occurs when insulin is administered: (1) at bedtime the previous night, (2) before breakfast the previous day, (3) before breakfast the same day.

CAUSES OF INSULIN REACTIONS

An insulin reaction is likely to occur (1) if the amount of insulin given exceeds the patient's need, (2) if the patient misses a meal or part of a meal, or (3) if the patient vomits or develops diarrhea. In these examples the patient does not absorb as much food as was planned for him and the reaction occurs.

Symptoms

Reactions to insulin may cause (1) a fall in blood sugar to below 70 mg per 100 ml of blood, (2) acute hunger, (3) trembling, nervousness, and restlessness, (4) sweating and sudden weakness, and (5) hypotension and unconsciousness, if the first symptoms are not treated at once.

Treatment

To treat a patient with insulin reactions, the nurse should remember the following:

1. Give 2 to 4 oz (60 to 120 ml) of orange juice or sweet fruit juice, a lump of sugar, or a piece of candy.
2. Repeat the treatment in 15 to 20 minutes if relief from symptoms does not occur.
3. Notify team leader, head nurse, or supervisor as soon as symptoms are observed, who will then notify the physician for orders concerning this and any further treatment.

TYPES OF INSULIN

There are several forms of insulin. The type used will determine the time it takes to lower the blood sugar level and how long it will be maintained at that level. The type and amount of insulin to be used are always prescribed by the physician (see Table 9-2).

Many patients will need to be informed about their insulin requirements and their special diet. Nurses and patients should realize that they must never discontinue or change the physician's orders in any way. The physician will do this and will inform the nurse and the patient. A physician, nurse, or pharmacist should be willing to discuss the insulin dosage and diet with the patient whenever the need arises.

MEASUREMENT OF INSULIN*

Insulin is ordered by prescription, just as other medicines are. Its dosage is exact and individualized, so great care should be taken to measure the amount correctly.

*For the next part of the lesson the instructor will pass out to the class several types of insulin syringes and insulin bottles of different strengths.

Insulin solutions are made in two concentrations. These concentrations vary according to the number of units (U) of insulin in each cc (ml). One kind of insulin solution, called U-40, has 40 units in each cc (ml). The other solution, called U-100, has 100 units in each cc (ml).

The label on each bottle of insulin states whether that bottle contains 40 U or 100 U in each cubic centimeter. Always read the label. Pay particular attention to the concentrations of insulin when two types are used in one syringe. Draw up the regular insulin first to avoid contamination of the regular bottle. The most prevalent today is 100 U.

Every bottle of insulin holds 10 cc (10 ml). Therefore, a bottle of U-100 insulin contains a total amount of 1,000 units of insulin, or 100 × 10. A bottle of U-40 contains 400 units of insulin (40 × 10).

Some common insulin syringes

1. One kind of insulin syringe is measured in 40 units to a cc (ml) (Fig. 9-2, *A*).
   a. This is used to measure U-40 insulin only.
   b. This means that the bottle of insulin should be a strength of 40 U of insulin to 1 cc (ml).
   c. The patient may receive any fraction of this U-40 strength.
2. Another kind of insulin syringe is measured in 100 units to a cubic centimeter (Fig. 9-2, *B*).
   a. This syringe is used for U-100 insulin only.
   b. This means that the bottle of insulin should be a strength of 100 U to 1 cc (1 ml).
3. The type of insulin syringe most commonly used today is 100 units.
   a. Standardized concentrations in 1973 simplified dosage calculations.
   b. Fast, intermediate, and long-acting insulins are available in 10-ml vials of 100 units per milliliter strength.
   c. The patient and his family may find this conducive to self-administration.
   d. It is used only for U-100 insulin.
   e. The 100 U mark on the syringe equals 1 cc (1 ml).

ADMINISTRATION OF INSULIN

Insulin is given by hypodermic injection into the loose connective tissues of the body (Fig. 9-1). Arms or thighs are the usual sites or locations. The site of injection should be changed often in order not to use the same site more often than once a month. The dose of insulin is individualized. It is ordered for one patient and his special needs. There is no average dose of insulin.

Insulins are given subcutaneously or intravenously. Careful attention must be given to determine whether an insulin ordered can be given intravenously or not. Some insulins are stable at room temperatures, and clinical pharmacists suggest they be administered at this temperature to reduce tissue damage from multiple injections.

The skin must be pinched firmly between the thumb and forefinger before injection to ascertain that the insulin will be injected into the subcutaneous tissue. Massage after injection is contraindicated.

Watch the expiration date on all bottles of insulin. Do not use insulin from any bottle past the expiration date marked on it.

Procedure: measuring insulin

Materials needed
4 to 8 insulin bottles, regular type, 100 U per cc (ml)
4 to 8 insulin bottles, Lente, 100 U per cc (ml)
4 to 8 insulin bottles, NPH, 100 U per cc (ml)
These bottles can be collected from the wards or pharmacy when empty. The instructor can inject 10 cc of water into each bottle, mark each bottle "placebo—classroom practice," and thus give students adequate experience in withdrawing different doses of insulin. The bottles should always be kept in the classroom.
About 4 to 8 students can be taught at a time, or as many as the instructor thinks can be observed. Each student should have at the table 1 100 U per cc insulin syringe.

Most hospitals and physicians' offices use sterile packed, disposable syringes with needle attached. Since the contents inside the packaged syringe are sterile and used only once and discarded, the possibility of contamination, hepatitis, and other infections is greatly re-

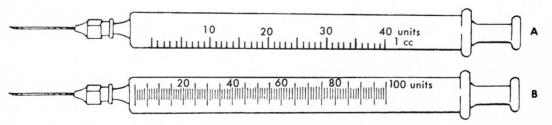

Fig. 9-2. Insulin syringes. **A,** Syringe measured in 40 units per cubic centimeter. **B,** Syringe measured in 100 units per cubic centimeter. (The U-40 syringe is used only for U-40 insulin, or 40 units of insulin in 1 cc. The U-100 syringe is used only for U-100 insulin, or 100 units of insulin in 1 cc.)

duced. Most syringe and needle paper containers are opened by either peeling off or tearing off one end.

1. The physician ordered your patient to receive by hypodermic injection 5 units of U-100 regular, or unmodified, insulin.

Instructions

1. Read label, name of drug, and strength. Compare with medicine ticket order and physician's order in patient's chart. If in doubt, ask!
2. It is unnecessary to rotate a bottle of regular insulin. Rotate only cloudy insulin. Do not shake or allow drug to foam.
3. Cleanse bottle's rubber cap with alcohol sponge or any other disinfectant your hospital uses for skin cleansing.
4. Read label on paper package containing syringe. Is it the right type of insulin syringe for you to use for your insulin and dosage?
5. Open package containing syringe and needle. Be careful not to touch the inside of the paper package except at the extreme edges. Spread it flat on the counter, sterile inside surface up, handling extreme edges only. This provides a sterile surface if you should need to put the syringe down during this procedure.
6. Remove protector from needle. Place protector on counter beside you. Be careful not to touch plunger or needle; touch only head of plunger.
7. Notice that the syringe is measured so that each line represents 1 unit of the whole 100 units.
8. Draw back the same amount of air into the syringe as the amount of drug you intend to draw up. Read the order again: the physician ordered 5 units of U-100 regular insulin.
9. Push the needle, still attached to the syringe, into the bottle's rubber cap.
10. Push 5 units of air into the bottle of insulin to ease withdrawal of the drug.
11. Notice the longer line on the syringe that marks the half point between 0 and 10 units. This indicates 5 units of the entire 100 units.
12. Draw back on the plunger, drawing the drug slowly into the syringe until the lower end of plunger is on the long line for 5 units. Be sure the needle is in the drug while withdrawing the drug or too much air will be obtained.
    a. Place little finger on narrow neck of plunger, wedging plunger against the barrel. This will hold the plunger tight and prevent losing the drug as the syringe is removed from the bottle.
13. Withdraw syringe with needle attached from bottle, maintaining wedging plunger against barrel with little finger.
14. Hold syringe with needle pointing up at eye level. Expel any air if necessary. If drug amount is then too little, draw up more drug until right amount is obtained.
15. Place needle container over needle. Be careful not to touch needle.
16. Check the dose, medicine ticket, bottle of insulin for type of insulin and strength, and physician's order from chart again.
17. Always have an RN, team leader, head nurse, supervisor, or instructor check your dose of insulin. Show the following to the RN:
    a. Medicine ticket containing the order
    b. Physician's order for this particular drug and dose from the chart
    c. Bottle from which you drew the insulin
    d. Insulin syringe containing the dose for that patient
18. Always maintain the rule described in 17, even as a graduate nurse. Better to be safe than sorry.
19. Was your syringe measured in any other amounts beside U-100? Always check the measurements on insulin syringes carefully. Use the U-100 for U-100 strength and the U-40 for U-40 strength. Your instructor will show you some insulin syringes measured in two different insulin units. Turn these syringes around and notice what amount of error you would be making if you read the wrong side of the syringe. Be careful!

2. The physician ordered your patient to receive by hypodermic injection 10 units of U-100 regular, or unmodified, insulin.

Follow the instructions just given to you and prepare this insulin dosage, using another packaged, sterile syringe. Use the measurements and dosage for this problem and the instructions discussed under the first insulin problem.

3. The physician ordered your patient to receive by hypodermic injection 15 units of U-40 NPH insulin. Use a U-40 syringe.

What strength insulin dose does physician want?
   15 units

What strength insulin is on hand? 40 U/cc

What volume of insulin is drawn into the syringe?

$$\frac{40 \text{ U}}{1 \text{ cc}} = \frac{15 \text{ U}}{x}$$

$$x = 0.37 \text{ cc (ml)}$$

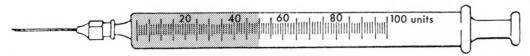

Fig. 9-3. Example of insulin dose: 50 units.

Administer 0.37 cc or 15 units of the 40 U per cc. (REMEMBER: Every line on the syringe measurement is 1 unit.)

Find 10 units and count 5 more lines or 15 units.

If you have two measurement strengths on your syringe, did you measure on the U-40 strength side of the syringe?

What amount of error would you have made if you did not measure on the U-40 strength side of the syringe?

4. The physician ordered your patient to receive by hypodermic injection 60 units of U-100 Lente insulin. Use a U-100 syringe.

What strength insulin dose does the physician want? 60 units

What strength is on hand? 100 U/cc

What volume of insulin is drawn into the syringe?

$$\frac{100 \text{ U}}{1 \text{ cc}} = \frac{60 \text{ U}}{x}$$

$$x = 0.6 \text{ cc (ml)}$$

Administer 0.6 cc or 60 units of the 100 U/cc.

5. The physician ordered your patient to receive by hypodermic injection 35 units of U-100 regular insulin. Use a U-100 syringe only.

$$\frac{100 \text{ U}}{1 \text{ cc}} = \frac{35 \text{ U}}{x}$$

$$x = 0.35 \text{ cc (ml)}$$

Administer 0.35 cc or 35 units of the 100 U per cc.

6. Using unsterile syringes for dosage practice, draw up the following doses of insulin. For practice in technique do not touch needles or plunger (except head and narrow neck of plunger).
   a. U-20 of U-40
   b. U-12 of U-40
   c. U-8 of U-100
   d. U-7 of U-40
   e. U-12 of U-100
   f. U-14 of U-100

Did you select the correct syringe for your dosage? (U-100 syringe for divisions of U-100 dosage; U-40 per cc for divisions of U-40 strength.)

If you have a syringe that has two measurement strengths, did you read on the correct side for drawing your dose?

The physician prescribes the medicine and treatment.
The nurse carries out the physician's orders.
Self-medication is dangerous. Consult your physician first.
There is in every medicine a possible danger.
When in doubt—ASK!

ASSIGNMENT

Review previous lessons and questions according to the direction of your instructor.

1. What organ of the body is most involved in diabetes? Locate this organ.
2. Name the cells in the pancreas that supply insulin to the body.
3. What does insulin help the body do?
4. Which organ of the body changes and stores sugar?
5. In diabetes, is the supply of insulin adequate or inadequate?
6. What is the result of the insufficient supply of insulin?
7. When sugar cannot be stored by the body, what happens to it?
8. How is diabetes treated?
9. Give several characteristics of a diabetic diet.
10. Who discovered insulin? When was it first made available to the public?
11. What is the route of administration of insulin? Can it be administered by mouth?
12. Name four oral hypoglycemic agents used for diabetes in the United States.
13. Name the commercially available forms of insulin. What is the duration of hours of each? When does glycosuria and hypoglycemia occur for each type?
14. List the possible causes of diabetes mellitus.
15. List some common symptoms of diabetes. Know these well.
16. List some complications of diabetes.
17. Define acidosis. Explain its causes. List its symptoms and learn these well. What is the treatment for acidosis?
18. What are the causes of insulin reactions? What are the symptoms and treatment for these reactions?
19. Give two examples of the kinds and strengths of insulin.
20. Work all the problems given to you in class practice. Use the correct insulin syringe to practice the dosage if insulin syringes are available to you from your instructor. Be sure you are measuring from the correct side of the syringe for your dosage. Check your bottle label strength for this. Your instructor may give you additional insulin doses to measure, using various strengths.

CHAPTER 10

Drugs affecting the central nervous system

THE CENTRAL NERVOUS SYSTEM

All human functions, from the most complex (abstract reasoning and creative thought) to the most basic (elimination and respiration), require coordination to perform as a whole. The main coordinator of these functions is the central nervous system.

The central nervous system consists of the brain, spinal cord, and many nerve cells called neurons. It is often called the cerebrospinal or somatic nervous system. The primary concerns of the central nervous system are reasoning and memory of the brain and striated muscle control.

The central nervous system functions similar to a computer. External world information, such as sound, sight, smell, touch, and taste, and internal world information, such as oxygen or carbon dioxide blood levels, body temperature, and muscle tension, are integrated. Instructions are relayed to the appropriate cells or tissues to produce the necessary actions and environmental adjustments. Information concerning these actions and adjustments is again relayed to the central nervous system. This permits continuous adjustment in the instructions sent to various tissues for efficient control of body functions.

THE EFFECT OF DRUGS ON THE CENTRAL NERVOUS SYSTEM

Drugs act to decrease or increase the activity of nerve centers and conducting pathways. Many stimulants and depressants for the brain, the spinal cord, or specific centers of each have been developed, and the effects of such drugs can be accurately predicted.

The cerebral cortex makes up the outer layer of gray matter covering each of the two hemispheres of the brain and the four lobes into which each hemisphere is divided. Drugs that depress cortical activity may decrease sharpness of sensation and perception, lessen or slow motor activity, decrease alertness and concentration, and even promote drowsiness and sleep. Drugs that stimulate the cortical areas may cause greater awareness of the surrounding environment, more vivid impulses to be received, increased muscle activity, and restlessness. The specific response caused by a drug may depend on fac-

tors other than the drug itself, such as the personality of the individual.

The thalamus is made up of sensory nuclei and acts as a relay center for impulses to and from the cerebral cortex and as a center of unlocalized sensations. It is a mass of gray matter at the base of the brain projecting into and bounding the third ventricle. The thalamus enables the individual to have impressions of agreement or disagreement about a sensation. Drugs that depress cells in the various portions of the thalamus may interrupt the free flow of impulses to the cerebral cortex. This is how pain is relieved.

The hypothalamus lies below the thalamus and contains centers that regulate water balance, carbohydrate and fat metabolism, and possibly a center for sleep and wakefulness. Some of the sleep-producing drugs are believed to depress centers in the hypothalamus. Others, such as aspirin, are known to affect the heat-regulating center. The thalamus and the hypothalamus together are known as the diencephalon.

The cerebellum, which contains centers for muscle coordination, equilibrium, and muscle tone, is important in the maintenance of posture. Drugs that disturb the cerebellum or vestibular branch of the eighth cranial nerve cause dizziness and loss of equilibrium.

The medulla oblongata, or the lower portion of the brain, is a cone of nerve tissue continuous above with the pons and below with the spinal cord. It lies ventral to the cerebellum (division of the brain behind the cerebrum), and its back forms the floor of the fourth ventricle. The medulla oblongata contains the vital respiratory, vasomotor, and cardiac centers. Stimulation of the respiratory center will cause it to discharge an increased number of nerve impulses over nerve pathways to the muscles of respiration. Depression of the respiratory center will cause it to discharge fewer impulses, and respirations will be correspondingly affected. Other centers in the medulla that respond to certain drugs are the cough center and the vomiting center.

The spinal cord is a center for reflex activity and also transmits impulses to and from the higher centers in the brain. It may be affected by drugs; for example, large doses of spinal stimulants may cause convulsions, and smaller doses may increase reflex excitability. When a drug is said to have *central action* it means that it acts on the brain or the spinal cord.

The reticular formation is made up of cells and fine bundles of nerve fibers that extend from the spinal cord forward through the brainstem to the diencephalon. This formation exhibits both inhibitory and excitatory functions. It relays impulses to the cortex to promote wakefulness and alertness, which affects many cerebral functions such as consciousness and learning. Depression of the reticular formation produces sedation and loss of consciousness. Many drugs seem to exert an effect on the reticular formation; it is particularly sensitive to certain depressant drugs, such as the barbiturates.

Transmission of impulses at synapses in the central nervous system is probably chemical rather than electrical. Some parts of the central nervous system contain acetylcholine and acetylcholinesterase. The presence of acetylcholine in the central nervous system is for transmission of nerve impulses. High concentration areas of acetylcholine, such as the motor cortex, thalamus, hypothalamus, and anterior spinal roots, are considered responsive to acetylcholine levels. Increased acetylcholine levels can cause nausea, vomiting, muscle tremors, and convulsions. Atropine blocks the action of acetylcholine and is used in treating some of the symptoms of Parkinson's disease, such as muscle rigidity, tremors, and disturbance of voluntary and involuntary movements. Areas with high concentrations of acetylcholine are considered cholinergic, and areas with low concentrations are considered noncholinergic.

Lower motor neurons release acetylcholine at the neuromuscular junction. This causes contraction in voluntary striated muscle. The concentration of acetylcholine must be high because acetylcholine is rapidly destroyed by the enzyme cholinesterase and because a large number of muscle fibers must respond synchronously for striated muscle contractions to occur. This is probably a protective mechanism that prevents the body from becoming a constantly quivering organism.

Serotonin and catecholamines (dopamine, norepinephrine, and epinephrine) are synthesized, stored, and metabolized in the brain. These substances do not easily penetrate the blood-brain barrier, but their precursors do. The effect of injected catecholamines on the central nervous system is slight compared to the effect on the autonomic nervous system, but an increase in catecholamines and serotonin causes cerebral stimulation. Chapter 11 contains further details about acetylcholine and the catecholamines. Reserpine and other drugs that release catecholamines and reduce amine concentration in the brain produce a depressing or sedative action. The serotonin level is lowered by methyldopa, thus causing a cerebral depressing effect.

A few examples of other drugs causing depressing action on the central nervous system are the analgesics (narcotic and nonnarcotic), hypnotics and sedatives, and general anesthetics.

Stimulants are classified on the basis of where they exert their major effects in the nervous system; for example, on the cerebrum, the medulla, the brainstem, or the spinal cord. Amphetamine is primarily a stimulant of the cerebral cortex, as is caffeine. Nikethamide acts mainly in the medulla and the brainstem. Strychnine is a spinal stimulant. Central nervous system stimulants used to antagonize depressant drugs are known as analeptics. They restore consciousness and mental alertness. However, some pharmacologists believe analeptics should not be used for this purpose.

CEREBROSPINAL STIMULANTS
Caffeine (kaf'een)

1. Caffeine is a white crystalline powder obtained from tea leaves. It is an active alkaloid found in a number of plants used as beverages, such as coffee and tea. Coffee contains about 1% to 2% caffeine and tea about 1% to 6%. A cup of coffee in the United States has about 2 to 3 grains of caffeine.

2. In large doses, caffeine stimulates the entire central nervous system, including the spinal cord. Caffeine particularly stimulates the cerebral cortex. Small doses stimulate the cerebrum and larger doses stimulate the medullary centers and spinal cord. Ordinary oral therapeutic doses have no effect on medullary centers. Large parenteral doses will stimulate the respiratory center.

3. Respirations are quickened and deepened because of the strong stimulation of the respiratory center in the medulla.

4. Caffeine stimulates the myocardium (heart muscle). It brings about an increase in both cardiac rate and cardiac output. This effect is antagonized by an increase in vagal tone, so a slight slowing of the heart may be observed in some individuals and a slight increase in others. The increased rate is usually noticed after large doses.

5. It has diuretic action (increases the flow of urine). The mode of action seems to be that of depressing the tubule cells and preventing reabsorption of fluid.

6. The output of both pepsin and hydrochloric acid from the stomach is increased by caffeine. Coffee, for this reason, is usually restricted or eliminated from the diet of patients with gastric and duodenal ulcer.

7. Since it is readily excreted and tolerance is easily developed, fatal doses are rare. Overdose can cause nervousness, inability to sleep (insomnia), heart palpitation, headache, and increased flow of urine.

The best treatment is to stop coffee drinking or to reduce the daily intake.

8. Caffeine is used with one or more analgesic drugs or with ergotamine tartrate for the relief of headache. Some authorities believe that caffeine constricts the intracranial blood vessels and causes some lowering of intracranial pressure, thus relieving headache.
9. Usual dose: 65 to 200 mg.
10. Forms of caffeine include:
    a. *Caffeine and sodium benzoate injection*
       Usual dose: 0.5 g intramuscularly.
    b. *Citrated caffeine*
       Usual dose: 60 to 120 mg orally.
    c. *Ergotamine tartrate* (er-got'ah-min tahr'trate) *with caffeine (Cafergot)* (ka'fehr-got)
       This drug is administered orally, two tablets at onset of migraine headache, followed by one tablet every half hour (not to exceed six tablets per episode). Each tablet contains 1 mg of ergotamine tartrate and 100 mg of caffeine.

The amphetamines (am-fet'ah-min)

1. The amphetamines are a class of sympathomimetic amines that stimulate the central nervous system. Therapeutic use should be limited to patients with narcolepsy, certain children with minimal brain dysfunction, and for the short-term treatment of obesity in conjunction with caloric restriction.
2. The amphetamines have a high potential for abuse. They give a feeling of well-being and exhilaration, lessen fatigue, and increase confidence, alertness, and concentration. They also cause irritability, insomnia, nervousness, tremor, and headache. If used continuously tolerance to dosage, psychologic dependence, personality changes, and social dysfunction may occur.
3. Preparations of amphetamine include:
    a. *Amphetamine sulfate (Benzedrine)* (ben'zedrin). This drug is available in tablets of 5 and 10 mg and in 15 mg sustained-release capsules (Spansules). It is given orally in divided doses during the day. The final dose should not be given after 4 PM to prevent interference with sleep. Usual dosage range: 5 to 30 mg daily in divided doses.
    b. *Dextroamphetamine sulfate* (dek-stro-am-fet'ah-min) *(Dexedrine)* (dek'se-drin). This drug is available in a variety of forms and dosage: 5 and 10 mg tablets, as an elixir (5 mg per 5 ml), and in sustained-release capsules (Spansules) containing 5, 10, or 15 mg of drug. Usual dose: 5 mg twice a day. Range of dose: 2.5 to 30 mg daily.
    c. *Methamphetamine hydrochloride* (meth-amfet'ah-min) *(Desoxyn)* (des-ok'sin). The CNS stimulant is available in 2.5-, 5-, 10-, and 15-mg

tablets. Usual dose: 2.5 mg orally three times daily, increasing to 20 to 25 mg daily.

Methylphenidate hydrochloride (meth-il-fen'i-date) *(Ritalin Hydrochloride)* (rit'ah-lin)

1. Methylphenidate is a CNS stimulant that may be used in narcolepsy. It may also be effective in certain types of minimal brain dysfunction in children, mild depression, and apathetic or withdrawn senile behavior.
2. Chronic abuse may cause tolerance and psychologic dependence.
3. Methylphenidate should not be used in patients with marked anxiety, tension, agitation, or glaucoma.
4. Usual dosage: 10 mg orally two or three times daily. Patients with minimal brain dysfunction may require 60 mg daily. To prevent insomnia, the last dose should be given in the late afternoon (not later than 6 PM).

Phenmetrazine hydrochloride (fen-met'rah-zeen) *(Preludin)* (preh-loo'din)

1. This drug is a mild stimulant of the central nervous system resembling amphetamine pharmacologically, especially in its ability to depress the appetite.
2. It rarely causes changes in pulse rate or blood pressure. As with other stimulants, psychologic dependency can occur.
3. Preludin is administered orally in 25 mg doses two or three times a day, an hour before meals, or in an oral extended-release form that contains 75 mg of the drug and is taken once daily.

HYPNOTICS AND SEDATIVES

A *hypnotic* is a drug that produces sleep. A *sedative* quiets the patient and gives a feeling of relaxation and rest, not necessarily accompanied by sleep. Hypnotics and sedatives are not always different drugs; it depends on the dose and the condition of the patient. A small dose of a drug may act as a sedative. A larger dose of the same drug may act as a hypnotic and produce sleep.

The nurse should realize that there are many other measures that can be employed *before giving a patient a sedative or hypnotic*. If the nurse takes time to carry out these measures, a hypnotic many times will not be needed. These measures include eliminating environmental and human noises and providing the patient with such comforts as backrubs, better ventilation, clean linens, bedpan, or urinal if needed, a change of position, extra pillows if needed, an extra blanket for warmth or removal of a blanket if weather is hot, light nourishment (such as warm milk, hot chocolate, and one or two crackers), and reassurance (listening to the patient's worries).

A good hypnotic should provide action within a fairly

short period, a restful natural sleep, a duration of action that will allow the patient to awaken at his usual time, a natural awakening with no hangover effects, and no danger of habit formation.

A sedative is a drug that allays activity and excitement. Many of the so-called tranquilizers such as meprobamate and related drugs and the benzodiazepines (represented by chlordiazepoxide and its congeners) are viewed today by some pharmacologists as sedative-hypnotics rather than as tranquilizers. They cause the characteristic dose-related progression of effects from sedation through hypnosis, coma, and death, just as do other members of the hypnotic group of drugs. In addition, they are addictive; their sudden withdrawal can lead to hyperexcitability and convulsions. This does not occur with the true tranquilizers, such as the phenothiazines.

Barbiturates (bar-bit'your-ayts)

The main action of barbiturates is to depress the sleep centers, but they do act on many levels of the central nervous system. Their main effect is to depress, and the extent of action varies, depending on the drug used, from mild sedation to light sleep to deep sleep. Barbiturates are not analgesic so will not usually cause sleep if severe pain is present. When barbiturates are combined with an analgesic, the sedative action of the barbiturate seems to reinforce the action of the analgesic and lessen the patient's emotional reaction to pain. All of the barbiturates used clinically depress the motor cortex of the brain, but phenobarbital, mephobarbital, and metharbital are particularly effective as anticonvulsants. Death from overdosage of barbiturates is usually caused by respiratory failure accompanied by hypotension. Barbiturates in the usual hypnotic dose do not affect the heart and respiratory centers to any great extent.

Since barbiturates can cause unusual effects in some patients, nurses should watch for depression, hangover sensations, nausea, and emotional disturbances. The nurse should especially watch the aged patient, for he may become confused, try to get up at night, and fall. Further effects include skin rash, hives, bad dreams, and restlessness. General adverse effects of barbiturates include lethargy, drowsiness, agitation, headache, mental depression, and muscle or joint pain.

Barbiturates cross the placental barrier and appear in fetal circulation and in breast milk, resulting in sedation of the infant.

Barbiturates may potentiate the CNS depressant effects of analgesics, anesthetics, antihistamines, tranquilizers, and sedative-hypnotics.

Barbiturates, especially phenobarbital, may enhance the metabolism of warfarin (Coumadin), digitoxin, corticosteroids (prednisone), phenytoin (Dilantin), chlorpromazine (Thorazine), and doxycycline (Vibramycin).

Therapeutic uses of barbiturates

1. As hypnotics, to produce sleep.
2. As sedatives, to overcome anxiety states, nervous tension, and menopausal nervousness.
3. As anticonvulsants, to control convulsions in tetanus, epilepsy, brain injury, and strychnine poisoning.
4. As anesthetics, to produce anesthesia in very brief operations. Thiopental sodium (Pentothal Sodium) is used intravenously for brief operations and to initiate anesthesia.
5. As preanesthetic medications, the night before and the morning of surgery.
6. As obstetric medications, to produce sedation during labor. The drug affects the baby as well, so its respirations may be depressed.

Barbiturate poisoning treatment

Treatment for acute barbiturate poisoning will vary with the condition and needs of the patient. Perhaps little more than such supportive treatment as keeping the patient warm, turning him often, and providing adequate fluids and nutrition will suffice.

If the patient is deeply comatose and unresponsive, greater effort will be required to save his life. If the physician believes that the drug has been swallowed and most of it still remains in the stomach, a prompt gastric lavage may be done. There is danger of aspiration of stomach contents during lavage. If depression is severe and there is trouble with respiration, an open airway is of vital importance. The physician may plan to use an endotracheal tube and respirator to administer oxygen.

Extensive use of analeptic drugs is contraindicated, according to most clinicians, because many of these drugs are capable of producing toxic symptoms. Levarterenol, dopamine, and phenylephrine may be used to combat circulatory collapse. Parenteral fluid volume should be maintained and the urine alkalinized with sodium bicarbonate to enhance the excretion of phenobarbital.

Amobarbital sodium (am-o-bar'bi-tal) (Amytal) (am'i-tol)

1. Amobarbital is a short- to intermediate-acting barbiturate. Sedative and hypnotic effects last from 3 to 6 hours when administered orally.
2. Amobarbital may also be used as an anticonvulsant and preoperative medication when administered intravenously.
3. It is available in several strengths of tablets and capsules for oral administration. Amobarbital sodium is available for intramuscular or intravenous administration.
4. Usual hypnotic dose: 100 to 200 mg.

Pentobarbital (pen-to-bar′bi-tal)
(Nembutal) (nem′byou-tal)

1. Pentobarbital is an intermediate-acting barbiturate. It is used as a hypnotic, sedative, and preanesthetic medication.
2. Preparations include an elixir, capsules, suppositories, and ampules for parenteral injection.
3. Usual hypnotic dosage: 120 to 200 mg.

Phenobarbital (fee-no-bar′bi-tal)
(Luminal) (loo′mi-nal)

1. Phenobarbital requires 45 minutes for an onset of sedative activity when taken orally; however, the duration of activity is 6 hours or more. Phenobarbital is classified as a long-acting barbiturate.
2. Although phenobarbital may be used as a sedative-hypnotic, it often causes excess drowsiness and hangover the next day. Its primary use now is as an anticonvulsant.
3. Usual anticonvulsant dosage: 100 to 200 mg daily, given orally at bedtime.
4. Dosage forms available include an elixir, tablets, capsules, suppositories, and ampules for parenteral injection.

Secobarbital (se-ko-bar′bi-tal)
(Seconal) (sek′o-nol)

1. Secobarbital is a short-acting barbiturate used as a sedative-hypnotic and preanesthetic medication.
2. Hypnotic dose: 100 to 200 mg.
3. Secobarbital is available in a variety of oral, rectal, intramuscular, and intravenous dosage forms.

Benzodiazepines (ben-zo-dye-a-zep′eens)
(antianxiety drugs)
Chlordiazepoxide (klor-dye-a-ze-pok′side)
(Librium, Libritabs) (lib′ree-um)

1. In low oral doses this sedative is effective in the treatment of mild to moderate anxiety and tension, such as premenstrual tension, menstrual stress, tension headache, and pre- and postoperative apprehension.
2. In higher oral doses, chlordiazepoxide may be effective in treating more severe anxiety and tension, phobias, obsessive-compulsive reactions, schizoid behavior, chronic alcoholism, or alcohol withdrawal symptoms.
3. Side effects may include drowsiness and ataxia, especially in aged and debilitated persons. Skin rash, nausea, constipation, and menstrual irregularities may occur.
4. Withdrawal symptoms are rare but possible if patients have been taking large doses for 5 months or more. Caution should be observed in administering this drug to addiction-prone individuals.

5. Paradoxic reactions may occur in some individuals: excitement and stimulation rather than the usual sedative effects. These symptoms should be watched for during early stages of treatment.
6. Usual dose for mild to moderate symptoms: 5 to 10 mg three or four times daily; for severe symptoms: 20 to 25 mg three or four times daily. Librium Injectable is used chiefly for acute states. Patients receiving the drug by injection should remain under observation for several hours after administration. Ambulatory patients should not be permitted to operate a vehicle or machinery after an injection. Oral and intravenous administration are the best methods of administration. Administration by intramuscular route results in slow and erratic absorption.
7. Benzodiazepines may be potentiated by other central nervous system depressants, such as barbiturates, narcotics, phenothiazines, antidepressants, and antihistamines.

Clorazepate dipotassium (klor-az′eh-payt)
(Tranxene, Tranxene-SD) (tran′zeen)

1. Clorazepate is an effective antianxiety drug; its most common side effects are drowsiness and ataxia. Other adverse effects are the same as for other benzodiazepine compounds.
2. This drug is available in 3.75-, 7.5-, and 15-mg capsules. Oral dose for adults: 15 to 60 mg daily in divided doses. Elderly patient dosage: 7.5 to 15 mg daily.
3. Tranxene-SD (22.5-mg tablets) may be administered as a single dose (SD) every 24 hours to those patients stabilized on a dose of 7.5 mg three times daily.

Diazepam (dy-az′ee-pam)
(Valium) (val′e-um)

1. This drug is useful in the control of anxiety and tension states caused by stressful circumstances or in treating psychosomatic complaints that are exacerbated by emotional factors.
2. Valium, or diazepam, has muscle relaxant properties that make it effective in the treatment of muscle spasms of cerebral palsy and athetosis. It is the treatment of choice for status epilepticus.
3. This drug has beneficial sedative and amnesic effects when administered parenterally prior to minor dental and surgical procedures, endoscopy, and cardioversion of atrial fibrillation.
4. Side effects may occur, such as drowsiness, dizziness, blurred or double vision, headache, incontinence, slurred speech, tremor, nausea, and vomiting.
5. Abrupt withdrawal of the drug after prolonged administration may cause convulsions, tremor, muscle and abdominal cramps, vomiting, sweating, and

other symptoms similar to those seen following withdrawal of barbiturates, meprobamate, and chlordiazepoxide.

6. Patients should be instructed about the dangers of driving cars, working around machinery, or working in conditions where they must be mentally alert while taking diazepam.
7. Diazepam is contraindicated in patients with acute narrow-angle glaucoma.
8. As with the other benzodiazepines, treatment for overdosage may include maintenance of an airway and administration of oxygen. Methylphenidate (Ritalin) or caffeine may be effective against severe CNS or respiratory depression. Hypotension may occur and severe hypotensive effects may be reversed with administration of levarterenol (Levophed), metaraminol (Aramine), or dopamine (Intropin).
9. Diazepam should be used with caution in pregnant women. Small amounts are found in breast milk.
10. Average adult dose: 2 to 5 mg two or three times daily, 5 to 10 mg three or four times daily for severe or acute symptoms. Oral and IV methods of administration are best; IM injections are not absorbed well and are painful. IV injection vary in dosage between 2 to 40 mg and should be given very slowly, taking at least 1 minute for each 5 mg (1 ml) given.
11. When diazepam must be given with a narcotic, the dose of the narcotic should be reduced by one third. Diazepam should not be mixed in the same syringe with other drugs. Diazepam may be potentiated by other CNS depressants such as phenothiazines, barbiturates, antihistamines, and antidepressants.

Flurazepam (floor-az'ee-pam)
(Dalmane) (dal'main)

1. Flurazepam is a benzodiazepine derivative used specifically for inducing and maintaining sleep. It is useful in the treatment of all types of insomnia: difficulty in falling asleep, frequent night awakening, and early morning awakening. This drug is effective in acute or chronic conditions requiring restful sleep.
2. Insomnia is usually transitory, so prolonged administration is generally not necessary or recommended.
3. Side effects, including dizziness, drowsiness, lightheadedness, staggering, ataxia, and falling, have occurred in elderly or debilitated patients. Other symptoms reported are headache, heartburn, digestive disturbances, nausea, vomiting, diarrhea, constipation, nervousness, talkativeness, apprehension, irritability, weakness, chest pains, palpitations, body and joint pains, and genitourinary complaints. Rare symptoms that may appear are blurred vision, sweating, burning

eyes, faintness, hypotension, shortness of breath, skin rash, dry mouth or excessive salivation, slurred speech, confusion, and hallucinations. These symptoms are not apt to occur with occasional usage unless there is hypersensitivity or overdosage.

4. Symptoms of overdosage, such as somnolence, confusion, and coma, are treated as usual, with respiration, pulse, blood pressure monitoring and gastric lavage and by providing intravenous fluids, adequate airway, and oxygen if necessary.
5. Flurazepam is contraindicated in patients with known hypersensitivity to the drug or with impaired kidney or liver function.
6. Patients taking fluorazepam should be instructed about possible combined effects with alcohol and other CNS depressants and should be cautioned against driving a car, working around machinery, or being employed in any other occupation requiring mental alertness shortly after taking the drug.
7. The safety of this drug during pregnancy has not yet been established.
8. Dosage: individualized. The usual adult dose is 30 mg before retiring; for elderly or debilitated patients, 15 mg. Capsules of 15 and 30 mg are available.

Oxazepam (oks-az'ee-pam)
(Serax) (ser'aks)

1. Oxazepam exhibits properties similar to those of diazepam and is used for the control of similar symptoms.
2. Usual dosage: 30 to 60 mg daily; however, dosages of 120 mg daily may be required in severe cases.

Other sedative-hypnotic agents
Chloral hydrate (klor'al)
(Somnos) (som'nos), *(Noctec)* (noc'tek)

1. Chloral hydrate is the oldest of the hypnotic group of drugs and is still commonly used today.
2. It depresses the cerebrum and, to a certain extent, the spinal reflexes.
3. It causes sleep in a short time and lasts 5 to 8 hours.
4. Large doses depress the respiratory and vasomotor (circulatory) centers.
5. It should not be given to patients with severe liver or heart disease or severe inflammation of the stomach (gastritis).
6. Toxic reactions include slow pulse, slow respirations, deep stupor, fall in blood pressure, cyanosis (bluish color to face), and vasodilation. Watch *respiration, pulse, blood pressure, and color of face and lips.* Treatment is essentially the same as that for acute poisoning with the barbiturates or benzodiazepines.
7. A major metabolite of chloral hydrate is trichloroacetic acid. This metabolite displaces warfarin from

protein-binding sites, thus increasing anticoagulant activity and lengthening the prothrombin time. Ethanol may potentiate the sedative effect of chloral hydrate. Chloral hydrate may be potentiated by other CNS depressants such as narcotics, barbiturates, phenothiazines, antihistamines, and other antidepressants.

8. Usual dosage as a hypnotic for adults: 500 mg. Larger doses can be given if ordered: 250 mg to 2 g. Adult sedative: 250 to 500 mg three times a day after meals. The liquid solution has a very unpleasant taste. The liquid should be well diluted with water or given in a syrup or milk to disguise the taste. Soft gelatin capsules containing 250 and 500 mg for oral use and suppositories for rectal use are also available.

Ethchlorvynol (eth-klor′vin-ol)
(Placidyl) (plas′i-dil)

1. Ethchlorvynol is effective as a mild hypnotic in the management of most forms of insomnia or as a daytime sedative in the management of mild anxiety or tension states.
2. It is particularly valuable when barbiturates cannot be given.
3. Such side effects as nausea, urticaria, dizziness, aftertaste, and mild hangover feelings may occur.
4. This drug should not be given over a long period since it may cause dependency. Sudden withdrawal of the drug may cause convulsions.
5. Ethchlorvynol should not be given to patients with suicidal tendencies.
6. This drug is not recommended during the first and second trimester of pregnancy.
7. Ethchlorvynol may enhance the metabolism of oral anticoagulants, such as warfarin (Coumadin), resulting in a decreased prothrombin time. It also may be potentiated by other CNS depressants such as narcotics, barbiturates, phenothiazines, antihistamines, and alcohol.
8. Usual dose as a hypnotic: 500 mg orally at bedtime; as daytime sedation: 100 or 200 mg orally two or three times a day.

Glutethimide (gloo-teth′i-myd)
(Doriden) (dor′i-den)

1. Glutethimide is an orally effective sedative-hypnotic for nighttime, daytime, and preoperative sedation. It is well tolerated by elderly patients and those with chronic illness.
2. Its greatest use is for patients who cannot tolerate the barbiturates and for relief of simple or nervous insomnia in the absence of severe pain or agitation.
3. The principal side effects are nausea and skin rash.
4. Glutethimide enhances the metabolism of warfarin (Coumadin), so prothrombin times should be performed frequently. Glutethimide may be potentiated by other CNS depressants, such as narcotics, barbiturates, phenothiazines, antihistamines, and alcohol.
5. Glutethimide is effective in 15 to 30 minutes. Duration of action is 4 to 8 hours.
6. Usual dose for adults: 500 mg given orally at bedtime. Daytime dose: 125 to 250 mg orally three times daily after meals. Preoperative sedation: 500 mg the night before surgery and 500 to 1,000 mg 1 hour before anesthesia.

Meprobamate (mep-ro-bam′ate) or (me-pro′bahmate)
(Equanil) (ek′wan-il), (Miltown) (mil′town)

1. Meprobamate is a synthetic drug chemically related to mephenesin, a skeletal muscle relaxant.
2. When used in large doses, the drug acts as an antianxiety agent and muscle relaxant. In small doses, the drug acts mainly as a sedative.
3. Meprobamate has been effective in relieving anxiety, tension, some psychosomatic disorders, some behavior disorders, and insomnia. Relief of tension aids in promoting sleep. It may be used to treat musculoskeletal disorders.
4. This drug causes side effects and untoward reactions such as skin rash, urticaria, itching, and drowsiness.
5. Habituation, tolerance, and physical dependence can develop. Withdrawal symptoms, including convulsions, can occur after prolonged administration and abrupt withdrawal of the drug. Gradual withdrawal over 2 or 3 weeks is essential to prevent these symptoms.
6. Meprobamate may potentiate the CNS depressant effects of analgesics, anesthetics, and other tranquilizers and sedative-hypnotics. This drug may enhance the metabolism of warfarin (Coumadin), corticosteroids (prednisone), digitoxin, doxycycline (Vibramycin), phenytoin (Dilantin), and chlorpromazine (Thorazine).
7. Usual doses for meprobamate: 400 mg tablets orally three times a day; 800 mg for sleep.

Methyprylon (meth-ee-pry′lon)
(Noludar) (nol′you-dar)

1. Methyprylon is a mild hypnotic used to relieve insomnia.
2. When taken at bedtime, methyprylon induces sleep within 45 minutes that continues for 5 to 8 hours.
3. Patients should be warned not to perform tasks requiring mental alertness shortly after ingesting this drug.
4. Dependency may develop in patients who use this

drug on a nightly basis for a long time. Withdrawal symptoms may occur if the drug is discontinued too rapidly.

5. Usual dose: 300 to 400 mg at bedtime. Doses of 50 to 100 mg three or four times daily for sedation.

Paraldehyde (par-al'dee-hyd)

1. Paraldehyde depresses the central nervous system as much as chloral hydrate does.
2. This drug is used for its hypnotic-sedative effects in treatment of nervous hyperexcitability, possible convulsions, delirium tremens, mania, tetanus, and strychnine poisoning.
3. Paraldehyde acts rapidly, producing sleep in 15 to 20 minutes.
4. It has an unpleasant, clinging odor and a disagreeable taste, so should not be spilled on counters, in sinks, and in bedding.
5. It can be used in patients with renal disease but should be used with caution in patients with liver disease.
6. Overdosage is rare, but symptoms are similar to those of chloral hydrate. Treatment is the same.
7. This drug may be potentiated by other CNS depressants such as narcotics, barbiturates, antihistamines, phenothiazines, and alcohol. It will appear in fetal circulation in quantities sufficient to cause respiratory depression.
8. Usual oral dose: 10 to 30 ml. It should be given in syrup. If given rectally, it should be mixed with a thin oil. Paraldehyde must be drawn up in a glass (not plastic) syringe for measuring and any unused drug must be discarded.

Bromides

These drugs are not commonly used today because of the appearance of better drugs. They have been used for their sedative, hypnotic, and anticonvulsant effects. They have a depressant action on the central nervous system and relieve nervousness, worry, and anxiety. They may be cumulative and taken over a long period of time, they may cause skin eruptions that may form ulcers, commonly on the legs. These ulcers may take weeks or months to heal. The student may be familiar with **sodium bromide** and **potassium bromide.** Bromo-Seltzer no longer contains bromide.

ALCOHOL

Ethyl alcohol (eth'il), Ethanol (eth'ah-nol)

1. Ethyl alcohol contains not less than 92.3% by weight, which corresponds to 94.9% by volume, of C_2H_5OH.
2. It produces an effect of *progressive* and *continuous depression* on the central nervous system. This includes the cerebrum, cerebellum, medulla, and spinal cord.

3. Alcohol is contraindicated in the following conditions: diseases of the liver and kidneys, ulcers of gastrointestinal tract, acute genitourinary infections, pregnancy, epilepsy, and susceptibility (low tolerance).
4. Some available forms include:
   a. **Dehydrated alcohol (absolute alcohol)**
      This contains no less than 99% of ethyl alcohol by weight.
   b. **Diluted alcohol**
      This contains 41% to 42% (no more, no less) of ethyl alcohol by weight.
   c. **Whiskey (spiritus frumenti)**
      This contains no less than 47% and not more than 53% of ethyl alcohol by volume. The fermented mash of whole or partly malted cereal grains is distilled for this liquid and stored for at least 2 years in charred wood containers.
   d. **Brandy (spiritus vini vitis)**
      This contains no less than 48% and no more than 54% of ethyl alcohol by volume. The fermented juice of ripe grapes is distilled for this liquid and stored in wood containers for at least 2 years.
   e. **Wines**
      Wines are fermented liquors made from grapes or other fruit juices. Dry wines contain about 10% alcohol, sweet wines about 15% alcohol, and red wines about 14.5% to 22% alcohol.

• • •

Alcohol is *not* considered a stimulant. This surprises many people, who remember the cheerful confidence and talkativeness it gives in its early effects. Small amounts of alcohol impart a feeling of confidence, well-being, talkativeness, and gay, lively manner. Large amounts of the drug cause laughter, extreme talkativeness, speech without previous consideration about the effect of what is being said, excitement, and sometimes a desire to fight someone. Even with small amounts, people lose the keen power of discrimination or choosing, ability to concentrate, use of good judgment, and memory. What seems to be stimulation results from the depression of the higher faculties of the brain and represents the loss of learned inhibitions acquired by civilization.

Problem drinking among teenagers has reached epidemic proportions, even outranking other drug abuse as a teenage problem in this drinking society. In the United States approximately 1.3 million boys and girls between the ages of 12 and 17 have serious drinking problems. Of those killed in drunken-driving accidents, 60% are teenagers. The number of teenagers arrested for drunkenness has tripled since 1960. The popular beverage is beer—the initial alcoholic beverage used by many who proceed to heavier drinking. Education concerning the need for limitation and problems of drinking is necessary for all ages, since this is a problem concerning all age levels and not teenagers alone. (For a more detailed discussion of alcohol see Index.)

The *National Safety Council* regards concentrations of alcohol in the blood up to 0.05% as evidence of sobriety, concentrations between 0.051% and 0.149% as suspicious and demanding performance tests, and more than 0.15% evidence of unquestionable intoxication. The states differ as to what is accepted as a legal limit.

A number of doses of alcohol will cause diminished visual acuity, especially peripheral vision, slowed reaction time, impairment of judgment and self-control, and a feeling of complacency and being well pleased with one's self. Many drivers of automobiles or workers with machinery will take chances when under the influence of alcohol they would not ordinarily take. As statistics show, this can lead to disaster.

After consuming large amounts of alcohol, some people become progressively melancholy and sentimental. The speech may become thick and slurred, the special senses are much more sluggish, and drowsiness or stupor may result. The vomiting that usually occurs at this point is a lifeguard, since it rids the system of much of the alcohol.

There is little effect on the respiratory center except when alcohol is taken in very large doses. Alcohol acts as a depressant on the tone of the vasomotor center and dilates peripheral vessels. This causes a flushing of the skin and a feeling of warmth. It also depresses the heat-regulating center in the brain, just as antipyretics do, and was used many years ago to reduce fever. Today we have antipyretics for this purpose.

Small doses of alcohol will stimulate the secretion of hydrochloric acid from the stomach glands. This explains why ulcer patients should not drink alcohol. Large doses of alcohol lessen gastric juice secretion but may cause gastritis or malnutrition, the latter because the person drinks and does not eat properly.

Alcohol is metabolized in the liver. It produces an increased flow of urine, generally because of the increased amount of fluids consumed with the alcohol and because of suppression of antidiuretic hormone (ADH). It is known that large and concentrated doses of alcohol consumed over long periods may injure the liver. Persons with liver disease should not drink alcohol since it may cause further damage to the liver.

Acute alcoholic poisoning

Symptoms. Symptoms of acute alcoholic poisoning include cold, clammy skin, stupor or coma, slow, noisy respirations, dilated pupils (sometimes pupils are normal), and alcoholic breath.

Treatment. The treatment of acute alcoholic poisoning should include the following:

1. Establish and maintain an airway, using artificial respirations if necessary.
2. Emesis should be initiated *unless* the patient is comatose, convulsing, or has lost the gag reflex.
3. If emesis cannot be initiated, insert a tube and perform a gastric lavage. If patient is comatose, some physicians insert an endotracheal tube before stomach lavage to prevent aspiration of stomach contents into the lungs.
4. Forced diuresis should be instituted using parenteral fluids and diuretics if necessary.
5. Keep the patient warm; headache and nervous irritability may be treated with acetaminophen and chlordiazepoxide. Encourage the patient to drink fluids.

Chronic alcoholic poisoning

Symptoms. Symptoms of chronic alcoholic poisoning include gastroenteritis, redness of face, nose, and conjunctiva of eye, malnutrition, liver damage, kidney damage, arteriosclerosis, dulling of mental faculties, nerve degeneration, tremors, muscular weakness, moral deterioration, and delirium tremens.

Treatment. The treatment of chronic alcoholic poisoning should include the following:

1. Withdrawal of the alcohol gradually within a 1-week period.
2. Use of chlordiazepoxide or paraldehyde during this period for sedation.
3. Maintenance of an adequate diet.
4. Use of paraldehyde or chlordiazepoxide (Librium) during delirium tremens. Characteristics of delirium tremens include marked trembling, inability to sleep, and terrifying hallucinations: snakes crawling on the patient or bed, "pink elephants" climbing the walls, and so on. Death may occur during this period.
5. Reeducation of the patient. This is vital to permanent success. Reeducation should include obtaining psychiatric help concerning the reasons for drinking, utilizing the help of Alcoholics Anonymous (an organization composed of former alcoholics who have been rehabilitated), and establishing an unpleasant conditioned-reflex association with drinking by using disulfiram (Antabuse). Vomiting usually follows alcohol consumption by the person taking Antabuse.

Other uses of alcohol

Other uses of ethyl alcohol include use as a solvent for many medicines, such as spirits, elixirs, and fluidextracts; as a preservative for specimens; for its astringent antiseptic action in prevention of bedsores and in skin cleansing; in wet dressings for wounds; in 60% to 70% strength, as a solution for disinfection of skin and thermometers; and as a treatment to relieve pain in severe, chronic neuralgia, or pain in nerves, such as trigeminal neuralgia (tic douloureux), or pain caused by inoperable cancer, with 80% alcohol being injected to produce destruction of nerve fibers. This may last from 1 to 3 years. Pain is relieved during this interval. Alcohol is also used as an appetizer for patients with poor appetite. Alcohol has been used by oral administration to produce vasodilation in peripheral vascular disease, such as Buerger's disease.

Methyl alcohol (meth'il) (wood alcohol)

1. This form of alcohol should *not be taken internally.* Several doses give a much greater toxic reaction than does ethyl alcohol. Its use in proprietary medicines is illegal.
2. Its main use is in shellacs and varnishes.
3. If taken internally, it affects the central nervous system, especially the optic nerve of the sense of sight. It can cause permanent blindness after as small a dose as 60 ml (about 2 ounces). Larger doses (2 to 8 ounces) may be fatal.
4. It can cause nausea, vomiting, and severe abdominal cramps.

Isopropyl alcohol (i-so-pro'pil)

1. Isopropyl alcohol is a clear, colorless liquid with the usual alcohol odor and taste. It is used for skin disinfection and in rubbing compounds and backrub lotions.
2. The stronger its concentration, the greater its bactericidal effect. The ideal bactericidal effect of alcohol is 60% to 70%.

PARKINSON'S DISEASE

Parkinson's disease, or paralysis agitans, is a chronic disorder of the central nervous system. Characteristic symptoms are muscle tremors, slowness of movement, and muscle rigidity and weakness, with alterations in posture and equilibrium. The cause of Parkinson's disease is unknown. It is believed that it reflects an imbalance between dopaminergic and cholinergic mechanisms in the central nervous system.

Dopamine, a catecholamine, is the precursor of norepinephrine. Dopamine is normally present in the corpus striatum. In patients with postencephalitic or idiopathic parkinsonism there is a depletion of dopamine. One theory is that the dopaminergic and cholinergic mechanisms are antagonistic—the cholinergic mechanisms innervated by acetylcholine are excitatory; the dopaminergic mechanisms innervated by dopamine are inhibitory. The symptoms of parkinsonism therefore reflect cholinergic dominance resulting from low levels of dopamine in the brain. (For more details concerning this theory, see the discussion that follows shortly on the drugs Larodopa, levodopa, and carbidopa.)

Treatment of parkinsonism remains palliative rather than curative. Goals are to provide maximal relief of symptoms and to maintain some independence of movement and activity.

Drug therapy includes the use of anticholinergic drugs to inhibit the cholinergic mechanisms, levodopa to replenish dopamine levels and enhance dopaminergic mechanisms, and the antihistaminic drugs to assist in anticholinergic action. Examples of the antihistamines include diphenhydramine hydrochloride (Benadryl), orphenadrine citrate and chloride (Disipal), and chlorphenoxamine hydrochloride (Phenoxene). Antihistamines are most useful in mild forms of the disease, in early stages, in the elderly, and in conjunction with levodopa. Levodopa is still the most effective drug available for treating parkinsonism.

Drugs used to treat Parkinson's disease
Trihexyphenidyl hydrochloride (try-hek-see-fen'i-dil) (Artane) (ar'tayn)

1. Trihexyphenidyl is a synthetic drug that acts as an antispasmodic on smooth muscle tissue and skeletal muscles. This is a result of its action on the brain.
2. It is used as a muscle relaxant and is especially useful in reducing the muscle rigidity and spasm of Parkinson's disease (palsy). It also has been used to control extrapyramidal disorders induced by phenothiazines and butyrophenones (haloperidol).
3. Minor side effects, such as mouth dryness, blurring of vision, dizziness, mild nausea, or nervousness, will occur in 30% to 50% of all patients taking this drug. Side effects occurring less often include constipation, drowsiness, urinary hesitancy or retention, tachycardia, dilation of the pupils, increased intraocular tension, weakness, headache, and vomiting.
4. Usual dose: individualized; initially, 1 mg, taken orally near mealtime. Dose can be increased to 12 to 15 mg daily or given in divided doses.

L-dopa
(Larodopa) (lar-ah-do'-pah), (levodopa) (le-vo-do'pah), (Dopar) (do'par)

1. Late in 1970 the Food and Drug Administration approved the marketing of L-dopa (Dopar, Larodopa).
2. Physicians have been warned to thoroughly familiarize themselves with all information concerning the drug before starting therapy. Accurate diagnosis is imperative since the drug may be harmful to other neurologic diseases and seems to be ineffective in their treatment. Clinical and laboratory facilities should be available and adequate for accurate moni-

toring of treatment. Long-term safety and efficacy for L-dopa have not yet been established.

3. L-dopa action is explained as follows:

   a. The brain-induced nerve impulses that control the voluntary movements in a healthy person are regulated by an interplay of neurochemicals that include dopamine.

   b. In the person with Parkinson's disease, dopamine deficiency destroys or injures this most important interplay. The results are muscle rigidity, tremors, postural abnormalities, and akinesia (absence, loss, or weakness of motor function). Persons dying of parkinsonism show a marked dopamine depletion in the basal ganglia of the brain.

   c. Improvement is most marked in such symptoms as bradykinesia (abnormal slowness of movement) and rigidity. Tremor, postural instability, and salivation may also improve, but often only after prolonged therapy. Improvement in gait, finger dexterity, facial expression, speech, and mobility may also occur.

   d. Some patients who have had limited physical exercise for years may find themselves suddenly more active.

   e. About one third of parkinsonism patients do not show any improvement.

4. The type of involvement, severity of the disease, and duration of disease do not seem to affect the response. Some advanced severe cases seem to respond better than some milder cases, for unknown reasons.

5. L-dopa is not a cure, so it must be administered indefinitely. Maximum benefits may not be obtained for 3 months or more.

6. All patients undergoing L-dopa therapy experience some side effects, so careful medical supervision is essential. The most frequently occurring side effects include nausea, vomiting, anorexia, dizziness, sedation, confusion, delusions, and nightmares. Cardiovascular complications include flushing, postural hypotension, palpitation, and arrhythmias. The drug must be discontinued if severe arrhythmias occur. Neurologic complications include involuntary chewing, lack of control of voluntary movement (dose should be lowered), agitation, depression, possible suicidal tendencies, insomnia, and complications involving the skin, urogenital tract, special senses, respiration, and endocrine system.

7. Contraindications include bronchial asthma, emphysema, myocardial infarction with residual atrial or ventricular arrhythmias, active peptic ulcer, diabetes, certain cases of glaucoma, and psychoses or severe psychoneuroses.

8. Other drugs for treating Parkinson's disease may be used with L-dopa, perhaps reducing the dose of each, yet in some cases, increasing the effectiveness. Such drugs as benztropine (Cogentin) and trihexyphenidyl (Artane, Tremin) have proved useful.

9. Pyridoxine slows or blocks the effect of L-dopa, so patients should avoid ordinary multiple vitamin preparations that contain this drug.

10. Therapy is started with small doses, usually 0.5 to 1 g daily in three divided doses, taken orally with meals or food to lessen the possibility of nausea. Dose is increased gradually to 4 to 6 g daily in divided doses. Dose is individualized.

Amantadine hydrochloride (ah-man'tah-deen) ***(Symmetrel)*** (sim'eh-trel)

1. This antiviral drug was administered by Dr. Robert S. Schwab of Harvard Medical School to a parkinsonism patient to prevent Asian flu. This is its primary use. The patient showed definite improvement in parkinsonism symptoms.

2. Amantadine seems to slow the destruction of dopamine, thus making the small amount present more effective. It may also aid in the release of dopamine from its storage sites.

3. Its most important use may be to lower the required dose of L-dopa, therefore reducing the possibilities of side effects. Its use with L-dopa is still being studied.

4. Dose is individualized and depends on the dose of L-dopa. Usual dosage: 100 to 200 mg daily.

Carbidopa (kar'bi-do-pah), ***levodopa*** ***(Sinemet)*** (sin'eh-met)

1. Sinemet is a combination of carbidopa and levodopa used for treating the symptoms of idiopathic Parkinson's disease, postencephalitic parkinsonism, and symptomatic parkinsonism, which may follow injury to the central nervous system by manganese intoxication and carbon monoxide intoxication.

2. Carbidopa reduces the amount of levodopa required by approximately 75%. When administered with levodopa, it increases both plasma levels and the plasma half-life of levodopa.

3. Carbidopa is indicated to allow the administration of lower doses of levodopa. Patients with irregular, "on and off" responses to levodopa do not show benefit from carbidopa or Sinemet, so certain CNS effects may occur sooner and at lower dosage than they do with levodopa.

4. Sinemet, as is true of levodopa, may cause involuntary movements, mental disturbances, hepatic, renal, or endocrine disease, and asthma. Other symptoms that may occur include depression, psychotic disturbances, nausea, anorexia, vomiting, development of a

duodenal ulcer, gastrointestinal bleeding, hypertension, phlebitis, hemolytic anemia, leukopenia, and agranulocytosis. The last six cited are rare. More common symptoms are abdominal distress, numbness, weakness, faintness, malaise, confusion, burning tongue, muscle twitching, urinary incontinence or retention, blurred vision, dilated pupils, constipation, and nausea and vomiting. Watch the patient carefully for blepharospasm or spasm of the orbicular muscle of the eyelids. This is an early sign of overdosage.

5. Dosage: levodopa must be stopped at least 8 hours before Sinemet is started. Most patients can be maintained on three to six tablets of Sinemet 25/250 mg given in divided doses. The maximum dose should not exceed eight tablets. Available: oral tablets of 10 mg carbidopa plus 100 mg levodopa, and 25 mg carbidopa plus 250 mg levodopa.

• • •

Other drugs that may be useful in the treatment of parkinsonism include *atropine sulfate, belladonna tincture, ethopropazine hydrochloride (Parsidol Hydrochloride), procyclidine hydrochloride (Kemadrin), cycrimine hydrochloride (Pagitane Hydrochloride), benztropine methanesulfonate (Cogentin), orphenadrine hydrochloride (Disipal),* and *chlorphenoxamine hydrochloride (Phenoxene).*

TRICYCLIC ANTIDEPRESSANTS

The tricyclic antidepressants have become the most widely used medications in the treatment of depression. They produce antidepressant and mild tranquilizing effects. After 2 to 3 weeks the tricyclic antidepressants elevate the mood, improve the appetite, and increase alertness in about 80% of patients with endogenous depression. These drugs may be administered in the evening because their sedative effect may aid in sleep.

Side effects include blurred vision, tachycardia, dry mouth, constipation, urinary retention, tremor of the hands, numbness and tingling of the arms and legs, temporary confusion, nausea, vomiting, peculiar taste, drowsiness, hypotension, hypertension, palpitations, and arrhythmias.

Combination therapy with phenothiazine derivatives may be beneficial in the treatment of the depression of schizophrenia or moderate to severe anxiety and depression observed with psychosis.

The tricyclic antidepressants should not be administered with monoamine oxidase inhibitors such as Marplan, Niamid, Nardil, or Parnate, and they should not be administered less than 2 or 3 weeks after the discontinuation of the monoamine oxidase inhibitors. Patients using tricyclic antidepressants should be observed closely for adverse effects when these drugs are used in conjunction with barbiturates, anticholinergic agents, vasopressors, thyroid products, and CNS depressants.

Table 10-1. Tricyclic antidepressants and their dosage

Generic name	Trade name	Dosage
Amitriptyline hydrochloride	Elavil, Endep, Amitril	Usual initial dose: orally, 75 mg daily in divided doses, gradually increasing dose to 150 to 250 mg daily Maximum dose: 300 mg daily
Desipramine hydrochloride	Norpramin, Pertofrane	Usual initial dose: orally, 75 mg daily in divided doses Maintenance dose is 75 to 100 mg in divided doses Daily doses should not exceed 200 mg
Doxepin hydrochloride	Sinequan, Adapin	Usual initial dose: orally, 25 mg three times daily Maintenance dose: no less than 150 mg daily Maximum daily dose: 300 mg
Imipramine hydrochloride	Tofranil, Presamine, SK-Pramine	Initial dose: orally, 30 to 75 mg daily in divided doses, gradually increasing to 150 or 250 mg daily; do not exceed 300 mg daily IM solution for injection: 12.5 mg/ml
Nortriptyline hydrochloride	Aventyl	Usual initial dose: orally, 25 mg daily in three to four divided doses Usual maintenance doses: 30 to 75 mg daily Daily doses should not exceed 100 mg
Protriptyline hydrochloride	Vivactil	Initial dose: orally, 5 to 10 mg three or four times daily Maintenance dose: 20 mg to 40 mg daily Maximum daily dose: 60 mg

ANTICONVULSANTS

Phenytoin sodium (fen'i-toe-in)
(Dilantin) (dil-an'tin)

1. Phenytoin sodium is an efficient drug in the treatment of epilepsy. It is more effective for grand mal seizures than for petit mal seizures.
2. It is also effective in controlling convulsions caused by brain injury and is used following brain operations for the same purpose.
3. It may cause infrequent, untoward actions such as dermatitis, dry skin, sedation, drowsiness, swollen gums, lethargy, fever, hallucinations, apathy, or indifference to surroundings.
4. Usual dose: 0.1 g (gr iss) three times a day. Dose may be doubled if necessary. It can be administered after meals if it causes gastric upsets. It is available in 30- and 100-mg capsules, in 50-mg scored tablets, in oral suspension (30 mg/5 ml and 125 mg/5 ml), and in ''Steri-Vials'' for parenteral administration, containing 50 mg/ml of the drug (2- and 5-ml vials).

Primidone (pri'mi-doan)
(Mysoline) (my'so-leen)

1. Primidone (Mysoline) is an effective anticonvulsant with a relatively wide margin of safety that is used to treat grand mal and psychomotor seizures.
2. This drug is said to have few toxic and side effects. Side effects such as sedation tend to disappear within a few days or after the drug dose is adjusted.
3. Primidone is chemically related to the barbiturates. One of its metabolites is phenobarbital.
4. Usual dose: individualized. Oral tablets, 0.25 g and scored, are available. Dose should not exceed 2 g daily.

Carbamazepine (kar-bah-maz'e-peen)
(Tegretol) (teg'reh-tol)

1. Carbamazepine may be effective in the control of grand mal epilepsy in those patients in whom phenytoin, phenobarbital, primidone, or any therapy combining these has failed.
2. Carbamazepine should be used with caution in women of childbearing age, in patients with glaucoma, and in those with psychiatric disturbances manifested by acute psychotic reactions.
3. Side effects from carbamazepine therapy include dizziness, drowsiness, urinary retention, mental confusion, blurred vision, hallucinations, and tinnitus (ringing in the ears). Periodic red and white blood cell counts are recommended.
4. Dosage range: 200 to 1,600 mg, with most patients being controlled at 800 to 1,200 mg daily. Carbamazepine is available in 100- and 200-mg tablets.

Trimethadione (try-meth-ah-dy'own)
(Tridione) (try-dy'own)

1. Trimethadione is used to control petit mal epilepsy. It is not effective for grand mal seizures. It seems to be more effective in children than in adults.
2. It may cause skin eruptions, blurring of vision, nausea, and gastric disturbances.
3. It should be administered with caution to patients with severe liver or kidney damage, diseases of the optic nerve, anemia, or certain other blood diseases.
4. This drug is available in 150-mg tablets and 300-mg capsules. It is also available in solution 40 mg/ml for oral administration. Usual dose for children: 300 to 900 mg daily; for adults, 900 to 2,400 mg daily in divided doses.

Ethosuximide (eth-o-suk'si-myd)
(Zarontin) (zah-ron'tin)

1. Many neurologists regard ethosuximide (Zarontin) as the first drug of choice in the treatment of petit mal epilepsy.
2. It is at least as effective as trimethadione, and the toxic effects are no more frequent and are of a less serious nature.
3. Usual adult dose: orally, 250 to 500 mg twice daily. It is available in 250-mg capsules.

Paramethadione (par-ah-meth-ah-dy'own)
(Paradione) (par-ah'dy-own)

1. Action and side effects are similar to those of trimethadione.
2. Usual dose: 900 to 2,400 mg daily in divided doses.

Phensuximide (fen-suk'si-myd)
(Milontin Kapseals) (mil-on'tin)

1. Phensuximide is an anticonvulsant succinimide that reduces the frequency of epileptiform attacks. It is indicated in the control of petit mal seizures.
2. The drug may be administered in combination with other anticonvulsants when other forms of epilepsy coexist with petit mal.
3. It should not be used in patients with a history of sensitivity to succinimide or in pregnancy. Blood dyscrasias are possible, so periodic blood counts are necessary. This drug should be administered with caution to patients with known liver or renal disease. All patients receiving the drug should have periodic urinalysis and liver function studies.
4. Phensuximide may impair the mental or physical abilities required for the performance of possibly hazardous tasks, so patients should be cautioned concerning driving a car, working around machinery, or other activities requiring alertness.

5. Side effects include nausea, vomiting, anorexia (that may result from overdosage), drowsiness, dizziness, ataxia, dream-like states, headache, lethargy, urinary frequency, renal damage, and hematuria.
6. Usual dose: 0.5 to 1 g orally three times a day. Dose is adjusted to suit individual requirements. It is available in liquid form for pediatric use.

Clonazepam (klo-nah′zee-pam)
(Clonopin) (klo′no-pin)

1. Clonazepam may be effective in the control of petit mal seizures.
2. This drug should be used with caution in women of childbearing age and in those patients with glaucoma. Abrupt discontinuation may result in grand mal seizures.
3. Clonazepam is a central nervous system depressant, so patients should be instructed about the danger of driving cars or working in conditions where they must be mentally alert. Patients should also be warned that they are particularly susceptible to the depressant effects of barbiturates, chlordiazepoxide, diazepam, meprobamate, and alcohol.
4. Side effects include drowsiness, nausea, blurred vision, confusion, hallucinations, slurred speech, and urinary retention.
5. Initial dosage: 1.5 mg per day with an individualized daily maintenance dose. Maximum daily dose should not exceed 20 mg.
6. Clonazepam is available in 0.5-, 1-, and 2-mg tablets.

Valproic acid (val-pro′ik)
(Depakene) (dep′ah-keen)

1. Valproic acid is an anticonvulsant structurally unrelated to any other agent used to treat seizure disorders. It is most effective in treating petit mal seizure activity; however, it may be effective in treating other types of seizures when used in combination with other agents.
2. Side effects include ataxia, dizziness, diplopia, nystagmus, "spots before the eyes," and headache. Patients should be warned against engaging in activities requiring mental alertness.
3. Initial oral dose: 5 mg/kg every 8 hours. The maximum recommended daily dose is 30 mg/kg per day. Valproic acid may be given with food to minimize gastric irritation.

TRANQUILIZERS

Tranquilizers are drugs that can suppress anxiety and modify disturbed behavior in doses that are not profoundly hypnotic. Anxiety is reduced without subsequent impairment of consciousness. Hyperactivity is controlled. Delusions, hallucinations, and confusion associated with psychopathology are decreased to a tolerable level. Nervousness and apprehension are also decreased. Tranquilizers are also used in the treatment of mental illness.

Tranquilizing and antianxiety drugs are often placed in one of two categories: the major tranquilizers and the minor antianxiety drugs. The major tranquilizers have characteristic effects on behavior and autonomic functions. They are important in the management of major psychoses. A few examples are Thorazine, Sparine, Compazine, Mellaril, and Stelazine from the phenothiazine derivatives. The minor antianxiety drugs are used in less serious illnesses and have less effect on central autonomic regulations. They resemble sedative-hypnotics. Some pharmacologists place meprobamate, chlordiazepoxide, and diazepam in this group; others place them in the sedative group.

Tranquilizers are also used in mental disease treatment to quiet a noisy, uncooperative patient.

America has become tranquilizer conscious. These drugs are of benefit to many people, but they are so new that their effects on the human body after long-term use, especially on the brain and nervous system, are not as yet fully known. Such drugs should be taken under medical supervision only. They should not be taken for occasional nervousness or merely to feel well.

Chlorpromazine hydrochloride (klor-pro′mah-zeen)
(Thorazine Hydrochloride) (thor′ah-zeen)

1. Chlorpromazine affects the central and autonomic nervous systems.
2. It relieves anxiety and apprehension, controls nausea and vomiting, and overcomes persistent hiccups. Chlorpromazine's primary use is treating mental and emotional disturbances and severe anxiety.
3. It should be administered with caution in combination with CNS depressants such as alcohol, barbiturates, opiates, and other tranquilizers, since these drugs would increase the CNS depression.
4. If administered intramuscularly, the drug should be injected slowly over 1 minute. The patient should be kept recumbent for $1/2$ hour to prevent postural hypotension. When preparing many hypodermic injections of chlorpromazine, it is advisable to wear rubber or plastic gloves to prevent possible skin irritation from a contact dermatitis reaction to this drug.
5. The drugs has some side effects, such as drowsiness, postural hypotension, nasal congestion, dryness of the mouth, low fever, urticaria or hives, and rarely, leukopenia (decrease in white blood cells) or jaundice. Patients receiving long-term therapy may develop symptoms similar to Parkinson's disease.
6. Usual dose: individualized, 200 to 800 mg per day,

depending on severity of symptoms and needs of patient.

7. It is available in:
   a. Tablets: 10, 25, 50, 100, and 200 mg.
   b. Syrup: 10 mg/5 ml in lightproof bottles.
   c. Sustained-release capsules (Spansules): 30, 75, 150, 200, and 300 mg.
   d. Concentrate: 30 mg and 100 mg/ml. Dilute each dose to at least 60ml with fruit juice or milk just prior to administration.
   e. Suppository: 25 and 100 mg.
   f. Ampule: 25 mg per ml.

Prochlorperazine (pro-klor-per′ah-zeen) *(Compazine)* (komp′ah-zeen)

1. Prochlorperazine is an antipsychotic agent used in schizophrenia, manic-depression, and anxiety and tension associated with various neuroses. Its most frequent use, however, is in the prevention and control of severe nausea and vomiting.
2. Usual dosages:
   a. Nausea and vomiting: 5 to 10 mg every 4 to 6 hours.
   b. Psychiatric disorders: up to 150 mg daily.

Thioridazine hydrochloride (thy-o-rid′ah-zeen) *(Mellaril)* (mel′ah-ril)

1. Thioridazine administration results in improved tranquilization, with minor sedative effects.
2. It has value in the treatment of mental and emotional disturbances, such as acute and chronic psychoneuroses, preoperative and postoperative apprehension and agitation, agitated geriatric patients, uncontrollable pain, and alcoholism.
3. Side effects may occur and include drowsiness, dryness of mouth, nasal stuffiness, skin eruption, nocturnal confusion, and retinitis. Pseudoparkinsonism symptoms may occur, but less frequently than with other antipsychotic drugs.
4. Thioridazine is contraindicated in severely depressed or comatose states.
5. Usual dose in nonpsychotic patients: 10 or 25 mg three or four times a day. Psychotic patients may require 100 mg three or four times a day. Dose is individualized.

Trifluoperazine (tri-floo-o-per′ah-zeen) *(Stelazine)* (stel′ah-zeen)

1. This drug is a tranquilizer-antiemetic that relieves apathy, anxiety, nausea, and vomiting and increases physical and mental energy. It has low sedating effects.
2. Usual dose: individualized. Initial dose: 1-mg tablet twice a day.

Haloperidol (hah-lo-per′i-dol) *(Haldol)* (hal′dol)

1. Haloperidol is used to help control agitated states associated with schizophrenia, manic-depressive psychoses, and mental retardation.
2. This drug should not be used in patients with severe mental depression or in those patients with CNS depression from other drugs or alcohol.
3. Side effects more commonly seen include drowsiness, nasal stuffiness, dry mouth, constipation, urinary retention, parkinsonism symptoms, tachycardia, headache, confusion, and rash.
4. Dosages: 1 to 6 mg daily in those patients with mild symptoms to 20 mg daily in those patients with severe symptomatology.
5. Haloperidol is available in 0.5-, 1-, 2-, 5-, and 10-mg tablets, a concentrated solution of 2 mg/ml, and injections of 5 mg/ml.

Molindone hydrochloride (mo-lin′doan) *(Moban)* (mo′ban)

1. Molindone is a product available for the treatment of schizophrenia. It is used to control disorientation, hallucinations, emotional withdrawal, and tension associated with this psychiatric disorder.
2. Side effects include drowsiness, restlessness, dizziness, blurred vision, hyperactivity, dry mouth, tachycardia, nausea, and pseudoparkinsonism symptoms.
3. Dosages: 50 to 225 mg daily, depending on the severity and the side effects of the disease.
4. Molindone is available in 5-, 10-, and 25-mg tablets.

• • •

Some other tranquilizing agents are *acetophenazine maleate (Tindal Maleate), chlorprothixene (Taractan), fluphenazine hydrochloride (Permitil, Prolixin), perphenazine (Trilafon),* and *triflupromazine hydrochloride (Vesprin).*

ANALGESICS

Analgesics are drugs that relieve pain without producing loss of consciousness or reflex activity. They act in several ways: (1) by producing sedative and soporific effects, (2) by altering the attitude or mood of the patient from one of concern to one of detachment, promoting a mild euphoria, or sense of well-being, and (3) by elevating the pain threshold. The pain threshold varies from individual to individual, and tolerance to pain appears to be far more variable than pain threshold.

The search for an ideal analgesic continues, since it is difficult to find one that does all desired of it. An ideal analgesic should (1) not cause dependence, (2) be potent, so that it will give maximum relief of pain, (3) not cause tolerance to develop, (4) have minimal side effects, (5) act quickly and over a long period with minimum sedation, so that the patient remains conscious and responsive, and (6) be relatively inexpensive.

Nonsynthetic narcotic analgesics
Opium (o'pee-um)

1. The source of opium is the hardened, dried juice of the unripe seed capsules of the Oriental white poppy, which is grown mostly in China, India, Iran, and Turkey.
2. Opium was used in its crude form until the nineteenth century, when its chief alkaloid, morphine, was discovered. There are twenty active principles of opium. Three of these are morphine, codeine, and papaverine.
3. Preparations containing opium, given orally, are:
   a. *Opium tincture (laudanum)* (law'dah-num) (deodorized opium tincture)
      This drug is seldom used today. It is effective in checking intestinal peristalsis. It is a solution containing 10% opium (1% morphine) and 18% ethanol. Average adult dose: 0.6 to 1.5 ml (6 to 15 mg of morphine).
   b. *Paregoric* (par-e-gor'ik) *(camphorated opium tincture)*
      Paregoric is effective to check diarrhea and intestinal peristalsis. Each teaspoon (5 ml) contains 20 mg opium (2 mg morphine). Usual dose: 4 ml. Range of dose: 4 to 10 ml.
4. Side effects of opium are similar to those of morphine (see following section).

Morphine sulfate (mor'feen sul'fayt)

1. Morphine is a CNS depressant that produces analgesia, drowsiness, and mental cloudiness. Its most important use is in the relief of severe pain. It is a more effective analgesic if it is given to patients before pain begins or becomes severe. Patients should not be allowed to toss restlessly or suffer with severe pain if there is an order for morphine.
2. Action of morphine in other tissues include:
   a. Increased muscle tone of the gastrointestinal tract, reducing peristalsis and gastric, biliary, and pancreatic secretions. Emptying of the stomach and small intestine is slowed, occasionally resulting in constipation.
   b. Increased tone in the sphincter muscle of the bladder, resulting in difficulty in urination. Use with caution in patients with prostatic hypertrophy or urethral stricture.
   c. Peripheral dilation, resulting in relaxation of small blood vessels in the face, neck, and upper chest, causing a patient to feel warm and flushed. Reac-

tions such as itching, urticaria, and erythema are probably caused by morphine's ability to release tissue histamine.
   d. Pupillary contraction or miosis. In higher doses morphine may produce "pinpoint" pupils.
   e. Stimulation of the chemoreceptor trigger zone, which may result in nausea and emesis.
   f. Depression of the cough reflex. This may be advantageous in patients with a severe, nonproductive cough.
3. The most frequently observed adverse reactions to morphine include lightheadedness, dizziness, sedation, nausea, vomiting, and sweating. Vomiting may be reduced by requiring the patient to remain recumbent for 30 minutes after the administration of morphine.
4. A major hazard of all narcotic analgesics is respiratory depression. Morphine should be used with caution in patients with bronchial asthma or chronic pulmonary disease.
5. Usual dose: 10 mg (gr $\frac{1}{6}$), subcutaneously. Range of dose: 4 to 20 mg (gr $\frac{1}{8}$ to $\frac{1}{3}$). Common doses available for IM an IV administration are 8, 10, and 15 mg (gr $\frac{1}{8}$, $\frac{1}{6}$, and $\frac{1}{4}$).

Codeine sulfate (ko'deen sul'fayt)
Codeine phosphate (ko'deen fos'fayt)

1. Codeine is another natural alkaloid of opium. It is used for its analgesic and cough suppressant effects. About 60 mg of codeine provides the same analgesic potency as 10 mg of morphine. Codeine has an advantage of being effective when given orally.
2. This drug may cause constipation and respiratory depression, although generally less so than morphine. It is less habit-forming than morphine, but drug dependence may occur.
3. Codeine is available in a variety of forms as tablets or capsules, in solution for injection, and in elixir and syrup form for coughs. Codeine is also prepared in combination with other analgesics, such as aspirin and acetaminophen, and expectorants, such as terpin hydrate (terpin hydrate with codeine elixir), and antihistamines, such as promethazine (Phenergan expectorant with codeine).
4. Usual dosage:
   a. For cough suppression: 10 to 15 mg.
   b. Analgesia: 30 mg; dosage range: 15 to 60 mg.

Hydrocodone (hi-dro-ko'don)
(Dihydrocodeinone Bitartrate) (di-hi-dro-ko'de-i-noan bi-tar'trayt), *(Dicodid)* (dik'o-did)

1. This drug is similar in action to codeine sulfate and codeine phosphate. It is used primarily as an antitussive agent (cough suppressant).

2. Usual dose: 5 to 15 mg. It is available in oral tablets.
3. It is often used in combination with antihistamines and other antitussive agents (Hycodan, Tussionex).

Hydromorphone hydrochloride (hi-dro-mor'foan) (Dilaudid) (di-law'did)

1. Hydromorphone is prepared from morphine and may be used as an analgesic and antitussive.
2. It may cause respiratory depression, nausea, vomiting, and constipation.
3. Both drug dependence and tolerance can occur.
4. Usual dose: 2 mg. It may be given orally, subcutaneously, intramuscularly, or by suppository.

Synthetic narcotic analgesics
Oxycodone hydrochloride (ok-se-ko'doan)

1. Oxycodone is an opium derivative used as an oral analgesic for the treatment of moderate pain. It is approximately equivalent in analgesic potency to morphine and is five to six times more potent than codeine when similar doses are administered.
2. In the United States oxycodone is available only in combination with aspirin, phenacetin, and caffeine (Percodan) or with acetaminophen (Percocet, Tylox). It should be used with caution in patients with known idiosyncrasies to aspirin, phenacetin, and acetaminophen. Oxycodone is usually well tolerated but may cause nausea, vomiting, and constipation.
3. Oxycodone may be habit-forming.
4. Usual dosage: one to two tablets every 4 to 6 hours.

Oxymorphone hydrochloride (ok-se-mor'foan) (Numorphan) (new-mor'fan)

1. Oxymorphone is a semisynthetic narcotic with a pharmacologic action resembling that of morphine.
2. It is a potent drug used for relieving severe pain.
3. This drug effectively relieves preoperative and postoperative pain, chronic and acute pain, obstetric pain, cancer, renal and biliary colic, traumatic injuries, and some heart conditions, such as myocaradial infarction.
4. Oxymorphone provides tranquility and a slight drowsy effect. Patients usually remain alert and cooperative to treatment and care.
5. Such side effects as respiratory depression, drowsiness, restlessness, malaise, nausea, vomiting, sweating, itching, and headache may be overcome with the use of nalorphine (Nalline), levallorphan (Lorfan), or naloxone (Narcan).
6. Oxymorphone is habit-forming.
7. Usual dose, for SC or IM injection: 1 to 1.5 mg every 4 to 6 hours. Oral: one 10-mg tablet every 4 to 6 hours, when necessary. Rectal: one 2- or 5-mg suppository every 4 to 6 hours.

Butorphanol tartrate (byou-tor'fay-nol) (Stadol) (stay'dol)

1. Butorphanol is a powerful parenteral narcotic analgesic.
2. Duration of analgesia is generally 3 to 4 hours and is approximately equivalent to the analgesia of morphine. This drug is recommended for the relief of moderate to severe pain.
3. Butorphanol should not be given to patients with a drug dependence history, to emotionally unstable patients, to patients with severe liver and kidney conditions or head injuries (it elevates cerebrospinal fluid pressure), or in patients with respiratory disease, since it causes some respiratory depression.
4. The safety of usage of butorphanol in pregnancy, during labor and delivery, to nursing mothers, and in pediatrics has not been well established.
5. The most frequent adverse reactions are sedation, nausea, and clammy sweating. Less frequent reactions are headache, vertigo, dizziness, a floating feeling, lethargy, confusion, lightheadedness, agitation, euphoria, hallucinations, flushing and warmth, dry mouth, sensitivity to cold, palpitation, increase or decrease of blood pressure, vomiting, slow and shallow respirations, diplopia or blurred vision, and rash or hives.
6. The immediate treatment of butorphanol overdosage is intravenous naloxone. The respiratory and cardiac status should be continuously evaluated, and supportive measures such as oxygen, intravenous fluids, vasopressors, and assisted or controlled respiration should be initiated when necessary.
7. Usual IM dose: 2 mg every 3 to 4 hours as necessary. Range of IM dose: 1 to 4 mg every 3 to 4 hours as necessary. IV dose, single: 1 mg every 3 to 4 hours as necessary. Range of IV dose: 0.5 to 2 mg every 3 to 4 hours if necessary.

Meperidine hydrochloride (me-pair'i-deen) (Demerol Hydrochloride) (dem'er-ol)

1. Meperidine is a synthetic analgesic with a potency similar to morphine. It is recommended for the relief of moderate to severe pain in postoperative and cancer patients. The onset of analgesia is slightly more rapid than morphine, but the duration (2 to 3 hours) is slightly less than that of morphine. It is also frequently used as a preanesthetic medication.
2. Meperidine resembles morphine in some of its effects on smooth muscle. It promotes spasm of muscle in the biliary and gastrointestinal tract, although generally to a lesser extent than morphine. Meperidine has a rather weak antispasmodic effect on the bronchial musculature and can be more safely used than morphine for the asthmatic patient who needs an anal-

gesic. Frequent side effects are nausea and vomiting.
3. Overdose symptoms include dizziness, dryness of mouth, nausea, vomiting, face flushing, sweating, slow pulse, fainting, and fall in blood pressure.
4. Prolonged use (2 to 3 weeks) of meperidine may result in drug dependence.
5. Analgesic dose: 50 to 100 mg, IM or IV. Range of dose: 50 to 150 mg. Give by IM injection, not subcutaneously, to prevent injury to tissues.

Anileridine hydrochloride (an-i-ler′i-deen)
(Leritine Dihydrochloride) (ler′i-teen)

1. Anileridine is a synthetic narcotic analgesic drug that also has sedative, spasmolytic, and antitussive action.
2. It is effective for relieving pain in the treatment of angina pectoris, biliary colic, renal colic, extensive burns, fractures, carcinoma, and acute congestive heart failure, during oral surgery and childbirth, and for preoperative apprehension.
3. It has little hypnotic effect, although rest and sleep may follow its use because of pain relief.
4. Anileridine should be given with caution when respiratory failure is a possibility, as in patients with head injuries or respiratory disease. Respiratory failure can be treated with naloxone (Narcan).
5. In addition to circulatory and respiratory depression, untoward reactions might include nausea, vomiting, hypotension, dizziness, slow pulse, perspiration, a sense of warmth, dry mouth, vision impairment, itching, euphoria, restlessness, excitement, and nervousness.
6. Anileridine is an addictive drug. It should be given with caution over prolonged periods or to people who seem to be unusually responsive to narcotics.
7. Initial dose: 25 to 50 mg orally, subcutaneously, or by IM injection, every 4 to 6 hours. The total 24 hour dose should not exceed 200 mg.

Methadone hydrochloride (meth′ah-doan)
(Dolophine) (do′lo-feen)

1. Methadone is a synthetic narcotic analgesic that is particularly effective in cancer patients and posttrauma patients who require a prolonged duration of analgesia. It is effective when administered orally or parenterally.
2. Methadone is most frequently used as a substitute for heroin or other narcotic addictives. Each dose is given under supervision, often in orange juice. It does not cure the addict, since it is also addictive. However, it does control the ''habit'' and does allow the addict to work at gainful employment. Withdrawal symptoms from methadone are less severe than those of morphine and heroin. Some addicts do obtain freedom from use of the original narcotic and methadone

by very gradual withdrawal from each drug under close medical supervision.
3. Side effects are similar to those of meperidine.
4. Usual dose: 2.5 to 10 mg, depending on the severity and cause of the pain. It is often given orally but may be given intramuscularly every 3 to 6 hours as needed. It should not be given intravenously.

Alphaprodine hydrochloride (al-fa-pro′deen)
(Nisentil Hydrochloride) (ny′sen-til)

1. This drug is a rapid-acting synthetic analgesic with a potency similar to meperidine but with a shorter duration of action. Pain is relieved within 5 to 10 minutes for about 2 hours after sc injection.
2. It is useful for obstetric analgesia, urologic examinations and procedures, especially cystoscopy, and preoperatively in major and minor surgery.
3. Alphaprodine is well tolerated, with side effects similar to those of meperidine. Overdoses of alphaprodine may result in respiratory depression. Naloxone (Narcan) may be used as an antidote. Alphaprodine may be addicting with long-term use.
4. Usual dose: 20 to 40 mg, subcutaneously or intravenously only.

Pentazocine (pen-taz′o-seen)
(Talwin) (tal′win)

1. Pentazocine is a potent, effective, well-tolerated synthetic analgesic for moderate or severe pain. In larger doses it exerts CNS depression similar to that of morphine. Hypertension and tachycardia may be produced rather than the classic hypotension and bradycardia produced by morphine.
2. Prolonged use of pentazocine may result in drug dependence.
3. Naloxone (Narcan) can be given parenterally to reverse respiratory depression caused by pentazocine.
4. Usual dosages:
   a. Oral: 50 to 100 mg every 3 to 4 hours.
   b. IM: 30 to 60 mg every 3 to 4 hours.
   c. IV: 30 to 60 mg every 3 to 4 hours.

Levorphanol tartrate (le-vor′fah-nol)
(Levo-Dromoran) (le-vo-dro′mo-ran)

1. Levorphanol is a potent synthetic narcotic-analgesic with uses similar to morphine or meperidine. It is used preoperatively and postoperatively and in biliary and renal colic, myocardial infarction, and severe trauma, and for intractable pain from cancer.
2. Side effects such as nausea, emesis, and dizziness are more likely to be observed in the ambulatory paient. Pruritus and sweating rarely occur. Levorphanol is less likely to cause constipation that morphine.
3. Its use is contraindicated in patients with acute alco-

holism, bronchial asthma, increased intracranial pressure, and respiratory depression.

4. Levorphanol is an addictive drug, so the usual precautions should be observed.
5. Naloxone (Narcan) is an effective antidote for overdosage.
6. Usual dose: 2 mg orally or subcutaneously every 6 to 8 hours. Dose may be increased to 3 mg if necessary.

NARCOTIC ADDICTION

Addiction to opiates is a very serious problem to the individual as well as to relatives, friends, business associates, and community. The cause of addiction varies. The greatest underlying cause is an unstable personality. Other causative factors include prolonged use of an opiate for relief of pain, easy access to drugs, inability to deal with frustrations in daily life, and curiosity about the effects of drugs.

Symptoms of addiction are at times difficult to observe, unless the individual is deprived of the drug. When the drug is withheld about 4 to 12 hours, the following symptoms occur: marked craving for the drug, trembling, sweating, chilliness, vomiting, yawning, inability to sleep, sneezing, muscular aches and pains, and mental depression. The individual feels acutely ill and will do anything to obtain another dose of the drug, including resorting to crime, lying, cheating, stealing, and sacrificing money, social position, family, food, and self-respect. The great expense of the drug adds to this burden.

It is difficult to cure an addict; only about 1% to 2% are cured. Treatment is best carried out in a hospital or sanitarium. United States Public Health Service hospitals (federal hospitals), many medical center chemical-dependence units, and privately operated clinics are providing intensive treatment of the addict of any age for a nominal sum or without charge.

Before administering any narcotic, the nurse should observe the pupil of the eye for constriction or pinpoint appearance and note the rate and depth of the respirations, along with other symptoms already discussed. The nurse should use various measures for comfort prior to administering the medication. Many times, however, a physician will order a lighter dose, a tranquilizer, or a less habit-forming drug to gradually replace the narcotic.

Every nurse should realize the great responsibility of such easy access to drugs. The nurse should consider the symptoms and effects of addiction to self, patient, relatives, and community and should never be tempted to take such drugs. The nurse never self-medicates but takes drugs only on the advice and supervision of a personal physician.

The manufacture and distribution of narcotic drugs are controlled by federal legislation, primarily the Drug Abuse Control Act of 1970.

NARCOTIC OVERDOSAGE AND NARCOTIC ANTAGONISTS

Narcotics are CNS depressants. They should be administered with caution and with the following points in mind.

Symptoms of narcotic overdosage include CNS depression that progresses into deep sleep with eventual coma and slow, shallow respirations (ten to twelve per minute or slower), possibly with Cheyne-Stokes respirations. The pupils of the eyes at first are moderately constricted and later are pinpoint. As the asphyxia deepens, the pupils of the eyes dilate. In early stages the skin is warm and moist and the color fairly normal. In later stages the body temperature falls, the skin becomes cold and clammy, and skin color is cyanotic or gray. The effect on heart action is not apparent at first, but later the pulse becomes weak and irregular. Limited change in blood pressure is noted until the lack of oxygen is pronounced. A drop in blood pressure with shock then develops. Death usually results from respiratory failure. Respiratory depression must be treated quickly with oxygen and ventilatory support if the patient is to survive. Treatment with antagonists should be initiated immediately after respiratory support has been established. The patient should be kept warm and dry and turned often to prevent pneumonia. If the patient is in a stupor, food and fluids must be given by tube. A fluid intake and output record should be maintained. Distention of the bladder can be prevented by catheterization.

Antidotes to narcotic poisoning include naloxone hydrochloride, nalorphine hydrochloride, and levallorphan tartrate.

Naloxone hydrochloride (nal-oks'own) (Narcan) (nar'can)

1. Naloxone is a so-called pure narcotic antagonist because it has no effect of its own, other than its ability to reverse the depressant effects of narcotics. Nalorphine and levallorphan are both partial antagonists. They have effects of their own, such as mild analgesia, mood sedation to dysphoria, respiratory depression, and parasympathetic side effects.
2. Naloxone reverses CNS depression induced by pentazocine (Talwin), propoxyphene (Darvon), and the narcotics related to heroin, morphine, codeine, and meperidine. Naloxone is not effective in CNS depression induced by tranquilizers or sedative-hypnotics.
3. Naloxone may precipitate symptoms of withdrawal when administered to patients addicted to narcotics.
4. It is available for IV, IM, or sc administration in

ampules containing 0.4 mg/ml and 0.02 mg/ml. Usual adult dose: 0.4 mg, repeated as needed.

Nalorphine hydrochloride (nal-or'feen)
Nalorphine hydrobromide
(Nalline Hydrochloride) (nal'leen)

1. Nalorphine is a derivative of morphine that acts as an antagonist of morphine, meperidine, methadone, and all other natural or synthetic narcotics.
2. It reverses the respiratory depression caused by these drugs, but it is not effective in the treatment of respiratory depression caused by barbiturates, other hypnotics, and general anesthetics. It may cause further respiratory depression.
3. Usual dose: subcutaneously, intramuscularly, or intravenously, 5 mg/ml ampules. A dose of 5 to 10 mg can be given and repeated in 5 to 10 minutes if respirations are not deeper and somewhat faster.

Levallorphan tartrate (lev-al-lor'fan)
(Lorfan) (lor'fan)

1. Levallorphan is a morphine antagonist similar in indications to nalorphine.
2. Usual dose: 0.3 to 1.2 mg by injection.

NONNARCOTIC ANALGESICS

Acetaminophen (as-eet-ahm'ino-fen)
(Tylenol) (ty'len-ol), *(Datril)* (day'tril)

1. Acetaminophen is a synthetic nonnarcotic analgesic used in the treatment of mild to moderate pain. Its antipyretic effectiveness and analgesic potency are similar to that of aspirin in equal doses. This drug has no antiinflammatory activity and is therefore ineffective (other than as an analgesic) in the relief of symptoms of rheumatoid arthritis.
2. It is an effective analgesic-antipyretic for fever and discomfort associated with bacterial and viral infections, headache, dysmenorrhea, and conditions involving musculoskeletal pain.
3. Acetaminophen is a good substitute for patients who cannot take products containing aspirin because of allergic reactions, hypersensitivities, hemostatic disturbances (including anticoagulant therapy), or possible bleeding problems for gastric or duodenal ulcers, gastritis, and hiatus hernia.
4. Blood dyscrasias, including leukopenia, thrombocytopenia, and pancytopenia, are rare side effects that may occur from prolonged administration of large doses.
5. Usual dose: 325 to 650 mg every 4 to 6 hours, as necessary. Daily dose should not exceed 2.6 g. The drug is available in a variety of oral liquids, tablets and capsules, and rectal suppositories. It is also available in combination with codeine for greater analgesic potency.

Ethoheptazine citrate (eth-o-hep'tah-zeen)
(Zactane) (zak'tayn)

1. Ethoheptazine is a synthetic nonnarcotic analgesic structurally similar to meperidine.
2. It is without antipyretic and sedative effects and apparently has no effect on cough and respiration.
3. Ethoheptazine is used for mild to moderate pain, musculoskeletal disorders, and postpartum and postoperative patients. It is not particularly effective for headaches.
4. Side effects are rare but may include dizziness, epigastric distress, and pruritus.
5. Usual dose: 75 to 150 mg three or four times daily. It is available in 75-mg tablets for oral administration. Ethoheptazine is also available combined with aspirin (Zactirin) and in another compound containing ethoheptazine citrate, aspirin, phenacetin, and caffeine (Zactirin Compound-100). Dosage for this compound form of the drug is one or two tablets three or four times a day.

Propoxyphene hydrochloride (pro-poks'i-feen)
(Darvon) (dar'von)

1. Propoxyphene is an effective, well-tolerated synthetic nonnarcotic analgesic equal to aspirin in potency and duration of analgesic effect.
2. It is used for the relief of mild to moderate pain associated with muscular spasm, premenstrual cramps, dysmenorrhea, bursitis, minor surgery and trauma, headache, and labor and delivery.
3. Propoxyphene has low toxicity and side effects are unusual, but nausea, vomiting, constipation, and respiratory depression can occur. Large doses may cause drowsiness and dizziness. The narcotic antagonist naloxone (Narcan) may be used to overcome the respiratory depression.
4. Orphenadrine (Norflex, Disipal) and propoxyphene may cause mental confusion, tremors, and anxiety if used together.
5. Darvon Compound contains propoxyphene, acetylsalicylic acid (aspirin), phenacetin, and caffeine for the added benefits of antipyretic and antiinflammatory action. Dosage is one or two capsules three or four times a day, as needed.
6. Usual dose, propoxyphene hydrochloride (Darvon): one or two capsules three or four times a day, as needed. Capsules are available in 32- and 65-mg dosage. Propoxyphene napsylate (Darvon-N): one or two tablets three or four times daily, as needed. Available in 100-mg tablets.

ANALGESIC, ANTIPYRETIC, AND ANTIINFLAMMATORY AGENTS
The salicylates

The natural source of salicylic acid is willow bark. Today it is made synthetically from phenol, which is less expensive and just as effective as the natural product. The salicylates were introduced into medicine in the later nineteenth century because of their three primary pharmacologic effects as analgesic, antipyretic, and antiinflammatory agents.

The salicylates are the most commonly used analgesic for relief of slight to moderate pain. Salicylates provide relief by affecting both the hypothalamus of the central nervous system and the peripheral pain receptors at the site of the pain. Analgesic doses of salicylates do not dull the conscious level and do not cause mental sluggishness, memory disturbances, euphoria, or sedation.

The antipyretic effect of the salicylates is centrally mediated. The salicylates act on the thermoregulatory centers in the hypothalamus to increase the elimination of heat by peripheral blood vessel vasodilation. Heat is lost from the body by radiation and by evaporation of increased perspiration.

Salicylates exert antiinflammatory effects by inhibition of prostaglandin synthesis. Prostaglandins are released when tissues are damaged, causing inflammation and pain in the area.

The combination of pharmacologic effects make the salicylates drugs of choice for symptomatic relief of discomfort and pain associated with bacterial and viral infections, headache, myalgia, rheumatoid arthritis, and neuritis. Salicylates can be taken to relieve pain on a chronic basis without inducing drug dependence; however, the salicylates have no effect on progression of the underlying disease process.

As beneficial as the salicylates are, they are not without adverse effects. In normal therapeutic doses, aspirin may produce gastrointestinal irritation, occasional nausea, and gastric hemorrhage. Gastrointestinal side effects can usually be reduced by administering aspirin with food, milk, antacids, or large amounts of water. Extreme caution should be used with administration to those patients with a history of peptic ulcer, liver disease, or coagulation disorders.

Patients receiving higher dosages on a continuing basis are susceptible to developing salicylate intoxication (salicylism). Symptoms included tinnitus (ringing in the ears), impaired hearing, dimness of vision, sweating, fever, lethargy, dizziness, mental confusion, nausea, and vomiting. This condition is reversible on reduction of dosage. Massive overdoses may lead to respiratory depression and coma. There is no antidote; primary treatment is discontinuation of the drug, gastric lavage, forced IV fluids, and alkalinization of the urine with IV sodium bicarbonate.

Salicylates also interact with other drugs, altering the response to these therapeutic agents. Patients taking salicylates and the following agents should be monitored closely for subtherapeutic or toxic effects: warfarin, heparin, chlorpropamide, tolbutamide, phenytoin, methotrexate, sulfinpyrazone, and probenecid.

Acetylsalicylic acid (as-ee-til-sal-i-sil′ik) (Aspirin)

1. Acetylsalicylic acid is the most commonly used analgesic, antipyretic, and antiinflammatory agent. It is a most popular and effective agent for relief of mild to moderate pain.
2. Patients who are hypersensitive to salicylates should be warned to read the labels of over-the-counter products carefully, since aspirin is a common ingredient in many cold, allergy, and analgesic products.
3. Usual dose: 650 mg every 4 hours, as necessary. This drug is available in tablet, capsule, and suppository form.

Acetylsalicylic acid, phenacetin (fe-nas′e-tin), and caffeine (A.P.C. [aspirin compound])

1. This is a common combination of a stimulant and two analgesics.
2. Usual dose: one to two tablets every 4 hours as needed.
3. REMEMBER:
   Asp. comp. means aspirin with other ingredients.
   A.S.A. means aspirin or acetylsalicylic acid alone.
   A. & C. means aspirin and codeine.
   A.P.C. means aspirin, phenacetin, and caffeine.
   Two aspirin-compound drugs well known by trade names are Anacin and Excedrin.

Indomethacin (in-do-meth′ah-sin) (Indocin) (in′do-sin)

1. Indomethacin is a potent, nonsteroidal drug with antiinflammatory, antipyretic, and analgesic properties with a mode of action not fully known. It is thought that indomethacin inhibits the biosynthesis of prostaglandins, which contribute to inflammation.
2. Indomethacin relieves pain and stiffness and reduces fever, swelling, and tenderness of joints. It is used in rheumatoid and degenerative joint disease, gout, moderate to severe degenerative hip joint disease, and moderate to severe rheumatoid spondylitis.
3. Side effects include headache, dizziness, nausea, skin rashes, and bone marrow depression.
4. Because of the possibility of serious adverse effects, the drug should not be used casually; other analgesics should be tried first.

5. It is not recommended for children under 14 years of age, pregnant women, nursing mothers, and patients with gastrointestinal problems, peptic ulcer, ulcerative colitis, allergies to indomethacin and aspirin, corneal and retinal disturbances of the eye, psychiatric disturbances, epilepsy, and parkinsonism.

6. Concurrent administration with salicylates, corticosteroids, or phenylbutazone may enhance the ulcerogenic properties of indomethacin. This drug must be used with caution in patients receiving anticoagulants because of possible drug-induced bleeding and displacement of oral anticoagulants from protein-binding sites. Probenecid blocks the renal tubular secretion of indomethacin. This results in the accumulation and prolongation of the half-life of indomethacin.

7. Usual dose: 25 mg two or three times a day, increasing gradually if no adverse symptoms develop until a total daily dose of 150 to 200 mg is reached. Higher doses are ineffective. The drug should be given after meals or with food or antacids.

Phenylbutazone (fen-il-byou′tah-zoan) (Butazolidin) (byou-tah-zol′i-din), (Azolid) (az′o-lid)

1. Phenylbutazone is a nonsteroidal, antiinflammatory, antipyretic analgesic used for the symptomatic relief of rheumatoid arthritis, osteoarthritis, rheumatoid spondylitis, and gout. It does not alter the course of the disease process.

2. This drug has many serious side effects, so it should be used only after other drugs have failed. The drug should be discontinued within 7 days if no significant improvement is observed. Some of these side effects are: serious and fatal blood dyscrasias, including agranulocytosis, hemolytic anemia, aplastic anemia, creation and reactivation of ulcers, occult bleeding, nausea, vomiting, abdominal distention, sodium and chloride retention (that may result in congestive heart failure, edema, or hypertension), various dermatoses, possible fatal hepatitis, visual disturbances, and renal impairment. Butazolidin inhibits the thyroid uptake of iodine and may result in hypothyroidism.

3. Biweekly blood counts with differential are absolutely essential. The patient should be checked periodically for signs of fluid retention in ankles, feet, and sacrum.

4. Such symptoms as fever, sore throat, lesions (sores) in the mouth, or black, tarry stools should be reported immediately to the physician.

5. Phenylbutazone should not be given to nursing mothers or to pregnant women.

6. Phenylbutazone displaces warfarin (Coumadin) from protein-binding sites; enhancing the anticoagulant activity of warfarin; inhibits the metabolism of acetohexamide (Dymelor) and tolbutamide (Orinase); and may also displace tolbutamide from protein-binding sites, thus enhancing the hypoglycemic effects of these drugs. The metabolism of phenytoin (Dilantin) may be inhibited by phenylbutazone, leading to phenytoin toxicities.

7. Usual dose: initially, 300 to 600 mg daily, orally, divided into three or four equal doses; maintenance doses: 200 to 400 mg daily. The drug should be taken with food or milk or given after a meal to avoid gastric irritation. Low-sodium antacids help to minimize irritation without increasing the ingestion of sodium. The diet should be restricted in sodium chloride while the patient is receiving this drug.

Ibuprofen (i-byou′pro-fen) (Motrin) (mo′trin)

1. Ibuprofen is a representative of a relatively new class of compounds used in the treatment of rheumatoid arthritis, osteoarthritis, and dysmenorrhea.

2. Ibuprofen may be considered an alternative to aspirin therapy in those patients who cannot tolerate the side effects of salicylates.

3. Clinical studies indicate that the antiinflammatory and analgesic effects are similar to those of salicylates and significantly less than indomethacin and phenylbutazone.

4. Gastric irritation causing nausea and heartburn are the most common side effects of ibuprofen. The drug should be used with caution in patients with a history of ulcer disease.

5. Possible interactions include displacement of oral anticoagulants (Coumadin) from protein-binding sites, enhancing the effects of the anticoagulant, and increased potential of the ulcerogenic effects of salicylates, indomethacin, phenylbutazone, and corticosteroids when administered with ibuprofen.

6. Usual dosage: 1,600 mg daily in divided doses. Maximum daily dose: 2.4 g. Ibuprofen is available in 300- and 400-mg tablets.

• • •

Other nonsteroid antiinflammatory agents indicated for the relief of rheumatoid arthritis are **naproxen (Naprosyn), fenoprofen (Nalfon), tolmetin sodium (Tolectin),** and **sulindac (Clinoril).**

> **The physician prescribes the medicine and treatment.**
> **The nurse carries out the physician's orders.**
> **Self-medication is dangerous. Consult your physician first.**
> **There is in every medicine a possible danger.**
> **When in doubt—ASK!**

ASSIGNMENT

Review previous lessons and questions according to the directions of your instructor.

1. Drugs that depress cerebral cortex activity may
   a. Cause greater awareness of the surrounding environment
   b. Decrease sharpness of sensation, perception, alertness, and concentration, and lessen motor activity
   c. Increase sharpness of sensation and perception
   d. Increase motor activity and promote drowsiness and sleep
2. What are the purposes for the centers found in the thalamus, hypothalamus, medulla oblongata, cerebellum, and spinal cord? (See this chapter, the Glossary, and a medical dictionary.)
3. What is the purpose for the presence of acetylcholine in the central nervous system?
4. What effect does caffeine have on the entire central nervous system, the spinal cord, respirations, the myocardium, and pepsin and hydrochloric acid output from the stomach? Give one good reason for the administration of caffeine to a patient, stating the condition for which it might be used.
5. If you drank a cup or two of coffee shortly before a nursing examination, this might be considered a good use of caffeine because caffeine (more than one are correct)
   a. Depresses the higher centers and so relieves tension and worry
   b. Stimulates the cerebral cortex
   c. Stimulates the myocardium and thus improves circulation
   d. Stimulates fatigued muscles
6. What is one of the main uses of Cafergot? What is the generic name for Cafergot?
7. What effect do the amphetamines have on the central nervous system? List the effects the amphetamines have on the human body. Why does amphetamine have a high potential for abuse? If used continuously over long periods, what symptoms are apt to occur? Name three preparations of amphetamine. Can amphetamine be taken without medical supervision for weight-reducing purposes? Explain the dangers of this.
8. What are the main uses of methylphenidate (Ritalin) and phenmetrazine (Preludin)?
9. A hypnotic is a drug that
   a. Is a specific to relieve severe cancer pain
   b. Causes severe addiction that is most difficult to cure
   c. Produces sleep
   d. Merely overcomes restlessness
10. A sedative
    a. Always produces deep sleep
    b. Quiets the patient and gives a feeling of relaxation and rest
    c. Causes severe addiction that is most difficult to cure
    d. Is a specific drug used to relieve severe cancer pain
11. Could a hypnotic ever be a sedative or a sedative ever be a hypnotic? Explain.
12. List and discuss the nursing measures that may be used before giving a patient a sedative or hypnotic. Why are these measures important?
13. What effects should a good hypnotic provide? A good sedative? Some pharmacologists view meprobamate and related drugs and the benzodiazepines as sedative-hypnotics rather than tranquilizers. Why? Are they addictive? What symptoms occur with sudden withdrawal after long periods of administration? Is this the same for true tranquilizers?
14. List the main effects of barbiturates. What are some of the therapeutic uses of barbiturates?
15. Outline the treatment for barbiturate poisoning.
16. Barbiturates
    a. Do not enhance the analgesic action of salicylates
    b. Are not effective analgesic agents when used alone
    c. Have as their chief effect a mildly stimulating action on the entire central nervous system
    d. Depress the central nervous system, with the exception of the motor areas of the cerebral cortex
17. What are the main uses of amobarbital sodium? What is its trade name?
18. What are the main uses of pentobarbital? What is its trade name?
19. Phenobarbital is an effective barbiturate to prevent convulsive seizures because it
    a. Depresses the entire cerebral cortex
    b. Rarely causes drowsiness and hangover the next day
    c. Acts as an anticonvulsant in ordinary doses
    d. Has a duration of activity of only 3 to 4 hours and is classified as a short-acting barbiturate
20. What is the trade name for phenobarbital? Learn well the trade names for phenobarbital and pentobarbital, so that you will not confuse them. What is the adult dose of phenobarbital given for its hypnotic effect? Is it given orally or by injection only?

21. What are the main effects of secobarbital? What is its trade name? Is it long-acting or short-acting?

22. Give two trade names for one of the benzodiazepines—chlordiazepoxide.

23. List the uses of chlordiazepoxide in low-oral and high-oral doses. What instructions should be given to patients taking chlordiazepoxide (Librium) or any other sedative or hypnotic because of the possible drowsy effects? What other effects may chlordiazepoxide or any other sedative or hypnotic have on the patient that makes these instructions so essential? What is the usual adult dose during the day and at night for its hypnotic effect?

24. Name five other depressants that may potentiate the effects of benzodiazepines.

25. Clorazepate is used for what medical conditions? What is the trade name for clorazepate?

26. List the uses of diazepam (Valium). Diazepam is the treatment of choice for what medical condition? This drug is often effective for treatment of what kind of seizures? Explain each type of seizure. List several side effects of diazepam. Why should abrupt withdrawal of this drug be avoided? What instructions should be given to the patients because of its possible drowsy effect? Outline the treatment of overdosage. What is the average adult dose? Diazepam may be potentiated by what othehr CNS depressants?

27. What is the main use of flurazepam? List several of its side effects and contraindications. What instructions should be given to patients taking this drug? Why? What is the usual adult dose when retiring?

28. What is the main use of oxazepam (Serax)?

29. Chloral hydrate is a hypnotic member of which group? What is its effect on the cerebrum? Is it fast- or slow-acting? What is its duration of effect? List the toxic reactions. Tell its usual adult hypnotic dose and best method of administration when given in liquid oral form. What are its contraindications? What toxic reactions should be watched for? What is the treatment of chloral hydrate poisoning? (See section on Barbiturate poisoning for treatment of overdosage; also see Index.)

30. What are the main effects of ethchlorvynol (Placidyl)? Why should this drug *not* be given over a long period? Discuss interaction of this drug with certain other drugs.

31. What is glutethimide's greatest use? Why should prothrombin-time testing be performed periodically? Discuss possible drug interactions if glutethimide is used with other drugs.

32. Give two trade names for meprobamate. In which group of drugs is meprobamate discussed: sedatives or tranquilizers, and why? List the main effects of meprobamate, including the effect on skeletal muscles. List the side effects and dangers in taking this drug in large doses over prolonged periods. Are habituation, tolerance, and physical dependence possible when taking meprobamate for extended periods? How can such dangers be overcome? What is the usual dosage if taken three or four times daily? What is the bedtime dosage? Discuss possible interactions if meprobamate is taken with certain other drugs for longer than brief periods.

33. In which group of drugs does methyprylon (Noludar) be-

long? What instructions should be given to patients who take this drug occasionally and over long periods? Can dependency occur with long-dosage therapy?

34. List five main effects or uses of paraldehyde and tell its average oral dose. How should the unpleasant taste be disguised for oral administration? If given rectally, how should it be mixed? What precautions should be taken while mixing it and during its administration? Paraldehyde may be potentiated by what other drugs?

35. Paraldehyde
   a. Is a member of the barbiturate hypnotic group
   b. Depresses the central nervous system, much as chloral hydrate does
   c. Stimulates the central nervous system much as amphetamine does
   d. Should always be given undiluted and by mouth

36. Bromides are rarely used today for their sedative, hypnotic, and anticonvulsant effects. They may be cumulative and may cause what medical condition?

37. Ethyl alcohol is
   a. A stimulant of the central nervous system
   b. A depressant of the central nervous system
   c. A stimulant to some persons and a depressant to others
   d. None of these

38. There are *several* choices correct in this question. Notice *what* the question asks. Of the following conditions or evaluations, which ones would you think indicate that alcohol should *not* be used as a beverage? Why, in each case?
   a. Epilepsy
   b. Liver and kidney diseases
   c. Slightly high blood pressure
   d. Ulcers of the gastrointestinal tract
   e. Individuals stable and seemingly able to control alcohol intake
   f. Individuals in normal health

39. Another name for whiskey is
   a. Spiritus frumenti
   b. Spiritus vini vitis
   c. Methyl alcohol
   d. Ethyl alcohol

40. What effect does alcohol have on the central nervous system, including the cerebrum, cerebellum, medulla, and spinal cord?

41. List the main steps in treatment of *acute* alcohol poisoning and *chronic* alcohol poisoning.

42. Name two drugs helpful in the treatment of delirium tremens of alcoholism.

43. Explain Alcoholics Anonymous and how it achieves its results. What is the effect of Antabuse in the treatment of alcoholism? Explain other uses of ethyl alcohol and tell the strength used in skin cleansing, back rubs, and thermometer disinfecting. What are the main uses of ethyl alcohol, isopropyl alcohol, and methyl alcohol? What complications might develop from taking isopropyl alcohol or methyl alcohol internally? What is the ideal bactericidal effect of ethyl alcohol?

44. List the characteristic symptoms of Parkinson's disease. What is the theory of how levodopa works on the brain?

Give some examples of drugs used in the treatment of Parkinson's disease. What is the drug of choice in treating Parkinson's disease? List the warnings for physicians in the use of levodopa and be familiar with them. What symptoms does levodopa (Laradopa, Dopar) relieve? About what fraction of patients show no relief from symptoms in the use of levodopa for Parkinson's disease? List the side and toxic effects of levodopa. What are some of the contraindications? Name three other drugs that might be used with levodopa, lessening levodopa's dosage and side effects. Be familiar with both generic and trade names. What has been the main use of amantadine? How was it discovered to be useful in the treatment of Parkinson's disease? List five other drugs useful in the treatment of Parkinson's disease, using both generic and trade names. Can Parkinson's disease thus far be cured?

45. What are the main effects and uses of the tricyclic antidepressants? List several side effects. Which drugs should tricyclic antidepressants *not* be given with? Why? List four tricyclic antidepressants and become familiar with their generic and trade names and main effects.

46. Phenytoin sodium is most effective in the treatment of
    a. Petit mal seizures in epilepsy
    b. Central nervous system depression
    c. Grand mal seizures in epilepsy and the control of convulsions following brain accidents or brain surgery
    d. General stimulation of the patient

47. Name four anticonvulsants by generic and trade names and indicate the type of convulsion for which each seems particularly effective. What is the name of a possible drug of choice in the treatment of petit mal epilepsy? What are some of the side effects of phenytoin, carbamazepine, trimethadione, phensuximide, clonazepam, and valproic acid?

48. What effect do tranquilizers have on the human body? Tranquilizers are often placed in one of two categories. Name these categories. Give five examples of drugs from the phenothiazine derivatives and belonging to the major tranquilizer category. Name three minor antianxiety drugs that some pharmacologists place in the sedative group.

49. Tranquilizer drugs should be taken
    a. When a person feels nervous or is occasionally overly anxious
    b. When a person is in any kind of pain
    c. Under a physician's supervision and order only
    d. When a person thinks mental symptoms may be developing
    e. To be "happy" and "relaxed" and "free from care"

50. Chlorpromazine (Thorazine) is a drug that is effective
    a. For its stimulating action and for giving increased energy and alertness
    b. As an antiemetic, to relieve anxiety and fear, to overcome persistent hiccups, and primarily, in the treatment of mental and emotional disturbances and severe anxiety
    c. Mainly in the relief of convulsions
    d. Mainly as a mild sedative

51. When chlorpromazine is given by injection it should be
    a. Given intramuscularly slowly over 1 to 2 minutes to prevent reactions
    b. Given rapidly to hasten absorption
    c. Injected with an extra amount of force
    d. Injected with a very short needle to avoid contact with muscle tissue

52. List the side effects, contraindications, and average injectable dose of chlorpromazine. What precautions should the nurse take in preparing many injections of this drug at once?

53. What are the two chief uses of prochlorperazine (Compazine)?

54. What is the chief advantage of Mellaril when used as a tranquilizer? What are the main uses of trifluoperazine (Stelazine), haloperidol (Haldol), and molindone (Moban)? What are side effects for haloperidol and molindone? Your instructor will tell you which tranquilizers are used most commonly in your hospital. Become familiar with them.

55. Define analgesics. Discuss the various ways in which they act. What are the desirable characteristics of an analgesic?

56. The source of opium is the
    a. Purple foxglove
    b. White foxglove
    c. Hardened, dried juice of the unripe capsules of the Oriental white poppy
    d. A serpent-shaped shrub

57. Paregoric is effective in the treatment of
    a. Terminal stages of cancer
    b. Diarrhea
    c. Drowsiness
    d. Overweight

58. What narcotic does paregoric contain?

59. What effect does morphine have on the cerebral cortex, respiratory center, cough center, vomiting center, muscle tone of the stomach and intestines, peristalsis, ability to cause constipation, and eye pupil? List the common sc or IM doses of morphine sulfate. What is a fatal dose? Before you administer a dose of morphine, what signs should you observe in the patient that might indicate previous overdosage that this dose is contraindicated?

60. Morphine poisoning can be observed by
    a. Hypertension
    b. Abnormally slow respiration rate with shallow depth and pinpoint eye pupils
    c. Increased respiration rate and dilated eye pupils
    d. Tachycardia

61. What are adverse reactions to morphine? What is a major hazard of morphine and all narcotic analgesics? Is it habit-forming? Addictive?

62. What type of pain does codeine relieve? Is it more or less habit-forming than morphine? What is its chief use other than to relieve pain? Name two cough medicines containing codeine. What is the average dose of codeine for relief of pain and how often may it be given?

63. Hydrocodone (Dicodid) is similar in action to what other analgesic you have recently learned? What is its primary use?

64. Hydromorphone (Dilaudid) is a drug prepared from morphine. List and discuss several of its main uses and disadvantages. Can drug dependence and tolerance occur?

65. Oxycodone is an opium derivative available in the United

States only in combination with what other drugs? It is approximately equivalent in analgesic potency to what other drug? Is it habit-forming?

66. What are the chief uses for the potent drug oxymorphone (Numorphan)? What side effects should be watched for and what drugs may overcome these side effects? What are the usual doses: orally, sc or IM injection? Is it habit-forming?

67. What type of pain does butorphanol (Stadol) relieve? Make a list of some of the contraindications for butorphanol. Make a list of some of the commonly observed adverse reactions in butorphanol overdosage. What is the immediate treatment for butorphanol overdosage? What is the usual dose and route of administration?

68. Meperidine (Demerol) (several choices are correct for this question)
    a. In therapeutic doses depresses the respirations
    b. Is definitely more effective than morphine in relieving pain
    c. Is a synthetic substitute for morphine whose analgesic effect is not nearly as strong as morphine
    d. Is not habit-forming
    e. Promotes spasm of muscle in the biliary and gastrointestinal tract, although generally to a lesser extent than morphine
    f. Should not be used for the asthmatic patient since it has a very strong antispasmodic effect on the bronchial musculature
    g. Has 10 mg as a usual dose for relief of pain in adults
    h. Has frequent side effects of nausea and vomiting
    i. Has overdose symptoms, including dry mouth, dizziness, nausea, vomiting, sweating, face flushing, slow pulse, fainting, and fall in blood pressure
    j. Should be given by IM injection to prevent injury to the tissues
    k. Has as its usual dose, IM 2 mg every 3 to 4 hours, as necessary

69. Explain the source and main uses of methadone (Dolophine). Does methadone have fast or slow action in the relief of pain? Is it cumulative? What symptoms should be watched for in patients receiving this drug? Explain methadone's use in the treatment of morphine or heroin addicts. Methadone is a morphine derivative effective for what type of pain?

70. Explain the pain-relief effects of alphaprodine (Nisentil). Why should this drug *not* be given with barbiturates?

71. Discuss the main uses and duration of action of pentazocine (Talwin). Is it a narcotic or nonnarcotic type of analgesic? Can prolonged use cause dependence? What drug can be given parenterally to reverse the respiratory depression caused by pentazocine? What is the usual oral dosage?

72. What are some of the chief uses for the powerful synthetic narcotic levorphanol (Levo-Dromoran). Its use is contraindicated in what conditions? Is it an addictive drug? What drug is an effective antidote for overdosage of this drug?

73. Let us review the drugs thus far learned under the topic Analgesics. Make two columns, one with the heading *Nonsynthetic narcotic analgesics* and the other with the heading *Synthetic narcotic analgesics*. List all the drugs you have learned under their correct heading. Place after each drug a key word or phrase such as "powerful," "mild or moderate pain," or "habit-forming or addictive." Did you find any drugs that were *not* habit-forming, addictive, or caused dependencies? In making your lists, be careful: do *not* name narcotic antagonists. You may start with opium (an example of a drug containing opium), and you may place codeine with morphine, using a key word or phrase to distinguish the type of pain controlled by each drug.

Become familiar with the names and chief effects of these narcotics and the average dose of each, especially the ones commonly used in your hospital.

74. What are the causes of nacotic addiction, and what is probably the greatest underlying cause? What are the symptoms of addiction? What percent of addicts can be cured? Which act regulates all these addictive narcotics, and is this a federal, state, city, or county law?

75. What are the symptoms and treatment of narcotic overdosage? What is the nursing treatment of narcotic overdosage?

76. Name three antidotes or antagonists to narcotic poisoning and tell the symptoms they overcome.

77. Name five drugs in which naloxone (Narcan) reverses the CNS depression. Is naloxone effective in overcoming the depression induced by tranquilizers or sedative-hypnotics?

78. What is the source of nalorphine (Nalline)? Which drugs is it, and is it not, effective against in overcoming respiratory depression?

79. What type of analgesic is acetaminophen (Tylenol)—narcotic or nonnarcotic? Is it effective against severe or mild, moderate pain? Acetaminophen is an effective drug for what medical conditions? Unlike aspirin, it has no antiinflammatory activity; therefore, is it *ineffective* or *effective* (other than as an analgesic) in the relief of symptoms of rheumatoid arthritis or other conditions in which a good degree of inflammation is present? In regard to drug interactions and acetaminophen, name several blood conditions that may occur and explain each. List the drugs that, if given with acetaminophen for long periods, may show alteration in their effects. Acetaminophen may lengthen the prothrombin time when given with what oral anticoagulant? What is the usual dose of acetaminophen?

80. What is the source of ethohepatzine (Zactane)? Does it act as an antipyretic or a sedative? Does it relieve cough, impaired respiration, or headache? What are its main uses? When combined with aspirin, what is its trade name? What is the usual dose?

81. What type of analgesic is propoxyphene (Darvon)? List some of its chief uses. Side effects are rare, but which ones may you observe? If respiratory depression occurs, what drug may be used to overcome the depression? What is the average dose? Darvon Compound contains which other drugs? What is the usual dose? Give the generic and trade names of a drug that should *not* be used with propoxyphene and tell why.

82. Define antipyretic.

83. What is the natural source of salicylates? Today, what is its source? What type of agents are the salicylates? Salicylates are the most commonly used analgesic for relief of what

type of pain? Salicylates provide relief from pain by their effects on what parts of the central nervous system? Do analgesic doses dull the conscious level and cause mental sluggishness, memory disturbances, euphoria, or sedation? How do salicylates reduce fever? The salicylates are the drug of choice for symptomatic relief of discomfort and pain associated with what type of conditions? List the adverse effects of salicylates. How can gastrointestinal side effects usually be reduced? What are symptoms and treatment of salicylate intoxication (salicylism)? Patients taking salicylates and a number of other drugs should be monitored closely for drug interactions. Name these other drugs.

84. Give the generic and trade names for aspirin. What type of a drug is acetylsalicylic acid? It is a most popular and effective drug for the relief of what kind of pain? What are some of its many uses? What is the usual dose of acetylsalicylic acid in mg and grains? Memorize this. What are some of the side effects of this drug, salicylates in particular? Explain what the following abbreviations mean and what drug or drugs each contains: Aspirin Compound, A.S.A., A. & C., A.P.C. Know these abbreviations and meanings well, since you may often administer these drugs and chart them.

85. What type of drug is indomethacin? Its mode of action is not fully known, but what is the theory for this action? Name several serious side effects. Why should other analgesics be used before administering this drug? What is the usual adult dose and what is the best time and method of administration? Discuss drug interactions in connection with this drug.

86. What type of analgesic is phenylbutazone (Butazolidin)? It is used for the symptomatic relief of what medical conditions? Name as many of the serious side effects as you can. What symptoms should you observe in patients taking this drug? How often should a blood examination be made and why? Is phenylbutazone a first-choice drug in the treatment of arthritis? Discuss drug interactions for this drug.

87. Ibuprofen (Motrin) is used in the treatment of what medical conditions? It may be used as a substitute for what drug?

Why? List some common side effects of ibuprofen. The drug should be used with caution in patients with a history of what disease? Drug interactions have not as yet been reported, but what are some possible reactions that may occur with drugs administered with ibuprofen?

88. Name three additional nonsteroid antiinflammatory agents indicated for the relief of rheumatoid arthritis.

89. **A helpful review suggestion:** Select a large piece of paper (tape several pieces together if necessary) wide enough and long enough for thirteen columns. Head the columns as follows:

Cerebrospinal stimulants	Tranquilizers
Cerebrospinal depressants	Nonsynthetic narcotic analgesics
Bromides	Synthetic narcotic analgesics
Alcohol	Narcotic antagonists
Parkinson's disease drugs	Nonnarcotic analgesics
Tricyclic antidepressants	Analgesic antipyretic and anti-
Anticonvulsants	inflammatory agents

Now go through the entire CNS drugs, selecting the proper ones and placing them in the correct column. Use key words or phrases beside each drug name, such as "mild to moderate pain," "addictive," "habit-forming," and "severe pain." Then study the drugs that belong in each group to help familiarize you with which drugs are narcotics, narcotic analgesics, nonnarcotic analgesics, tranquilizers, hypnotics, sedatives, and so on, also giving you a chief use or effect of the drug.

90. The physician orders the patient to receive 0.25 g of a drug orally. The medicine bottle label strength of each tablet in the bottle is 0.5 g. How many tablets will you give?

91. The physician orders the patient to receive 0.5 g of a drug orally. The medicine bottle label strength of each tablet in the bottle is 0.25 g. How many tablets will you give?

92. The physician orders the patient to receive 0.1 g of a drug orally. The bottle label strength of each tablet in the bottle is 100 mg. How many tablets will you give? *Remember:* this is a conversion problem. How do you convert from gram to milligram? (See Index for conversion.) How do you convert from milligram to gram, using this same problem?

CHAPTER 11

Drugs affecting the autonomic nervous system

The sympathetic nervous system can be considered an emergency protective system operating for mass response and the expenditure of large amounts of energy. The parasympathetic nervous system is a stabilizing force with functions that are constructive, conservative, creative, and reparative.

The autonomic nervous system is an efferent motor system. Efferent nerves conduct messages from the central portions of the nervous system to the periphery. The transmission of the impulse from one neuron to another takes place at a synapse, or junction. The peripheral synapses of the autonomic nervous system are found in groups of nerve cells, called ganglia, situated at the periphery. Preganglionic neurons conduct the impulse from the central nervous system to the peripheral ganglion; postganglionic neurons transmit the impulse from the ganglion to the effector organ.

Studies have shown that transmission of nerve impulses at myoneural junctions and synaptic connections occurs because of the activity of chemical substances called mediators. A mediator is liberated by the end of one nerve activating the next nerve in the chain or the smooth muscle, heart, or gland. These mediators are called acetylcholine and the catecholamines. The nerve fibers that synthesize and liberate acetylcholine are called *cholinergic* fibers, and the ones that synthesize and secrete norepinephrine (noradrenalin) are called *adrenergic* fibers.

Drugs that cause effects in the body similar to those produced by acetylcholine are called *cholinergic* drugs or, to use an older term, parasympathomimetic, because they seem to mimic the action produced by stimulation of the parasympathetic division of the autonomic nervous system. Drugs that cause effects similar to those produced by the adrenergic mediator are called *adrenergic,* or sympathomimetic, drugs.

Acetylcholine is important in transmission of nerve impulses in both the parasympathetic and the sympathetic divisions of the nervous system. It has two major actions on the autonomic nervous system: (1) stimulant effects at postganglionic nerve endings in cardiac muscle, smooth muscle, and glands and (2) stimulant effects on the ganglia, adrenal medulla, and skeletal muscle.

One theory is that acetylcholine is released by all postganglionic fibers and that the principal function of acetylcholine is to liberate norepinephrine, not to act directly. Another theory is that acetylcholine is involved at adrenergic nerve endings as an intermediary transmitter for the release of norepinephrine. Still another theory is that acetylcholine acts by making the fiber membrane permeable to calcium. The rise in calcium concentration within the fiber causes a release of norepinephrine.

Acetylcholine is released from the vagal nerve endings in the heart at the sinoatrial and atrioventricular nodes and the bundle of His. It slows the heart rate by inhibiting impulse formation and atrioventricular conduction, as well as by other methods. It is rapidly destroyed in the blood. The antagonist for acetylcholine is atropine.

CATECHOLAMINES

Epinephrine is a catecholamine. It was discovered in the mid-1940s that epinephrine had a twin called norepinephrine. These are separate substances that occur naturally in the body. Two more catecholamines have been identified: dopamine and isoproterenol (isoprenaline). Dopamine is a precursor of norepinephrine and epinephrine. Norepinephrine acts as a hormone, a transmitter of nerve impulses, and an intermediary in epinephrine formation. Epinephrine acts mainly as a hormone.

The catecholamines norepinephrine and epinephrine are neurohormones that serve important functions in neural and endocrine integration. They are synthesized in the sympathetic ganglia, in the brain, in nerve endings, and in the adrenal medulla. These two catecholamines are secreted into the circulation from the adrenal medulla. Norepinephrine is released locally as a neurotransmitter by sympathetic nerve endings. Norepinephrine and epinephrine influence the heart, liver, adipose tissue, vascular smooth muscle, and uterine muscle. The synthesis of norepinephrine is controlled by nervous impulses from the central nervous system. Norepinephrine increases myocardial contraction and heart rate, causes a rise in blood pressure, and is less likely to produce severe tachycardia, arrhythmias, and fibrillation than epinephrine. It has many effects similar to epinephrine.

Norepinephrine and epinephrine are continuously present in arterial blood. The amount varies widely during any one day. Physiologic stimuli such as stress and exercise definitely increase catecholamine blood levels. Most of the catecholamine secreted by the human adrenal medulla is norepinephrine. Only a small amount is epinephrine. Most epinephrine in the blood comes from the adrenal glands. The release of catecholamines from the adrenal gland probably occurs in spurts in response to proper stimuli. The greatest amount of catecholamines occurs in organs that receive a large fraction of blood and contain large numbers of sympathetic nerve endings, such as the heart and blood vessels.

The catecholamines are stored in specialized subcellular particles called granules, granulated vesicles, or storage granules. These storage granules take up dopamine from cytoplasm, oxidize it to norepinephrine, bind and store the norepinephrine to prevent its diffusion out of the cell and its destruction by enzymes, and release norepinephrine after proper physiologic stimuli.

Norepinephrine is a powerful vasoconstrictor, and this effect tends to impede coronary flow.

The autonomic nervous system controls function of all tissues with the exception of striated muscle. The word *autonomic* means self-governing; thus, the autonomic nervous system has also been called the involuntary nervous system because we have little or no control over it. The voluntary nervous system controls skeletal muscle, and we do have control of it.

The autonomic nervous system is composed of sympathetic and parasympathetic nerve systems. This system includes nerves of the body, nerve cell bodies in groups usually located outside the brain and spinal cord (ganglia), and networks of nerves that interlace or intertwine (plexus). This system regulates the heart, glands, digestion, respiration, circulation, and metabolism.

ADRENERGIC DRUGS

These drugs produce effects that are similar to the effects of epinephrine. Some adrenergic drugs that are discussed elsewhere are amphetamine sulfate, methamphetamine hydrochloride, isoproterenol hydrochloride, and mephentermine sulfate (see Index).

Dobutamine hydrochloride (do-byou′tah-meen)
Dobutrex (do′byou-treks)

1. Dobutamine is a synthetic catecholamine.
2. This drug has been found effective when parenteral therapy is necessary in the short-term treatment of adults with cardiac decompensation caused by depressed contractility resulting either from organic heart disease or from cardiac surgical procedures. Patients who have atrial fibrillation with rapid ventricular response should be given a digitalis preparation before therapy with dobutamine. Dobutamine facilitates atrioventricular conduction.
3. Both dobutamine and isoproterenol will increase the cardiac output to a similar degree for patients with depressed cardiac function. With dobutamine this increase is not accompanied by marked increases in heart rate, as is produced with isoproterenol. However, in about 10% of the cases a marked increase in heart rate and blood pressure, especially systolic, has been noted with dobutamine. Reduction of dosage or temporary termination is the suggested therapy.
4. This drug is contraindicated in patients with idiopathic hypertrophic subaortic stenosis.
5. Adverse reactions include increased heart rate, blood pressure elevation, and ventricular ectopic activity. A 10- to 20-mm increase in systolic pressure and an increase in heart rate of 5 to 15 beats per minute have been noted in most patients. In 1% to 3% of the patients the following adverse symptoms have been noted: nausea, anginal pain, headache, nonspecific chest pain, shortness of breath, and palpitations.
6. Treatment for adverse symptoms or overdosage: reduce the rate of administration or temporarily discontinue administration of dobutamine until the patient's condition stabilizes. Duration of action is short, so usually no other treatment is necessary.
7. During administration of dobutamine, as with any adrenergic drug, ECG and blood pressure should be continuously monitored. In addition, the physician should monitor pulmonary wedge pressure and cardiac output.
8. This drug is given intravenously and is reconstituted with Sterile Water for Injection, or 5% dextrose injection, and must be further diluted. It is an exact and complex process and should be done by your hospital pharmacist. Observe it if possible. Slight discoloration of the drug does not affect its potency. Do not mix with any other drug. The rate of infusion needed to increase cardiac output ranges from 2.5 to 10 μg/kg/min. Onset of action is 1 to 10 minutes.

Dopamine hydrochloride (do′pah-meen)
(Intropin) (in-tro′pin)

1. Dopamine may be used effectively as a selective vasodilator and vasoconstrictor. In low doses, dopamine selectively dilates blood vessels in the kidneys, abdomen, brain, and heart. In larger doses, dopamine may be effective in maintaining blood pressure by vasoconstriction. Dopamine is used in patients with shock resulting from myocardial infarction, trauma, renal failure, and infection.

2. It is administered by IV infusion diluted in dextrose 5% solution. Initial dose: 2.5 to 5 μg/kg/min. Maximum dose: 50 μg/kg/min.

Ephedrine (e-fed'rin)

1. Ephedrine is the name of an active principle found in the Ma Huang plant that has been used as a drug in China for several thousand years.
2. In addition to its adrenergic effects, it stimulates the central nervous system, primarily the cortex and medulla, but also the respiratory center.
3. It is used to control low blood pressure caused by some spinal anesthetics, and it aids in prolonging the effects of spinal anesthetics.
4. Ephedrine is useful in preventing acute attacks of bronchial asthma, although epinephrine is more effective because of its rapid action. It is also a common ingredient in both prescription and nonprescription nasal decongestants.
5. It may also be occasionally effective in the treatment of the muscle weakness of myasthenia gravis, but it is most effective for this purpose when combined with neostigmine methylsulfate.
6. Toxic doses may cause nervousness, dizziness, tremor, headache, insomnia, heart palpitation, and sweating. A barbiturate or some type of sedative is sometimes prescribed with ephedrine to counteract its central stimulating effect. Repeated administration brings diminished response. Tolerance develops, but the drug does not cause addiction.
7. It is available in the following forms:
   a. **Ephedrine sulfate capsules; ephedrine sulfate tablets.** Usual dose: 25 mg (gr $^3/_8$). It is available in 25 and 50 mg for oral administration.
   b. **Ephedrine sulfate injection.** Usual dose: 25 mg. This is available in 1-ml ampules containing 25 or 50 mg of drug in solution for injection.
   c. Local application is in the form of drops or sprays to shrink mucous membranes, in the form of aqueous solution, or as a jelly or ointment. A 1% to 3% solution is for nasal use. These are all salts of ephedrine.

Epinephrine (ep-i-nef'rin)
(Adrenalin) (ah-dren'ah-lin)

1. Epinephrine is one of the primary catecholamines of the autonomic nervous system. It is a powerful heart stimulant that increases heart rate and cardiac output. It is also a potent dilator of bronchial smooth muscle. It inhibits bronchial secretions and constricts pulmonary blood vessels, resulting in easier respiratory effort after allergic or asthmatic attacks.
2. Epinephrine constricts small arterioles and capillaries, making it useful for topical application in stopping bleeding from small vessels. Epinephrine is often added to local anesthetic solutions to delay their absorption from the site of injection by promoting local vasoconstriction. Epinephrine is such an intense vasoconstrictor, however, that it should not be applied to lacerations of the fingers, nose, penis, or toes. Tissue necrosis may result.
3. Common side effects of epinephrine include palpitations, tachycardia, tremor, weakness, and dizziness. Serious arrhythmias, angina pectoris, hypertension, and hypotension may also occur. Patients should be kept in a recumbent position until adverse effects have dissipated.
4. Products available and dosage:
   a. **Epinephrine injection 1:1,000.** Usual dose: 0.2 to 1 mg (0.2 to 1 ml) sc every 5 to 15 minutes as needed.
   b. **Epinephrine injection 1:10,000.** Usual dose: 0.2 to 1 mg (2 to 10 ml) IV every 5 to 15 minutes as needed.
   c. **Epinephrine aqueous suspension (sus-phrine).** Shake well. Initial adult dose: 0.5 mg (0.1 ml) subcutaneously. Do not inject intravenously.
5. Be extremely cautious of dosage calculations. Have prepared doses checked by team leader, head nurse, or instructor.

Isoproterenol (i-so-pro-te-re'nol)
(Isuprel Hydrochloride) (i'soo-prel)

1. Isoproterenol is a synthetic drug with potent cardiovascular properties. It has greater action in some respects than epinephrine. It is useful in shock.
2. Results of its many uses include increased stroke volume, cardiac output, cardiac work, and coronary flow.
3. Improved atrioventricular conduction and enhancement of the rhythmicity of the sinoatrial and ventricular pacemakers make it the drug of choice by many physicians for the treatment of atrioventricular heart block induced by digitalis.
4. Isoproterenol is a more powerful bronchodilator than epinephrine. It shrinks swollen mucous membranes and reduces mucous secretions, making it a useful drug in the treatment of bronchial asthma and pulmonary emphysema.
5. Side effects and toxic effects include precordial pain, heart palpitation, anginal pain (pain down one or both arms), headache, nausea, tremor, arrhythmias, flushing of the skin, and possible fall in arterial blood pressure.
6. Contraindications include insufficient coronary blood flow. Precautions are valvular stenosis and severe hypotension.
7. Isoproterenol and propranolol are antagonistic to

each other because of their opposite actions. The effects of isoproterenol are increased when used with nitroglycerin. When isoproterenol and digitalis preparations are given together, cardiac arrhythmias may develop. If the patient has a tachycardia resulting from digitalis toxicity, isoproterenol is contraindicated.

8. *Isoproterenol hydrochloride (Isuprel Hydrochloride)* is available in 10- and 15-mg sublingual tablets, solution for inhalation in concentrations of 1:100, 1:200, and 1:400, and as a solution for injection in 1:5,000 concentration.

9. *Isoproterenol sulfate (Norisodrine Sulfate)* (nor-is'o-dreen) is available in the form of a powder for inhalation, 10% and 25% solutions.

10. Isoproterenol may be given intravenously, 0.5 to 5 μg/min, in a continuous drip.

Naphazoline hydrochloride (naf-az'o-leen)
(Privine Hydrochloride) (pri'veen)

1. Naphazoline is a synthetic drug that shrinks mucous membranes of the nose in head colds, hay fever, asthma, other nasal congestion, and sinusitis.

2. It has prolonged action. If nasal irritation is experienced to a marked degree, a weaker solution may be used.

3. Naphazoline is available for adults and children. Adult dose: 2 drops of 0.05% solution in each nostril every 4 to 6 hours.

Norepinephrine (nor-ep-i-nef'rin)
(Levarterenol Bitartrate) (lev-ar-te-re'nol), *(Levophed)* (lev'o-fed)

1. Norepinephrine increases myocardial contraction and heart rate, but it is less likely to produce severe tachycardia, fibrillation, and arrhythmias than epinephrine. It can cause a reflex bradycardia.

2. It causes vasoconstriction, an increase in total peripheral resistance to blood flow, and a rise in blood pressure. It may be used to maintain blood pressure in hypotensive patients, in patients with hemorrhage, and during spinal anesthesia.

3. Many effects of norepinephrine are similar to those of epinephrine. However, norepinephrine is less effective than epinephrine in relieving bronchospasm, causing hyperglycemia, and inhibiting intestinal activity; oxygen consumption by the heart is increased to a lesser extent with norepinephrine than with epinephrine, and norepinephrine is a more powerful pressor agent than epinephrine. Its vasoconstricting effects are not as easily reversed with adrenergic blocking agents as are those of epinephrine.

4. Watch for overdosage by monitoring blood pressure. Check blood pressure every 2 minutes from beginning of treatment until desired blood pressure is maintained.

5. *Do not leave a patient alone while he is receiving this drug. It is powerful and dangerous.*

6. It is given intravenously in 5% glucose in distilled water. Average dose: 2 to 4 μg of base per minute.

Phenylephrine hydrochloride (fen-il-ef'rin)
(Neo-Synephrine Hydrochloride) (nee-o-sin-ef'rin)

1. Phenylephrine is a synthetic drug chemically related to epinephrine and ephedrine, but unlike ephedrine, it has little effect on the central nervous system. Its effects are longer lasting than those of epinephrine and ephedrine.

2. This drug is used primarily as a nasal decongestant, a mydriatic for examination of the fundus, and in the relief of paroxysmal atrial tachycardia.

3. It has few toxic effects and side actions.

4. It is available in IV form, oral form, nose drops, eye drops, and nose spray. Usual dose: nose drops, 0.25% to 1% solution in each nostril every 3 to 4 hours.

BETA BLOCKING AGENT
Propranolol (pro-pran'o-lol)
(Inderal) (in'der-al)

1. Propranolol is a drug that blocks the beta adrenergic receptors.

2. It inhibits cardiac response to sympathetic nerve stimulation by blocking the beta receptors. As a result, it slows the heart rate and has an antiarrhythmic effect, although most of the antiarrhythmic effect results from incidental quinidine-like action.

3. Uses of propranolol include the following:

   a. The drug has been found effective in the treatment of various ventricular arrhythmias. It inhibits atrioventricular conduction, thus slowing the ventricular rate.

   b. It also has been found effective in treating certain digitalis-induced arrhythmias. Caution must be used in producing severe bradycardia.

   c. Propranolol also has been found effective in the treatment of some cases of angina. It may act by preventing an increase in cardiac activity in response to exercise. Some patients treated with propranolol can take a greater amount of exercise before having anginal pain.

   d. Propranolol is beneficial in the long-term treatment of hypertension, although the mechanism of action is not fully known. It is generally used in combination with other antihypertensive agents.

   e. Propranolol is also being used experimentally to treat migraine headache.

4. Side effects include nausea, vomiting, lightheaded-

ness, mild burning, prickling, or numbing skin sensations, hallucinations, nightmares, insomnia, and lassitude.

5. Propranolol may produce hypoglycemia, particularly in patients with diabetes mellitus. Propranolol may also prevent the appearance of signs and symptoms (tachycardia, sweating) of acute hypoglycemia.

6. This drug must be used with extreme caution in patients with congestive heart failure, asthma, hypotension, and atrioventricular heart block.

7. Propranolol may be given orally or intravenously.
   a. Oral administration is most readily absorbed in the fasting state, so it should be given before meals. It is effective within 1 to 4 hours; duration of effect is about 6 hours. Usual oral dose: 30 to 120 mg daily. Much higher doses may be required in hypertension, however.
   b. With IV administration, maximum effects occur within 10 minutes. Range of dose: 1 to 5 mg. The drug *must* be given slowly (1 mg/min) and discontinued when a change of heart rate or rhythm is observed.

CHOLINERGIC DRUGS

Cholinergic drugs produce effects that are similar to those of acetylcholine. These effects include slowing of the heart, increased gastrointestinal peristalsis and secretion, increased contractions of the urinary bladder, sweating, increased power of contraction of skeletal muscle, and sometimes a rise in blood pressure. Some cholinergic drugs discussed elsewhere are neostigmine methylsulfate and bethanechol chloride (see Index).

Cholinergic drugs stimulate the intestines and bladder postoperatively, promote salivation, lower intraocular pressure in glaucoma, and dilate peripheral blood vessels in conditions of vasospasm.

Neostigmine methylsulfate (nee-o-stig′min)
(Prostigmin) (pro-stig′min)

1. Neostigmine is a synthetic drug of the autonomic nervous system useful in the treatment of postsurgical urinary retention and abdominal distention. It is also used in the symptomatic control of myasthenia gravis.

2. a. Usual dose for abdominal distention: 1 ml of the 1:4,000 solution (0.25 mg), subcutaneously or intramuscularly every 4 to 6 hours for 2 or 3 days postoperatively. Dose can be increased for abdominal distention to 1 ml of the 1:2,000 solution (0.5 mg), subcutaneously or intramuscularly, every 4 to 6 hours as required.
   b. Symptomatic control of myasthenia gravis: 1 ml of the 1:2,000 solution (0.5 mg) subcutaneously or intramuscularly. Dosage often must be based on the patient's response.

   c. Urinary retention: 1 ml of the 1:2,000 solution (0.5 mg), subcutaneously or intramuscularly. If urination does not occur within an hour, the patient should be catheterized. After the patient has voided or the bladder has been emptied, continue the 0.5 mg injections every 3 hours for at least five injections.

Pilocarpine hydrochloride (pi-lo-kar′pin)
Pilocarpine nitrate

1. The original source of pilocarpine was the leaf of *Pilocarpus jaborandi,* a South American plant. It is now produced synthetically.

2. Pilocarpine contracts the eye pupil (miosis) and increases tear secretion—it reduces tension within the eyeball. It is used to treat glaucoma, a disease of the eye in which there is increased tension and pressure within the eyeball.

3. It is sometimes used to treat corneal ulcer of the eye.

4. Pilocarpine increases secretions of glands controlled by parasympathetic nerves: saliva, sweat, and mucus in nose and bronchi.

5. It increases contraction of all involuntary muscles in stomach, intestines, bladder, uterus, and bronchi.

6. Average dose: when applied to the eye conjunctiva, 0.25% to 4% solution. Pilocarpine is available in 0.25%, 0.5%, 1%, 1.5%, 2%, 3%, 4%, 5%, 6%, 8%, and 10% solutions

Physostigmine salicylate (fi-so-stig′min)
(Eserine Salicylate) (es′er-in), (Antilirium) (an-til-eer′ee-um)

1. The source of physostigmine was originally an African seed called the Calabar bean.

2. Its main action is on the eye, skeletal muscle, and bowel.

3. It constricts the eye pupil and relieves intraocular tension in glaucoma.

4. It increases the tone and motility of the gastrointestinal tract and relieves gastric distention and postoperative gas pains.

5. Physostigmine may be effective as an antidote for reversing most of the cardiovascular and CNS effects of overdosage with tricyclic antidepressants and atropine.

6. Average dose: as an antidote, 2 mg intramuscularly or intravenously is administered. To treat eye diseases, including glaucoma, solutions varying from 0.25% to 0.5% are used.

ANTICHOLINERGIC DRUGS

Anticholinergic drugs block the effects of acetylcholine. Some anticholinergic drugs discussed elsewhere include trihexyphenidyl hydrochloride, methantheline bromide, and propantheline bromide (see Index).

Scopolamine hydrobromide (sko-pahl′ah-meen)
(Hyoscine; Hyoscine Hydrobromide) (hy′o-sin)

1. Scopolamine belongs to the atropine or belladonna group.
2. It acts similar to atropine in its effects on nerve endings, but it has a depressing effect on the brain, whereas atropine has a stimulating effect.
3. It causes little change in respirations, and it slows the heart, if given in small doses.
4. Morphine and scopolamine occasionally are combined for a single preanesthetic injection to quiet the patient and remove fear and apprehension.
5. Usual dose: topically, 0.2% solution; orally or hypodermically, 0.3 to 0.6 mg.

Atropine sulfate (at′ro-pin)

1. A number of plants belonging to the potato family contain similar alkaloids. Some of these plants are *Atropa belladonna* (deadly nightshade), Jimson weed or thorn apple, and several species of scopola. The principal alkaloids found in these plants are atropine, scopolamine (hyoscine), and hyoscyamine.
2. The name *Atropa belladonna* was given to one of these plants by Linnaeus in 1753. The first part of the name was chosen because of the poisonous qualities of the plant and was derived from Atropos, the eldest of the Greek Fates who was supposed to have cut the thread of life. Belladonna means beautiful lady; it was the custom of Roman women to place belladonna preparations in their eyes to make them appear larger and more lustrous.
3. Atropine and scopolamine resemble each other closely in effects and chemical structure.
4. Atropine is the prototype of the anticholinergic drugs and has been used for more than a half of a century. It is the chief alkaloid of the plant *Atropa belladonna,* which is grown for commercial purposes in Germany, Austria, America, and England. It is also synthesized.
5. Effects include the following:
   a. Atropine in aqueous solution dropped into the conjunctival sac of the eye quickly produces dilation of the pupil, diminished secretion of tears, and impaired ability to focus on objects close to the eyes. If the eye is normal, there is little change in intraocular tension, but it may increase the tension already existing in glaucoma.
      (1) The muscle of accommodation is paralyzed. The sphincter muscle of the iris and the ciliary muscle are both innervated by cholinergic nerve fibers and are therefore affected by atropine. Since the sphincter muscle cannot contract normally, the radial muscle of the iris causes the pupil to dilate.
      (2) Photophobia occurs after the pupil is dilated.

When the drug has reached its full effect, the usual reflexes to light and accommodation disappear.
      (3) Atropine and related alkaloids are usually contraindicated for patients with glaucoma for the reason in this discussion.
   b. Atropine is said to have a depressant effect on motor mechanisms that affect muscle tone and movement. This is the reason atropine and especially scopolamine have been used to lessen tremor in Parkinson's disease. The exact mechanism of this action is unknown.
   c. Therapeutic doses of atropine stimulate the respiratory center and make breathing faster and sometimes deeper. If respiration is seriously depressed, atropine may not be a reliable stimulant; it may even act as a depressant. Large doses stimulate respiration but can also cause respiratory failure and death.
      (1) Secretions of the nose, pharynx, and bronchial tubes are decreased, and the mucous membrane is made more dry. The muscles of the bronchial tubes relax, and the airway widens and aids breathing.
      (2) Atropine is especially useful as a preliminary medication before surgical anesthesia, for the reasons and effects just described.
   d. Small doses of atropine (0.1 to 0.4 mg) stimulate the vagus center in the medulla, causing primary slowing of the heart. The vasoconstrictor center is stimulated for a short period, then depressed. Because depression follows so soon after stimulation, atropine often has been called a borderline stimulant of the central nervous system.
      (1) Moderate to large doses (0.6 to 1 mg) accelerate the heart by interfering with the response of the heart muscle to vagal nerve impulses. This is a peripheral action.
      (2) Atropine's ability to interfere with vagal stimuli explains its use in the treatment of sinus bradycardia and atrioventricular heart block.
   e. Therapeutic doses have little or no effect on blood pressure. Large doses, and sometimes ordinary doses, cause vasodilation of vessels in the skin of the face and neck. This may result from histamine release or a direct dilator action, especially after large or toxic doses. Young children who are given atropine (or scopolamine) as a preanesthetic medication often have a pronounced flushing of the face and neck, which is a transient side effect.
   f. Atropine and other belladonna alkaloids decrease motility, tone, and peristalsis in the stomach and small and large intestines. Secretion of bile is not affected, but atropine does have a mildly antispasmodic effect in the gallbladder and bile ducts

and exerts a relaxing effect on the ureter, especially when it has been in spasm. Therapeutic doses decrease the tone of the fundus of the urinary bladder.

    g. Sweat gland activity is decreased or abolished by atropine. This causes the skin to become hot and dry. Dryness of the mouth, nose, pharynx, and bronchial mucous membranes occurs. Patients complain of dryness and thirst when given the drug preoperatively. Rinsing of the mouth may relieve the complaint.

6. Uses of atropine include the following:

    a. It may be given as a preoperative medication before surgical anesthesia (see Index).

    b. Atropine may be used as a mydriatic to dilate the pupil for eye examination and as a treatment for certain conditions of the eye. It is used especially for eye examination of children, whereas homatropine, a shorter-acting mydriatic, can be used for adults.

    c. Atropine is sometimes given with morphine to relieve biliary and renal colic. It tends to relieve the muscular spasm induced by morphine.

    d. It has antispasmodic effects in conditions such as pylorospasm, spastic colon, renal and biliary colic, and hypertonicity of the urinary bladder and ureters. In such conditions preparations of belladonna or its alkaloids are usually used.

    e. Preparations of belladonna or its derivatives also are found in certain cough remedies (antihistaminic mixtures) to relieve mild conditions of bronchial spasm and excessive secretions.

    f. Belladonna derivatives are sometimes used for the relief of painful menstruation.

    g. Symptoms such as tremor and possibly muscular rigidity of selected cases of Parkinson's disease are sometimes relieved by belladonna derivatives. Some synthetic anticholinergic drugs are thought to be superior to atropine for this use.

7. Atropine is a powerful alkaloid, but it has a wide margin of safety. Poisoning can occur. Typical symptoms of poisoning are dry mouth, great thirst, difficulty in swallowing and talking, blurred vision, dilated pupils, photophobia, rash (chiefly on face, neck, and upper trunk), elevation of temperature, rapid weak pulse, urinary urgency and difficulty in emptying the bladder, restlessness, excitement, talkativeness, confusion, giddiness, staggering, stupor, delirium, mania, coma, and respiratory and circulatory failure.

8. Treatment of overdosage includes a stomach lavage with activated charcoal slurry, if the atropine was taken by mouth, to inhibit further absorption of the drug. Physostigmine is sometimes given intravenously in life-threatening overdoses. Artificial respiration and oxygen may be necessary. If the patient is stuporous, cautious use of CNS stimulants is recommended. Ice bags aid in reducing the fever.

9. Preparations of atropine include the following:

    a. **Atropine sulfate tablets** containing 0.3, 0.4, and 0.6 mg are available. The drug is also available in multiple dose vials (0.1, 0.3, 0.4, 0.5, 0.6, 1.0, and 1.2 mg/ml) for injection and prefilled syringes for immediate use. Atropine sulfate is available in the form of atropine sulfate ophthalmic ointment. Atropine sulfate is usually administered orally, subcutaneously, or topically (in the eye). The usual subcutaneous or oral dose is 0.5 mg, although 0.4 mg often is ordered. The ophthalmic solution and the ointment are usually used in a 0.5% to 1% concentration.

    b. **Belladonna extract.** The extract is prepared from belladonna leaf and contains alkaloids of the leaf. It is given orally, usually in doses of 15 mg three or four times daily.

    c. **Belladonna tincture**

       (1) Tincture of belladonna, an autonomic nervous system drug, decreases gastrointestinal muscle tone and peristalsis and exerts a relaxing effect on the ureters (two tubes connecting the kidneys to the bladder). It has a mild antispasmodic effect on the gallbladder and the bile ducts and gives some degree of relaxation in muscle spasm of the bladder.

       (2) It may be given to patients with peptic ulcer to decrease secretions of the stomach and therefore to relieve ulcer pain.

       (3) Toxic symptoms that should be watched for include dry throat, dilated pupils, dim vision, and possible body rash.

       (4) Belladonna is a form of atropine.

       (5) Usual dose: 0.6 ml. Dose can be increased gradually, so that it may vary between 0.3 and 2.4 ml.

Dicyclomine hydrochloride (di-si'klo-meen) (Bentyl) (ben'til)

1. Dicyclomine is said to relieve smooth muscle spasm of the gastrointestinal tract.

2. It may be useful in conditions such as irritable colon, spastic colon, mucous colitis, gastrointestinal disorders, acute enterocolitis, neurogenic bowel and colon, and splenic flexure syndrome.

3. It is contraindicated in bladder neck obstruction resulting from prostatic hypertrophy, obstructive uropathy, obstructive diseases of the gastrointestinal tract

such as pyloroduodenal stenosis, paralytic ileus, intestinal atony of elderly or debilitated patients, severe ulcerative colitis, unstable cardiovascular status in acute hemorrhage, and myasthenia gravis. In very hot climates heat prostration (fever and heat stroke) can occur with this drug use because of decreased sweating.

4. Usual dose: one or two capsules or teaspoonfuls of the syrup three or four times daily. It is available in capsules, tablets, syrup, and prefilled syringe for injection.

Donnatal (don'nah-tahl)

1. Donnatal, a gastrointestinal antispasmodic drug, is a mixture of atropine, hyoscyamine, hyoscine, and phenobarbital.
2. It is effective in treating hypertonic and spastic conditions, peptic ulcer, gastrointestinal spasm such as pylorospasm, gastritis (inflammation of the stomach), colitis (inflammation of the colon or large intestine), biliary colic (spasm of the gallbladder, hepatic ducts, common bile duct, and cystic duct), genitourinary tract and renal (kidney) spasm, motion sickness, and Parkinson's disease (palsy).
3. Contraindications include glaucoma, advanced renal or hepatic disease, or hypersensitivity to any of the drug's ingredients.
4. Side effects include dry mouth, blurred vision, flushing, dry skin, and painful urination.
5. Usual dose: two tablets or teaspoonfuls of the elixir with meals and at bedtime, adjusting the dosage as necessary.

Homatropine hydrobromide (ho-mat'ro-pin) (Isoptohomatropine)

1. Homatropine is a synthetic alkaloid of atropine.
2. Homatropine is used mainly in place of atropine to dilate the pupil. The pupil dilates and returns to normal size more quickly when homatropine is used.
3. Usual dose: 1% to 2% aqueous solution, or 5 drops of a 1:500 solution, given a drop at a time about every 5 minutes. Complete dilation of the pupil occurs in about 45 minutes.

Mepenzolate bromide (me-pen' zo-late) (Cantil) (kan' til)

1. This drug is a postganglionic, parasympathetic inhibitor. Mepenzolate diminishes gastric acid secretion and suppresses spontaneous contractions and spasm of the colon.
2. It is probably effective for use as adjunctive therapy in peptic ulcer, irritable bowel syndrome, splenic flexure syndrome, and the neurogenic colon.

3. Mepenzolate may possibly be effective in the treatment of mild ulcerative colitis, diverticulitis, and several forms of diarrhea, such as functional, postgastrectomy, drug-induced, diarrheas with ileostomies, and diarrhea in acute enteritis, intestinal viral infection, and colitis.
4. Contraindications include obstructions of the gastrointestinal tract, glaucoma, obstructive uropathy such as bladder neck obstruction, paralytic ileus, severe ulcerative colitis, intestinal atony in the elderly or debilitated, acute hemorrhage, and myasthenia gravis. The drug is to be used with caution in cases of hyperthyroidism, congestive heart failure, coronary heart disease, hypertension, cardiac arrhythmias, complications of biliary tract disease, and any tachycardia.
5. Adverse reactions include blurred vision, dilation of the pupil, cycloplegia, dryness of the mouth, increased ocular tension, urinary hesitancy and retention, palpitations, tachycardia, loss of taste, headache, nervousness, weakness, drowsiness, insomnia, dizziness, nausea, vomiting, impotency, constipation, bloated feeling, severe allergic reactions, including anaphylaxis and urticaria, mental confusion, or excitement, especially in elderly persons.
6. Drug interactions: concomitant administration of anticholinergic drugs and any other drugs that would increase the anticholinergic effects of mepenzolate should be avoided.
7. Usual adult dose: one or two tablets three times a day, preferably with meals, and one or two tablets at bedtime. Each tablet contains 25 mg mepenzolate.

Methantheline bromide (me-than'the-lin) (Banthine Bromide) (ban'thyn)

1. Banthine is an autonomic nervous system drug effective in the treatment of peptic ulcer and hypertrophic gastritis, or inflammation of the stomach.
2. It lessens excess movements of the stomach and reduces hyperacidity, which almost always accompanies peptic ulcer.
3. It also is used in the treatment of chronic and acute pancreatitis (inflammation of the pancreas) and diverticulitis (an inflammation in the small outpouchings of the colon). These may be acquired or congenital.
4. Banthine also is used to relieve genitourinary spasm and is sometimes used to control salivation, such as during dental surgery.
5. It may cause blurring vision, dryness of the mouth, and gastric fullness.
6. Usual dose: 50 to 100 mg orally approximately every 6 hours throughout the day and night. It is available for IM and IV injection, but oral administration is preferred whenever possible.

Propantheline bromide (pro-pan'the-leen)
(Pro-Banthine Bromide)

1. The action of Pro-Banthine is similar to that of Banthine.
2. It has fewer side effects or toxic reactions in some persons.
3. It should not be given to patients with glaucoma or to elderly patients with enlarged prostates.
4. Usual dose: 15 mg with meals and 30 mg orally at bedtime. The dose can be increased if necessary. It is available in IV and IM forms.

Methscopolamine bromide (meth-sko-pol'ah-min)
(Pamine Bromide) (pah'meen)

1. Pamine, an autonomic nervous system drug, inhibits gastric secretion and decreases acidity. It also decreases gastrointestinal motility, reducing tone and peristaltic activity. This may cause constipation.
2. It is useful as an aid in the treatment of peptic ulcer and gastric disorders associated with hyperacidity and hypermotility and in the treatment of excessive sweating and excessive salivation.
3. A common side effect is dryness of the mouth. This may be overcome to some degree by the use of chewing gum. Blurred vision may occur, restricting patients from operating machinery and automobiles. Rarely observed are dizziness, skin dryness or flushing, drowsiness, or nausea.
4. This drug should be used with caution, if at all, for patients with pyloric obstruction, prostatic hypertrophy, or glaucoma.
5. Usual dose: 2.5-mg tablets orally 30 minutes before meals and at bedtime.

• • •

Other autonomic nervous system drugs discussed elsewhere in this text are **phenoxybenzamine hydrochloride (Dibenzyline), ergotamine tartrate,** and such cholinergic drugs as **bethanechol chloride (Urecholine Chloride).** See Index.

**The physician prescribes the medicine and treatment.
The nurse carries out the physician's orders.
Self-medication is dangerous. Consult your physician first.
There is in every medicine a possible danger.
When in doubt—ASK!**

ASSIGNMENT

Review previous lessons and questions according to the direction of your instructor.

1. The autonomic nervous system is an efferent motor system. What do efferent nerves do? What do the following do and where are they found: peripheral synapses, preganglionic neurons, and postganglionic neurons? How does transmission of nerve impulses at myoneural junctions and synaptic connections occur? Define mediator. Name two mediators. What are the nerve fibers that synthesize and liberate acetylcholine called? What are the nerve fibers that synthesize and secrete norepinephrine (noradrenalin) called? What are drugs that cause effects in the body similar to those produced by acetylcholine called (both names)? What are drugs that cause effects similar to those produced by the adrenergic mediator called (both names)?
2. Explain the three theories concerning the action of acetylcholine.
3. Name four catecholamines discussed and tell the important action of each.
4. Several of these choices are correct. Dobutamine (Dobutrex)
   a. Is a synthetic catecholamine
   b. Is a synthetic acetylcholine
   c. Has been found effective in the short-term treatment of adults with cardiac decompensation caused by depressed contractility resulting either from cardiac surgical procedures or organic heart disease
   d. Should not be used if the patient has cardiac decompensation
   e. Is effective for patients who have atrial fibrillation with rapid ventricular response, but a digitalis preparation should be given before dobutamine therapy
   f. Decreases cardiac output
   g. Is a powerful drug, so ECG and blood pressure should be continuously monitored during its administration
   h. Is given intravenously and should not be mixed with any other drug
   i. Has as an onset of action 1 to 2 to 10 minutes
5. List the contraindication and adverse reactions of dobutamine.
6. What type of drug is dopamine (Intropin)? What effect does dopamine have on blood vessels and where in the body? What is the chief use of dopamine, and how is it administered?

7. What is the source of ephedrine? What effect does it have on the central nervous system? On the respiratory center? List two of its chief uses. What symptoms may occur in toxic doses?

8. See how many correct choices you can find for this question. Epinephrine
   a. Is one of the primary catecholamines of the autonomic nervous system
   b. Is a powerful heart depressant useful in slowing the heart rate and decreasing cardiac output
   c. Is a powerful heart stimulant and increases heart rate and cardiac output
   d. Is a potent dilator of bronchial smooth muscle, inhibits bronchial secretions, and constricts pulmonary blood vessels, resulting in easier respiratory effort after allergic or asthmatic attacks
   e. Dilates blood vessels and so may increase capillary bleeding
   f. Is often added to local anesthetic solutions to delay absorption from the site of injection by promoting local vasoconstriction
   g. Is such an effective vasoconstrictor that it can be applied to lacerations of fingers and toes to stop bleeding

9. List common side effects of epinephrine. Why should prepared doses be checked by your instructor, team leader, or head nurse? Remember, for checking dose, have ready medicine card, bottle from which you withdrew the dosage, and syringe containing this medication.

10. What is the source for isoproterenol (Isuprel)? List several of its many uses. Which is the more powerful bronchodilator, epinephrine or isoproterenol? What effect does isoproterenol have on swollen mucous membranes and mucous secretions, which makes it a useful drug in the treatment of what medical conditions? List the side and toxic effects of isoproterenol. Discuss drug interaction and isoproterenol.

11. What is the source of naphazoline (Privine)? What effect does it have on the mucous membranes and for what conditions is it effective?

12. Several choices are correct in this question. Norepinephrine (Levophed)
    a. Lessens myocardial contraction and heart rate and reduces blood pressure
    b. Is powerful and dangerous, so the patient should not be left alone during administration of this drug
    c. Increases myocardial contractions and heart rate and is less likely to produce severe tachycardia, fibrillation, and arrhythmias than epinephrine
    d. Causes vasoconstriction, an increase in total peripheral resistance to blood flow, rise in blood pressure, and may be used to maintain blood pressure in hypotensive patients, patients with hemorrhage, and during spinal anesthesia
    e. Causes vasodilation and a definite lowering of blood pressure
    f. Is less effective than epinephrine in relieving bronchospasm, causing hyperglycemia, and inhibiting intestinal activity
    g. Is not as powerful a pressor agent as epinephrine

    h. Has as a sign of overdosage a sudden lowering of blood pressure

13. Phenylephrine hydrochloride (Neo-Synephrine) is a synthetic drug chemically related to which two drugs? What is its effect on the central nervous system? Are its effects of shorter or longer duration than the effects of epinephrine and ephedrine? List the main uses of phenylephrine. What is the usual dose for nose drops?

14. To which group does propranolol (Inderal) belong? To which drug is it chemically related? What effect does it have on the heart? Explain the main uses of this drug. List its side effects and contraindications. This drug must be used with extreme caution in what types of conditions? Describe methods of administration, onset of effect, and duration of effect.

15. What is meant by cholinergic drugs? In general, what is their effect on various parts of the body? Give the generic and trade names of two cholinergic drugs. Explain their chief effects and uses. What is the source of each of the two drugs discussed as cholinergics?

16. What are the main uses of neostigmine methylsulfate (Prostigmin)? What is the usual dose for abdominal distention? What is the usual dose for symptomatic control of myasthenia gravis? Describe the treatment and dosage for urinary retention.

17. State the source of pilocarpine. What effect does it have on the eye pupil? Pilocarpine is used to treat what two medical conditions? What effect does it have on glands controlled by parasympathetic nerves? What effect does it have on all involuntary muscles in the stomach, intestines, bladder, uterus, and bronchi? What is the average dose when applied to the eye conjunctiva?

18. What is the source of physostigmine salicylate? What are its main effects on the eye, skeletal muscle, and bowel? Physostigmine may be effective as an antidote for what conditions if caused by what two drugs?

19. What effect do anticholinergic drugs have? Give three examples of anticholinergic drugs.

20. Scopolamine hydrobromide (Hyoscine) belongs to what drug group? It acts similar to which drug in its effects on nerve endings? What effect does this drug have on the brain? Is this effect similar, or in contrast, to the effect of atropine? Why are morphine and scopolamine sometimes combined for a single preanesthetic injection? What is the usual dose hypodermically?

21. Several of these choices are correct. Atropine
    a. Is an alkaloid and belongs to the potato family
    b. Has as its name the potato family plant it comes from, *Atropa belladonna* (deadly nightshade), and is the chief alkaloid of the plant
    c. In effect and chemical structure resembles scopolamine very little
    d. Can now be synthesized
    e. Causes the pupil to contract
    f. Is used chiefly in the treatment of glaucoma to decrease or relieve the tension in the eye
    g. Is said to have a depressant effect on motor mechanisms that affect muscle tone and movement and will lessen tremors in Parkinson's disease

h. In therapeutic doses stimulates the respiratory center and makes breathing faster and sometimes deeper, but if respiration is seriously depressed, atropine may not be a reliable stimulant and may even act as a depressant

i. Is the specific drug to use to stimulate the respiratory center because of its sustained and consistent stimulant effect

j. Decreases secretions of the nose, pharynx, and bronchial tubes, dries mucous membranes, and relaxes the muscles of the bronchial tubes that aid breathing, making the drug very useful as a preliminary medication before anesthesia

k. Has the ability to interfere with vagal stimuli, which explains its use in the treatment of sinus bradycardia and atrioventricular heart block

l. Dilates the pupil for eye examinations for a temporary period, especially in children, and produces an impaired temporary ability to focus on objects close to the eyes

m. Has a spasmodic effect on the stomach and intestines, increasing motility, tone, and peristalsis

22. As a good review question of this most important and often used drug, list the many uses of atropine and learn them well.

23. Poisoning from atropine is rare in therapeutic doses but can occur. List the symptoms and treatment. Name three atropine preparations and tell the chief use for each. What are the effects and usual doses of belladonna extract and belladonna tincture? What effect does belladonna tincture have on peptic ulcer? What is the usual dose of belladonna tincture? Can the dose be increased? How?

24. Dicyclomine hydrochloride (Bentyl) has what effect on the smooth muscle of the gastrointestinal tract? It may be useful in treating what conditions? List the contraindications for this drug. What is the usual dose of Bentyl and how often daily is it administered?

25. Donnatal is what type of drug? It is a mixture of what drugs? List the conditions for which Donnatal may be effective. List the contraindications and the side effects for this drug. What is the usual dose, and how often daily is it given?

26. What is the source of homatropine? What is its chief use? What is the advantage of homatropine over atropine in its use in the eye for eye examinations?

27. What effect does mepenzolate bromide (Cantil) have on gastric acid secretion and on the colon? Name the conditions for which mepenzolate (Cantil) is probably effective? List the contraindication for this drug. List adverse reaction for Cantil. Discuss drug interactions in connection with this drug. What is the usual dose?

28. List the main uses of Banthine and Pro-Banthine. Does Banthine increase or decrease salivation? List several side effects of these two drugs. What are the advantages of Pro-Banthine compared to Banthine? What are contraindications in the use of both drugs? What is the action of both drugs? What is the usual dose of each drug?

29. What are the main uses of Pamine? What is its generic name? List some common side effects of this drug. Pamine should be used with caution in what medical conditions?

30. Review, using your Index, some of the additional drugs of the autonomic nervous system mentioned at the close of this chapter and discussed elsewhere in your text. Which are cholinergics, and which are anticholinergics?

31. The physician orders the patient to receive 1.5 g of a drug in oral tablet form. The medicine bottle label strength is 0.5 g. How many tablets will you administer?

32. The physician orders the patient to receive 0.250 g of a drug in oral tablet form. The medicine bottle label strength is 250 mg. How many tablets will you administer? *Remember:* this is a *conversion* problem. Convert from grams to milligrams. Then try converting from milligrams to grams, using the same problem. (See conversion in the Index for help in working this problem.)

CHAPTER 12

Drug abuse

During the past two decades there has been an alarming increase in drug abuse by people of all ages. The drug problem is a total community concern and should not be the sole responsibility of law enforcement officers, teachers, or professional workers. Parents have a responsibility to be informed and to be able to discuss the drug problems with their children. Both parents and children should be alert to recognize signs and symptoms of the drug and the drug user. Information about drug abuse and determination to control the use of these dangerous drugs could be a strong influence in assisting children, teenagers, and adults to avoid involvement with drug abuse.

Since far back in history man has turned to drugs in his search for relief from physical and psychosocial problems. Drug abuse refers to self-medication or self-administration of a drug in chronically excessive quantities, which results in psychic or physical dependence, functional impairment, or deviation from approved social norms.

In the abuse of consciousness-altering drugs there are two types of drug dependence: psychic and physical. Psychic dependence, ranging from mild desire to "craving" or compulsive use, is an emotional reliance on a drug in order to maintain the drug-induced state the psychically dependent individual prefers. Physical dependence on a drug can be demonstrated only by production of a withdrawal syndrome. This syndrome can be relieved by readministering the drug or by administration of a pharmacologically related drug.

There are three major categories of commonly abused drugs. These are central nervous system depressants, central nervous system stimulants, and mind-altering drugs (hallucinogens).

Cannabis drugs (marijuana, or marihuana, hashish), opiates, ethyl alcohol, barbiturates, and minor tranquilizers act as CNS depressants. All of these are likely to lead to physical or psychic dependence. All except *cannabis* cause withdrawal symptoms on discontinuation after long-term use.

Amphetamines, cocaine, and hallucinogenic agents such as LSD, mescaline, phencyclidine, and psilocybin act as CNS stimulants. None, so far as is known, produces physical dependence, and none causes withdrawal symptoms following discontinuance of the drug. Strong psychologic dependence is often evident.

The depressant opiates (heroin, opium, morphine, codeine, meperidine, alphaprodine, and others), ethyl alcohol, barbiturates, and minor tranquilizers such as meprobamate (Equanil, Miltown), diazepam (Valium), and chlordiazepoxide (Librium) have been discussed in previous chapters (see Index). One depressant drug not as yet discussed is marijuana.

CENTRAL NERVOUS SYSTEM DEPRESSANTS

Tetrahydrocannabinol (THC) (tet-rah-hi-dro-kah-nab'i-nol), *(Marijuana, Marihuana)* (mar-i-wahn'ah)

1. It is perhaps inadequate to describe marijuana solely as a depressant because it possesses properties of a euphoriant, sedative, and hallucinogen.
2. The botanical name for the plant is *Cannabis sativa*. It is also known as devil weed, Indian hemp, Mary Jane, and grass.
3. A slang term often heard is the word hash. It is a term used for the substance known as *hashish*, which is the resin of the marijuana plant. The term *hashish* is derived from Hasan ibn al-Sabbah, the old man of the mountain of the eleventh century and leader of religious and political ideas. He used the drug to induce and maintain his hold over his followers. Hashish contains the physiologically active element, THC, and can be referred to as concentrated marijuana. The substance is usually dark brown in color and comes in powder form or is compressed in small squares or balls.
4. Marijuana grows over the entire world, but the potency of the plant depends to some extent on where it is grown. The most potent marijuana is grown in parts of tropical countries such as India, Africa, and Mexico. The plant is a stout, erect annual ranging in height from 4 to 20 feet. The leaves are found at the end of its branches and are always odd in number. Tops of the leaves are light green, bottoms a duller green; edges of the leaves are saw-

toothed. Fibers from the stem (or "trunk") are still used commercially to produce hemp rope.

5. Marijuana leaves are usually dried and smoked.
   a. The most common way is in a cigarette form, or "joint." The user inhales the smoke deeply into the lungs and holds it there as long as possible before exhaling, in order not to waste the euphoric effect. Often, one cigarette is lighted at a time and passed from person to person in a group of people to obtain the maximum effect of the smoke.
   b. "Roach clips" are used to smoke the entire cigarette to the end without burning the fingers. These clips can be any device to hold the cigarette, such as an alligator clip or a large bobby pin. A "crutch" can be any small piece of cardboard, such as a matchbook cover, that is wrapped around the butt, or "roach."
   c. Water pipes, or "hooka" pipes of Eastern origin, as well as conventional pipes, are also used.

6. Ways in which marijuana is sold include:
   a. Cigarette, or "joint." A hand-rolled cigarette is made of dried and crushed marijuana leaves, using common white or wheat straw cigarette papers.
   b. Matchbox. This is exactly what it implies—a small matchbox full of crushed marijuana.
   c. Lid. A lid of marijuana is about 1 ounce of the dried, crushed leaves. The term *lid* or *tin* comes from the practice many years ago of selling marijuana in a well-known tobacco container closed by a metal lid. Today, about the same amount of marijuana is wrapped in an ordinary plastic sandwich bag.
   d. Kilo. The term kilo, key, or brick is an abbreviation for a kilogram (2.2 pounds) in dry weight of marijuana. It is most commonly packed in brick form, compressed to an approximate size of 4 by 8 inches. It is in this form that marijuana is transported or sold in large quantities. The weights and qualities of the drug vary greatly since there are no supervising governing agents and no regulation of ethics among drug peddlers.

7. The immediate physiologic effects of marijuana use include an increase in pulse rate, some loss in limb coordination, abnormal lowering of body temperature, increased hunger, and inflammation of bronchial tubes and mucous membranes.

8. Psychologic effects include exhilaration of mood, fantasy, the feeling of being above reality, space disorientation, loss of timing, hilarity over something that may not be particularly amusing to a nonuser, extremely vivid hallucinations (when larger doses are used), panic, unreasonable fear of death, delusions, and periods of paranoia. For most individuals a "high" from use of marijuana is pleasurable; and for others it can be a fearful experience, depending on the mood of the individual or the group of smokers. Whether a "trip" is pleasurable or fearful, there may be memory loss, erratic behavior, a distorted sense of space and time, and the possibility of becoming accident-prone, risking injury to self and others.

9. Marijuana users tend to become advocates of the drug among nonusers. Effects of the drug are not predictable and depend on the psychologic susceptibility of the user. There is mind disorientation, impaired perception, and uncoordination. A few users tend to be emotionally unstable and can be unpredictably violent. Their personal habits and appearance may deteriorate. They may withdraw from family life, have little respect for authority and discipline, and have little self-discipline. Their attitude toward school and work may be "so what," and their behavior may be furtive and questionable.

10. The drug is the center of much confusion and controversy. Prominent people in politics, education, and the arts are outspoken in their emotional support of legalizing its use and are urging social acceptance on the same terms as tobacco and alcohol. Others are attempting to reduce the crime of possession from felony to the lesser charge of misdemeanor.

11. Several researchers who have specialized in the study of these hallucinogens and the study and care of addicts using these drugs have these opinions to present:
   a. With a drug such as marijuana, with potency varying from batch to batch and reaction varying from user to user and from time to time in an individual, the fact of unpredictability must be given most serious consideration in any attempt to legalize its use.
   b. There are many differences between the effects of tobacco and marijuana. Tobacco has no apparent effect on emotional and mental responses, but marijuana does. The harmful effects of tobacco only affect the user, but the uncertain behavior of a marijuana user may endanger not only himself but others as well.

12. It will be of interest to note what the future brings in regard to the legal possibilities in the use of this drug. In recent years one philosophy regarding the effects of marijuana smoking is that its dangers have been exaggerated and the laws regarding marijuana smoking should be lightened, allowing its use in small amounts with guests in the privacy of the home. Meanwhile, the controversies regarding effects and laws concerning marijuana continue.

CENTRAL NERVOUS SYSTEM STIMULANTS
Amphetamine (am-fet′ah-min)

1. The amphetamines produce an elevation of mood, a reduction of fatigue, invigorating aggressiveness, and a sense of increased alertness. Amphetamines do not create extra mental and physical energy. On the contrary, they promote expenditure of present resources, sometimes to a dangerous point of fatigue that is often unrecognized.
2. Intravenous injection causes marked euphoria, a sensation or feeling known as a "flash" or "rush," a sense of great physical strength and capacity, and a sense of sharp, clear thinking.
3. The user feels little or no need for food, sleep, or rest, and may continually engage in vigorous activity. To the observer, this activity may seem an inefficient, stereotyped, and repetitious behavior common during an amphetamine "high."
4. Discontinuation of the drug is followed by long periods of sleep, and on awakening, hunger, lethargy, and profound depression, occasionally ending in suicide attempts.
5. The stimulant properties of amphetamines can cause marked cardiorespiratory effects, such as dyspnea, tachycardia, and chest pain.
6. Amphetamines do not appear to lead to physical dependence, although psychic dependence is well documented. Tolerance to amphetamines can occur.
7. For further discussion of specific amphetamines, see Index.

Cocaine (ko′kayn)

1. Cocaine is used largely as a local anesthetic (see Anesthetics, local, in the Index).
2. When used for its stimulant effects, it produces euphoria and increased expenditure of energy similar to the action of amphetamines.
3. Cocaine may be administered by sniffing the white, fluffy powder that resembles snow, hence the name "snow," or by injection.
4. Chronic use may cause nausea, weight loss, gastrointestinal disturbances, insomnia, twitching or spasm of muscles, or convulsions. Prolonged sniffing may result in vasoconstriction and perforation of the nasal septum.
5. Physical dependence does not seem characteristic of cocaine abuse, but strong psychologic dependence does.

HALLUCINOGENS
Lysergic acid diethylamide (LSD) (li-serg′ik as′id di-eth-il′ah-myd)

1. This is a powerful man-made chemical generally called "acid" or LSD. A single ounce is enough to provide 300,000 average doses.
2. It was first developed in 1938 from one of the ergot alkaloids. Ergot is a fungus that grows as a rust on rye, a common grain plant.
3. LSD has been tested widely as a possible treatment for mental and emotional illnesses and for alcoholism, but no usefulness has been established.
4. The drug is legally classed as a hallucinogen—a mind-affecting drug.
5. The hallucinogen seems to affect the levels of certain chemicals in the brain and to produce changes in the brain's electric activity. Exactly how LSD works in the body is not yet known.
6. According to animal experiments with LSD, the brain's normal filtering and screening process becomes blocked, causing it to become flooded with unselected sights and sounds.
7. LSD is noted mainly for producing strong and bizarre mental reactions in people and causing marked distortions in their physical senses: what and how they see, touch, smell, and hear. All effects are apparently reversible. However, the user may have "flashbacks" that are uncontrollable as to when and where they occur.
8. An average dose may last for about 8 to 10 hours. It can be taken in a sugar lump, a cracker, or a cookie, licked off a stamp impregnated with the drug, or taken in other ways.
9. Physiologically, it increases the pulse and heart rate and causes a rise in blood pressure and temperature, dilated pupils, shaking of the hands and feet, flushed face or pallor, cold, sweaty palms, tightness in the chest and abdomen, shivering, chills, irregular breathing, nausea, loss of appetite, and increased salivation.
10. Psychologic effects include the following:
    a. First effects are likely to be sudden changes in the user's physical senses:
       (1) Walls may appear to move.
       (2) Colors seem stronger and more brilliant.
       (3) Unusual patterns are seen.
       (4) Flat objects seem to stand out in three dimensions.
       (5) Taste, smell, hearing, and touch seem more acute.
    b. One sensory impression may be translated or merged into another: music may appear as a color; colors may seem to have a taste.
    c. A most confusing yet common reaction is the feeling of two strong and opposite emotions at the same time. For example, a user can feel both happy and sad at the same time, or elated and depressed, or tense and relaxed. Arms and legs may feel both heavy and light.
    d. The normal feeling of boundaries between body

and space are lost. This sometimes gives the user the impression that he can fly or float with ease or step in front of a speeding automobile without harm.

e. Effects can be different at different times in the same individual. Responses to the drug cannot be predicted. It is this reason that users refer to "bad trips" or "good trips" to describe their experience with this drug.

f. There may be loss of a sense of time, although the user remains conscious.

g. The LSD user can usually remember much of what happened to him after the drug wears off.

h. Creativity is *not* increased with LSD's use; it often is noticeably poorer than before use of the drug.

i. Many medical authorities think that chronic or continued use of LSD changes values, impairs the user's ability to think, and weakens powers of concentration.

j. Medical authorities emphasize that the overwhelming sense of worry and fear that can accompany the LSD experience is sometimes disturbing enough to cause acute and even long-lasting mental illness.

11. Summary of dangers in the use of LSD:

a. Panic—the user may grow frightened because he cannot stop the drug's action. He may fear he is losing his mind.

b. Paranoia—the user may become increasingly suspicious, feeling that someone is trying to harm him or control his thinking.

c. Recurrence—the things the user saw and felt while on the drug may recur days, weeks, or even months after taking LSD ("flashback").

d. Accidental death—the user may cause himself bodily harm because of a sense of detachment and the conviction that he is magically in control.

12. The drug is *not* physically addicting, as are the narcotics; the body does not develop a physical need for LSD or physical sickness when it is withdrawn.

13. Reasons why healthy people take LSD include:

a. Curiosity

b. "For kicks"

c. "To understand myself better"

d. In quest of religious or philosophic insights

e. Emotional problems and inability to cope with life's problems

14. Hopefully the drug's popularity may decrease as its potential ill effects become better known.

15. Use of LSD is closely regulated by the Drug En-forcement Agency of the Justice Department. The law provides strict penalties for anyone who illegally possesses, produces, sells, or distributes such drugs as LSD. Conviction can bring heavy fines of several thousand dollars and imprisonment of several years.

Mescaline (mes'kah-lin)

1. Mescaline is the chief alkaloid extracted from the peyote cactus.

2. It produces hallucinogenic effects similar to LSD.

3. The usual dose is about 500 mg. The effects appear within 2 or 3 hours and may last 4 to 12 hours or longer.

4. Initial effects may be characterized by prodromal abdominal pain, nausea, vomiting, and diarrhea but are followed by vivid and colorful visual hallucinations.

Psilocybin (si-lo-si'bin)

1. This is a drug derived from Mexican mushrooms.

2. Effects produced are similar to those of mescaline but are of shorter duration.

THE NURSE'S ROLE

1. The nurse must relate to and treat the whole patient in a nonjudgmental way.

2. A knowledge of mind-altering drugs is essential to the nurse in the course of the patient's treatment and the education of the patient, the patient's family and friends, and the community.

3. The nurse has a responsibility in identifying persons who are dependent on drugs in order that she may refer them to appropriate sources for help. She should be aware of such signs as needle marks and scars of abscesses along intravenous routes, pupillary dilation or constriction, striking changes in personality, interest patterns, and social relations, the presence of some drugs in the blood or urine, and other symptoms already described in this chapter. Conclusive evidence of drug abuse is the appearance of withdrawal symptoms.

4. The nurse is often called on to give nonjudgmental nursing care and support to the patient receiving drug withdrawal treatment. When withdrawal of the drug is completed, the nurse must be consciously aware that treatment is *not* completed. Continued nonjudgmental friendly care, firm support and encouragement, and discussion of emotional problems and how to solve them are vital, or relapse into the abuse of drugs is almost inevitable.

The physician prescribes the medicine and treatment.
The nurse carries out the physician's orders.
Self-medication is dangerous. Consult your physician first.
There is in every medicine a possible danger.
When in doubt—ASK!

ASSIGNMENT

Review previous lessons and questions according to the direction of your instructor.

1. The drug abuse problem is a total community concern; it should not be the sole responsibility of law enforcement officers. Who else should be responsible?
2. Explain the meaning of psychic dependence and physical dependence.
3. Name the three major categories of commonly abused drugs.
4. Name several opiates and several other depressants that may lead to drug abuse.
5. Name several stimulants that may lead to drug abuse.
6. What type of CNS drug is marijuana, stimulant or depressant? Why is it difficult to place marijuana in a proper category, such as depressant, stimulant, or hallucinogen?
7. What is "hash"? What is its concentration?
8. Describe the marijuana plant and tell where it grows, including where it grows best. What is the most common way marijuana is used? What are the chief effects of marijuana? Discuss in detail the controversy regarding the effects and legalizing the use of marijuana. What are your opinions, and why?
9. What type of CNS drug is amphetamine, depressant or stimulant? What are the chief effects of amphetamine? What are the dangers of these effects? Withdrawal of amphetamine is followed by what symptoms? How does the drug abuser attempt to control the disturbing symptoms caused by the stimulant properties of amphetamine? Does overuse of amphetamines appear to lead to physical dependence? Can tolerance occur?
10. Cocaine is an example of what type of CNS drug, depressant or stimulant? When used for its stimulation in drug abuse, what effects are produced? What is a common method of administration of cocaine used by the drug abuser? What is a complication of this method of use? What syptoms may occur from chronic use of cocaine?
11. What type of CNS drug is LSD, depressant, stimulant, or hallucinogen? What is the source of LSD? Make two separate lists: one of the physical effects and one of the psychologic effects of LSD. List the definite dangers of LSD from the summary of these dangers. Is LSD physically addicting? What is meant by this? Discuss the federal law's view and penalties regarding LSD. List the reasons, including your own, why people take LSD.
12. What is the source of mescaline? Its effects are similar to what other abused drug? What are the initial effects?
13. What is the source of psilocybin? Its effects are similar to what other abused agent?
14. Outline the nurse's role in caring for the drug-abuse patient. Emphasize the nonjudgmental type of nursing care you must give and list some examples of how you may accomplish this.

Some basic information concerning some of the more commonly employed anesthetics

DISCOVERY OF GENERAL ANESTHETICS

Before the discovery and use of anesthetics, agents used to relieve pain were limited to opium, belladonna preparations, and alcoholic beverages. Surgeons were limited by time and the physical and psychic trauma tolerated by the patient. Nitrous oxide was discovered in 1772 by Joseph Priestley, but he and others did not understand the significance of the anesthetic properties of the gas, and it was not used for many years.

Three hundred years passed after the discovery of ether before it began to be used for the relief of pain during surgery. In 1842 Dr. Crawford Long of Georgia had a patient inhale ether for a removal of a neck tumor, but he failed to publish his report in medical literature and thus did not receive full credit for being the first to discover the value of ether as an anesthetic agent.

Horace Wells, a dentist, began to use nitrous oxide in connection with his dental practice. In 1845 he tried unsuccessfully to demonstrate its use to relieve pain for a surgical operation. In that day it was not realized how difficult it is to produce a good level of anesthesia with nitrous oxide alone and for a period of time necessary for surgical operations.

William Morton, a dentist who later studied medicine, successfully demonstrated the use of ether for a surgical operation in 1846 at Massachusetts General Hospital in Boston. This success began a new era in surgery.

In 1831 chloroform was discovered, and in 1847 James Simpson of England successfully proved its usefulness. Queen Victoria knighted him for this contribution to the relief of pain. It is said that she permitted its use on herself during the birth of one of her children.

Most of the drugs used in the operating room are administered by anesthetists. The nurse, however, does have the responsibility of knowing important details concerning these drugs, since the nurse aids in the care of the patient during anesthesia, postoperatively in the recovery room, and during convalescent care on the hospital ward. The nurse should not give anesthetics unless especially educated for this purpose and adequately supervised by a physician.

GENERAL ANESTHETICS

Anesthetics fall into two large groups: general and local. A general anesthetic is any agent that produces unconsciousness (coma) from which the patient may not be awakened until the effects of the anesthetic have been eliminated from the body system. General anesthetics may be administered rectally, intravenously, or by inhalation. Inhalation is the most common method of use. Any means of administration and combination of drugs may be used. For example, an anesthetic may be started intravenously, and when the patient is asleep, inhalation may be used. Local anesthetics block pain impulses without producing unconsciousness.

Most general anesthetic drugs produce the same stages. The length of these stages may vary widely with different agents. The first and second stages may be very short or almost absent as a result of the types of anesthetic given and the types and amounts of preanesthetic medication. Stages of anesthesia are usually divided into four, with subdivisions in the third stage.

The first stage, or beginning induction, is one of analgesia, with some mucous membrane irritation, increasing loss of awareness of pain, a feeling of warmth, asphyxia, and vague sensations. There is little or no change in pulse, respiration, or pupil size. Amnesia for this period may or may not occur. When consciousness is lost, the patient has progressed to the second stage.

The second stage of anesthesia is the stage of excitement or delirium. Consciousness is lost as a result of depression of the higher cerebral centers. The lower areas are unaffected, so the patient may struggle and cry out. Respirations and pulse are often irregular. Pupils are usually normal. Movement of the eyeballs may occur. Muscular tone is increased and tense. This stage may be absent if the proper premedications have been given, and induction is rapid and smooth. Reflex dilation of the pupils may occur occasionally in children and emotionally upset adults, but a rapid, smooth induction often prevents this. Pupil size is not a reliable factor concerning the stage of anesthesia because of the effect of the preoperative medications.

The third stage, often divided into four levels, is the stage of surgical anesthesia. It covers all depths or levels from light anesthesia to unconsciousness so deep as to cause respiratory failure. During surgical anesthesia, at a level without toxic symptoms, pulse rate is increased with the rhythm, volume is normal, and respirations are deep, regular, and slightly increased in rate. Reflexes of eyelids are absent, eyeball activity continues, and pupils are normal and respond to light, though less rapidly than is normal.

As the third stage deepens, several adverse symptoms occur. The pupils dilate because of loss of pupillary reflexes, activity of the eyeballs ceases, pulse is thready and weak with low volume, respirations are irregular and shallow, blood pressure drops, and the skin becomes cold and clammy.

The fourth or toxic stage is characterized by paralysis of the respiratory center and often an imperceptible pulse. The anesthetist must constantly check vital signs throughout anesthesia and be prepared for any danger signals.

When anesthetics were first used, only one drug was given at a time, such as chloroform or ether. Today, however, most anesthetists use two or more drugs for each patient. An anesthesiologist must be an expert, highly educated, skilled physician to administer most agents now in use. A good anesthesiologist can maintain a safe surgical stage of anesthesia for hours by using small amounts of two or more drugs at a time or, depending on the anesthetic employed and length of the operation, using small amounts at a time of one particular anesthetic.

Inhalatory anesthetic methods

Open method. Liquid anesthetics such as ether can be given by dropping the anesthetic on gauze or cotton placed on a wire mask that fits over the patient's nose and mouth. This is known as the open-drop method. There is free access to air, there is no rebreathing of the anesthetic mixture, and the vapor is not confined. Another form of the open method is when a gaseous agent such as nitrous oxide (laughing gas) flows over the patient's face. This method is now rarely used. The open system wastes anesthetic, the amount of anesthetic administered is difficult to control, and the possibility of explosion is increased when a flammable agent is used. There is also no method of mechanical ventilation if an emergency should arise.

Semi-open method. Semi-open refers to the use of some means to decrease the escape of the anesthetic vapor. The patient inhales from a closed mask that communicates with a reservoir or breathing bag a mixture containing gases or vapors combined with air or oxygen. Valves prevent the recirculation of expired gases. Exhalations pass through a valve located on the top of the mask. A higher concentration of anesthetic vapor is provided by this method, although there is a greater retention of carbon dioxide than with the open method. This method also tends to tire the patient more, since the patient's respiratory effort is increased because of the valves that increase the resistance to gas flow.

Closed method. The closed method can be used for both volatile liquids and gases. An anesthetic machine is used. An apparatus fits over the nose and face of the patient, or an endotracheal tube connects the respiratory tract of the patient with the anesthetic machine, forming a closed system. The removal of carbon dioxide, absorption of moisture, and regulation of the intake of the anesthetic agent or agents and oxygen are all provided for. The anesthetist can regulate respirations by periodic rhythmic compression of the breathing bag. The closed method has the advantages of better control of the anesthetic state and greater economy of the anesthetic, since rebreathing of the mixture occurs.

Some general anesthetics
Chloroform (klo′ro-form)

1. Chloroform is a highly volatile, light-sensitive liquid.
2. It is not flammable.
3. It is administered by the open-drop method in minute amounts and very slowly.
4. Induction is rapid, 2 to 3 minutes.
5. The anesthesia produced is good.
6. Muscular relaxation is good.
7. Undesirable side effects include immediate cardiac disorders and delayed hepatotoxic reactions.
8. It is used outside the United States for obstetrics and surgery, but it is rarely used in the United States.

Cyclopropane (si-klo-pro′pane)

1. Cyclopropane is a gas given with 85% to 90% oxygen.
2. It is flammable and explosive. Avoid all sparks.
3. Administration is by the closed method.
4. Induction is rapid.
5. Anesthesia produced is good.
6. Muscular relaxation is good.
7. It has low toxicity when used by a skilled anesthetist, but it may cause cardiac arrhythmais.
8. Its use is in general surgery and obstetrics. It is effective for patients with respiratory difficulties because of the high concentration of oxygen administered.

Ether
(Diethyl ether) (di-eth′il e′ther)

1. Ether is a volatile liquid. An opened can should not be used after 48 hours.

2. Ether is flammable. The vapor is explosive in 2% concentration.
3. Administration is by the open, semi-open, and closed methods.
4. Induction is medium to long, 10 to 15 minutes, and is unpleasant.
5. Anesthesia produced is good.
6. Muscular relaxation is excellent.
7. It may cause excitement, restlessness, and choking during anesthesia induction and nausea and vomiting after anesthesia.
8. Ether is a good emergency and general anesthetic with a wide margin of safety when used alone or with other anesthetics to give good muscular relaxation. It is now used infrequently, however, because of flammability and patient discomfort during recovery.

Ethylene (eth'i-leen)

1. Ethylene is a gas with an objectionable odor.
2. It is flammable and explosive.
3. Administration is by the semi-open and closed methods.
4. Induction is rapid.
5. Anesthesia produced is good.
6. Muscular relaxation is moderate.
7. Ethylene has practically the same pharmacologic effects as nitrous oxide, but it has a slightly greater potency.
8. Two characteristics make it a poor substitute for nitrous oxide. It is explosive in concentrations used clinically, and it has an unpleasant odor. For these reasons, it is rarely used today.

Enflurane (en'floo-rane)
(Ethrane) (eth'rane)

1. Enflurane is a new, nonflammable anesthetic.
2. Anesthesia is maintained with 1.5% to 3% enflurane.
3. Analgesia is slightly better than halothane, muscle relaxation is good and postoperative emergence is rapid.
4. Postoperative nausea, vomiting, and headache do occur.

Halothane (hal'o-thane)
(Fluothane) (floo'o-thane)

1. Halothane is a volatile liquid.
2. It is not flammable and not explosive.
3. Administration is by the semi-open and closed methods. A special inhaler is used.
4. Induction is rapid.
5. Anesthesia produced is good.
6. Muscular relaxation is fair to medium.
7. Undesirable side effects are hypotension, arrhythmias, and hepatotoxicity.

8. It is used in general surgery with the addition of synthetic muscular relaxants. Levarterenol and epinephrine must be used with extreme caution.

Ketamine hydrochloride (keet'ah-meen)
(Ketalar) (ket'ah-lar)

1. Ketamine is a nonbarbiturate used to induce a dissociative anesthesia characterized by amnesia and analgesia without complete loss of consciousness.
2. It is administered intravenously or intramuscularly.
3. It is particularly effective in short procedures, such as skin grafting and dressing changes. It may also be used as an induction agent, following by inhalation anesthetics.

Nitrous oxide ("laughing gas") (ni'trus ok'side)

1. Nitrous oxide, a gas, is always given with oxygen. The highest safe concentration is nitrous oxide 75%, oxygen 25%.
2. It is not explosive and not flammable. At sufficiently high temperatures it will dissociate, release oxygen, and support combustion. Thus, it can increase the explosiveness of other anesthetics, such as ether and ethylene.
3. Administration is by the semi-open and closed methods.
4. Induction is short to medium.
5. Anesthesia produced is fair.
6. Muscular relaxation is poor when this gas is used alone.
7. Undesirable side effects include hypoxia in higher concentrations and even in lower concentrations in some patients.
8. It is relatively nontoxic and should be given only by a skilled anesthetist.
9. It is used in short surgery and obstetrics and with other anesthetics for longer surgery. It is now one of the most commonly used inhalatory anesthetic agents.

Thiopental sodium (thi-o-pen'tahl)
(Pentothal) (pen'to-thol)
Thiamylal sodium (thi-am'i-lal)
(Surital) (sur'i-tal)
Methohexital sodium (meth-o-hek'si-tahl)
(Brevital) (brev'i-tahl)

1. These are all short-acting barbiturates. They are hygroscopic powders dissolved in water.
2. They are not flammable and not explosive.
3. They are generally administered intravenously; some can be given rectally.
4. Induction is rapid.
5. Anesthesia produced is fair.

6. Muscular relaxation is poor.
7. Toxicity is low in light, short anesthesia.
8. It is used for very short anesthesias, for short duration but repeated anesthesia, and for labor pains in childbirth.

• • •

The nurse should be aware of the patient's natural dread of anesthesia and operative procedures and should try with an unhurried, confident, pleasant attitude to allay this fear.

When the surgical operation is completed, the patient is usually taken to a recovery room adjoining the operating rooms for nursing care and close supervision during recovery from the anesthetic. Recovery from anesthetics proceeds in reverse order: from the stage of surgical anesthesia through the stages of excitement and analgesia before consciousness returns. It is vitally important to make sure that the patient's face is turned to the side to prevent aspiration of mucus or vomitus. Vital signs must be accurately and frequently checked, according to the routine orders of the recovery room and the condition of the patient. Many patients will cry, shout, scream, toss about, and talk restlessly and incoherently. The nurse should understand that this is all a result of the effects of the anesthetic and cannot be controlled by the patient until the effects of the anesthetic are eliminated and the patient is fully conscious. No patient should ever be left alone until fully conscious. The sense of hearing returns comparatively early during recovery from the anesthetic. Nurses should realize this and be careful of what is said and of any discussion of the patient's medical status in the hearing range of a seemingly unconscious patient, who may hear what is said, misunderstand it, and remember it later.

Postanesthetic doses of morphine or similar narcotics should not be given until the swallowing, gagging, and coughing reflexes have returned fully, which is usually with the return of consciousness.

LOCAL ANESTHETICS

Local anesthetics are those that produce insensitivity to pain without loss of consciousness. These agents may be used for topical or surface anesthesia, in local infiltration, or to produce nerve block, caudal, spinal, saddle, and paravertebral anesthesia.

Topical or surface anesthesia. In topical anesthesia the drug is applied directly to the skin or mucous membrane and acts by deadening the nerve endings.

Infiltration anesthesia. Infiltration anesthesia is obtained by putting the medication into the tissues surrounding the operative area. This blocks the transfer of pain sensation from the wound to the nervous system.

Nerve block anesthesia. The drug is placed around the main nerve supplying the area of operation, blocking the conduction of the impulses to the brain. It is sometimes called conduction anesthesia and is often combined with infiltration anesthesia.

Caudal anesthesia. The drug is placed in the caudal or sacral canal. It prevents the transfer of impulses from the lower part of the body to the spinal cord. It is also similar to the nerve block, since it is directed to the nerves of the cauda equina. It anesthetizes the pelvic region and is often used for obstetric patients.

Spinal anesthesia. The anesthetic drug is introduced into the subarachnoid space. A needle is inserted into the spinal canal, usually between the third and fourth lumbar vertebrae, and a specified volume of anesthetic is injected into the spinal canal. The area anesthetized is determined by the amount of drug and the position of the patient. Its use for operations above the diaphragm is rare because of the danger of respiratory depression. Procaine, tetracaine, lidocaine, and dibucaine are the most commonly used drugs for spinal anesthesia.

Saddle anesthesia. Saddle block is sometimes used in obstetrics and surgery involving the perineum, rectum, genitalia, and upper parts of the thigh. The patient sits upright while the anesthetic is injected after a lumbar puncture has been done. The patient remains upright for a short period to allow the anesthetic to become effective in the desired areas. The parts of the body that would come in contact with a saddle when riding are anesthetized, hence the name.

Paravertebral anesthesia. The drug is placed near the point at which the nerves enter the spinal canal. Since it prevents the conduction of nerve impulses through the main spinal nerves supplying the operative area, paravertebral anesthesia is similar to nerve block anesthesia.

• • •

Some local anesthetic drugs are used only topically, such as ethyl chloride which anesthetizes by freezing when sprayed on; benzyl alcohol and phenol, usually combined in ointments and lotions with other drugs; and cocaine hydrochloride, used only for ophthalmic topical anesthesia, since it is too toxic to be introduced into the body tissues. Many derivatives of cocaine can be used below the surface. Procaine hydrochloride (Novocain) is used extensively for all types of local anesthesia.

Local anesthetics can cause severe toxic symptoms. Idiosyncrasy to these drugs may occur, causing severe reactions. Toxic symptoms may be mild or severe and include mental confusion, drug delirium, anxiety, blurred vision, tremors irregular jerking movements, dizziness, palpitation, irregular pulse and respiration, tachycardia, dilated pupils, and diaphoresis. The use of one of the short-acting barbiturate drugs before administration of the local anesthetic will often prevent occurrence of these symptoms. Treatment is symptomatic. Spinal anesthetics tend to cause hypotension; this is why patients recovering from spinal anesthesia are placed flat or in shock position. They also sometimes cause postoperative headache, which may be of short duration or may be intermittent and persist.

From the viewpoint of the patient, local anesthetics can cause several problems. He cannot move voluntarily during surgery. He can hear but often cannot understand what is being said by physicians and nurses and may misunderstand and become apprehensive. He also is fearful that the anesthetic may not cause complete freedom of pain. The patient feels helpless and alone and needs considerable emotional and physical support from the nurse, attendants, physician, and anesthetist during anesthesia and surgery.

Examples of injectable local anesthetics are procaine (Novocain), chloroprocaine (Nesacaine), hexylcaine (Cyclaine), lidocaine (Xylocaine), mepivacaine (Carbocaine), piperocaine (Metycaine), etidocaine (Duranest), bupivacaine (Marcaine), prilocaine (Citanest), tetracaine (Pontocaine), and dibucaine (Nupercaine), the latter two having long duration action. Many of these are also available in topical form.

Examples of topical anesthetics are cocaine, benzocaine (Americaine), piperocaine (Metycaine), hexylcaine (Cyclaine), tetracaine (Pontocaine), dibucaine (D-caine, Nupercainal), lidocaine (Xylocaine), cyclomethycaine (Surfacaine), and dyclonine (Dyclone). Many of these are also available in injectable form.

**The physician prescribes the medicine and treatment.
The nurse carries out the physician's orders.
Self-medication is dangerous. Consult your physician first.
There is in every medicine a possible danger.
When in doubt—ASK!**

ASSIGNMENT

Review previous lessons and questions according to the directions of your instructor.

1. Before the advent of anesthetics, what drugs were used in an attempt to relieve pain for surgery?
2. Who first discovered nitrous oxide and when? Was it immediately of practical use?
3. Who first discovered the use of ether in surgery and when? Did he receive full credit for his discovery? If not, why?
4. What dentist began to use nitrous oxide in his dental practice? Why was it unsuccessful at that time for surgery?
5. What dentist in what year successfully demonstrated the use of ether for a surgical operation? Where was this operation performed? What were the implications of this success?
6. When was chloroform discovered? In what year and by whom was it successfully proved useful in anesthesia?
7. Explain the difference between general and local anesthetics.
8. Explain the four stages of general anesthesia, beginning with the first stage.
9. In modern anesthesia is it usual to employ one anesthetic for a patient or two or more anesthetics?
10. Why should nurses not give anesthetics?
11. Explain the open, semi-open, and closed methods of inhalatory anesthesia.
12. For the following anesthetics, list whether flammable or explosive or both, method of administration, induction, anesthesia and muscular relaxation produced, and general uses: cyclopropane, ether, enflurane, halothane, ketamine, nitrous oxide, and thiopental sodium (Pentothal).
13. The next time you are on duty in the hospital, look at the anesthetic and operations forms for several of the surgical patients on your ward. They are in the chart for each patient. List the preanesthetic and anesthetic medications given. Tell the advantages and disadvantages of each of these medications.
14. Plan an imaginary conversation between you and a preoperative patient, indicating his fears and worries and how you would attempt to relieve those worries. Explain the care of the patient in the recovery room in your study notes for your instructor and give the reasons for restlessness, crying, talkativeness, screaming, and similar behavior observed in the recovery room.
15. The sense of hearing returns early after anesthesia. Explain precautions the nurse and physician should take regarding this.
16. When should postanesthetic doses of narcotic be given following surgery? Why, in addition to the relief of pain?
17. Explain each of the following terms for local anesthesia: topical anesthesia, infiltration, nerve block, caudal, spinal, saddle, and paravertebral anesthesia.
18. Name one spray-on local anesthetic drug that anesthetizes

by freezing. Name two local anesthetic drugs usually combined in ointment with other drugs.

19. Cocaine hydrochloride is used only for what type of anesthesia? Procaine hydrochloride (Novocain) is used extensively for what type of anesthesia? For what conditions has it been used in weak intravenous solutions?

20. List the toxic symptoms that may be caused by local anesthetics. How may these symptoms be prevented?

21. Name two postoperative symptoms that may be caused by spinal anesthetics. How may these symptoms be prevented?

22. Why does a local anesthetic present several problems to a patient during anesthesia and surgery from his own viewpoint? How can nurses, attendants, physicians, and anesthetist overcome many of these problems?

23. Mrs. H. is going to surgery for an appendectomy, or removal of the appendix. The physician orders 50 mg of Nembutal Sodium, 20 mg of Demerol, and 0.3 mg of scopolamine to be given by hypodermic injection, intramuscularly, 1 hour before surgery. You have on hand the following strengths: Nembutal Sodium ampule, 100 mg (gr iss)/2 cc; Demerol, 50 mg (gr ³/₄)/1 cc; and scopolamine, 0.5 mg (gr ¹/₁₂₀)/1 cc. Work the problems for each medication and explain the procedure for drawing up into the syringes and mixing what drugs can be mixed. Tell the main uses and effects of each drug. Explain the reasons for giving these medications preoperatively. (See Index for help in working these problems: Fractional dosage, for preoperative hypodermic medications, first problem.)

CHAPTER 14

Drugs affecting the respiratory system

OXYGEN

Oxygen is a colorless, odorless, and tasteless gas that is not flammable but supports combustion more actively than does air. This gas constitutes 21% of ordinary air and is necessary to maintain life. Oxygen must be continuously supplied to tissue cells to maintain life, especially to organs such as the brain, heart, lungs, and kidneys. It is compressed and marketed in steel cylinders that are fitted with reducing valves for the delivery of the gas. It is under considerable pressure, and care should be taken to avoid jarring, dropping, and bumping cylinders into one another.

Purposes for giving oxygen

The chief use of oxygen in medicine is to treat hypoxia (lack of oxygen) and hypoxemia (diminished oxygen tension in the blood). Following are some of the conditions for which oxygen is indicated:
1. Cardiac failure or threatened cardiac decompensation and coronary occlusion
2. Lobar and bronchial pneumonia, severe asthma, pulmonary edema, poisoning from gases such as carbon monoxide, and other conditions associated with inadequate oxygenation in the lungs
3. During anesthesia to increase the safety of general anesthesia
4. Certain types of headache
5. In certain conditions involving injury to the nervous system and threatened respiratory difficulty or failure
6. Abdominal distention from intestinal ileus

The gas causing the gastrointestinal distention is mainly nitrogen. When the patient inhales a high concentration of oxygen or pure oxygen, the nitrogen dissolved in the blood gradually leaves by way of the lungs. The blood can then absorb the nitrogen from body cavities such as the intestine, discharge it into the expired air, and thus relieve distention and gas pain.

Administration

There are a number of ways oxygen can be administered. Each has its advantages and disadvantages.

Endotracheal intubation. Intubation is the placement of a catheter from the mouth or nose directly into the trachea. A cuff at the tracheal end is inflated enough to lodge against the walls of the trachea, thus forming a seal to prevent air leakage. Intubation is advantageous (1) to prevent an unconscious patient from aspirating regurgitated stomach contents, (2) to allow maximum oxygen content directly into the lungs, and (3) to provide mechanical ventilatory support to patients who cannot maintain adequate respiratory effort.

Nasal catheter. The nasal catheter, lubricated with a water-soluble jelly, is passed through the nose until the tip is just above the epiglottis. Measurement for this is the same as the distance from the patient's external nares to the tragus of the ear minus 1 cm. If the catheter is inserted too far, the patient will swallow oxygen and have stomach distention and abdominal discomfort. The catheter is fastened with tape to the nose and forehead.

Oxygen is drying to the mucous membrane, so frequent daily nasal and oral hygiene is essential to maintain intact mucous membranes, remove nasal encrustations and obstructions, maintain cleanliness, prevent infection and discomfort, and aid breathing by removing nasal obstructions of mucus. The flow rate of oxygen depends on the patient's need, but the usual rate is from 2 to 4 liters (1 liter = 1000 cc) of oxygen per minute.

Nasal cannulae. Nasal cannulae fit into the nostril, cannot be passed, and are more comfortable for the patient than nasal catheters. They are less likely to become obstructed with nasal secretions than nasal catheters, but nasal and oral mucosa still need frequent daily attention. The usual rate of flow is 3 liters of oxygen per minute.

Oxygen masks. This method is still one of the most effective means of delivering needed oxygen. Oxygen concentrations of 90% to 100% can be given by a mask that must fit well over the nose and mouth for full effect. The patient tolerates the mask better when intermittent use of it can be made or when a clear, plastic, disposable type is used. If rubber masks are used, they should be absolutely clean and uncontaminated or they will be a source of infection from the last patient or some hospital source.

Oxygen tents and hoods. These have the advantage of temperature and humidity regulation. Oxygen concentration in a tent rarely reaches 50%; in a hood it may reach 90% to 100%. Periodic testing of the tent and hood with an oxygen analyzer for oxygen concentration is important. The usual rate of oxygen flow is 15 liters per minute for the first 15 to 30 minutes after the patient is in the tent and 10 to 12 liters per minute thereafter.

Make sure that the tent is securely tucked under the mattress and around the patient to avoid leakage. Open and remove the tent as little as possible to prevent leaking. Cover the mattress with plastic or a rubber sheet to prevent oxygen saturation of the mattress and loss of oxygen. The use of a croup tent with an open top will give adequate oxygen concentration for a child with a respiratory infection. The top can be covered to increase the mist, if desired.

Dangers of administration

Oxygen supports combustion. Combustible material such as bed linens and wooden furniture burn more easily and with greater intensity. This is why smoking, use of matches, or use of electric equipment that may cause sparks is absolutely forbidden in rooms where oxygen is being administered. This is the reason for notices to this effect on the patient's door, or by the patient, or on an oxygen tent. The nurse must see that these notices are obeyed.

High concentrations of oxygen given over prolonged periods are toxic. The result may be hypoventilation, acidosis, possible paresthesias, confusion, and visual disturbances.

Use of oxygen for the premature baby

The nurse must constantly be aware of the potential damage to the retina of the premature baby exposed to high concentrations of oxygen. Blindness may result. Oxygen should only be administered as needed in low concentrations, and the infant should be closely monitored during treatment. Some incubator models are equipped with a safety valve that automatically releases the excess oxygen outside the chamber. Often the removal of a very small plug of mucus will clear the baby's airway and enable it to inhale oxygen without assistance.

CARBON DIOXIDE

Carbon dioxide is the chief respiratory stimulant. The respiratory center is directly stimulated by an increase in the carbon dioxide tension of the blood, increasing both the depth and the rate of breathing. Patients with chronic pulmonary disease are particularly dependent on the oxygen content in the blood to maintain their respiratory effort. If the oxygen content provided to these patients is too high, they may develop apneic episodes that may be fatal.

NEBULIZATION THERAPY

Nebulization therapy is used to deposit medication in the respiratory tract in the form of droplets that have been suspended in air. The medication is inhaled as a fine mist. The finer the mist, the greater the degree and extent of penetration into the respiratory tree.

Nebulization therapy is used to promote loosening of secretions, bronchodilation and pulmonary decongestion, moistening, cooling, or heating of inspired air, and topical application of antibiotics, steroids, and antifoaming agents.

Drugs used for nebulization therapy include bronchodilators, mucolytic agents, antibiotics, and steroids.

Respiratory agents
Bronchodilators

Bronchodilators, which are adrenergic agents or sympathomimetic drugs, relax the smooth muscle of the tracheobronchial tree. This allows an increase in lumen or opening size of the bronchioles and alveolar ducts and a decrease in resistance to air flow. These drugs also decrease congestion in the respiratory tract through vasoconstriction and decrease mucous membrane swelling. Aerosol therapy varies from 3 to 15 minutes.

Aminophylline (ah-mee-no-fil′in)

1. Aminophylline is a theophylline derivative that acts directly on the smooth muscle of the bronchi and pulmonary blood vessels to cause bronchodilation. It has about 80% of the potency of theophylline.
2. Aminophylline is one of the most commonly used bronchodilators in asthma, emphysema, and other forms of chronic obstructive lung disease.
3. Common side effects associated with aminophylline therapy include nausea, vomiting, headache, flushing, cardiac palpitations, arrhythmias, and tachycardia.
4. Usual adult maintenance dose: 200 to 300 mg orally every 6 to 8 hours. Aminophylline is available in 100-, 200-, and 300-mg tablets; 100 mg/15 ml, 250 mg/15 ml, and 315 mg/15 ml liquids; 125-, 250-, 300-, 350-, and 500-mg suppositories; and 250- and 500-mg ampules for injection.

Isoproterenol (i-so-pro-te-re′nol)
(Isuprel) (i′soo-prel)

1. Isuprel is chemically related to epinephrine. It relaxes the spasm of bronchial smooth muscle and is effective in the treatment of bronchial asthma.
2. It eases expectoration of pulmonary secretions, has a wide margin of safety, and is frequently effective when epinephrine and other drugs fail.
3. Large sublingual doses produce direct myocardial stimulation with an increase in heart rate.

4. It is available in 10- and 15-mg glossets for sublingual use and in 1:100 and 1:200 solution for nebulization.
5. It should be used with caution in cardiovascular disorders, diabetes, hyperthyroidism, and persons sensitive to sympathomimetic amines.

Oxytriphylline (ok-see-tri'fil-in)
(Choledyl) (kol'eh-dil)

1. Oxytriphylline is a theophylline derivative that is about 65% as potent as theophylline. When compared with theophylline or aminophylline, it is less irritating to the gastric mucosa and more readily absorbed orally.
2. Oxytriphylline is used in long-term therapy to reduce bronchospasm in patients with acute bronchial asthma, chronic bronchitis, and emphysema.
3. Side effects are similar to those of aminophylline and theophylline.
4. Usual adult dose: 200 mg orally four times daily.

Tedral (ted'rahl)

1. Tedral contains theophylline, ephedrine hydrochloride, and phenobarbital. Theophylline relaxes smooth muscle bronchial tissue, thus relieving bronchospasm. It also reduces local edema. Ephedrine reduces congestion, and phenobarbital provides a mild sedation.
2. Tedral provides quick, prolonged action in relief of bronchial asthma and hay fever.
3. It should be used with caution in cardiovascular disease, severe hypertension, circulatory collapse, glaucoma, hyperthyroidism, and prostatic hypertrophy.
4. Usual dose: one or two tablets every 6 hours. Tedral is available in a variety of forms: Tedral Expectorant tablets, Tedral Pediatric Suspension (licorice flavored), Tedral SA (sustained), and Tedral-25. The latter contains 25 mg of butabarbital instead of phenobarbital.

Terbutaline sulfate (ter-bu'tah-leen)
(Brethine) (breh'thine), (Bricanyl) (bri'kan-il)

1. Terbutaline is a synthetic drug that relaxes the smooth muscle of the bronchial tree. It is used as a bronchodilator in the treatment of asthma and emphysema.
2. Usual dose: 2.5 to 5 mg three times daily. Maximum daily dose should not exceed 15 mg. Terbutaline is available in 2.5 and 5 mg tablets and for parenteral injection.

Theophylline (the-o-fil'in)
(Elixophyllin) (ee-lik-so-fil'in), (Slo-Phyllin)

1. Theophylline is the parent compound of the methylxanthine derivatives. It is an effective bronchodilator,

myocardial stimulant, and mild diuretic; however, it causes gastrointestinal irritation, and oral absorption is poor unless it is administered in an elixir (Elixophyllin). Consequently, aminophylline is more frequently used.
2. Side effects are common and include nervousness, insomnia, irritability, nausea and vomiting, tachycardia, arrhythmias, flushing, and hypotension.
3. Usual adult dose: 200 to 250 mg every 6 hours.

The major aerosol bronchodilators are epinephrine (1:100 concentration, 1% solution), isoproterenol (1:100 or 1:200 concentration), and isoetharine (1% solution).

Bronchodilators can be given by aerosol, oral tablets, elixirs, injections, and suppositories. A few examples of these are **Alupent, Asmolin, Bronkephrine Hydrochloride Injection, Dilor, Lufyllin, Medihaler-Epi, Norisodrine Aerohalor** and **Aerotrol, Quibron, Sudafed,** and **Ventaire.**

Mucolytic agents

Mucolytic agents lessen the thickness and stickiness of purulent and nonpurulent pulmonary secretions. This eases the removal of the secretions by suction, postural drainage, or coughing. The mucolytic agents are most effective in removing mucous plugs obstructing the tracheobronchial airway and in the treatment of patients with acute and chronic pulmonary disorders, prebronchoscopy and postbronchoscopy, following chest surgery, and as a part of the treatment in tracheostomy care. Some examples are **acetylcysteine (Mucomyst)** and **tyloxapol (Alevaire).**

RESPIRATORY DEPRESSANTS OR SEDATIVES

The most important respiratory depressants are the central depressants of the opium group and those of the barbiturate group. It is seldom desirable to depress respirations, but sometimes this is a side effect in otherwise very useful drugs. Sometimes a cough is so painful or so exhausting that an opiate such as codeine is administered to slow the rate and depth of respiration. Codeine's greater value, however, lies in its action to depress the cough reflex.

DRUGS THAT AFFECT THE COUGH CENTER AND THE RESPIRATORY MUCOSA
Preparations to relieve cough (antitussives)

Ordinarily, a cough is a protective reflex that operates to clear the upper part of the respiratory tract of irritants. A variety of stimuli can start a cough, such as a foreign substance, excessive mucus, cold air, inflammatory exudates, or the present of nonmalignant and malignant growths. When the irritating agent is expelled, the cough is helpful and called productive. A nonproductive cough produces no mucus or foreign material and is both irritating and exhausting. This type of cough is typical of asthmatic patients. The sinusitis cough is caused by excess secretions draining into the respiratory tract and occurs particularly in the sleeping or lying-down position. Treatment of the cough is, of course, of secondary importance; primary treatment is aimed at the underlying disorder. Antitussives should not be given in situations in which retention of respiratory secretions may be harmful.

Medications that may be used to relieve the cough include narcotic and nonnarcotic antitussives, demulcents, antiseptics, expectorants, and others.

Narcotic antitussives

Narcotics such as morphine, dihydromorphinone, and levorphanol are powerful suppressants of the cough reflex but only have limited use for this purpose because of their respiratory depressant action, bronchial constriction, especially in allergic or asthmatic patients, and their habit-forming nature. They also inhibit the ciliary activity of the respiratory mucous membrane, an aid in the suppression of cough.

Codeine and dihydrocodeinone have less pronounced antitussive effects but have fewer side effects than the more powerful narcotics. They are widely used to suppress cough. Dihydrocodeinone is more active than codeine, but its addiction possibility is greater. The usual antitussive dose for codeine is 10 to 20 mg every 4 to 6 hours.

Nonnarcotic antitussives

Dextromethorphan hydrobromide (dek-stro-meth'-or-fan hi-dro-bro'myd)
(Romilar) (ro'mil-ar)

1. Dextromethorphan is a synthetic derivative of morphine but is employed only as an agent to relieve cough.
2. It has no analgesic properties, does not depress respirations, does not cause addiction, and has low toxicity and few side effects.
3. Usual adult dose: 20 to 30 mg every 6 to 8 hours orally. It is available in 5- and 10-mg lozenges and 15-mg capsules and as a syrup (3 mg/ml). Higher doses may be required in patients with severe cough.

Demulcents

Demulcents are sticky substances that check coughing by protecting the lining of the respiratory tract from the irritation of contact with air. They are also used as vehicles for other drugs such as the syrups acacia, citric acid, glycyrrhiza, and tolu.

Cough syrups are soothing mainly because of their local action on the throat. For this reason, they should not be diluted, and no fluids or food should be taken for

15 to 30 minutes after administration. Smoking should be avoided since it increases the irritation and coughing. Simple syrups, honey, or hard candy may have soothing effects to lessen coughing. Steam inhalations also may be helpful.

There are many cough medicine preparations available under proprietary names: **Syrup of Cherry, Cheracol, Syrup of White Pine,** and **Syrup of Tolu Balsam.**

Expectorants

Expectorants are drugs that reduce the viscosity of mucus or increase the production of secretions in the bronchi and ease the expulsion of sputum. They are used in the treatment of coughs, bronchitis, and pneumonia. The respiratory passages are lined with cilia that normally carry secretions of the tract toward the exterior. Mucus that is thick and sticky probably interferes with these ciliated movements, and coughing results. The exact mode of action of expectorants is not known. Adequate fluid intake and inspiration of humidified air are also important factors in production of liquid sputum.

Ammonium chloride (ah-mo'nee-um)

1. Ammonium chloride is believed to increase the amount of respiratory tract fluid by irritation of the gastric mucosa.
2. Dose: 300 mg every 2 to 4 hours in water or thin fruit juice.

Guaifenesin (gwi-fe-ne'sin)
(Robitussin) (row-bi-tus'sin)

1. Guaifenesin, formerly known as glyceryl guaiacolate, is an expectorant that acts by enhancing the output of respiratory tract fluid. The increased flow of secretions promotes ciliary action that facilitates the removal of mucus.
2. Usual dose: 200 to 400 mg every 4 hours.
3. Robitussin is available as guaifenesin alone or in combination with other products.
   a. **Robitussin A-C.** In 5 cc (ml) contains 100 mg of guaifenesin and 10 mg of codeine phosphate as a cough suppressant. It may be habit-forming because of its codeine content.
   b. **Robitussin CF.** In 5 cc contains 100 mg of guaifenesin, 10 mg of dextromethorphan as a nonnarcotic cough suppressant, and 12.5 mg of phenylpropanolamine to reduce mucosal congestion and edema in the nasal passages.
   c. **Robitussin DAC.** In 5 cc contains 100 mg of guaifenesin, 10 mg of codeine phosphate, and 30 mg of pseudoephedrine for nasal congestion.
   d. **Robitussin DM.** In 5 cc contains 100 mg of guaifenesin and 15 mg of dextromethorphan.
   e. **Robitussin PE.** In 5 cc contains 100 mg of guaifenesin and 30 mg of pseudoephedrine.

4. Side effects are infrequent, but gastrointestinal upsets, nausea, and vomiting can occur, or side effects may be caused by phenylpropanolamine or pseudoephedrine such as tremors, insomnia, or palpitations.
5. These agents should be used with caution in patients with hypertension, cardiac disorders, diabetes, hyperthyroidism, or peripheral vascular disease.

Terpin hydrate (ter′pin hi′drate)

1. Terpin hydrate is believed to act by direct stimulation of lower respiratory tract secretory glands.
2. Usual dose: 200 mg every 4 hours.
3. Terpin hydrate is frequently used in combination with codeine for a combined antitussive-expectorant effect.

NASAL DECONGESTANTS

Many adrenergic or vasoconstricting drugs are commonly used for their capacity to shrink the engorged mucous membranes of the nose in mild upper respiratory infections and to relieve nasal stuffiness. Misuse by patients, including too large a dose or a dose too often, may cause a "rebound" swelling of the mucous membranes; the nose feels more stuffy or congested than before treatment. Antihistamines are sometimes added to the decongestant. Sprays and nose drops are of benefit when used correctly under the advice of a physician, but improper use and dosage may spread the infection deeper into the sinuses or the middle ear.

Examples of some commonly used nasal decongestants are **naphazoline hydrochloride (Privine), phenylephrine hydrochloride (Neo-Synephrine),** and **phenylpropanolamine.**

USE OF ANTIHISTAMINES FOR COLDS

There is much difference of opinion at present concerning the usefulness of antihistaminic drugs for the treatment of the common cold. Such antihistaminic drugs as **diphenhydramine hydrochloride (Benadryl)** and **tripelennamine hydrochloride (PBZ)**, as well as other antihistamines, may be used. Very few, if any, investigators since 1950 believe that these drugs taken early during the onset of a cold may relieve any allergic symptoms of the cold such as watery eyes, sneezing, and continuous discharge from the nasal mucous membrane. Indiscriminate use of these drugs can be dangerous since they cause drowsiness, and prolonged use may cause dry mouth, blurred vision, urinary retention, and constipation. The drying effect on respiratory secretions may be particularly bothersome in producing a nonproductive cough.

The physician prescribes the medicine and treatment.
The nurse carries out the physician's orders.
Self-medication is dangerous. Consult your physician first.
There is in every medicine a possible danger.
When in doubt—ASK!

ASSIGNMENT

Review previous chapters and questions according to directions of your instructor.

1. Describe the characteristics of oxygen. How is it marketed? It is under considerable pressure, so what precautions should be taken with oxygen tanks? What is the chief use of oxygen? List the conditions for which oxygen is indicated. What is the name of the gas that causes gastrointestinal distention during administration of oxygen (high concentration or pure oxygen)? Tell how the nitrogen leaves the body and distention and gas pains are relieved.
2. Tell five ways oxygen can be administered and describe each.
3. List the reasons frequent daily nasal and oral hygiene is essential for the patient receiving oxygen, in addition to the fact that oxygen is drying to the mucous membrane.
4. What is the usual flow rate of oxygen: by nasal catheter, nasal cannulae, oxygen masks, and oxygen tents and hoods?
5. What precautions must you take in making the tent-bed and checking it throughout the day?
6. Describe the two types of croup tents for a child with croup.
7. Explain the dangers of oxygen administration and how each of these can be prevented. Is oxygen flammable? Combustible?
8. Explain the correct use of oxygen and the dangers of high concentrations of oxygen for the premature baby.

9. Tell the uses of carbon dioxide and its effect on the respiratory center.
10. What are the advantages of nebulization therapy? Name four drug *groups* used for nebulization therapy.
11. Explain the effects of bronchodilators. Aerosol therapy for these drugs varies for what length of time?
12. Aminophylline (several choices are correct)
    a. Is a theophylline derivative
    b. Acts on the smooth muscle of the bronchi and pulmonary blood vessels to cause bronchoconstriction
    c. Acts on the smooth muscle of the bronchi and pulmonary blood vessels to cause bronchodilation
    d. Has about 80% of the potency of theophylline
    e. Is one of the most commonly used bronchodilators in asthma, emphysema, and other forms of chronic obstructive lung disease
    f. Fortunately, rarely has any side effects
    g. Has as some common side effects nausea, vomiting, headache, flushing, cardiac palpitations, arrhythmias, and tachycardia
    h. Has as a usual adult maintenance dose 200 to 300 mg orally every 6 to 8 hours
    i. Is only available in oral form
13. Isoproterenol (several choices are correct)
    a. Is chemically related to epinephrine
    b. Relaxes the spasm of bronchial smooth muscle and is effective in the treatment of bronchial asthma
    c. Eases expectoration of pulmonary secretions
    d. Lessens expectoration of pulmonary secretions
    e. Has a wide margin of safety
    f. Is frequently effective when epinephrine and other drugs fail
    g. Unfortunately, has a narrow margin of safety, which limits its use in bronchial asthma
    h. In large sublingual doses may produce direct myocardial stimulation with an increase in heart rate
    i. Should be used with caution in cardiovascular disorders, diabetes, hyperthyroidism, and persons sensitive to sympathomimetic amines
    j. Is available for sublingual use only
14. Oxytriphylline (Choledyl) (several choices are correct)
    a. Is an epinephrine derivative
    b. Is an theophylline derivative
    c. Is about 65% as potent as theophylline
    d. When compared with theophylline or aminophylline is less irritating to the gastric mucosa and more readily absorbed orally
    e. Has its usefulness in short-term therapy only because of its powerful effects on bronchospasm and emphysema
    f. Has side effects similar to those of aminophylline and theophylline
    g. As an example of long-term therapy is effective to reduce bronchospasm in patients with acute bronchial asthma, chronic bronchitis, and emphysema
15. What drugs does Tedral contain and what is the effect of each drug? Tedral provides quick, prolonged action in the relief of what two medical conditions? Name the conditions for which Tedral should be used with caution. List the forms in which Tedral is available. What is meant by Tedral SA? What drugs does Tedral-25 contain?

16. What is the origin of terbutaline (Brethine)? What is its action? Tell it main uses. What is the usual dose?
17. Name the conditions for which theophylline is effective. Tell the two disadvantages of this drug. As a result of these disadvantages, what drug is more commonly used than theophylline? List the common side effects. What is the usual adult dose?
18. Name the three major aerosol bronchodilators. Tell the way in which bronchodilators can be given. Name six of these major aerosol bronchodilators.
19. Explain the effects of mucolytic agents and tell the conditions for which they are used. Give two examples of mucolytic agents.
20. Name two groups that are important respiratory depressants. What effect does codeine have on the respirations? What is codeine's greater value?
21. What is the purpose of a cough? Name the stimuli that can start a cough. Explain the difference between a productive and nonproductive cough. Which type of cough is typical of asthmatic patients? What causes the sinusitis cough and how is it treated?
22. When should antitussives *not* be given?
23. List the *groups* of medications that may be used to relieve cough.
24. Narcotics such as morphine, dihydromorphinone, and levorphanol are powerful suppressants of the cough reflex. Tell the reasons why their use to relieve cough is limited. Do codeine and dihydrocodeinone have more or less pronounced antitussive effects than morphine and other more powerful narcotics? Do they have more or less side effects than the more powerful narcotics? Which is possibly more addictive, dihydrocodeinone or codeine? What is the usual dose of codeine, and how frequently may it be given per day?
25. What is the source of dextromethorphan hydrobromide (Romilar)? In which group of antitussives does it belong? Does it have analgesic properties, depress respirations, cause addiction, have many side effects, and have low or high toxicity? What is its main use? What is the usual adult dose? In what forms is it available for dosage?
26. Define demulcents. What is the main reason cough medicines are soothing? Tell the correct administration of cough medicines and instructions to be given to the patient for 15 to 30 minutes after administration and throughout the day. Give four examples of cough medicines, using proprietary names.
27. Define and explain the effect of expectorants. What are important factors in production of liquid sputum? How is ammonium chloride believed to increase the amount of respiratory tract fluid?
28. How is the commonly used guaifenesin (Robitussin) thought to act? What is the usual dose? Name five types of Robitussin and tell what each contains and what effects these drugs are supposed to obtain (see Index for some of these drugs). Which type of Robitussin is more apt to be habit-forming than the others? List the side effects that may infrequently occur and the side effects that may be caused by phenylpropanolamine or pseudoephedrine. Robitussin should be used with caution in what medical conditions?

29. What is thought to be the action of terpin hydrate? What is the usual dose? Terpin hydrate is frequently used in combination with what other drug?

30. What is the common use of many nasal decongestants? What may misuse by patients cause? Name a drug that is sometimes added to decongestants. What may improper use and dosage cause? Give three examples of nasal decongestants.

31. Discuss the use of antihistamines for colds and the consensus of opinion concerning this use. What are the undesirable effects that may be caused by indiscriminate use of antihistamines for the treatment of the common cold?

32. The physician asked you to administer to the patient terbutaline sulfate (Brethine) for its bronchodilator action in the treatment of asthma. The dose the physician wanted given was 5 mg. The only strength of the drug available was 2.5 mg. How many tablets will you administer?

CHAPTER 15

Drugs affecting the muscular system

CENTRALLY ACTING SKELETAL MUSCLE RELAXANTS

The centrally acting skeletal muscle relaxants are a class of compounds used to relieve acute muscle spasm of local origin. They are used in conjunction with physiotherapy in the treatment of strains, sprains, or trauma to ligaments. They are often used with other drugs, such as adrenal corticosteroids and other analgesics in the treatment of arthritis, bursitis, fibrositis, myositis, and spondylitis. These drugs have been used in the treatment of certain neurologic disorders, such as cerebral palsy, and in other diseases characterized by increased muscle tone, involuntary movements, and incoordination.

Muscle spasm is a symptom associated with many conditions and is the result of several processes. These processes include inflammation of the tissues around muscles resulting in muscular spasm, injury to the muscle itself, and damage to the nerve fibers responsible for the control of motor activity of muscles.

The exact mechanism of the centrally acting skeletal muscle relaxants is not known. They have been shown to depress nerve transmission through several spinal and supraspinal nerve pathways that control muscle tone by prolonging synaptic recovery time and by reducing the frequency of repetitive interneuron discharges. They do not have any direct effect on muscles, myoneural junctions, or neuronal conduction. All muscle relaxants produce some degree of sedation, and most physicians think that the benefits of these drugs come from their sedative effects rather than from actual muscle relaxation.

There are many side effects and precautions for these drugs. Mild symptoms include drowsiness, blurred vision, headache, dizziness, lightheadedness, feelings of weakness, lethargy, and lassitude. These symptoms often occur during initial drug therapy and resolve after proper dosage adjustment. Patients should be cautioned to avoid activities that require mental alertness, physical coordination, and judgment, such as operating dangerous machinery and driving an automobile. Such activities can be resumed when symptoms have disappeared. Gastrointestinal discomfort such as nausea, vomiting, abdominal distress, heartburn, diarrhea, and constipation are common.

Centrally acting skeletal muscle relaxants may produce hepatotoxicity and blood dyscrasias. Periodic laboratory tests, including blood counts and liver function tests, are recommended to avoid complications.

This group of drugs is contraindicated in patients with myasthenia gravis or muscular dystrophy, since the drugs may reduce the strength of remaining active muscle fibers and produce further impairment and debilitation. These drugs are contraindicated in patients with severe liver disease and are used with great caution, if at all, during pregnancy. See Table 15-1 for additional comments on specific centrally acting muscle relaxants.

Baclofen (bak′lo-fen)
(Lioresal) (ly-or′e-sahl)

1. Baclofen is a skeletal muscle relaxant that apparently acts somewhat differently than the centrally acting musculoskeletal agents. Its complete mechanism of action is unknown, although reflex activity at the spinal cord is partially inhibited.
2. Baclofen is used in the management of spasticity resulting from multiple sclerosis, spinal cord injuries, and other spinal cord diseases. It is not recommended for use in spasticity associated with Parkinson's disease, cerebral palsy, stroke, or rheumatic disorders.
3. The most common side effects associated with baclofen therapy are drowsiness, fatigue, nausea, mental depression, headache, and muscle weakness. These side effects are usually transient and may be minimized by starting therapy with low dosages. Increases in dosage should be made as tolerated.
4. Baclofen therapy should not be abruptly discontinued. Severe exacerbation of spasticity and hallucinations may result.
5. Use with caution in patients who must use spasticity to maintain an upright posture and balance in moving.
6. Baclofen has additive CNS depressant effects when used with other CNS depressants such as antihistamines, tranquilizers, and alcohol.
7. Initial dosage: 5 mg three times daily. Increase dosage by 5 mg every 3 to 7 days based on response. Optimum effects are usually noted at dosages of 40 to 80 mg daily but may take several weeks to achieve.

127

Table 15-1. Centrally acting muscle relaxants

Generic name	Brand name	Usual dosage (po)	Comments
Carisoprodol	Rela, Soma	350 mg four times daily	Onset of action—30 minutes; duration—4 to 6 hours
Chlorphenesin carbamate	Maolate	400 to 800 mg three to four times daily	Recommended only for short-term treatment (8 weeks) of muscle spasm induced by trauma or inflammation; may cause blood dyscrasias
Chlorzoxazone	Paraflex	250 to 750 mg three to four times daily	Commonly causes gastrointestinal discomfort; may be hepatotoxic
Cyclobenzaprine	Flexeril	10 mg three times daily; do not exceed 60 mg daily	Recommended only for short-term treatment (2 to 3 weeks) of painful musculoskeletal conditions
Metaxalone	Skelaxin	800 mg three to four times daily	Use with caution in patients with liver disease; causes false-positive Clinitest reaction
Methocarbamol	Robaxin, Delaxin, Robamol, others	1 to 1.5 g four times daily	Parenteral forms also available
Orphenadrine citrate	Norflex, Flexon, Myolin	100 mg two times daily	Also has analgesic properties; do not use in patients with glaucoma or prostatic hypertrophy

DIRECT ACTING SKELETAL MUSCLE RELAXANT

Dantrolene (dan′tro-leen)
(Dantrium) (dan′tree-um)

1. Dantrolene is a muscle relaxant that acts directly on skeletal muscle. It is used to control the spasticity of chronic disorders such as cerebral palsy, multiple sclerosis, spinal cord injury, and stroke syndrome. Dantrolene produces generalized mild weakness of skeletal muscles and decreases the force of reflex muscle contractions, hyperflexia, clonus, muscle stiffness, involuntary muscle movements, and spasticity.
2. Side effects:
   a. Common side effects include muscle weakness, drowsiness, dizziness, lightheadedness, and diarrhea. These common side effects occur early in treatment and may be prevented by initiating treatment with low doses and increasing gradually. If symptoms persist or recur after temporary discontinuance of the drug, dantrolene may have to be permanently discontinued.
   b. Neurologic side effects include speech and visual disturbances, difficulty in swallowing, alteration of taste, confusion, mental depression, increased nervousness, and insomnia.
   c. Digestive system side effects include gastric irritation, gastrointestinal bleeding, anorexia, and constipation.
   d. Urogenital side effects include incontinence, urinary frequency, difficult urination, urinary retention, nocturia, crystalluria, and difficult erection.
   e. Blood changes may occur, such as increased or decreased white blood cell count; increased serum uric acid, SGOT, BUN, alkaline phosphatase, and serum bilirubin; decreased serum phosphate and proteinuria.
   f. Other side effects rarely observed include tachycardia, phlebitis, erratic blood pressure, dermatitis, backache, chills, fever, abnormal hair growth, excessive tearing, and a feeling of suffocation.
3. Dantrolene must be used with caution in patients with chronic lung disease, liver disease, and impaired myocardial function. Dantrolene has been implicated as a causative factor in reported cases of hepatitis.
4. It should not be used in pregnancy or given to nursing mothers.
5. Patients taking dantrolene should be warned against engaging in activities requiring skill and alertness.
6. Dantrolene is contraindicated for patients whose spasticity is used to obtain or maintain an upright posture and balance or body function.
7. Drug-induced photosensitivity may occur, so patients should refrain from excessive or unnecessary exposure to sunlight.
8. Dantrolene should be used with caution in patients on tranquilizer therapy because of additive CNS depressant effects.
9. Usual adult dose: 25 mg daily initially, may be increased to 25 mg two, three, or four times daily at 4- to 7-day intervals, then by gradually increasing dosage up to 100 mg two, three, or four times daily. A few patients may require 200 mg four times daily.

SKELETAL MUSCLE RELAXANTS USED DURING SURGERY

Neuromuscular blocking agents are important skeletal muscle relaxants. These drugs are used to (1) produce adequate muscle relaxation during anesthesia to reduce excessive use of general anesthetics, (2) ease endotracheal intubation and prevent laryngospasm, (3) decrease muscular activity in electroshock therapy, and (4) aid in the management of tetanus.

Neuromuscular blocking agents have no effect on consciousness or the pain threshold. Reassurance by nursing personnel is essential to paralyzed patients (such as those on respirators), and analgesics must be administered on schedule. These patients may not understand what is happening and may suffer extreme pain without being able to ask for analgesics. This is true of other powerful neuromuscular blocking agents.

Side effects shared by all neuromuscular blocking agents are residual muscle weakness, hypersensitivity reactions, and interference with respiratory function. Neuromuscular blocking agents can cause hypotension, bronchospasm, and cardiac arrhythmias. The hypotension is thought to be caused by sympathetic ganglionic blockade and histamine release. Both of these cause peripheral vasodilation. Bronchospasm is perhaps caused by the histamine release.

These drugs are usually given intravenously but may also be given intramuscularly. They are potent drugs, not without danger, so they should be used only by persons thoroughly familiar with their effects and under conditions where the patient can receive constant, close attention for signs of respiratory failure or difficulties. Adequate equipment for artificial respiration, antidotes, and other measures for prompt treatment of toxicity must be readily available.

These drugs should be administered only by adequately trained individuals who are familiar with their actions, characteristics, and hazards and who are experienced in the technique of artificial respiration under positive pressure. Facilities for these procedures should be available close to the patient at all times.

Neuromuscular blocking agents; curariform blocking agents

Curare (koo-rah′re)

1. Curare is a generic name for a number of arrow poisons obtained from tropical vines used by South American Indians.
2. The clinical use of curare has been replaced by tubocurarine.

Tubocurarine chloride (too-bow-koo-rah′rin)
(d-Tubocurarine), (Tubarine) (too′bah-rin), (Tubodil) (too′bow-dil)

1. Tubocurarine is the active principle of curare.
2. This drug is used as (a) an adjunct to anesthesia to induce skeletal muscle relaxation, (b) a diagnostic agent for myasthenia gravis when results with anticholinesterases have been inconclusive, and (c) to de-

crease the intensity of muscle contractions in electroshock therapy.

3. Side effects, toxic effects, and precautions:
   a. Tubocurarine can cause hypotension because of its sympathetic ganglionic blocking ability and its capacity to release histamine from storage sites. The resulting peripheral vasodilation produces a drop in blood pressure. Diminished venous return caused by loss of skeletal muscle tone also contributes to the hypotension. The histamine release may cause bronchospasm and tachycardia.
   b. This drug should be used with extreme caution in myasthenia gravis patients, since they are very sensitive to tubocurarine blocking effects. The blocking effect of this drug is enhanced by acidosis and decreased by alkalosis.
   c. Depression of the muscles of respiration can cause hypoxia and death.
   d. Thirty-three to seventy-five percent of the drug is eliminated unchanged in the urine. Some of the drug is eliminated through the intestinal tract via the bile. Action may be prolonged in patients with renal or liver disease and in elderly or debilitated patients because of altered drug excretion.
4. Treatment of overdosage includes artificial respiration with oxygen and antidotes such as neostigmine methylsulfate (Prostigmin Methylsulfate) and edrophonium chloride (Tensilon Chloride).
   a. The antidotes inactivate cholinesterase and permit acetylcholine to be accumulated. This increased level of acetylcholine tends to overcome the paralysis.
   b. Overdosage with the antidote can also produce untoward effects.
   c. Effective doses of neostigmine may produce slowing of the heart, increased flow of saliva, hypotension, and increased motility of the intestine. Atropine is sometimes given to overcome some of these effects.
5. Drug interactions:
   a. The general anesthetics, such as halothane, ether, and cyclopropane, potentiate the action of tubocurarine. This necessitates reduction of the dose of tubocurarine.
   b. Drugs that potentiate the neuromuscular blocking action of tubocurarine include many antibiotics, such as streptomycin, neomycin, gentamicin, kanamycin, and amikacin; diuretics, particularly the thiazides; monoamine oxidase inhibitors; and quinidine.
   c. Drugs that inhibit the action of tubocurarine include the anticholinesterases, such as neostigmine, pyridostigmine, and edrophonium.
   d. There have been reports of recurarization occurring postoperatively when patients were given

antiarrhythmic drugs such as quinidine or lidocaine.

6. A single IV dose of tubocurarine produces muscle relaxation in 3 to 5 minutes, which may persist for 20 to 30 minutes. After IM injection, paralysis occurs within 10 to 25 minutes. Additional doses will have longer durations of action than the initial dose.
   a. Muscles are affected in the following order:
      (1) Those innervated by the cranial nerves—facial muscles
      (2) Muscles of the trunk and extremities
      (3) Muscles of respiration, with the diaphragm affected last
   b. Usual dosage for adults, as an adjunct to general anesthesia: 0.1 to 0.3 mg/kg is given intravenously over 60 to 90 seconds. Subsequent doses depend on the patient's response, intensity and duration of action, and the anesthetic used. Additional doses, $1/4$ to $1/2$ of the initial dose, may be given every 45 to 60 minutes, when necessary.

Dimethyltubocurarine iodide (Metubine) (me-tu'bin)

1. This drug is similar to the parent compound, tubocurarine.
2. Uses, side effects, toxic effects, and precautions are the same as those for tubocurarine.
3. Dimethyltubocurarine iodide should not be used in patients sensitive to iodides.
4. Dimethyltubocurarine causes respiratory depression, hypotension, and bronchospasm resulting from histamine release.
5. Drug interactions are similar to those of tubocurarine.
6. Dosage must be individualized, based on the type of surgery, surgical premedication used, duration of surgery, and the type of anesthetic to be used. It is administered intravenously.

Decamethonium bromide (dek-ah-me-tho'ne-um) (Syncurine) (sin'koo-reen)

1. Decamethonium is a potent relaxant of skeletal muscle, with rapid onset of action but short duration of effect. It is used infrequently, however, because its effects are somewhat unpredictable with the rapid development of tachyphylaxis.
2. Bronchospasm resulting from the release of histamine is minimal.
3. Decamethonium has been used to produce marked, but short-term, muscle relaxation in such procedures as endoscopy, endotracheal intubation, and closure of the peritoneum during surgical procedures.
4. The chief side effect is respiratory depression. As always, artificial respiration with oxygen equipment should be on hand. No antidotes are available.

Succinylcholine chloride (suk-si-nil-ko'leen) (Anectine) (an-ek'tin), (Quelicin) (kwel'i-sin), (Sucostrin) (soo-kos'trin), (Sux-Cert), (Suxamethonium chloride) (suk-sah-me-tho'ne-um)

1. Succinylcholine produces good muscular relaxation during anesthesia and electroshock therapy and is quite effective for such procedures as endotracheal intubation and endoscopy because of its short duration. It does not seem to produce significant effects on the circulatory system and autonomic ganglia when used in therapeutic doses.
2. Succinylcholine in normal dosage has a low level of toxicity.
   a. Large doses produce respiratory depression, so facilities to combat respiratory paralysis must be at hand.
   b. Succinylcholine can cause vagal stimulation, hypotension, bradycardia, cardiac arrhythmias, and increased gastric and salivary secretions. Release of histamine may induce bronchospasm.
   c. This drug should be used with caution in patients with liver disease, severe dehydration, severe anemia, nutritional disturbance, or a deficiency of cholinesterase as a result of genetic defect. These patients are highly sensitive to even small doses of the drug.
   d. Cholinesterase levels can also be decreased by topical administration of long-acting anticholinesterases, such as echothiophate (Phospholine Iodide), which is used in the treatment of wide-angle glaucoma. These drugs should be discontinued 2 to 4 weeks before surgery if succinylcholine is to be given. Succinylcholine causes a rise in intraocular pressure and is dangerous to patients with glaucoma, with penetrating wounds of the eye, and those patients undergoing eye surgery.
   e. This drug may also increase intragastric pressure, especially if the patient was unable to fast before surgery.
3. There is no antagonist. Neostigmine and edrophonium prolong the effect of succinylcholine and therefore are contraindicated as antidotes in case of overdosage. Succinylcholine loses its activity rapidly when administration is discontinued, so it is a relatively safe drug. The patient must be observed closely to prevent undue respiratory depression, and artificial respiration equipment and oxygen must be at hand for immediate use.
4. The following drug interaction may occur.
   a. Phenothiazines reduce plasma cholinesterase levels and enhance the blocking effects of succinylcholine.
   b. Neostigmine and other anticholinesterase drugs, such as cyclophosphamide, isoflurophate, and

organophosphate insecticides, may prolong the action of succinylcholine.

   c. Quinidine potentiates the action of muscle relaxants.

   d. Procaine should not be given intravenously concurrently with succinylcholine, because it competes with succinylcholine for hydrolysis by cholinesterase. Prolonged apnea may result.

   e. Antibiotics, such as streptomycin, neomycin, gentamicin, and kanamycin, may potentiate the action of succinylcholine and prolong the recovery time.

5. Usual adult dose: 10 to 40 mg when used for short procedures. It is given intravenously, either in continuous drip infusion or separate repeated injections. Onset of action is in 1 minute, with a peak reached in 2 minutes. Rapid recovery occurs in about 5 to 10 minutes. Sustained relaxation is accomplished by continuous drip infusion, with 2.5 mg given per minute.

Gallamine triethiodide (gal'ah-meen tri-e-thi'o-dyd)

1. Gallamine triethiodide is a synthetic compound. Its actions, uses, contraindications, and drug interactions are similar to those of the curare drugs.
2. This drug is used as an adjunct to anesthesia for muscle relaxation. It is *not* used for electroshock therapy. This is because of its short duration of action and side effects.
3. Its advantages include causing little bronchospasm from histamine release, having no effect on autonomic ganglia, and having a high degree of flexibility because of rapid onset and short duration of action.
4. A major disadvantage is that it produces vagal blockade similar to that of atropine; therefore, it can cause blood pressure elevation and tachycardia.
5. It is antagonized by neostigmine and edrophonium.
6. Side effects and toxic effects:
   a. Gallamine may produce an allergic reaction in patients sensitive to iodine.
   b. This drug may produce a marked tachycardia.
   c. It crosses the placental barrier so must be used with great caution for cesarean sections, although no effects on the newborn have been reported.
   d. Gallamine is excreted unchanged by the kidneys and should not be administered to patients with impaired renal function.

7. Gallamine triethiodide is administered intravenously in an aqueous solution. Average adult dose initially is 2.5 mg/kg of body weight. Muscular relaxation begins immediately and reaches a maximum in about 3 minutes. Duration of action is 15 to 35 minutes. Dosage must be individualized.

Pancuronium bromide (pan-ku-ro'ne-um) (Pavulon) (pav'you-lon)

1. Pancuronium is a synthetic neuromuscular blocking agent that is used to produce skeletal muscle relaxation during surgery. It is compatible with all currently used general anesthetics. This drug is also used to ease mechanical respiration in patients with status asthmaticus and to facilitate endotracheal intubation.
2. Pancuronium has advantages over tubocurarine since pancuronium causes little or no release of histamine, with no resulting bronchospasm, and causes no ganglionic blockade, with no resulting hypotension.
3. Side effects, toxic effects, and precautions:
   a. Pancuronium has the same side effects as other nondepolarizing neuromuscular blocking agents.
   b. It should not be used in patients with tachycardia or when an increase of heart rate is undesirable.
   c. This drug is contraindicated in patients sensitive to bromides.
   d. Pancuronium should be used cautiously in children since there are only limited data on this age group. It has caused sweating and excessive salivation in children.
   e. Wheezing, transient skin rashes, and a burning sensation at the site of injection have been reported.
4. The following drugs may prolong the action of pancuronium: halothane, ether, quinine, neomycin, streptomycin, kanamycin, gentamicin, tobramycin, amikacin, and magnesium.
5. Antidotes for pancuronium include neostigmine methylsulfate, edrophonium chloride (Tensilon), and calcium gluconate.
6. Usual initial dosage: 0.1 mg/kg IV, followed every 20 to 60 minutes as needed by 0.04 mg/kg of body weight.

The physician prescribes the medicine and treatment.
The nurse carries out the physician's orders.
Self-medication is dangerous. Consult your physician first.
There is in every medicine a possible danger.
When in doubt—ASK!

ASSIGNMENT

Review previous lessons and questions according to the directions of your instructor.

1. Centrally acting skeletal muscle relaxants are often used with what other drugs in the treatment of what medical conditions? Know the meaning of the medical terms given to these conditions. Do centrally acting skeletal muscle relaxants have any direct effect on muscles, myoneural junctions, or neuronal conduction? Most physicians think that the benefits from these drugs come from what type of effect, rather than from actual muscle relaxation?

2. List the side effects and precautions for centrally acting skeletal muscle relaxants. What are the contraindications for these drugs?

3. Name by generic and trade names five centrally acting muscle relaxants and give the comments on each, as found in Table 15-1. Your instructor will tell you which ones are commonly used in your hospital.

4. Baclofen (Lioresal) (several choices are correct)
   a. Is an excellent example of a centrally acting skeletal muscle relaxant
   b. Acts somewhat differently than the centrally acting musculoskeletal agents
   c. Is the specific drug for the treatment of Parkinson's disease, stroke, cerebral palsy, and rheumatic disorders to relieve spasticity
   d. Is used in the management of spasticity resulting from multiple sclerosis, spinal cord injuries, and other spinal cord diseases
   e. Rarely has any side effects
   f. Causes such side effects as nausea, fatigue, drowsiness, headache, mental depression, and muscle weakness
   g. Has an advantage in that the most common side effects are usually transient and may be minimized by starting therapy with low dosages and increasing as tolerated
   h. May cause side effects that indicate the drug must be discontinued at once
   i. Should not be abruptly discontinued since hallucinations or severe exacerbation of spasticity may result
   j. Has increased depressant effects when used with other depressants such as tranquilizers, antihistamines, and alcohol
   k. Has an initial dose of 5 mg three times daily, increasing dosage by 5 mg every 3 to 7 days based on response
   l. Has optimum effects noticeable within 2 days

5. Dantrolene (Dantrium) (several choices are correct)
   a. Acts indirectly on skeletal muscle
   b. Acts directly on skeletal muscle
   c. Controls spasticity of chronic disorders such as cerebral palsy, multiple sclerosis, spinal cord injury, and stroke syndrome
   d. Produces generalized mild weakness of skeletal muscles and decreases the force of reflex muscle contractions, hyperflexia, clonus, muscle stiffness, involuntary muscle movements, and spasticity
   e. Rarely produces any side effects
   f. Has such common side effects as muscle weakness, drowsiness, dizziness, lightheadedness, and diarrhea, which may be prevented by low initial doses and increasing gradually
   g. May cause some of the side effects discussed in f, which may persist after temporary discontinuance of the drug, but the drug should be continued despite the persistent side effects
   h. Has many additional side effects such as neurologic, digestive system, urogenital, and blood changes
   i. Must be used with caution in patients with chronic lung disease, liver disease, and impaired myocardial function
   j. Never causes any decrease in skill activities or alertness
   k. May cause photosensitivity; patients should be cautioned to refrain from excessive or unnecessary exposure to sunlight
   l. Should be used with caution in patients on tranquilizer therapy because of additive CNS depressant effects

6. What are the main effects of the skeletal muscle relaxants used during surgery? What effect do these neuromuscular blocking agents have on consciousness or the pain threshold? List the side effects of all neuromuscular blocking agents. How are these drugs usually administered? These are powerful, dangerous drugs. Who should administer these drugs and why, in addition to the reasons already cited?

7. What is the source of curare? In clinical use, curare has been replaced by what other drug?

8. Tubocurarine is the active principle of what drug? List the uses of tubocurarine. List the side effects of this drug. Can this drug be used in myasthenia gravis patients? Why should caution be taken in administering this drug to myasthenia gravis patients? What is the treatment for overdosage? Discuss drug interactions in connection with tubocurarine. How soon does action occur after a single IV dose of tubocurarine? In what order are the muscles affected after administration of tubocurarine? Can the drug be repeated, and if so, in what dosage?

9. Dimethyltubocurarine iodide (Metubine) is similar to what parent compound drug? List its main side effects, toxic effects, and precautions. Drug interactions are the same as for what drug? Is this drug administered orally, subcutaneously, intramuscularly, or intravenously?

10. Since decamethonium bromide is a potent relaxant of skeletal muscle, with rapid onset of action and short duration of effect, why is it not used more frequently? What are its main uses? What is the chief effect? How should it be treated and where should the equipment and antidotes be kept?

11. Succinylcholine chloride (several choices are correct)
    a. Is not a stable drug of the skeletal muscle relaxant group and is seldom used
    b. Produces good muscular relaxation during anesthesia and electroshock therapy and is quite effective for endotracheal intubation and endoscopy because of its short duration
    c. Has a low level of toxicity in normal dosage, but large doses may produce respiratory depression, so facilities to combat respiratory paralysis must be at hand
    d. Can be used with complete safety in patients with liver

disease, severe dehydration, severe anemia, nutritional disturbance, or a deficiency of cholinesterase as a result of genetic defect

e. Causes a decreased intraocular pressure and so is safe to use for patients with glaucoma, with penetrating wounds of the eye, and for patients undergoing eye surgery

f. Has several effective antagonists, such as neostigmine and edrophonium

g. Interacts when administered with other drugs, such as quinidine, which potentiates the action of muscle relaxants; neostigmine and isoflurophate (Humorsol), which may prolong the action of succinylcholine; and antibiotics such as streptomycin, neomycin, gentamicin, and kanamycin, which may potentiate the action of succinylcholine and prolong the recovery time

12. What is the method of administration of succinylcholine? What is the onset of action, and how is sustained relaxation accomplished?

13. Gallamine has actions, uses, contraindications, and drug interactions similar to those of what drug group? This muscle relaxant is not used for electroshock therapy. Why? List the advantages of this drug. List two antagonists for gallamine. Make a list of side effects and toxic effects of gallamine.

14. What are the advantages of pancuronium over tubocurarine? List the side effects, the toxic effects, and precautions for this drug. List the drugs that may prolong the action of this drug. Is this generally an advantage or a disadvantage, or even a danger, for pancuronium?

15. The physician ordered Robaxin 0.5 g for your patient. The bottle label strength is 500 mg. How many tablets will you administer? *Remember:* This is a conversion problem. How do you convert from gram to milligram? Then use this same problem and convert from milligram to gram (see Index: Conversion).

16. The physician ordered 0.25 mg of a drug in oral tablet form, with scored tablets. Your bottle label strength is 0.5 mg. How many tablets will you administer?

CHAPTER 16

Cardiovascular drugs

THE DIGITALIS GLYCOSIDES

The digitalis group of drugs is among the oldest and most effective therapeutic agents for the treatment of congestive heart failure. It is also used in the treatment of atrial fibrillation and for the management of atrial flutter and paroxysmal tachycardia. Their use in medicine dates back to the eighteenth century. In 1785 William Withering, the English physician and botanist, published excellent observations on the treatment of various ailments with digitalis. Derived naturally from the dried leaves of *Digitalis purpurea,* or purple foxglove, the drug is now synthetically prepared.

Digitalis influences the mechanical performance of the heart by increasing the strength of myocardial contraction. The exact mechanism by which it does this is unknown. Important benefits for the failing heart result from this increased strength of myocardial contraction: the ventricles empty and fill more completely and there is a slower heart rate and more complete filling. The results of this include:

1. A fall in venous pressure
2. Reduced systemic and pulmonary congestion with symptoms either lessened or eliminated
3. Decrease in heart size toward normal
4. Excretion of excess salt and water by the kidneys—the "diuretic" effect; it is secondary to the effect on the heart and not a result of an effect on the kidney

Thus, digitalis and its preparations *slow* and *strengthen* the heart.

The aim in the treatment of heart failure is to give digitalis until the best cardiac effects are achieved and most of the signs and symptoms have disappeared. The patient is given a total amount of the drug over a period of hours or days necessary to produce the desired cardiac effect. This is known as digitalizing the patient. The amount of drug required for digitalization varies with each patient. A maintenance dose is then given, usually once daily. Many patients must continue to take digitalis preparations for the remainder of their lives.

Digitalis preparations are cumulative, especially digitoxin and digoxin. Since these drugs slow the pulse and are cumulative, the pulse is always counted before giving the drug in either oral or injectable forms.

Physicians may discontinue the drug for 2 or 3 days if the pulse beat is below 60 beats per minute. Physicians may also order the drug given regardless of pulse beat below 60 beats a minute if, in their opinion, no cumulative effects exist for the particular patient in question. Many physicians prefer the apical pulse beat as being more accurate, since some abnormal heartbeats (arrhythmias) are felt at the radial artery. The nurse should always consult the head nurse, team leader, instructor, or physician before giving any digitalis preparations if the pulse beat is below 60 beats a minute.

Common side effects and toxic effects of digitalis include nausea, vomiting, diarrhea, arrhythmias, and pulse rate below 60 beats a minute (bradycardia). Headache, visual disturbances, weakness, and restlessness may also occur. Discontinuance of the drug for 2 or 3 days usually causes the symptoms to subside, and then dosage may have to be reduced. These symptoms should be observed, reported, and charted.

The importance of reporting signs and symptoms of digitalis intoxication and the need for close observation are particularly important in the presence of any predisposing factor such as potassium loss. Causes of potassium loss include the loss of large amounts of body fluid through vomiting, diarrhea, or diuresis from drugs such as furosemide, ethacrynic acid, and the thiazide preparation; through major surgical procedures associated with severe electrolyte disturbances, such as colostomy, ileostomy, colectomy, and ureterosigmoidostomy; through poor dietary intake or severe dietary restrictions that decrease electrolyte intake; and through the use of adrenal steroids and potassium-free IV fluids.

Digitalis toxicity may be caused by kidney, liver, and severe heart disease. From 60% to 80% of the digitalis glycosides are excreted by the kidneys. Renal disease thus promotes digitalis cumulation and intoxication. The liver is the primary organ for inactivating digitalis, so any impairment of liver function decreases an individual's tolerance to digitalis. Severe cardiac disease impedes the function of all body organs and increases myocardial sensitivity to digitalis.

Elderly persons have a slowing of body functions and decreased tolerance to drug therapy. They often show signs of toxicity with small doses of digitalis.

Intravenous administration of digitalis and rapid digitalization may increase the risk of digitalis overdosage.

The most common treatment of digitalis intoxication is discontinuance of the drug for 2 or 3 days. Drugs such as potassium chloride (which tends to decrease myocardial excitability and abolish arrhythmias), procainamide, lidocaine, phenytoin, or propranolol may be administered to control arrhythmias. There is no specific antidote for digitalis intoxication.

Nursing implications

Nursing measures for patients on digitalis therapy include observation of the patient's electrocardiogram and monitoring of the heart rate. The pulse should be checked, apically if desired, before administering any dose of digitalis preparations by any route. This should be recorded and reported. The physician may wish the drug withheld if the pulse is below 60 beats a minute.

An understanding of the relationship between dosage and potency is vital to intelligent nursing care and safety of the patient. A mistake in dosage is paticularly dangerous. Much difference exists between a dosage of 1 mg and 0.1 mg; 1 mg is ten times the doage of 0.1 mg; 0.2 mg is twice the dosage of 0.1 mg. Check your dosage. When in doubt—ASK! Make sure of the exact name of the drug. Check spelling. Dig*it*oxin and digoxin are *not* the same drug; their dosages are also very different.

Good skin and mouth care should be given to the patient. He should have sufficient rest and sedation. The rest is usually in semi-Fowler's to full Fowler's position to aid breathing. Good pillow support is an aid to breathing; having the patient bend forward and rest his head on a pillow placed on an over-bed table sometimes helps.

Adequate, easily digested diet and fluids should be given according to the physician's order. Restriction of salt is an aid in control of edema.

Blood pressure and pulse readings should be taken daily. Diuretics, if ordered by the physician, help the body rid itself of excess fluid and salts. Oxygen, if necessary, aids breathing and relieves the apprehension caused by difficulty in breathing.

Intake and output should be recorded daily. Recording the patient's weight at the same time every day, with the patient in the same clothing and on the same scales, aids in watching for weight gain from edema or excess caloric intake or for undue weight loss.

Establishment of rapport between the nurse and the patient is vital in reassuring the patient and aiding in his convalescence or acceptance of his condition. Listen to the patient; make explanations simple. Explore any fears and concerns. Tell the physician of any of the patient's fears or home worries.

Assist the patient in any simple exercise or physical therapy approved by the physician. Persist in this, encourage the patient and help relieve his fears of another attack or of injuring the heart further.

Digitalis preparations

Acetyldigitoxin (ass-ee-til dij-i-tok′sin)
(Acylanid) (ass-il-an′id)

1. Acetyldigitoxin is a cardiac glycoside derived from lanatoside A. It resembles digitoxin in many ways, but it has a more rapid onset and a shorter duration of action than digitoxin.
2. This drug is available in 0.1-mg tablets for oral administration.

Digitoxin (dij-i-tok′sin)
(Crystodigin) (kris-to-dij′in), **(Purodigin)** (pu-ro-di′jin)

1. Maintenance dosage range: 0.05 to 0.3 mg daily.
2. Digitoxin tablets are available for oral use in amounts of 0.05, 0.1, 0.15, and 0.2 mg per tablet. It is also available in ampules for IV injection (0.2 mg/ml).
3. Note dosage and spelling of the word carefully: dig*it*oxin.

Digoxin (di-joks′in)
(Lanoxin) (lah-nok′sin)

1. Digoxin is a hydrolytic product formed from lanatoside C.
2. It digitalizes more rapidly than digitoxin. Oral administrations may digitalize within a few hours and IV injections within a few minutes.
3. It is available in oral dosages of 0.125-, 0.25-, and 0.5-mg tablets; in injectable solution of 0.5 mg/2 ml and 0.1 mg/ml; and in a pediatric elixir (0.05 mg/ml) for oral administration to children.
4. There is a distinct advantage to the proprietary or trade name of Lanoxin. It helps to differentiate digoxin and digitoxin. These are sometimes mistaken by both student nurses and graduate nurses. Notice the difference in dosage between digoxin and digitoxin.
5. *Remember:* Digitoxin and digoxin (Lanoxin) are *not* the same drug. Note spelling. Check your reading of names. Note usual dosage for each and memorize.
   Digitoxin: 0.1 to 0.2 mg (oral tablets)
   Digoxin: 0.125 to 0.25 mg (oral tablets)

Gitalin (amorphous) (jit′ah-lin)
(Gitaligin) (ji-tahl′i-jin)

1. Gitalin is a mixture of glycosides obtained from *Digitalis purpurea*.
2. The rate of elimination or destruction of gitalin is slower than that of digoxin but faster than that of digitoxin.
3. Gitalin is administered orally. It is available in tablets (0.5 mg).

Ouabain (wah-ba'in)
G-Strophanthin (stro-fan'thin)

1. This preparation is obtained from *Strophanthus gratus*.
2. It is not absorbed well from the gastrointestinal tract and so must be given parenterally, usually intravenously.
3. It has rapid action and its maximum effects appear within about 30 minutes after IV injection, with the peak of effect occurring in about 90 minutes. Most of the effects disappear within 24 hours.
4. It is available in 2-ml ampules containing 0.25 mg/ml of solution.

• • •

The digitalis preparations are poisonous and cumulative—they are dangerous. Digitoxin and digoxin are *not* the same drug, and the dosage is different. Check spelling of these and all drugs. Become familiar with side effects, toxic effects, and treatment. Have instructor, team leader, or head nurse check your dosage, amount taken, and bottle or ampule from which you withdrew it. When in doubt—ASK!

ANTIARRHYTHMIC DRUGS

Bretylium tosylate (bre-til'ee-um tahs'e-layt)
(Bretylol) (bre'til-ol)

1. Bretylium, an adrenergic blocking agent, inhibits the release of norepinephrine. It is used for suppression of life-threatening ventricular arrhythmias, primarily tachycardia and fibrillation, that have not responded to other widely used antiarrhythmic drugs. Bretylium is not a cardiac depressant, so it should be particularly useful in patients with poor myocardial contractility and low cardiac output.
2. Side effects include postural hypotension in most patients and nausea and vomiting often following rapid IV infusion. Other symptoms that may occur include vertigo, light-headedness, slow heart rate; syncope, increased premature ventricular contractions, increased arrhythmias, transient hypertension, substernal discomfort, anginal attacks, abdominal pain, diarrhea, renal dysfunction, hiccups, rash, hyperthermia, flushing, confusion, lethargy, anxiety, psychosis, shortness of breath, sweating, and nasal suffiness.
3. Precautions: the drug should be given slowly to patients with fixed cardiac output, such as severe aortic stenosis and pulmonary hypertension, and to patients receiving digitalis, since it may aggravate digitalis toxicity. The nurse should:
   a. Keep patients under constant ECG monitoring during therapy
   b. Expect a rapid suppression of ventricular fibrilla-

tion and a slower (20 minutes to 2 hours) suppression of other ventricular arrhythmias
   c. Keep the patient supine until tolerance to hypotensive effects develops, which may take several days
4. Dosage—parenteral: initial doses of 5 to 10 mg/kg of body weight may be given intramuscularly, with increments of 100 mg hourly up to a maximum of 2 g. A total dose of 9 g/day has been given without toxicity. Maintenance therapy of 5 mg/kg every 4 to 5 hours has been suggested.
   a. Since the drug is excreted by the kidney, the dose should be lower for patients with kidney impairment.
   b. The drug dosage should be reduced under ECG monitoring and the drug discontinued after 3 to 5 days.

Disopyramide (die-so-peer'ah-myd)
(Norpace) (nor'pace)

1. Disopyramide is effective in the treatment of primary cardiac arrhythmias and those that occur in association with organic heart disease, including coronary artery disease. It may be used in both digitalized and nondigitalized patients.
2. It is usually a useful drug as an alternative to quinidine or procainamide when patients develop an intolerance to or serious side effects or toxicity from these drugs.
3. Side effects may affect the gastrointestinal and urogenital systems, but these effects are usually transitory or may disappear on reduction of dose. Disopyramide is said to have fewer side effects than quinidine and is comparable to quinidine in treatment of atrial and ventricular arrhythmias.
4. There is no specific antidote for overdosage. Treatment is supportive and may include administration of isoproterenol and/or dopamine, hemodialysis, and mechanically assisted respiration.
5. Dosage is individualized. Usual adult dose: 400 to 800 mg/day, given in divided doses four times daily. Recommended adult dosage schedule is 150 mg every 6 hours. If the body weight is less than 110 pounds (50 kg), the recommended dose is 100 mg every 6 hours.

Lidocaine (li'do-kayn)
(Xylocaine) (zi'lo-kayn)

1. Lidocaine has become one of the most frequently used drugs in the treatment of ventricular arrhythmias.
2. This drug is also extensively used as a local and topical anesthetic agent.

3. Toxic effects may include CNS stimulation, heart block, and hypotension, especially with large doses.
4. Nursing measures include careful monitoring for cardiac depressant effects during infusions of lidocaine and checking blood pressure for hypotension.
5. Usual dose: intravenously, 1 mg/kg of body weight by slow IV injection followed by a continuous IV drip. Onset of action is within 2 minutes, duration of action 10 to 20 minutes, and 60 minutes after discontinuance of the drug, none of its effects persists. The drug is metabolized by the liver and rapidly excreted by the kidneys.

Phenytoin (fen′i-toe-in)
(DPH), (Dilantin) (di-lan′tin)

1. Phenytoin was introduced about 40 years ago for the treatment of epilepsy, but it is also effective in controlling ventricular arrhythmias, particularly those induced by digitalis toxicity.
2. Phenytoin has been discussed in detail elsewhere in the text (see Index).

Procainamide hydrochloride (pro-kane′ah-myd)
(Pronestyl) (pro-nes′til)

1. Procainamide is an effective antiarrhythmic synthetic drug with generally fewer side effects than quinidine but with many similar cardiac effects.
2. It is used to treat a wide variety of ventricular and supraventricular arrhythmias, atrial fibrillation, and flutter, but it is usually not as effective for the last two as quinidine.
3. Side effects and toxic effects include CNS disturbances, gastrointestinal system disturbances, hypotension, possible bone marrow depression, possible allergic reactions, blood changes, tachycardia, or other arrhythmias. These are treated by adjustment of dosage and vasopressor drugs, such as dopamine, phenylephrine, and levarterenol, to overcome hypotension, periodic blood studies, and possible withdrawal of the drug.
4. Procainamide is available in 250-, 375-, and 500-mg capsules and in solution for injection (100 mg/ml and 500 mg/ml). It can be given orally, intravenously, or intramuscularly.

Propranolol (pro-pran′o-lol)
(Inderal) (in′der-ahl)

Another widely used antiarrhythmic drug is propranolol. It inhibits cardiac response to sympathetic nerve stimulation by blocking the beta receptors. As a result, it slows the heart rate and has an antiarrhythmic effect, although most of the antiarrhythmic effect results from incidental quinidine-like action. Propranolol has been found effective in the treatment of various ventricular arrhythmias. It inhibits atrioventricular conduction, thus slowing the ventricular rate. Propranolol has also been found effective in the treatment of certain digitalis-induced arrhythmias.

Propranolol has been discussed in detail elsewhere in the text (see Index).

Quinidine sulfate (kwin′i-din)

1. Quinidine is obtained from cinchona bark, as is quinine.
2. It acts on the muscles of the heart, decreasing the irritability and the rate of conduction of impulses. It slows the heart and changes a rapid, irregular pulse to a slow, regular pulse.
3. Quinidine aids in correcting both auricular and ventricular arrhythmias, in restoring the normal rhythm of the heart, and in overcoming many types of arrhythmias.
4. Many physicians expect an apical or radial pulse to be counted and the drug to be withheld if the pulse is below 60 beats a minute, as is done with digitalis drugs.
5. Side effects and toxic effects include CNS disturbances, gastrointestinal system disturbances (nausea and vomiting), hypotension, bone marrow depression, allergic reactions, tachycardia or other arrhythmias, headache, face flushing, palpitation, and convulsions. Treatment of these effects includes administration of vasopressor drugs, such as dopamine, to overcome the hypotension, as well as discontinuance of the drug.
6. Quinidine is a potentially hazardous drug. It may cause cardiac arrest, since it is a depressant of myocardial excitability.
7. This drug should be given with caution to patients with a quinine idiosyncrasy, heart damage, including heart block, or hyperthyroidism.
8. Usual dose: orally, 0.2 to 0.4 g (gr iii to vi) every 6 to 8 hours.
9. The combination of quinidine and atropine or any anticholinergic drug can cause additive anticholinergic effects. Such a combination must be given with caution. Quinidine can potentiate the anticoagulant effect of warfarin by depression of prothrombin formation or by inhibition of the synthesis of vitamin K–sensitive clotting factors in the liver. The combination of quinidine and digoxin produces an additive effect with potential bradycardia, so must be used with caution. Quinidine combined with phenytoin, procainamide, or propranolol also produces an additive effect. Added effects may also occur between quinidine and lidocaine.

10. *Remember:* Observe the spelling of quinidine carefully. Quinidine and quinine are *not* the same. They have different purposes and dosage. They are both alkaloids of cinchona. Check the name of the drug, exact spelling, and dosage carefully. When in doubt—ASK!

VASOCONSTRICTORS

Vasoconstrictors are drugs that cause constriction of blood vessels. They usually exert their effects by causing contraction of the muscle fibers in the walls of the blood vessels or by stimulation of the vasomotor center in the medulla. They may be used to stop minor hemorrhage of small blood vessels, raise blood pressure, relieve nasal congestion, and sometimes increase the force of the heart action. Different vasoconstrictors have different purposes.

Ergotamine tartrate (er-got′ah-min tar′trayt) *(Gynergen)* (guy′ner-jen)

1. Ergotamine is an alkaloid of ergot, a mold on the grain rye that appears when the grain becomes damp.
2. Ergotamine is effective in treating migraine headache. It corrects dilation of cranial arteries, the cause of throbbing and migraine headaches. Its effect is thought to result from cerebral vasoconstriction that decreases the amplitude of the pulsations of cranial arteries.
3. The drug is cumulative, so the following symptoms should be watched for: tingling and numbness of fingers and toes, weakness and pain in muscles, gangrene of toes, and blindness.
4. Usual initial dose: 2 mg orally, or 0.25 mg to 0.5 mg intramuscularly.
5. Some other drugs for migraine headache are *Ergotamine with caffeine (Cafergot)* and *Dihydroergotamine (DHE 45)*.
   The latter is said to produce fewer side effects than ergotamine tartrate.

Methoxamine hydrochloride (me-thok′sah-meen) *(Vasoxyl)* (vas-ok′sil)

1. This vasoconstrictor is useful in treating hypotension and paroxysmal atrial tachycardia. It has no direct stimulating effect on the heart.
2. Side effects include severe hypertension, headache, urinary urgency, and vomiting.
3. This drug is available in solution form for IM or IV injection. Available are 1-ml ampules containing 20 mg and 10-ml vials containing 10 mg/ml.
4. Effects after IV injection occur almost immediately and last for 1 hour; after IM injection effects are seen within 15 minutes and last about 90 minutes. Slow IV infusion may also be used, which contain 60 to 70 mg of methoxamine in 500 ml of 5% dextrose.

• • •

For a discussion of the vasoconstrictor activity of *levarterenol (Levophed)* and *dopamine (Intropin)*, see Index.

Metaraminol bitartrate (met-ah-ram′i-nol) *(Aramine)* (ar′ah-myn)

1. Metaraminol, a vasopressor agent, is a valuable drug for the treatment of shock, since it constricts blood vessels, increases peripheral resistance, elevates both systolic and diastolic blood pressure, and improves cardiac contractility and cerebral, coronary, and renal blood flow.
2. It is used to overcome hypotension associated with myocardial infarction, surgical procedures, trauma, and barbiturate poisoning.
3. It may be given subcutaneously, intramuscularly, by IV drip, or by direct IV injection.

VASODILATORS
Antianginal drugs

Vasodilators are drugs that cause dilation of blood vessels and tend to lower the blood pressure. Drugs that bring about vasodilation have a number of uses in the treatment of hypertension, coronary disease (or angina pectoris pain), and peripheral vascular disease.

Angina pectoris occurs when the work load on the heart is too great and oxygen delivery is inadequate. Inadequate oxygenation may be caused by various disorders of the coronary vessels, such as vasomotor spasm, or by coronary atherosclerosis. Angina pectoris is characterized by chest pain that may radiate to one or both arms and the jaw. Specific types of stress and exercise may initiate this pain.

The nitrites seem to bring about a relaxation of abdominal smooth muscle, which causes a pooling of blood, reducing the amount of blood returning to the heart. This reduces the work load on the heart, which in turn reduces anginal pain.

Action and use

The nitrites have a direct action that causes relaxation of most smooth muscles in the body, including the bronchial, gastrointestinal, biliary, ureteral, and uterine. The most important pharmacologic effects are on vascular smooth muscle. The nitrites dilate all large arteries, such as the temporal, radial, and coronary arteries, as well as arterioles, capillaries, and venules. Because of this, they can be thought of as universal vasodilators. They are used extensively for patients with angina pectoris, and the rapid-acting nitrites remain the drug of choice for this condition.

Side effects

The side effects of the nitrites result from the vasodilator action. They include flushing of the skin, severe headache, nausea and vomiting, hypotension, and vertigo.

Tolerance to "long-acting" nitrites is easily developed, but usually does not develop with nitroglycerin. The smallest dose to give satisfactory results should be used in order that the dose may be increased as tolerance develops. Tolerance can appear within a few days and be well established within a few weeks. Tolerance is broken by withdrawal of the drug for a short period.

Following are some of the preparations of nitrites.

Amyl nitrite (am′il ny′tryt)

1. Amyl nitrite is a vasodilator volatile liquid that is available in small glass pearls, or ampules, containing 0.3 ml of the drug. The glass pearls are placed in a loosely woven material so that the pearl can be easily crushed under the patient's nostrils and inhaled.
2. The drug has a short onset of action (less than 1 minute), but its duration of action is also short (not more than 10 minutes).
3. It is very apt to cause cutaneous vasodilation, marked lowering of systemic pressure, syncope, and tachycardia. The odor is objectionable. For these reasons, nitroglycerin is preferred.
4. The patient should inhale the contents of the pearl no more than three times to prevent throbbing headache, facial flushing, nausea, and vomiting. Some facial flushing is normal as a result of cutaneous vasodilation.
5. Amyl nitrite is rarely, if ever, used today for angina pectoris.

Erythrityl tetranitrate (e-rith′ri-til tet-rah-ny′trayt) *(Cardilate)* (kar′di-layt)

1. This drug is available in 5-, 10-, and 15-mg tablets for oral or sublingual use.
2. Initial dose: usually 5 to 10 mg three times a day. Dosage may be increased to 30 mg three times a day.
3. Sublingual dosage onset of action is within 5 to 10 minutes; oral dosage onset is within 30 minutes. Duration of action for both routes is about 2 to 4 hours.

Isosorbide dinitrate (i-so-sor′byd) *(Isordil)* (i′sor-dil)

1. Isosorbide is available in 2.5- and 5-mg sublingual tablets; 5-, 10-, and 20-mg oral tablets; 5- and 10-mg chewable tablets, and 40-mg (long-acting) oral tablets and capsules.
2. Onset of action sublingually is 2 minutes; orally, on-set is 15 to 30 minutes. Oral effects last about 4 hours.
3. Sustained-release tablets of 40 mg are available. Onset of action is 30 minutes, with the effect lasting 12 hours.

Nitroglycerin (ny-tro-glis′er-in), *Glyceryl trinitrate tablets* (glis′er-il)

1. Nitroglycerin tablets are available in 0.15, 0.3 to 0.4, and 0.6 mg. The usual sublingual dose is 0.4 mg (gr 1/150). The dose may be repeated several times a day as needed.
2. A physician should be notified if pain persists after two or more tablets. Some patients can take as many as thirty tablets per day without harm, but a physician should be consulted before a patient takes more than a few tablets per day.
3. When taken sublingually, the drug appears in the blood in about 2 minutes, peak blood level is about 4 minutes, and the effects begin to disappear in 10 to 30 minutes.
4. Before undertaking any effort or strain that might induce an anginal attack, the patient should insert a nitroglycerin tablet sublingually.
5. Nitroglycerin deteriorates readily, being inactivated by light, heat, air, moisture, and time. Patients should be given these instructions:
   a. Keep a fresh supply of drug on hand, obtaining it at least every 3 months to assure freshness
   b. Keep the drug in the airtight, dark container it was dispensed in
   c. Avoid keeping the drug close to the body to protect it from body heat
6. Nitroglycerin also is available as a 2% topical ointment for prophylactic use, particularly at night. A chronic headache is a sign of overdosage, requiring the dose to be reduced.

Papaverine hydrochloride (pah-pav′er-in)

1. Papaverine acts directly on cardiac muscle, depresses conduction, and increases the refractory period. Relaxation of muscle in blood vessels occurs, especially if spasm is present.
2. Its effects are noticed in the coronary, peripheral, and pulmonary arteries.
3. The drug is occasionally used for angina but is not considered to be as reliable as nitroglycerin for this condition.

Pentaerythritol tetranitrate (pen-tah-e-rith′ri-tol) *(Peritrate)* (per′i-trayt), *(Pentritol)* (pen′tri-tol)

1. This drug is a vasodilator that may be effective in preventing angina pectoris attacks or in lessening the number and severity of attacks.

2. Some medical authorities believe that it is not as effective for relief of acute attacks as other angina agents but may lessen the number and the severity of the attacks.
3. It has few toxic or side effects but should be given with caution to patients with glaucoma, as is true of all nitrates.
4. Usual oral dose: 10 to 20 mg four times a day or one sustained-release tablet on arising and another 12 hours later.
5. Onset of action of the tablets is within 30 to 60 minutes and disappears in about 4 to 5 hours. Sustained-release preparations of 80 mg persist in effect for about 12 hours.
6. This drug also is available in sublingual preparations consisting of 10 mg of pentaerythritol and 0.3 mg of nitroglycerin.
7. Tolerance rapidly develops with continuous administration.

Peripheral vasodilators

The use of vasodilating drugs in chronic occlusive arterial disease or peripheral vascular disease has not been too encouraging to date. However, several drugs have been used with some success in the treatment of these diseases.

Cyclandelate (si-klan'de-layt)
(Cyclospasmol) (si-klo-spaz'mol)

1. Cyclandelate has a direct relaxation effect on the smooth muscles of peripheral arterial walls.
2. It increases peripheral circulation of the extremities and digits, which may elevate skin temperature of the extremities.
3. It is used for occlusive and vasospastic diseases of the vascular system associated with an impaired circulation, such as arteriosclerosis obliterans, thrombophlebitis (to control associated vasospasm and muscular ischemia), nocturnal leg cramps, local frostbite, Raynaud's disease, and certain cases of ischemic cerebral vascular disease, and as an aid to encourage healing of diabetic and trophic ulcers of the legs.
4. Side effects include flushing, tingling, sweating, dizziness, headache, feeling of weakness, and tachycardia.
5. The drug is available in 100-, 200-, 250-, and 400-mg capsules for oral use. The usual dose is 100 mg four times a day.

Isoxsuprine hydrochloride (i-sok'su-preen)
(Vasodilan) (vas-o-dy'lan)

1. Isoxuprine hydrochloride is a sympathomimetic agent that causes relaxation of vascular and uterine smooth muscle.

2. It is used in the treatment of peripheral vascular spasm, Raynaud's and Buerger's diseases, and arteriosclerotic vascular disease.
3. It produces noticeable uterine relaxation and is used by some physicians in the treatment of dysmenorrhea, threatened abortion, and premature labor.
4. Side effects are relatively mild and usually subside with reduction of dosage. They include nausea and vomiting, dizziness, lightheadedness, possible hypotension, and tachycardia.
5. This drug is available in 10- and 20-mg tablets. Oral dosage is 10 to 20 mg three or four times daily. Action occurs within 1 hour and persists for 3 hours after oral administration. Also available is an IM preparation of 5 mg/ml in 2-ml containers for acute and severe symptoms of arterial insufficiency.

Nicotine (nik'o-teen)

1. Nicotine is the chief alkaloid found in tobacco. It has no therapeutic use but has great pharmacologic interest and toxicologic importance.
2. The relation of excess tobacco smoking to lung cancer, mouth cancer, and coronary artery disease has now been clearly established.
3. Excessive smoking is known to cause irritation of the respiratory tract. Studies have shown a real possibility that tobacco smoke exerts effects that can cause lung cancer in humans.
4. It may increase secretion of hydrochloric acid from the stomach glands, so patients with gastric ulcers are instructed to reduce smoking or attempt to give up the habit.
5. Enough nicotine is absorbed by smokers to exert a variety of effects on the autonomic nervous system.
6. Nicotine is generally thought to be a contributing factor in causing thromboangitis obliterans (Buerger's disease). The drug may precipitate spasms of the peripheral blood vessels and thus reduce the blood flow through the affected vessels.
7. Vasospasm in the retinal blood vessels, associated with tobacco smoking, may be the cause of serious vision disturbances.
8. Most physicians recommend that patients with peripheral vascular disease or hypertension limit their smoking habits or discontinue smoking entirely. The adverse effects of tobacco smoking, especially cigarette smoking, on the cardiovascular system are being repeatedly emphasized to the public through many media.

Nicotinyl tartrate (nik-o-ti'nil tar'trayt)
(Roniacol) (ro-ny'ah-kol)

1. Nicotinyl tartrate is the tartrate salt of nicotinyl alcohol.

2. In the body it is converted to nicotinic acid, which produces direct peripheral vasodilation and increases blood flow to the extremities.

3. It has a more prolonged action than nicotinic acid since it oxidizes more slowly.

4. This drug is used in the treatment of Raynaud's disease, Buerger's disease, vascular spasm, blood vessel spasm, chilblains, and migraine associated with vascular spasm.

5. Nicotinyl tartrate is available in 50-mg tablets and as an elixir, 50 mg/ml. It is given in doses of 50 to 150 mg three times a day after meals.

Phenoxybenzamine hydrochloride
(fe-nok-se-ben'zah-meen)
(Dibenzyline) (di-ben'zi-leen)

1. Phenoxybenzamine increases peripheral blood flow, raises skin temperature, and relieves vasospastic pain.

2. It is used in vascular or blood vessel disorders, such as Raynaud's disease and ulceration of the legs.

3. Phenoxybenzamine lowers blood pressure when the patient is either lying down or erect.

4. This drug may aggravate coronary artery and renal vascular disease and respiratory infection symptoms. It is not used when the patient has compensated congestive heart failure or when a lowered blood pressure is not desired.

5. Dose is individualized. Dose range: 20 to 60 mg daily. Beginning dose for 4 days is 10 mg. It then may be increased until the desired effect is obtained. It takes about 2 weeks for the first observable improvement in the patient and several more weeks before full benefits occur.

Tolazoline hydrochloride (tol-az'o-leen)
(Priscoline) (pris'ko-leen)

1. Tolazoline hydrochloride dilates peripheral blood vessels and increases blood flow.

2. It is used to improve the circulation of patients with diabetes, Raynaud's disease, chronic ulcers, thrombophlebitis, saphenous vein ligation, and frostbite.

3. Tolazoline causes flushing of the face, neck, chest, and back as a result of dilation of blood vessels. This effect lasts about 20 to 30 minutes and is accompanied by a feeling of warmth.

4. The dose is individualized. In a parenteral form 10 to 50 mg is administered four times daily. The oral form is 25-mg tablets, and the parenteral form is 25 mg/ml in 10-ml vials.

ANTIHYPERTENSIVE AGENTS
General information on treatment of hypertension

Hypertension is a disease characterized by an elevation of the blood pressure above values considered normal for patients of similar racial backgrounds and environment. Statistics in North America show that blood pressures above 140/90 to 150/90 mm Hg are associated with premature death, which results from accelerated vascular disease of the brain, heart, and kidneys.

Primary, or *essential,* hypertension accounts for 80% to 90% of all clinical cases of high blood pressure. Its etiology is unknown; it is incurable at present but is certainly controllable. Twenty to twenty-five million Americans have hypertension. The prevalence increases steadily with advancing age. In every age group the incidence of hypertension is higher for black persons than for white persons of both sexes. Other factors associated with high blood pressure are a family history of hypertension, obesity, spikes of high blood pressure in young adult years, cigarette smoking, hyperglycemia, hypercholesterolemia, preexisting cardiovascular disease (angina, congestive heart failure), abnormal renal function, retinopathies, and a history of a previous stroke.

Secondary hypertension may be caused by renal or endocrine dysfunction or a number of other causes such as toxemia of pregnancy, CNS disorders, and coarctation of the aorta. Treatment of secondary hypertension is usually not necessary after the underlying disorder is corrected.

A patient is classified as having mild hypertension if the diastolic blood pressure is between 90 and 105 mm Hg and the patient has no indication of such tissue damage as retinopathies. This form of hypertension is usually treated with a thiazide diuretic. If necessary, clonidine, reserpine, or methyldopa may be added to the drug therapy.

Moderate hypertension is present when the diastolic pressure is between 105 and 130 mm Hg. Tissue damage may or may not exist. Treatment usually consists of a combination of hydralazine, clonidine, prazosin, methyldopa, and/or propranolol, plus a thiazide diuretic.

Severe hypertension exists when diastolic pressure is above 130 mm Hg. These patients have several symptoms and usually display tissue damage. The treatment is initiated with an oral diuretic, propranolol, and hydralazine. Guanethidine may be added if response is inadequate. Other combinations, such as clonidine, prazosin, and methyldopa, have also brought good results.

For patients suddenly developing hypertensive encephalopathy, as indicated by neurologic signs and symptoms, more rapid control of blood pressure is required. Boluses of diazoxide or a sodium nitroprusside infusion may be necessary to control the symptoms.

The goal of antihypertensive therapy is a prolongation of a useful life by preventing cardiovascular complications. To accomplish this goal, the blood pressure must be reduced and maintained at acceptable levels. Treatment schedules should be established so as to interfere with the patient's life-style as little as possible. However, some changes in life-style are absolutely essential.

The education of the patient is vitally important in treating hypertension. This education, which should include the following points, should be emphasized and reiterated frequently by the physician and the nurse.

1. The meaning of hypertension and its effects on blood pressure, brain, heart, and kidneys should be simply explained.
2. Hypertension cannot be cured at present but can be controlled by drugs, diet, moderate exercise, freedom from tension and worry, as well as other measures.
3. Hypertension often causes no symptoms until complications occur, so frequent physical checkups and blood pressure monitoring are of vital importance. With approval of his physician, the patient can be taught to take his own blood pressure.
4. Drug therapy is a main therapy of hypertension, but other measures are also vitally important, such as:
   a. Reduction of dietary sodium intake and weight (if necessary)
   b. Regular times for relaxation and the development of hobbies
   c. A plan of moderate exercise developed by the physician with his patient to improve the patient's physical condition
   d. Discontinuation of cigarette smoking, since it is an added risk factor in coronary artery disease
   e. Helping the patient realize that situations with feelings of anxiety, fear, anger, or annoyance aggravate hypertension, and that alterations in normal functions such as eating, sleeping, and elimination also increase the physiologic stress response and raise blood pressure
5. The patient's cooperation in changing much of his life-style is difficult but must be achieved.
6. Request the assistance of the patient, his spouse, family member, or close friend in planning these activities including a dietary plan, a reduction or cessation of smoking, a plan to lessen stressful, emotional activities, and a medication schedule with names of medications, times to be taken, and dosage. The patient should also be taught how to cope with such side effects as nasal congestion, loss of strength, fatigue, and anorexia.
7. Remind the patient to get up slowly to offset the feeling of dizziness or to lie down immediately if feeling faint.
8. Periodic encouragement and reminders of frequently forgotten "rules" will increase the patient's ability and desire to maintain the therapy.

Table 16-1. Ingredients of common antihypertensive combination products*

Product	Diuretic (mg)	Antihypertensive (mg)	Other (mg)
Aldoclor-150	Chlorothiazide (150)	Methyldopa (250)	
Aldoril-15	Hydrochlorothiazide (15)	Methyldopa (250)	
Apresazide 25/25	Hydrochlorothiazide (25)	Hydralazine (25)	
Apresoline-Esidrix	Hydrochlorothiazide (15)	Hydralazine (25)	
Butiserpazide-25	Hydrochlorothiazide (25)	Reserpine (0.1)	Butabarbital (30)
Combipres 0.1	Chlorthalidone (15)	Clonidine (0.1)	
Combipres 0.2	Chlorthalidone (15)	Clonidine (0.2)	
Diupres-250	Chlorothiazide (250)	Reserpine (0.125)	
Diutensen-R	Methylclothiazide (2.5)	Reserpine (0.1)	
Enduronyl	Methylclothiazide (5)	Deserpidine (0.25)	
Hydropres-25	Hydrochlorothiazide (25)	Reserpine (0.125)	
Hydrotensin-25	Hydrochlorothiazide (25)	Reserpine (0.125)	
Naturetin W/K	Bendroflumethiazide (5)		Potassium chloride (500)
Oreticyl	Hydrochlorothiazide (25)	Deserpidine (0.125)	
Rautrax	Flumethiazide (400)	Rauwolfia (50)	Potassium chloride (400)
Regroton	Chlorthalidone (50)	Reserpine (0.25)	
Renese-R	Polythiazide (2)	Reserpine (0.25)	
Salutensin	Hydroflumethiazide (50)	Reserpine (0.125)	
Ser-Ap-Es	Hydrochlorothiazide (15)	Reserpine (0.1)	Hydralazine (25)
Serpasil-Apresoline		Reserpine 0.1	Hydralazine (25)
Unipres	Hydrochlorothiazide (15)	Reserpine 0.1	Hydralazine (25)

*This is a representative listing. Other strengths of these products, as well as products not listed, are also available.

Many drugs are used in the treatment of hypertension, but generally, there are only three classes of drugs used: (1) direct vasodilators, such as hydralazine (Apresoline) and prazosin (Minipress); (2) diuretics, such as the thiazides, furosemide (Lasix), ethacrynic acid (Edecrin); and (3) sympathetic nervous system inhibitors, such as guanethidine (Ismelin), reserpine, methyldopa (Aldomet), metoprolol (Lopressor), propranolol (Inderal), and clonidine (Catapres). All of these drugs act either directly or indirectly to reduce the peripheral vascular resistance, therefore lowering blood pressure. It is routine practice to use two or more antihypertensive drugs at a time; using drugs that act by different mechanisms to reduce peripheral vascular resistance provides the benefit of using lower doses of each drug so that the patient suffers fewer side effects. See Table 16-1 for a list of the ingredients of common antihypertensive combination products.

Sympathetic nervous system inhibitors
Clonidine hydrochloride (klo'ni-deen)
(Catapres) (ca'tah-pres)

1. Clonidine is a potent antihypertensive agent that acts within the central nervous system to reduce both diastolic and systolic blood pressure.
2. It also causes bradycardia, which results in decreased cardiac output. After prolonged therapy the lowered blood pressure is a result mainly of reduced peripheral vascular resistance.
3. This drug is now used in the treatment of mild to moderate hypertension. Its effectiveness is generally improved when used in combination with diuretics and/or other antihypertensive agents.
4. Patients must be warned of the need to continue this drug therapy. Abrupt discontinuance of clonidine may cause a rapid increase in diastolic and systolic blood pressure, nervousness, agitation, restlessness, tremor, headache, nausea, and increased salivation.
   a. These symptoms are more pronounced after 1 to 2 months of therapy and begin to appear within a few hours after a dose is missed.
   b. Blood pressure rises markedly within 8 to 24 hours.
   c. Clonidine, therefore, when it must be discontinued, should be discontinued by gradually reducing the dose over 2 to 4 days, depending on the patient's response.
5. Most frequent adverse effects are dry mouth, drowsiness, sedation (caution patients about performing hazardous tasks), constipation, headache, and dizziness.
6. Patients on long-term clonidine therapy should have periodic eye examinations. Laboratory animals have developed degenerative retinal changes, although none has been reported in humans.

7. Those patients having a diagnosis of mental depression may be more susceptible to further depressive activity.
8. Clonidine should not be given during pregnancy, since embryo toxicities have been found at normal therapeutic doses. It should only be used in pregnancy if the potential benefit outweighs the potential risk. It is not known whether clonidine is found in breast milk.
9. Drug interactions include the following: the bradycardiac effects of clonidine may be enhanced by guanethidine, propranolol, and the digitalis glycosides; the sedative effects of clonidine may enhance the CNS depressant effects of barbiturates, tranquilizers, antihistamines, and alcohol; and desipramine (Norpramin, Pertofrane) blocks the antihypertensive effects of clonidine. Other tricyclic antidepressants may give similar effects. Clonidine may be administered together with methyldopa, hydralazine, guanethidine, reserpine, furosemide, spironolactone, and the thiazide diuretics without interactions, but the antihypertensive effects of these agents will be enhanced, requiring careful adjustment of dosage.
10. Usual adult dose: initially, 0.1 mg two times daily. Maintenance dose: add 0.1 to 0.2 mg daily until desired effect is achieved. Average daily doses range from 0.2 to 0.8 mg in divided doses daily. Maximum recommended daily dose is 2.4 mg.

Guanethidine sulfate (gwan-eth'i-deen)
(Ismelin) (is'meh-lin)

1. Guanethidine is an antihypertensive agent that causes a release and subsequent depletion of norepinephrine from postganglionic or adrenergic nerve endings. It is recommended for treatment of moderate to severe hypertension.
2. Side effects include fatigue, nausea, nasal stuffiness, abdominal distress, weight gain, bradycardia, diarrhea, lightheadedness, and weakness, especially when first getting out of bed. The cause of the last symptom is the arteriolar and venodilation that permits pools of blood to collect in the lower extremities, causing a reduction of cerebral blood flow. The lightheadedness and weakness often disappear during the day and can be lessened by rising slowly, sitting on the edge of the bed for a few minutes, and performing leg, foot, and toe exercises before standing.
3. Guanethidine should be used with caution in patients with severe coronary insufficiency, recent myocardial infarction, hypertension associated with renal disease, cerebral complications, or peptic ulcer.
4. Blood pressure should be taken daily when initiating therapy, in both lying-down and erect positions.
5. The dose is individualized and has long duration of action. Usual initial dose: 25 to 50 mg once daily.

Methyldopa (meth′il-do′pah)
(Aldomet) (al′do-met)

1. Methyldopa is an antihypertensive drug recommended for mild to moderate hypertension.
2. Some toxic effects resulting from methyldopa include sedation and orthostatic hypotension, often to an unpleasant degree. Methyldopa must be used with caution in patients with liver disease or a history of mental depression.
3. Side effects that may occur include sedation, dry mouth, nasal congestion, depression, fluid retention (edema), and possible fever. These can usually be controlled or eliminated by reduction of dosage.
4. Oral dosage: 250 to 500 mg three times a day. Maximum recommended dose is 3 g daily. **Methyldopate** (a methyl ester hydrochloride) injected intravenously in doses of 100 mg or more will cause a decline in blood pressure that may begin in 4 hours and extend for 10 hours or more.

Metoprolol tartrate (met′o-pro-lol)
(Lopressor) (lo-pres′or)

1. Metoprolol is a new antihypertensive agent that acts by selectively blocking specific adrenergic nerve receptors. It is used in the treatment of mild to moderate hypertension and is particularly effective when used in combination with thiazide diuretics and other antihypertensive agents.
2. The most common side effects of metoprolol are fatigue, headache, and diarrhea. Metoprolol should be used with caution in patients with diabetes mellitus, asthma, or heart disease. Metoprolol may exacerbate the symptoms of these diseases.
3. Usual initial dosage: 50 mg two times daily. Maintenance dosage range: 100 to 450 mg daily.

Propranolol
(Inderal)

1. Propranolol is a beta blocking agent used in combination with other antihypertensive therapy to treat moderate to severe hypertension.
2. Usual dosage range: 160 to 480 mg daily.
3. Propranolol is discussed in greater detail elsewhere (see Index).

Rauwolfia alkaloids
Alseroxylon (al-ser-ok′si-lon)
(Rauwiloid) (row′wi-loyd), (Rautensin) (raw-ten′sin)

1. Alseroxylon is an oral preparation extracted from the root of *Rauwolfia serpentina*.
2. Average adult dose: 2 to 4 mg daily.

Deserpidine (de-ser′pi-deen)
(Harmonyl) (har′mo-nil)

1. The action of deserpidine is similar to that of reserpine.
2. Average daily oral dose: 0.25 to 1.0 mg.

Rauwolfia serpentina
(raw-wol′fee-ah ser-pen-tee′nah)
(Raudixin) (raw-dik′sin)

1. This drug is the powdered whole root of *Rauwolfia serpentina*.
2. Daily oral dose for adults: 200 to 400 mg, usually divided into two doses.

Rescinnamine (re-sin′ah-min)
(Moderil) (mod′er-il)

1. The action of rescinnamine is similar to that of reserpine, except bradycardia and sedation are less common with rescinnamine.
2. Average initial oral dose: 0.5 mg once or twice daily for 2 weeks. Maintenance dose: 0.25 mg daily.

Reserpine (res′er-peen)
(Rau-sed) (raw′sed), (Reserpoid) (res′er-poyd), (Sandril) (san′dril), (Serpasil) (ser′pah-sil)

1. Reserpine is an alkaloid obtained from the root of a certain species of *Rauwolfia*. Reserpine is considered the most potent of the alkaloids of *Rauwolfia*.
2. Reserpine reduces norepinephrine levels in peripheral nerve endings (sympathetic postganglionic nerves). The reason for this action is not known. It is thought to result from an increased release of norepinephrine, which is rapidly destroyed by amine oxidases and related enzymes.
3. Reserpine also depletes norepinephrine from various organs, including the brain. Brain depletion of norepinephrine may be the cause of the sedative action of reserpine.
4. Side effects include nasal stuffiness, weight gain, diarrhea, dryness of the mouth, nosebleeds, itching, skin eruptions, insomnia, depression, and occasionally, gastric irritation and reactivation of old ulcers or formation of new ones.
5. The drug is administered orally or by IM or IV injection. Oral dose for mild hypertension is 0.1 to 0.5 mg once daily.
6. The blood pressure should be determined before administering any oral or injectable dose to avoid marked hypotension.

Direct vasodilators

Diazoxide (dy-az-ok′syd)
(Hyperstat IV Injection)

1. Diazoxide is used for emergency reduction of blood pressure in hospitalized patients with severe hypertension.
2. Diazoxide is available in 300-mg ampules. It is administered undiluted in a peripheral vein in a dosage of 300 mg in 30 seconds or less. The blood pressure must be monitored closely. If hypotension occurs, dopamine or levarterenol may be administered.

Hydralazine hydrochloride (hy-dral′ah-zeen)
(Apresoline) (ah-pres′o-leen)

1. This antihypertensive drug is used to treat moderate to severe essential hypertension and hypertension associated with renal disease and toxemia of pregnancy.
2. Blood pressure should be taken regularly to determine effects and possible change in dosage.
3. Early side effects that are sometimes observed and usually disappear as the drug is continued include nausea, vomiting, dizziness, palpitation, tachycardia, numbness and tingling of legs and feet, nasal congestion, and postural hypotension. The nasal congestion can be treated with an antihistamine such as pyribenzamine or diphenhydramine. If arthritic symptoms occur, the drug should be discontinued.
4. Hydralazine should be used with caution in coronary heart disease, advanced kidney damage, and possible cerebral accidents.
5. This drug is available in 10-, 25-, 50-, and 100-mg tablets for oral use and as a sterile solution for injection of 20 mg/ml. Initial oral dose: 10 mg after meals and at bedtime.

Nitroprusside sodium (ny-tro-prus′yd)
(Nipride) (ny′pryd)

1. Nitroprusside is a potent vasodilator that acts directly on the smooth muscle of blood vessels to produce vasodilation. It is used in patients with a sudden severe hypertensive crisis.
2. This drug is administered by slow IV infusion, usually starting at a rate of 0.5 to 1.0 μg/kg/min. Blood pressure must be taken every 3 to 4 minutes to avoid hypotension. The average infusion rate is 3 to 4 μg/kg/min.
3. Nitroprusside is highly light sensitive. A paper bag or foil wrap should be placed over the IV container to protect it from light. Solutions over 4 hours old should be discarded.
4. The drug is available as a 50-mg vial to be diluted in 500 to 1,000 ml of 5% dextrose and water.

Prazosin hydrochloride (prah′zo-sin)
(Minipress) (min′ee-pres)

1. Prazosin acts directly on smooth muscle of arterioles to produce peripheral vasodilation and a reduction in diastolic blood pressure. Prazosin is used in combination with other antihypertensive agents in the treatment of mild to moderate hypertension.
2. The most common adverse effects reported with prazosin include dizziness, headache, drowsiness, nausea, weakness, and lethargy. All are transient and disappear with continued therapy.
3. The initial doses of prazosin may cause dizziness, tachycardia, and fainting, but these adverse effects occur in less than 1% of patients starting therapy. Symptoms occur 15 to 90 minutes after initial dosages. This effect may be minimized by giving the first doses with food and limiting the initial dose to 1 mg. Patients should be warned that this side effect may occur, that it is transient, and that they should lie down immediately if symptoms develop.
4. Initial dose: 1 mg three times daily. Maximum recommended dose is 40 mg daily.

The diuretics

The diuretics, including the thiazides, chlorthalidone, metolazone, furosemide, and ethacrynic acid, are mainstays in antihypertensive therapy. The diuretics act as antihypertensive agents by causing volume depletion, sodium excretion, and direct vasodilation of peripheral arterioles. Diuretics are used to treat mild, moderate, and severe hypertension and are most effective when used in combination with other antihypertensive agents. The agents are discussed under the urinary system drugs (see Index).

Nursing care of patients receiving antihypertensive therapy

The following instructions should be given to patients receiving potent hypertensive agents to avoid or decrease orthostatic hypotensive effects.

1. The patient should rise slowly from a lying to a sitting or standing position to allow for physiologic adjustment of the vascular system and for vasoconstriction of lower extremity vessels to occur. This prevents pooling of blood, dizziness, and fainting.
2. If standing or sitting, the patient should flex his calf muscles, wiggle his toes, rise up on his toes, and allow his feet to return to flat position several times. The result is alternate vasoconstriction and vasodilation and prevention of blood pooling in the lower extremities. Demonstrate this to the patient, and have him practice it several times.

3. If weakness or dizziness occur, they can be relieved by muscular activity or recumbency.
4. Lying flat with the legs slightly higher than the head will promote cerebral flow and decrease pooling of blood in the legs. Instruct how this is accomplished; for example, two pillows under the legs.
5. The patient should not stand in long lines for extended periods, especially within 2 hours after taking the hypertensive drug. He should avoid standing still in theaters and church and waiting in line at ticket booths and supermarkets.
6. Hot baths, steam baths, or lengthy hot showers should be avoided, since they promote peripheral vasodilation and may cause a hypotensive reaction.
7. The patient *should not suddenly cease drug therapy*.
   a. If the drug is suddenly discontinued, blood pressure may rise higher because of increased sensitivity to pressor substances. Gradual withdrawal of the drug is therefore necessary.
   b. Explain this carefully in simple language to the patient, emphasizing the dangers of sudden discontinuance and the importance of maintaining a consistent drug therapy with periodic contact with his physician.
8. The patient should carry an identification card containing his name, address, phone number; the name, address, and phone number of his physician; and the name of the drug, dosage, and the times the drug is taken. Ask the patient to show this card on his next office visit.
9. Alcohol in moderation is acceptable. The physician or nurse should explain to the patient about the amount implied in the term "moderation."
10. In regard to the patient's diet:
    a. The physician may limit the patient's salt intake by ordering a salt-restricted diet. Patients should avoid eating foods high in sodium content, such as ham, bacon, crab meat, tuna, crackers, and various cheeses. Instruct the patient about low-salt foods available and ways to limit salt intake.
11. Diarrhea can be treated with Kaopectate, Lomotil, or similar preparations.
12. Dryness of the mouth caused by inhibition of sympathetic activity can be treated with good oral hygiene, including mouthwashes and lozenges, and dry nasal mucosa treated with nonirritating lubricants such as lanolin or glycerin.
13. Praise the patient for adhering to his diet, for making changes in his life-style to lessen tension and worry, for his success in losing weight and

the advantages of this to him, and for realizing the importance of remembering to follow his drug therapy consistently.
14. If the physician approves, teach the patient to take his own blood pressure, keeping a list of the times taken, dates, and his body position. Review the blood pressure procedure with the patient during his office visits or hospital stay to check on his accuracy and give him reassurance.
15. Make a booklet of several mimeographed pages listing the main points just described in this section. Have the physician approve of the booklet and give a copy to each hypertensive patient to read and study as reminders and for reassurance.

ANTICOAGULANTS

Diseases associated with abnormal clotting within blood vessels take a great toll of lives. Diseases caused by intravascular clotting include some of the major causes of death from cardiovascular sources, such as coronary occlusion and cerebral accidents. Drugs that inhibit clotting are therefore most important.

Nursing care of patients receiving anticoagulant therapy

1. Patients should be observed frequently each day for nosebleeds, bleeding gums, petechiae, purpura, ecchymosis, blood in the urine or stools, and symptoms of internal bleeding.
2. Patients on complete bed rest should be turned frequently each day, bathed and back-rubbed daily, encouraged to breathe deeply frequently, and aided in any limited movements or exercises the physician may prescribe.
3. Patients should be advised to protect themselves from injury. They should walk carefully up and down stairs and over street curbs and should shave with an electric razor.
4. Patients on long-term therapy should be instructed about the reasons and the importance in taking their medicines as prescribed and reporting when instructed for blood tests and prothrombin time.
5. Outpatients should carry cards stating their identity, the physician's name and phone number, and the drug's name, dosage, and time it is to be taken.
6. Antiembolic stockings should be worn if physician directs.

Bishydroxycoumarin
(bis-hy-drok-see-koo′mah-rin), *Dicumarol* (dy-koo′mah-rol)

1. Bishydroxycoumarin is a synthetic drug identical with the anticoagulant factor found in spoiled sweet clover.
2. It slows the formation of prothrombin in blood, thus

prolonging prothrombin time. Prothrombin is a substance in blood that aids blood to clot. This drug, then, prevents clot formation.

3. So far as is known, it does not help conditions in which clots have already formed, but it does help to prevent the formation of future clots.

4. This drug is used when treatment includes absolute bed rest for a long period, such as with a patient who has suffered a heart attack or a broken hip. Clots often form in the veins of the legs or the pelvis of an elderly patient at bed rest. If one of these clots breaks loose (embolus) and travels to the lungs, it is often fatal.

5. Bishydroxycoumarin is also used in the treatment of postoperative thrombophlebitis (inflammation of a vein caused by infection and a clot).

6. The dose depends on the prothrombin activity; laboratory specimens of blood are also necessary to determine daily dosage. It can be taken by mouth. The patient must be observed for bleeding from the nose, gums, rectum and for bruising on the skin. Report signs of bleeding immediately.

7. Vitamin K is effective as an antidote for overdosage of bishydroxycoumarin.

Heparin sodium injection (hep'ah-rin)

1. Heparin sodium is a natural substance found in the tissue, chiefly the gut and lungs, of food animals.

2. It prolongs the clotting time of blood.

3. Heparin must be administered by injection since it is inactive orally. The most common methods of administration are a single IV injection or a continuous IV drip.

4. The response to heparin occurs almost immediately and lasts for about 3 to 4 hours, unless the dose is repeated.

5. When administration is discontinued, the clotting time returns to normal within a few hours.

6. The dosage of this drug needs to be determined for each patient and maintained at a level that will keep the clotting time 1.5 to 2.5 times the normal clotting time. The potency of heparin sodium is expressed in units.

7. When heparin sodium is given intravenously at spaced intervals, 5,000 units may be administered at a time. For continuous IV drip, 10,000 to 20,000 units are added to 1,000 ml of 5% sterile glucose solution or to isotonic saline solution. The flow is started at about 500 to 750 units/hr and later adjusted based on the patient's response.

8. Heparin, warfarin, and other related anticoagulants must be used with caution in patients with blood cell disorders, liver or kidney damage, subacute bacterial endocarditis (because of the tendency of patients to bleed), hemophilia, recent brain and spinal cord surgery, or open lesions or wounds.

9. Blood specimens of the patient should be sent to the laboratory daily to obtain periodic determination of clotting time. The prothrombin time (PT) is used to monitor warfarin therapy, while the activated partial thromboplastin time (a-PTT) is generally used to monitor heparin.

10. Side effects or toxic effects can be overcome by reducing the dosage, frequency of injection, or both. The effects of heparin on the clotting mechanism can be reversed by the administration of protamine sulfate (see point 12 in this discussion).

11. Heparin is the drug of choice in treating thrombophlebitis occurring during pregnancy, since it does not cross the placental barrier and is not excreted in the mother's milk. It is the drug of choice for acute vascular occlusion because of its immediate action and its readily reversible quality if surgery is indicated for clot removal.

12. The heparin antagonist is **Protamine sulfate** injection. Protamine is itself an anticoagulant and will cause prolongation of clotting time when given alone, but when given in the presence of heparin, the two drugs are attracted to each other instead of to the blood elements, and each neutralizes the anticoagulant activity of the other. Overdosages of protamine, however, may result in further hemorrhage.

Warfarin sodium (war'fah-rin)
(Coumadin) (koo'mah-din), (Panwarfin) (pan-war'fin)

1. Warfarin is a powerful anticoagulant.

2. It prolongs prothrombin time and lessens the risk of emboli in thromboembolic disease, obstetrics, and surgery.

3. It takes about 3 to 5 days of use to obtain full therapeutic effect.

4. It can be given orally or intravenously. Tablets are available in 2, 2.5, 5, 7.5, 10, and 25 mg.

5. Drug interactions may be therapeutic or detrimental. A relatively minor undesirable drug interaction does not necessarily preclude the use of that combination in clinical practice.

   a. Drugs reported to increase the anticoagulant activity of warfarin include aspirin, quinidine, phenylbutazone, tolbutamide, phenothiazines, ethacrynic acid, indomethacin, allopurinol, chloral hydrate, and thyroid preparations.

   b. Drugs reported to decrease the anticoagulant activity of warfarin include alcohol, rifampin, phenytoin, oral contraceptives, and barbiturates.

6. A good rule to follow is that anytime patients start or stop a medication while continuing on warfarin, they should have their prothrombin time monitored closely for increased or decreased coagulation time.

COAGULANTS

Drugs that cause the blood to clot or hasten clotting are called coagulants. Some of these are useful in the treatment of bleeding caused by deficiency of prothrombin, in obstructive jaundice, as a preoperative preparation, in hemorrhagic conditions of the newborn, and, in special form, to control bleeding during surgical procedures.

Absorbable gelatin sponge (Gelfoam) (jel'foam)

1. Absorbable gelatin sponge is used to control capillary bleeding.
2. It can be left in surgical wounds and is completely absorbed in about 4 to 6 weeks.
3. It should be well moistened with isotonic salt solution or thrombin solution before it is placed in a bleeding surface.

Vitamin K

1. Vitamin K was found in hog liver and alfalfa by Dam of Copenhagen in 1935. It is also found in many foods and is synthesized by intestinal bacteria for body use.
2. This vitamin aids the blood in clotting, thus aiding the prevention of hemorrhage.
3. Vitamin K is useful only if the prolonged bleeding time is caused by low concentration of prothrombin factors in the blood. It is useful in preventing hemorrhage in newborn babies after delivery, so it is a drug commonly used on obstetric wards.
4. Some preparations of vitamin K are as follows:
   a. **Menadione** (men-ah-di'own). Usual dose: 5 to 10 mg daily. Do not administer to infants.
   b. **Menadione sodium bisulfite (Hykinone)** (hy'ki-nown). It may be administered subcutaneously, intramuscularly, and intravenously. Usual dose: 2.5 to 5 mg daily. Do not administer to infants.
   c. **Menadiol sodium diphosphate** (men-ah-di'ol) **(Synkayvite)** (sin'ka-vyt). This is a derivative of menadione. Oral dose is available in 5-mg tablets. Usual adult dose: 5 to 10 mg daily. An injectable form is available in 5 mg/ml, 10 mg/ml, and 37.5 mg/ml ampules.

Phytonadione (fy-toe-nah-di'own) (Aquamephyton) (ahk-wah-mef'i-ton), (Konakion) (kon-ah-ki'on), (Mephyton), (vitamin K₁)

1. Phytonadione can be obtained from natural sources or produced synthetically. It has a more prolonged effect than menadione.
2. Intravenous dose: as much as 10 mg for adults. Oral dose: 4 to 10 mg.
3. Infant: 1 mg intramuscularly at time of birth.

**The physician prescribes the medicine and treatment.
The nurse carries out the physician's orders.
Self-medication is dangerous. Consult your physician first.
There is in every medicine a possible danger.
When in doubt—ASK!**

ASSIGNMENT

Review previous lessons and questions according to the directions of your instructor.

1. Digitalis is used primarily in the treatment of
   a. Too slow a heart rate
   b. High blood pressure
   c. Congestive heart failure and atrial fibrillation
   d. Too low a blood pressure
2. What is the natural source of digitalis? Are most digitalis products produced synthetically today? Digitalis increases the strength of myocardial contraction of the heart. What are some important benefits of this action? What are some important results of these benefits? Do digitalis and its preparations speed and strengthen the heart, or slow and strengthen the heart? Learn this well. Give a brief definition of fibrillation, and name the drug of choice in the treatment of atrial fibrillation (see Glossary and medical dictionary).
3. Digitalization of the patient refers to
   a. A condition in which the heart has been speeded and strengthened
   b. A state in which the patient is completely free of symptoms of heart failure
   c. The first early symptoms of digitalis poisoning
   d. A state in which the failing heart is receiving maximum benefits from the digitalis preparation
   e. A condition in which the heart has been slowed to a completely normal rate without any irregularities in beat

4. Define cumulation and name two digitalis preparations that are cumulative. Why is it important to count the pulse before giving any digitalis preparations in any form? What is the treatment if the pulse beat is below 60 beats per minute? Explain how to take an apical pulse. What are some common side and toxic effects or cumulative effects of digitalis indicating digitalis toxicity? List predisposing factors to digitalis toxicity. What is the most common treatment for this condition? Why is the oral route of digitalis the safest to use?

5. Use full-size binder paper, $8^1/_2 \times 11$ inches, three or four pages. Outline briefly, but completely, all the nursing measures for patients receiving digitalis preparations. Check all the nursing measures from your text as you proceed to assure accuracy. Study these. Learn them well. They will be of great aid to you in more effectively nursing the patient taking digitalis and in preventing errors.

6. Name four digitalis preparations, using both generic and trade names.

7. Digitoxin (more than one choice is correct)
   a. Has as its trade name Lanatoside
   b. Has a maintenance dosage range of 0.05 to 0.3 mg daily
   c. Has as its trade name Digoxin
   d. Has as its trade names Crystodigin and Purodigin
   e. Is the same drug as digoxin

8. Digoxin (several choices are correct)
   a. Has trade names of Crystodigin and Purodigin
   b. Has a trade name of acylanid
   c. Has a trade name of Lanoxin
   d. Is a hydrolytic product formed from lanatoside C
   e. Is available in oral form only
   f. Digitalizes more rapidly than digitoxin
   g. Is available in oral doses of 0.125-, 0.25-, and 0.5-mg tablets
   h. Is the same drug as digitoxin
   i. Has one distinct advantage to its trade name in that it helps to differentiate digoxin and digitoxin
   j. May, as is true of other digitalis preparations, cause cumulative symptoms

9. The best way to prevent the possibility of confusion between digitoxin and digoxin is to (one choice is best)
   a. Ask a senior student nurse
   b. Ask your classmate
   c. Check the name of the medicine and dosage carefully with the medicine ticket, bottle label, and physician's order from the chart; then ask the team leader, head nurse, or instructor to check
   d. Give the drug but next time ask your instructor or team leader to check

10. Name the source and main effect of gitalin and ouabain.

11. Name four other digitalis preparations. Review the summary paragraph at the end of the discussion of digitalis preparations. Learn this well. Study again the entire discussion of digitoxin and digoxin. It will prevent you making errors when administering medications.

12. The nurse took an apical pulse rate with a stethoscope and found that the pulse rate was 52 beats per minute. The nurse should

   a. Administer $^1/_2$ tablet to the patient
   b. Administer the drug, but in twice as much water as usual
   c. Administer the drug
   d. Not administer the drug but report to the team leader

13. Bretylium (Bretylol) is what type of drug? It inhibits the release of what catecholamine autonomic nervous system drug? List the uses of bretylium. Is this drug a cardiac depressant? It should be particularly useful in patients with what particular heart condition? List the side effects. List the precautions to observe in administering this drug to patients with what medical conditions? What precautions should be observed in administering this drug to a patient already receiving digitalis and why? What points should the nurse remember during administration of this drug? Over how long a period is bretylium usually given?

14. What is the chief effect of disopyramide (Norpace)? Can it be used in digitalized as well as nondigitalized patients? Disopyramide is a useful drug as an alternative to what two drugs and why? Discuss the side effects of this drug. In overdosage, what is the best treatment?

15. What is the chief use of lidocaine (Xylocaine) in cardiovascular treatment? What is another common use of this drug? List toxic effects of lidocaine. List nursing measures to be followed during infusions of lidocaine. What are the onset and duration of action for this drug?

16. Give two uses of phenytoin (DPH, Dilantin).

17. What are the main uses of procainamide (Pronestyl)? List the side effects and toxic effects of this drug.

18. What effect does propranolol (Inderal) have on the heart?

19. The main effect of quinidine sulfate is to
   a. Raise the blood pressure
   b. Speed and strengthen the heart beat
   c. Control both auricular, or atrial, and ventricular arrhythmias, thus slowing the heart to a more regular beat
   d. Control auricular arrhythmia only

20. What is the source of quinidine? Should the pulse be counted before administering quinidine or is this rule for digitalis preparations only? List the side effects of quinidine. This drug is potentially hazardous. Why? This drug should be administered with caution to patients with what medical conditions? List and discuss drug interactions and quinidine. Reread point 10 of the quinidine discussion carefully—remember it.

21. To which group of drugs do the following belong: bretylium, disopyramide, lidocaine, phenytoin, procainamide, propranolol (in this study), and quinidine?

22. Define *vasoconstrictor*. Explain the effects of vasoconstrictors on blood vessels, muscle fibers in the walls of blood vessels, and the vasomotor center in the medulla. What are some of the uses of vasoconstrictors?

23. Give two examples of drugs that have come to be almost specifics for migraine headache. What is the effect on the cranial blood vessels in migraine headache? This effect is thought to result from what action? Is the drug cumulative? List symptoms that should be watched for during administration of this drug.

24. What effect do levarterenol (Levophed) and dopamine (Intropin) have on the blood vessels?

25. What are the chief uses of metaraminol (Aramine) and to which group does it belong, vasodilators or vasocontrictors?

26. Define *vasodilator* and tell some of the uses of vasodilator drugs.

27. What does *angina pectoris* imply? When does this condition occur? What are the causes of inadequate oxygenation? What are the symptoms of angina pectoris? What are the actions and effects of the nitrites on coronary smooth muscle, smooth muscle in the body, and all large arteries? Are the nitrites vasodilators or vasoconstrictors? Do they raise or lower blood pressure?

28. Name three of the nitrite drugs other than amyl nitrite used in the treatment of angina pectoris.

29. Nitroglycerin deteriorates readily, being inactivated by light, heat, air, moisture, and time. List the instructions to be given to patients receiving nitroglycerin tablets. How are these tablets to be given, orally or sublingually?

30. What is papaverine's effect on the heart? Is it as commonly used for angina as the nitrites?

31. What is the chief effect of Peritrate compared to the effectiveness of other angina agents?

32. Two peripheral vasodilators useful in the treatment of Raynaud's disease and other circulatory disease are
    a. Nitroglycerin tablets
    b. Cyclandelate
    c. Pentaerythritol (Peritrate)
    d. Papaverine
    e. Cardilate
    f. Isoxuprine (Vasodilan)

33. Patients with cardiovascular disease and hypertension are often told by their physicians to stop smoking for which one of the following reasons?
    a. Nicotine has a tendency to cause vasospasm
    b. Tobacco smoke contains substances thought to cause cancer
    c. Tobacco smoke is irritating to the respiratory mucous membrane
    d. Nicotine stimulates the central nervous system

34. Nicotine (several choices are correct)
    a. Has no therapeutic use and little pharmacologic interest and toxicologic importance
    b. Has not been clearly established as a causative factor relating excessive tobacco smoking and lung cancer
    c. Decreases the secretion of hydrochloric acid from the stomach glands
    d. Increases the secretion of hydrochloric acid from the stomach glands, so patients with gastric ulcers must reduce their smoking or give up the habit
    e. Does not affect the autonomic nervous system
    f. Is believed to be a contributing factor in causing Buerger's disease

35. If you smoke, write an honest objective account of why you smoke, when you are most apt to smoke and why, and how many cigarettes a day you smoke. List the harmful effects of tobacco smoking in excess. If you have stopped smoking, tell the class how you accomplished it and what differences there are in your health and respiratory system since overcoming the habit.

36. What effect does nicotinyl tartrate (Roniacol) have on the body? List the uses of this drug.

37. What effect does phenoxybenzamine (Dibenzyline) have on the body? It is used in which medical conditions?

38. What effect does tolazoline (Priscoline) have on the body? It is used in which medical conditions?

39. What is a characteristic of arterial hypertension, and what is the result of this characteristic? What is meant by *essential* or *primary* hypertension? How is it best treated? What factors may be responsible for essential hypertension? What is meant by *secondary* hypertension? Explain mild, moderate, and severe hypertension and tell the treatment of each. What is the goal of antihypertensive therapy? List the many ways this goal is accomplished. Many drugs are used in the treatment of hypertension, but generally, there are only three classes of drugs used. Name them.

40. What type of drug is clonidine (Catapres)? What is the main use of this drug? What is the danger of abrupt discontinuance of clonidine? What are the adverse effects of clonidine? Outline the drug interactions with this drug.

41. What is the main use of guanethidine (Ismelin)? List the side effects of this drug. What is the cause of weakness and possible lightheadedness when first getting out of bed? How can these symptoms be prevented? How often should blood pressure be taken and in what positions?

42. What is the main use of methyldopa in the treatment of cardiovascular disease? List the side effects that may occur with use of this drug and tell how they may be eliminated or controlled.

43. What type of drug is metoprolol (Lopressor) and what is its main use? What are the most common side effects?

44. What is the main use of propranolol (Inderal) in treating cardiovascular disease?

45. Name the first four *Rauwolfia* alkaloids discussed under that topic and tell their main effect.

46. Reserpine (several choices are correct)
    a. Raises the blood pressure
    b. Drops the blood pressure suddenly to a normal level
    c. Is considered the most potent of the alkaloids of *Rauwolfia*
    d. Greatly reduces norepinephrine levels in peripheral nerve endings
    e. May cause a subjectively unpleasant type of sedation similar to chlorpromazine
    f. Drops the blood pressure gradually
    g. May cause nasal congestion or ''stuffiness'' that can be treated with PBZ or Benadryl
    h. Is a specific in the treatment of Buerger's disease

47. Name and spell correctly four trade names for reserpine.

48. Diazoxide belongs to which group of drugs, vasoconstrictors or direct vasodilators? What is its main use? How is it administered? If hypotension occurs, name two drugs that can be used to overcome this problem.

49. Hydralazine (Apresoline) belongs to which group of drugs, vasoconstrictors or direct vasodilators? What is the main effect and use of this drug? List the side effects of hydralazine. What drugs can be used to overcome the nasal stuffiness of hydralazine? This drug should be used with caution in what medical conditions?

50. Nitroprusside (Nipride) belongs to which group of drugs, vasoconstrictors or direct vasodilators? What is its main use? How is it administered? Nitroprusside is highly light sensitive. What precautions are taken to protect it from light during administration?
51. To which group of drugs does prazosin (Minipress) belong, direct vasodilators or vasoconstrictors? What are its main effect and its use? List the most common adverse effects. What are the symptoms of the initial doses of prazosin, and how soon do they occur? What instructions should be given to patients concerning these symptoms?
52. Define *diuretic* (see Glossary) and name the drugs that are mainstays in antihypertensive therapy. Diuretics are used to treat which medical conditions? How are they most effective? Name several diuretics that your instructor says are commonly used in your hospital.
53. You are a graduate nurse employed by a physician who has the care of many hypertensive patients. Make an outline booklet to be given each hypertensive patient covering all the nursing measures for care of antihypertensive patients. Learn these well; it will help you give better nursing care to the hypertensive patient.
54. Define *anticoagulant*. Outline the nursing measures for patients on anticoagulant drug therapy.
55. Warfarin (Coumadin) (several choices are correct)
    a. Is a highly effective drug to thicken the blood and prevent hemorrhage
    b. Is a highly effective drug to prevent all clot formation, including those already formed
    c. Prevents clot formation, but as far as is known, does not help absorption of clots already formed
    d. Slows the formation of prothrombin in blood, thus prolonging prothrombin time
    e. Is used when patients are ambulatory only
    f. Is used when treatment includes absolute bed rest for a long period to prevent clots forming in leg veins, pelvis, or any part of the body
    g. Cannot be used in the treatment of postoperative phlebitis
    h. Is given by IV route only
    i. Patients must be observed for bleeding from nose, gums, and rectum and for and skin bruising; such symptoms must be reported at once
56. Heparin (several choices are correct)
    a. Is found in spoiled sweet clover
    b. Lessens the clotting time of blood
    c. Has as the best method of administration the IV route

d. Is an example of an anticoagulant
e. Is an example of a coagulant
f. Must be used with caution in blood disorders, liver or kidney damage, subacute bacterial endocarditis, hemophilia, recent brain and spinal cord surgery, or open lesions or wounds
g. Requires that daily blood specimens be sent to the laboratory to determine clotting time
h. Has protamine sulfate injection as its antagonist
i. Is the drug of choice in the treatment of open lesions or bleeding wounds
j. Is the drug of choice in treatment of thrombophlebitis occurring during pregnancy, since it does not cross the placental barrier and is not excreted in the mother's milk
k. Cannot be used as the drug of choice for acute vascular occlusion because its action is too slow and not reversible

57. Warfarin (Coumadin, Panwarfin) is a powerful anticoagulant or coagulant? What effect does it have on prothrombin time? It lessens the risk of emboli in what medical and surgical conditions? How long does it take to obtain full therapeutic effects for this drug? What are the routes of administration? List the drug interactions with this drug. What is a good rule to follow for patients who start or stop another medication while continuing on warfarin?
58. Define *coagulant*. List some of the uses of coagulants.
59. How is absorbable gelatin sponge used?
60. What is the action and what are the uses of vitamin K? What is its use in new mothers and newborn babies? Give three examples of vitamin K drugs, using both generic and trade names.
61. Does phytonadione (Mephyton, vitamin K_1) have a more, or less, prolonged effect than menadione?
62. Your patient is to receive 1.5 mg of an oral medication in tablet form. The medicine bottle label strength available is 0.5 mg. How many tablets will you administer?
63. The physician orders the patient to receive 0.25 mg of an oral medicine. The medicine bottle strength available for each tablet is 0.5 mg. How many tablets will you administer?
64. Your patient is to receive 0.5 g of an oral medication in tablet form. The medicine bottle label strength available for each tablet is 500 mg. How many tablets will you give? This is a conversion problem. How do you convert from gram to milligram? For further practice convert this same problem from milligram to gram (see Index: Conversion).

CHAPTER 17

Drugs affecting the urinary system

DIURETICS

Diuretics are drugs that increase the flow of urine. The purpose of a diuretic is to increase the net loss of water. To achieve this, there must also be a loss of sodium.

Diuretics act in several ways, for example:

1. Some inhibit tubular reabsorption of sodium by an indirect mechanism, such as competitive inhibition of aldosterone by spironolactone (Aldactone).
2. Some inhibit reabsorption of sodium by a direct action on the kidney tubules, such as the thiazides, furosemide, and ethacrynic acid.
3. Some increase glomerular filtration, such as the xanthines.

Acetazolamide (as-ee-tah-zol'ah-myd)
(Diamox) (dy'ah-moks), (Rozolamide) (rah-zol'ah-myd)

1. Acetazolamide is a rather weak diuretic that acts by inhibiting the enzyme carbonic anhydrase within the kidney, brain, and eye. As a diuretic, it promotes the excretion of sodium, potassium, water, and bicarbonate.
2. This drug is infrequently used as a diuretic but is occasionally used to reduce intraocular pressure in patients with glaucoma and to reduce seizure activity in patients with certain types of epilepsy.
3. Acetazolamide is available as 125- and 250-mg tablets, 500-mg long-acting capsules, and 500-mg vials for parenteral injection.
4. Usual dosage range, as a diuretic, 250 to 375 mg once daily; for glaucoma, 250 to 1,000 mg in divided doses daily; for epilepsy, 375 to 1,000 mg daily.

Ethoxzolamide (eth-oks-zol'ah-myd)
(Cardrase) (kar'drase), (Ethamide) (eth'ah-myd)

1. Ethoxzolamide has the same mechanism of action and use as acetazolamide.
2. Ethoxzolamide is available in 125-mg tablets.

Aminophylline (ah-mee-no-fil'in)

1. Aminophylline is a methylxanthine derivative used for its diuretic effects in cardiorenal disease and as a bronchodilator in patients with pulmonary diseases.

2. The methylxanthine derivatives include theophylline, caffeine, and theobromine, all of which display weak diuretic properties. All act by improving blood flow to the kidneys.
3. Aminophylline is rarely used now as a diuretic because of the availability of more effective diuretic agents. However, a diuresis is occasionally noted when aminophylline is used in the treatment of asthma. For discussion of aminophylline as a bronchodilator, see Index.

Ethacrynic acid (eth-ah-krin'ik)
(Edecrin) (e'deh-krin)

1. Ethacrynic acid is another diuretic more potent than the thiazides.
2. Its action is of short duration and its very potency may cause excessive diuresis with marked loss of water, sodium, and potassium, which limits its usefulness.
3. This drug must be initially administered only under medical supervision since it can cause severe loss of water and electrolytes, hepatic coma in cirrhotic persons, weakness, loss of appetite, tetany, hyperuricemia, dizziness, skin rash, and hypokalemia.
4. Ethacrynic acid is available in 25- and 50-mg oral tablets and 50-mg vials for parenteral injection.
5. Usual dose: 50 to 200 mg daily.

Furosemide (fu-ro'se-myd)
(Lasix) (lay'six)

1. Furosemide is one of the most potent and effective diuretics currently available.
2. Maximum effect occurs 1 hour after oral administration. Action lasts only about 4 hours.
3. The principal sites for action are the ascending limb of Henle's loop and the proximal tubule.
4. When used inappropriately, dehydration and reduction of blood volume can cause vascular collapse, thrombosis, embolism, and hepatic coma in cirrhotic patients. Potassium supplementation may be necessary.
5. This drug is available in tablets of 20, 40, and 80 mg. Usual dose: one to two tablets, preferably given as a

single dose in the morning. It is also available in 20-, 40-, and 100-mg ampules for IV injection.

The thiazides

The benzothiadiazides, better known as the thiazides, have been an important and useful class of diuretic and antihypertensive agents for the past two decades. As diuretics, thiazides act primarily on the distal tubules of the kidney to block the reabsorption of sodium and chloride ions from the tubule. The unreabsorbed sodium and chloride ions are passed into the collecting ducts, taking molecules of water with them, thus resulting in a diuresis. The thiazides are used as diuretics in the treatment of edema associated with congestive heart failure, renal disease, hepatic disease, pregnancy, obesity, premenstrual syndrome, and administration of adrenocortical steroids. The antihypertensive properties of the thiazides result from a direct vasodilatory action on the peripheral arterioles. (See Index for antihypertensive therapy.)

Mild side effects, such as gastrointestinal disorders, dizziness, weakness, fatigue, and rash, may occur. Use of thiazides may cause or aggravate electrolyte imbalance, so patients should be observed regularly for signs such as dry mouth, drowsiness, confusion, muscular weakness, and nausea. Hypokalemia (abnormally low potassium content of blood) may occur, especially in patients also receiving adrenocortical steroids and in patients with severe cirrhosis. (Supplementary potassium is used to prevent or treat hypokalemia.) The thiazides may induce *hyperglycemia* and aggravate cases of preexisting diabetes mellitus. Insulin requirements may need adjustment in patients with diabetes who also require diuretic therapy. The plasma uric acid is frequently elevated by the thiazides. Patients prone to *hyperuricemia* and acute attacks of gouty arthritis should be placed on thiazides with caution. Patients should also be observed for rare occurrences of leukopenia (reduction in the number of leukocytes in the blood, with the count being 5,000 or less), thrombocytopenia (decrease in the number of blood platelets), agranulocytosis (complete or nearly complete absence of the granular leukocytes [granulocytes] from the bone marrow and the blood), and aplastic anemia (a rare condition in which the bone marrow cells cease to produce red and white cells in sufficient amounts to compensate for their destruction).

Thiazide diuretics should be used with caution in pregnant patients, because depression of bone marrow and thrombocytopenia are possible effects on the newborn.

Tables 17-1 and 17-2 provide a list of thiazide diuretics and those diuretics chemically related to the thiazides. Most of the diuretics listed are administered in divided daily doses for the treatment of hypertension; however, single daily dosages may be most effective for mobilization of edema fluid. All patients placed on these products should be monitored for the potential adverse effects previously listed.

Table 17-1. Thiazide diuretic products

Thiazide	Brand name	Dosage range (mg)	Dosage forms available
Bendroflumethiazide	Naturetin	2.5-15	Tablets: 2.5, 5, and 10 mg
Benzthiazide	Exna, Hydrex, Urazide	50-150	Tablets: 25 and 50 mg
Chlorothiazide	Diuril, Ro-Chlorozide	1,000-2,000	Tablets: 250 and 500 mg Oral suspension: 250 mg/5 ml Injection: 500 mg/20 ml
Cyclothiazide	Anhydron	1-2	Tablets: 2 mg
Hydrochlorothiazide	Esidrix, HydroDiuril, Oretic, Hydromal	25-100	Tablets: 25, 50, and 100 mg
Hydroflumethiazide	Saluron, Diucardin	25-100	Tablets: 50 mg
Methyclothiazide	Enduron, Aquetensen	2.5-5	Tablets: 2.5 and 5 mg
Polythiazide	Renese	1-4	Tablets: 1, 2, and 4 mg
Trichlormethiazide	Naqua, Metahydrine, Aquex, Diurese	1-4	Tablets: 2 and 4 mg

Table 17-2. Thiazide-related products

Diuretic	Brand name	Dosage range (mg)	Dosage forms available
Chlorthalidone	Hygroton	50-200	Tablets: 25, 50, and 100 mg
Metolazone	Zaroxolyn, Diulo	2.5-10	Tablets: 2.5, 5, and 10 mg
Quinethazone	Hydromox	50-100	Tablets: 50 mg

The potassium-sparing diuretics

Spironolactone (spi-ro-no-lak'toan)
(Aldactone) (al-dak'toan)

1. Spironolactone is a diuretic that is particularly useful in relieving edema and ascites not responsive to the usual diuretics.
2. It blocks the sodium-retaining and potassium-excreting properties of aldosterone, resulting in a loss of water with the increased sodium excretion.
3. This drug may be given with thiazide diuretics to increase the effect of spironolactone and reduce the side effects of the thiazides.
4. Spironolactone is contraindicated in acute renal insufficiency. It should be given with caution in patients with deficiencies of sodium in the blood or with hyperkalemia (abnormally high potassium content in the blood). Potassium supplementation should not be used.
5. Side effects, such as drowsiness, mental confusion, and skin eruption, are rare.
6. Usual dose: 100 mg daily in divided doses. Dosage may range from 75 to 300 mg.

Triamterene (try-am'ter-een)
(Dyrenium) (dy-reen'ee-um)

1. Triamterene is a mild diuretic that acts by blocking the exchange of potassium for sodium in the kidney. Potassium is retained, making triamterene an effective agent to use in conjunction with the potassium-excreting diuretics such as the thiazides and furosemide.
2. Triamterene is available in 100-mg capsules.
3. Usual dosage: 100 to 300 mg daily.

Nursing measures for patients receiving diuretics

1. A recorded daily intake and output should be kept. Ambulatory patients can be taught to measure the intake and the output and maintain daily records.
2. Daily weight records should be taken for the first few days of therapy and once or twice weekly thereafter. Weight gain should be reported.
3. Daily observation should be made by the nurse for increase in tissue fluid swelling or pitting (edema) in common body areas, such as sacral, ankle, and pedal tissue. Edema can cause weight gain.
4. Diuretics should be administered early in the day to avoid nocturnal diuresis and disturbance of the patient's sleep.
5. Patients on diuretic therapy may be instructed by the physician to increase dietary intake of potassium to avoid undue potassium loss. A few foods high in potassium are oranges, tomatoes, grapefruit juice, and whole milk.

DRUGS THAT ACT ON THE BLADDER

Disturbance of bladder function in the hospitalized patient is usually caused by either too much muscle tone of the bladder or too little. In a hypertonic, irritable bladder the emptying reflex is easily stimulated and the bladder feels full, even though it may not be. Symptoms of this condition are usually frequency of urination, scanty or profuse urination, painful contractions during voiding, and possible burning sensation during voiding. Derivatives of belladonna are better for this condition than opiates. The preparation of choice is often oxybutynin chloride, which acts like belladonna derivatives to relax the hypertonic muscle of the bladder.

When a bladder lacks muscle tone, as occasionally occurs after spinal anesthesia, the patient is often unable to empty it completely. This condition may predispose the patient to the development of infection, particularly when he is catheterized. A drug that is used to improve this atonic condition, encourage voiding, and eliminate the need for catheterization is bethanechol chloride.

Oxybutynin chloride (ok-se-bu'ti-nin)
(Ditropan) (di'trow-pan)

1. Oxybutynin chloride is an antispasmodic drug that reduces the frequency of bladder contractions and delays the initial desire to void in patients with a neurogenic bladder.
2. Oxybutynin should not be used in patients with glaucoma, myasthenia gravis, bowel disease such as ulcerative colitis, or obstructive uropathy such as prostatitis.
3. Usual side effects include dryness of mouth, blurred vision, tachycardia, palpitations, and possible urinary retention.
4. Usual adult dose: 5 mg two or three times daily. Maximum recommended dose is 20 mg daily.

Bethanechol chloride (be-tha'ne-kol)
(Urecholine) (u-re-ko'leen)

1. Bethanechol is a parasympathetic nerve stimulant that causes contraction of the detrusor urinae muscle in the bladder, usually resulting in urination.
2. Side effects include increased salivation, abdominal cramping, and flushing of the skin. The drug should be used cautiously in patients with heart disease, peptic ulcer disease, asthma, epilepsy, parkinsonism, and hyperthyroidism.
3. Bethanechol is available in 5-, 10-, 25-, and 50-mg tablets and 5-mg ampules for subcutaneous injection.
4. Usual initial dose: 10 to 25 mg orally three or four times daily. Do not exceed 120 mg daily. Do not administer intramuscularly or intravenously.

A URINARY ANALGESIC

Phenazopyridine hydrochloride
(fen-ay-zo-peer′i-deen)
(Pyridium) (py-rid′ee-um)

1. Phenazopyridine produces an analgesic effect on the urinary tract within about 30 minutes after oral administration.
2. It relieves burning, pain, urgency, and frequency. It lessens bladder spasm, thus relieving the resulting urinary retention.
3. It is also used for preoperative and postoperative surface analgesia in urologic surgical procedures and after diagnostic tests in which instrumentation was necessary. Sometimes it is used to relieve the discomfort caused by the presence of an indwelling catheter.
4. Phenazopyridine is contraindicated in patients with renal insufficiency and severe hepatitis.
5. This drug causes the urine to be orange or red in color. Patients should be instructed about this to relieve apprehension.
6. Phenazopyridine is available in 100- and 200-mg tablets for oral administration. Usual adult dose: one to two tablets three times a day before meals.

URINARY ANTISEPTICS

Urinary antiseptics are substances that are excreted and concentrated in the urine in sufficient amounts to have an antiseptic effect on the urine and the urinary passages. Urinary antiseptics today include some of the older drugs, such as methenamine and mandelic acid, either alone or in combination, some of the sulfonamides, and a number of antibiotics. Which preparation to use is made on the basis of identification of the pathogens by Gram's stain or by urine culture in severe, recurrent, or chronic infections. Fluid intake should be encouraged so that there will be at least 2,000 ml of urinary output daily. Treatment should be continued for at least a week after symptoms have subsided or the results of cultures have been negative.

The most common organisms found in the urinary tract are gram-negative bacilli. Of this group, *Escherichia coli* is responsible for many urinary tract infections. Four other organisms also found frequently in the urinary tract are *Aerobacter aerogenes, Klebsiella pneumoniae*, and organisms of the genera *Proteus* and *Pseudomonas*.

Methenamine (meth-en-am′in)

1. Methenamine yields formaldehyde in the presence of an acidic urine. Methenamine is used in patients susceptible to chronic, recurrent urinary tract infections. The formaldehyde released helps suppress the growth and multiplication of bacteria that may cause the recurrent infection.
2. Methenamine is usually not potent enough to be effective in patients suffering from a preexisting infection. The infection should be treated with antibiotics until the urine is sterile; then methenamine is started to help prevent recurrence of the infection.
3. Many physicians order methenamine to be given with ascorbic acid (vitamin C) to make sure that the urine will be acidic. Methenamine can then act as a urinary antiseptic, which it cannot do if the urine is alkaline.
4. Usual dose: 0.5 g every 4 hours, but the dose can be increased to as much as 1 g.

Methenamine mandelate
(Mandelamine) (man-del-ah′min)

1. Methenamine mandelate combines the action of methenamine and mandelic acid. It is effective as a suppressant in recurrent urinary tract infections.
2. This drug, too, yields formaldehyde in the presence of free acid, helping it to act as a urinary antiseptic. It is effective only in acidic urine. Ascorbic acid (vitamin C) may be administered to assure urine acidity.
3. Mandelamine mandelate is available in 250- and 500-mg and 1-g tablets and as a suspension, 50 and 100 mg/ml, for oral administration. Average initial dose: 1 g four times a day with 500 mg of ascorbic acid four to eight times daily.

Nitrofurantoin (ny-tro-fu-ran′to-in)
(Furadantin) (fur-ah-dan′tin), (Macrodantin)
(mak-ro-dan′tin)

1. Nitrofurantoin shows antibacterial activity against many gram-positive and gram-negative organisms, such as *Streptococcus faecalis, Escherichia coli,* and *Proteus* species.
2. It is used to treat bacterial infections of the urinary tract that are caused by microorganisms sensitive to this drug.
3. This drug is rapidly and completely absorbed from the intestinal tract, and about 40% is excreted from the urine unchanged within 4 to 6 hours. Nitrofurantoin may tint the urine rust brown to yellow. The patient should be instructed about this.
4. Nitrofurantoin may cause nausea and vomiting. This may be prevented by administering the drug with food or milk or immediately after a meal. It should not be administered to patients with kidney damage or lessened secretion of urine.
5. Usual dose: children, 5 to 7 mg/kg of body weight daily, or 2.2 to 3.6 mg/pound of body weight, divided into four doses; adults, 50 to 100 mg four times daily. The drug is available in 50- and 100-mg tablets and as a suspension, 5 mg/ml for oral administration.

Nalidixic acid (nal-i-diks'ik)
(NegGram) (neg'gram)

1. Nalidixic acid is a urinary antiseptic chemically unrelated to other antimicrobial agents.
2. It is bacteriostatic or bactericidal against many gram-negative bacteria, especially those caused by strains of *Proteus*. It is not effective against most strains of *Pseudomonas* or enterococci.
3. Side effects include gastrointestinal and visual disturbances and occasionally, pruritus, rashes, confusion, and possibly convulsions. The drug should not be administered to epileptic persons.
4. The drug is available in 250-, 500-, and 1000-mg tablets for oral administration. Usual adult dose: 1 g four times daily.
5. Maximal doses are usually administered during initiation of therapy to lessen the possibility of bacterial resistance, which may develop within 48 hours.

Several other antiinfective agents may be used to treat urinary tract infections. These agents are effective in a variety of tissue infections against many microorganisms. Because of their use in multiple organ systems, they are discussed in detail in Chapter 23, which concerns antibiotics and chemotherapeutic agents.

URICOSURIC AGENTS

Uricosuric agents act on the tubules of the kidneys to enhance the excretion of uric acid. Uric acid is a normal metabolite of cellular metabolism and is excreted by the kidneys under normal circumstances. For several reasons, however, uric acid can accumulate, resulting in acute attacks of gout, gouty arthritis, and deposits of urate tophi in joints. Hyperuricemia may be treated by inhibiting the production of uric acid with an agent known as allopurinol (see Index) or by enhancing the excretion of uric acid by the kidneys. Two agents effective in enhancing the excretion of uric acid are probenecid and sulfinpyrazone.

Probenecid (pro-ben'eh-sid)
(Benemid) (ben'eh-mid)

1. Probenecid is a drug used to treat hyperuricemia and chronic gouty arthritis. It is not effective in acute attacks of gout and is not an analgesic.
2. This drug promotes renal excretion of a number of substances, including uric acid. It inhibits the reabsorption of urate in the kidney, which results in reduction of uric acid in the blood. This uricosuric action helps to prevent or retard joint changes often seen in chronic gouty arthritis.
3. When given with penicillin, probenecid raises and prolongs plasma concentrations (maintains high levels of the antibiotic in the blood).
4. Large doses of salicylates antagonize the uricosuric activity of probenecid. An occasional aspirin tablet for headache has no effect on probenecid, however.
5. A high fluid intake is recommended during administration of this drug to produce increased volume of urine, in order to minimize the formation of uric acid stones and the possibility of hematuria.
6. Side effects and toxic effects may include nausea, constipation, skin rash, liver necrosis, blood dyscrasias, and hypertensive reaction. Probenecid is generally well tolerated, and side effects are rare.
7. Usual dosage: 0.5 to 2 g daily; divided doses, orally.

Sulfinpyrazone (sul-fin-py'rah-zoan)
(Anturane) (an'tu-rayn)

1. This drug is structurally related to phenylbutazone. It is an effective uricosuric agent that acts by blocking renal tubular reabsorption of uric acid.
2. Side effects include nausea, vomiting, and abdominal discomfort. Use with caution in patients with a history of peptic ulcer disease. Hypersensitivity reactions, manifested by fever, pruritus, and rashes, occur in less than 3% of patients. If hypersensitivity reactions occur, discontinue therapy.
3. The frequency of gouty attacks may increase during the first year of therapy. During these attacks, continue sulfinpyrazone therapy without changing dosages. Treat the acute attack with full therapeutic regimens of colchicine or other antiinflammatory agents.
4. Large doses of salicylates may antagonize the uricosuric action of sulfinpyrazone. Occasional small doses of one or two tablets, however, will not effect sulfinpyrazone therapy.
5. Initial adult dose: 100 to 200 mg two times daily. Usual maintenance dose: 200 to 400 mg two times daily. Sulfinpyrazone may be administered with food or milk to diminish gastric irritation.

**The physician prescribes the medicine and treatment.
The nurse carries out the physician's orders.
Self-medication is dangerous. Consult your physician first.
There is in every medicine a possible danger.
When in doubt—ASK!**

ASSIGNMENT

Review previous lessons and questions according to the direction of your instructor.

1. Define and give the purpose of a diuretic. State the three ways in which diuretics act.
2. Acetazolamide (Diamox) (several choices are correct)
   a. Is a long-acting diuretic effective for 3 to 4 weeks after treatment
   b. Acts by inhibiting the enzyme carbonic anhydrase within the kidney, brain, and eye
   c. Decreases the excretion of sodium, potassium, and water
   d. Is infrequently used as a diuretic today
   e. Has occasional use in reducing intraocular pressure in Glaucoma
   f. Has occasional use to reduce seizure activity in certain types of epilepsy
   g. Is a rather weak diuretic
3. Give the two trade names for ethoxzolamide and tell its main use.
4. Give the main uses of aminophylline. How does it act? Is it commonly, or rarely, used as a diuretic? Why?
5. Ethacrynic acid (Edecrin) is a diuretic that is more, or less, potent than the thiazides? Is its duration of action short, or long? It may cause excessive diuresis with what results? Why must this drug be initially administered only under medical supervision?
6. Furosemide (Lasix) (several choices are correct)
   a. Is one of the most potent and effective diuretics available today
   b. Is slow-acting, with maximum effects occurring 12 hours after administration
   c. Never requires use of potassium supplementation
   d. Can cause dehydration and reduction of blood volume resulting in vascular collapse, thrombosis, embolism, and hepatic coma in cirrhotic patients
   e. Has as its principal sites of action the ascending limb of Henle's loop and the proximal tubule
   f. Is a weak diuretic
   g. Is so powerful that it may cause excessive diuresis, with marked loss of water, sodium, and potassium, which limits its usefulness
   h. Has a maximum effect occurring 1 hour after oral administration, and an action that lasts only about 4 hours
7. What is the main mechanism for diuretic action of the thiazides? What other actions do the thiazides have? List the side effects of thiazides. How can the loss of potassium be prevented when thiazide drugs are being administered? The thiazides may induce or aggravate what condition? Thiazides have what effect on the plasma uric acid? May patients with gouty arthritis receive thiazides? What blood conditions may occur from administration of thiazides? What are possible effects on the newborn with use of thiazides during pregnancy?
8. Name four thiazide preparations that your instructor tells you are commonly used in your hospital. (See Table 17-1 for aid in this selection.)
9. Spironolactone (Aldactone) (several choices are correct)
   a. Must not be administered with thiazide diuretics
   b. Is not particularly useful in relieveing edema and ascites
   c. Rarely has any side effects
   d. Is particularly useful in relieving edema and ascites resistant to or not responsive to the usual diuretics
   e. Has as a result of administration very little water loss and a definite decrease of sodium excretion
   f. Blocks the sodium-retaining and potassium-excreting properties of aldosterone, resulting in a loss of water with increased sodium excretion
   g. May be administered with thiazide diuretics to increase the effect of spironolactone and reduce the side effects of the thiazides
   h. May be administered safely in cases of acute renal insufficiency
   i. Has rare side effects such as mental confusion, drowsiness, and skin eruption
   j. Should be administered with caution in patients with hyponatremia or hyperkalemia, and potassium supplementation should not be used
10. Triameterene (Dyrenium) belongs to which group of diuretics? Is it a mild, or powerful, diuretic? How does it act?
11. List the nursing measures for patients receiving diuretics.
12. What are the two causes of disturbance of bladder function? What are the symptoms of a hypertonic, irritable bladder? What is the preparation of choice for this condition? Name one other choice for treatment of a hypertonic, irritable bladder. What symptoms occur when a bladder lacks muscle tone? This condition may predispose the patient to the development of infection, particularly when he is catheterized. What drug is used to improve this atonic condition and encourage voiding?
13. What type of drug is oxybutynin chloride (Ditropan)? What effect does it have on the bladder? What are the contraindications for this drug? What are the usual side effects?
14. What type of drug is bethanechol chloride (Urecholine)? What effect does it have on the bladder? List the side effects for this drug. Bethanechol should be used cautiously in what medical conditions?
15. What type of drug is phenazopyridine hydrochloride (Pyridium)? What effects does it have on the bladder? What are additional uses for this drug? What are the contraindications? This drug causes what changes in the color of urine? Should patients be instructed about this, and why?
16. Explain and give some examples of urinary antiseptics. Fluid intake should be encouraged to promote how many milliliters of urinary output daily? Treatment should be continued for how long?
17. Some of the most common organisms found in urinary tract infections are gram-negative bacilli. Of this group, one of the most commonly found is
   a. Hemolytic streptococci
   b. *Staphylococcus aureus*
   c. *Escherichia coli*
   d. *Streptococcus faecalis*
18. Two urinary antiseptics that act only in the presence of an acid urine are
   a. Bethanechol chloride (Urecholine)

    b. Phenazopyridine hydrochloride (Pyridium)
    c. Methenamine
    d. Oxybutynin chloride (Ditropan)
    e. Methenamine mandelate (Mandelamine)

19. What drug may be used with the urinary antiseptics discussed in question 18 to assure acidification of urine?

20. Nitrofurantoin (Furadantin) (several choices are correct)
    a. Is a mild antiseptic for the urinary tract
    b. Shows antibacterial activity against many gram-positive and gram-negative organisms, such as *Streptococcus faecalis, Escherichia coli,* and *Proteus* species
    c. Is especially useful in the treatment of fungi and virus infections
    d. Is slowly and incompletely absorbed
    e. May tint the urine rust brown to yellow; the patient should be instructed about this to avoid apprehension
    f. May cause nausea and vomiting, so the drug should be administered with food or milk or immediately after a meal
    g. Can be safely administered to patients with kidney damage or lessened secretion of urine

21. Nalidixic acid (NegGram) is bacteriostatic or bactericidal against which organisms? For which is it *not* effective? List several of its most common side effects.

22. What is the action of uricosuric agents? What is the result of the accumulation of uric acid? How is hyperuricemia treated? Name three agents that are effective in enhancing the excretion of uric acid.

23. Probenecid (Benemid) (several choices are correct)
    a. Is the specific drug highly effective in acute attacks of gout
    b. Is placed in the group of analgesics
    c. Has been for many years a specific for bladder infections
    d. Is a drug used to treat hyperuricemia and chronic gouty arthritis
    e. Promotes renal excretion of a number of substances, including uric acid

    f. Increases the reabsorption of urate in the kidney, which results in an increase of uric acid in the blood
    g. Raises and prolongs plasma concentrations (maintains high levels of the antibiotic in the blood) when administered with an antibiotic
    h. Should not be administered with large doses of salicylates since they antagonize the uricosuric activity of probenecid
    i. Requires the patient to have a restricted fluid intake during its administration in order to prevent hematuria and to minimize the formation of uric acid stones
    j. Has such side effects as nausea, skin rash, liver necrosis, blood dyscrasias, and hypertensive reaction, but these are rare

24. Sulfinpyrazone (Anturane) is structurally related to what drug? To which group of urinary drugs does it belong, and how does it act? List the side effects. Is it a safe drug to use for patients with peptic ulcer disease? Are there more frequent, or less frequent, attacks of gout during the first year of therapy with sulfinpyrazone? During the attacks of gout, what is the method of sulfinpyrazone therapy? What other drug is also used during acute attacks of gout? What is the effect of large doses of salicylates given during sulfinpyrazone therapy? How is sulfinpyrazone best administered?

25. The physician ordered the patient to have an oral medication in tablet form in the strength of 0.250 g. The label on the bottle of medicine says 250 mg, meaning the strength of each tablet in the bottle is 250 mg. How many tablets will you administer? *Remember:* This is a conversion problem. How do you convert from gram to milligram? Then try converting from milligram to gram, using this same problem (see Index: Conversion).

26. The physician ordered the patient to have an oral medication in tablet form in the strength of .0006 g. The label on the medicine bottle says the strength of each tablet in the bottle is 0.6 mg. How many tablets will you administer? This is also a conversion problem. How do you convert from gram to milligram? Try converting from milligram to gram for this same problem (see Index).

CHAPTER 18

Drugs affecting the digestive system

Drugs that affect the digestive tract exert their action mainly on glandular and muscular tissues. This may be indirect action via the autonomic nervous system or direct action on the smooth muscle and gland cells. Both divisions of the autonomic nervous system innervate the tissues of the digestive tract and discharge nerve impulses into these structures almost continuously. If conditions are normal, they maintain a delicate balance of control of functions.

Drugs may cause decreased or increased emptying time of this system, increased or decreased tone, or peristaltic action of the stomach or bowel. Drugs may also be used as diagnostic aids to counteract excess acidity or gas formation, to relieve enzyme deficiency, and to prevent or produce vomiting.

DRUGS AFFECTING THE MOUTH

Generally, good oral hygiene that includes mechanical cleansing of the mouth and teeth has more influence on the mouth than drugs.

Mouthwashes and gargles

A common personal need in the hospitalized patient is oral hygiene. The most effective treatment of oral discomfort is mechanical cleansing of the teeth with a brush and dentifrice. This may not be possible, however, in the patient who has undergone oral surgery or who has suffered from facial trauma. Although mouthwashes and gargles cannot be used in sufficient concentrations to ensure germicidal effects, they may be temporarily effective in removing disagreeable tastes and reducing halitosis.

Cēpacol mouthwash is used in many hospitals and is available commercially in liquid and lozenge form. It is used full strength. Chloraseptic mouthwash maintains oral hygiene and also provides surface anesthesia when needed to alleviate pharyngeal discomfort. It is to be diluted with equal parts of water or sprayed full strength.

Occasionally, certain mouthwashes are recommended for specific purposes. Products containing zinc chloride are used as astringents to temporarily decrease bleeding or irritation. A 0.9% sodium chloride solution is an effective gargle solution to be used to provide temporary soothing relief after pharyngeal irritation from nasogastric tubes, endotracheal tubes, sore throat, or oral surgery. Solutions containing hydrogen peroxide may be used to cleanse and debride minor oral lesions but should be limited to 7 to 10 days of use to prevent further tissue irritation.

Dentifrices

Most dentifrices contain one or more mild abrasives, a foaming agent, and flavoring materials in powder or paste form as an aid to the mechanical cleansing provided by a soft nylon toothbrush. The essential requirement of toothpowder or toothpaste is that it must not injure the teeth or surrounding tissues.

Dentifrices containing stannous fluoride are on the market and are efficient in reducing the incidence of dental caries or cavities. Drinking water that contains 1 part of fluoride to 1 million parts of water is effective against caries, is safe to use, and is said to cause no bodily harm. The American Dental Association recommends Crest, Colgate with MFP, and Macleans Fluoride as the only toothpastes having caries-inhibiting properties. Fluorigard (0.05% sodium fluoride) is the first nonprescription mouthwash available that has been proved effective in controlling caries in controlled clinical studies. It has not yet been evaluated for caries control when used by the general public.

DRUGS AFFECTING THE STOMACH
Antacids

Antacids are chemical substances used in the treatment of hyperchlorhydria and peptic ulcer disease. Peptic ulcer disease is thought to be the result of several pathogenic processes; the control of hyperacidity is one of the therapeutic measures used in its treatment.

The main digestive substances secreted by the stomach are hydrochloric acid and pepsin. Hydrochloric acid activates the secretion of pepsin, and pepsin then begins protein digestion. Oversecretion of hydrochloric acid may result in erosion, ulceration, and possible perforation of the gastric walls. Antacids are used to lower the acidity of gastric secretions by buffering the hydrochloric acid (normally pH 1 or 2) to a lower hydrogen ion concentration. Buffering hydrochloric acid to a pH of 3 or 4 is highly desired, since then the proteolytic action of pepsin is reduced and the gastric juice loses its corrosive effect.

Antacid products account for one of the largest sales volumes of medications that may be purchased without prescription. Antacids are commonly used for treatment of heartburn, excessive eating and drinking, and peptic ulcer disease. Nurses and patients must be aware, however, that all antacids are not alike and should be used judiciously, particularly by certain types of patients.

Long-term self-medication with antacids may also mask symptoms of serious underlying medical diseases, such as a bleeding ulcer.

The most effective antacids available are combinations of aluminum hydroxide, magnesium oxide or hydroxide, magnesium trisilicate, and calcium carbonate (see Table 18-1). All act by neutralization of gastric acid. Combinations of these compounds must be used because any compound used alone in therapeutic quantities may also produce severe systemic side effects. A common complaint of patients consuming large quantities of calcium carbonate or aluminum hydroxide is constipation, while excess magnesium results in diarrhea.

Other ingredients found in antacid combination products include simethicone, oxethazaine, alginic acid, and bismuth. Simethicone is a defoaming agent that breaks up gas bubbles in the stomach, reducing stomach

Table 18-1. Ingredients of commonly used antacids

Product	Form	Calcium carbonate	Aluminum hydroxide	Aluminum carbonate	Magnesium oxide or hydroxide	Magnesium trisilicate	Magnesium carbonate	Sodium bicarbonate	Simethicone	Other ingredients
Aludrox	Tablet, suspension		X		X					
Amphojel	Tablet, suspension		X							
Basaljel	Tablet, capsule, suspension			X						
BiSoDol	Tablet, powder	X			X		X	X		
Delcid	Suspension		X		X					
Di-Gel	Tablet, liquid		X		X		X		X	
Gelusil II	Tablet, suspension		X		X				X	
Kolantyl	Tablet, wafer, liquid		X		X					
Maalox	Tablet, suspension		X		X					
Maalox Plus	Tablet, suspension		X		X				X	
Mylanta	Tablet, suspension		X		X				X	
Mylanta II	Tablet, suspension		X		X				X	
Phillips' Milk of Magnesia	Tablet, suspension				X					
Phosphaljel	Suspension									Aluminum phosphate
Riopan	Tablet, suspension									Magaldrate
Riopan Plus	Tablet, suspension								X	Magaldrate
Rolaids	Tablet									Dihydroxyaluminum sodium carbonate
Soda Mint	Tablet							X		
Titralac	Tablet, suspension	X								Glycine
Tums	Tablet	X								
WinGel	Tablet, suspension		X		X					

distention and heartburn. It is effective for use in patients who have overeaten or who suffer from heartburn, but it is not effective in the treatment of ulcer disease. Oxethazaine is a local anesthetic that has been used in combination with antacids. It, however, requires a prescription and has no proved therapeutic benefit in the treatment of gastric disease. Alginic acid produces a highly viscous solution of sodium alginate that floats on top of the gastric contents. It may be effective only in the patient who suffers from esophageal reflux or hiatal hernia and should not be used in the patient with acute gastritis or ulcer disease. Bismuth compounds have little acid neutralizing capacity and are therefore poor antacids.

Several potentially significant drug interactions may develop when antacids are administered with other medications:

1. The absorption of tetracycline antibiotics, digoxin, digitoxin, and iron compounds is inhibited by antacids. These medications should be administered 1 hour before or 2 hours after the administration of antacids.
2. Levodopa absorption is increased by antacids. When antacid therapy is added, toxicity may result in the parkinsonian patient who is well controlled taking a certain dosage of levodopa. If the patient's parkinsonism is well controlled on levodopa *and* antacid therapy, withdrawal of antacids may result in a recurrence of parkinsonian symptomatology.
3. Frequent use of antacid therapy may result in increased urinary pH. Renal excretion of quinidine and aspirin may be dangerously altered if therapy is not monitored closely.

Health professionals are frequently asked by patients, friends, and neighbors to recommend antacid products.

Before recommending antacid therapy, several questions should be asked to help ascertain whether there is a serious underlying medical condition.

1. How long has the pain been present?
2. When and where does the pain occur? Immediately after meals or several hours after meals?
3. Have you vomited blood or black "coffeegrounds" material?
4. Have you noticed blood in the stool or have the stools been black?
5. Are you on any dietary restrictions, such as low-salt diet?
6. Are you under a physician's care?

If the answers to these questions suggest an underlying disease, patients should be referred immediately to a physician.

The following principles should be considered when antacid therapy is being planned:

1. Antacids for "indigestion" should not be administered for more than 2 weeks. If after this time the patient is still experiencing discomfort, a physician should be contacted.
2. Patients with edema, congestive heart failure, hypertension, renal failure, pregnancy, or salt-restricted diets should use "low-sodium" antacids. These products include Riopan, Maalox, and Mylanta II. Continued therapy should only be at the recommendation of a physician.
3. Antacid tablets should be used only for the patient with an occasional case of indigestion or heartburn. Tablets do not contain enough antacid to be effective in treating peptic ulcer disease.
4. Excessive use of antacids frequently results in either constipation or diarrhea. If a patient experiences these symptoms and is still suffering from stomach discomfort, a physician should be consulted.
5. Effective management of *acute* ulcer disease requires large volumes of antacids. The selection of antacid and the quantity to be taken depend on the neutralizing capacity of the antacid. Any patient with "coffee-grounds" hematemesis, bloody stools, or recurrent abdominal pain should seek medical attention immediately and must not attempt to treat himself.
6. Most antacids have similar ingredients (see Table 18-1). Selection of an antacid for occasional use should be determined by quantity of each ingredient, cost, taste, and frequency of side effects. Patients may need to try more than one product before reaching a happy medium between the advantages and disadvantages of each product.

Research has been continuous to develop drugs that will selectively inhibit gastric secretion or increase mucous secretion. As a result of this research, two new drugs with these actions have been developed that represent significant pharmacologic advances.

Selective gastric drugs
Cimetidine (si-me′ti-deen)
(Tagamet) (tag′ah-met)

1. Cimetidine is a histamine H_2 receptor antagonist. H_2 receptors mediate gastric acid secretion in response to various stimuli, including gastrin and histamine.
2. This drug blocks H_2 receptors, decreasing daytime and nocturnal secretions of gastric acid.
3. It appears to inhibit gastric secretion stimulated by food, caffeine, histamine, insulin, and pentagastrin. (Pentagastrin is a synthetic peptide that stimulates gastric acid without producing the undesirable side effects of histamine.)

4. Today, cimetidine is being used to treat acute acid-peptic disease of the esophagus, stomach, and duodenum.
5. The following side effects have occurred: muscle pain, dizziness, rash, and mild, transient diarrhea. Because of the relative newness of the drug, patients should report any suspected side effects to their physician, pharmacist, or nurse.
6. It is not known whether cimetidine can be used safely during pregnancy or in nursing mothers or children.
7. Usual adult dosage: Cimetidine is available for injection, in 300 mg/2 ml in 2- and 8-ml vials, and in 300-mg tablets.
   a. Intravenous administration is used for patients unable to take oral medications.
   b. Initial oral dose is 300 mg four times a day, with meals and at bedtime. Increase of dose is dependent on the patient's response.
   c. Healing of the ulcer may occur within the first 2 weeks of treatment, but therapy should continue for 4 to 6 weeks to ensure adequate healing.
   d. Antacid therapy should be used concomitantly with oral cimetidine.

Carbenoxolone (kar-ben-oks′o-loan)
(Biogastrone) (by-o-gas′troan)

1. Carbenoxolone, a derivative of licorice, is reported to be of benefit in the healing of gastric ulcers. It is *not* recommended in the treatment of duodenal ulcers.
2. Its mechanism of action is unknown, but it is believed that it acts locally on the gastric mucosa, increases the secretion of protective mucus, and increases the life span of gastric cells.
3. This drug is used primarily in Europe and Canada. It is as yet not available in the United States.
4. Adverse effects include water and sodium retention, resulting in headache, dyspnea, edema, and hypertension. Hypokalemia and EKG changes may occur. Adverse reactions occur most frequently in patients over 70 years of age and in those with renal, liver, or cardiovascular disease.
5. Precautions: Carbenoxolone should be used with caution in patients receiving digitalis therapy. Patients' weight, blood pressure, and serum electrolytes should be routinely checked. If marked increase occurs that does not respond to diuretics, carbenoxolone therapy should be discontinued.
6. Carbenoxolone is not recommended for pregnant patients or for treatment of duodenal ulcers.
7. Usual adult dose for adults: 100 mg after meals 3 times daily until the ulcer heals, which is usually in 4 to 6 weeks. It is available in 50-mg tablets. Treatment with this drug beyond 12 weeks is not recommended.

Digestants
Hydrochloric acid, diluted; dilute hydrochloric acid

1. Dilute hydrochloric acid is used to treat a condition in which there is a deficit, or too little, secretion of hydrochloric acid in the stomach—a state called hypochlorhydria.
2. Some possible causes for this condition are carcinoma (cancer) of the stomach, pernicious anemia, and gastric atrophy.
3. Too little secretion of hydrochloric acid may also be found in apparently normal persons.
4. Diluted hydrochloric acid contains 10% hydrochloric acid. It needs to be further diluted in a glass at least half-filled with water. It should be taken through a glass tube to avoid injury to the teeth. Food should be eaten after the last swallow of the acid.
5. The average dose is 5 ml diluted with water. It can be administered in a smaller dose, for example, in drops, in a glass half-filled with water.
6. It should be administered during or immediately after the meal, before digestion has begun, in order to control the symptoms of indigestion, gas, and bloating.

Glutamic acid hydrochloride (gloo-tam′ik)
(Acidulin) (ah-sid′u-lin)

1. Acidulin is a combination of glutamic acid and hydrochloric acid.
2. It is available in capsules to avoid exposure of dental enamel to the acid.
3. The hydrochloric acid is released when the drug comes in contact with water.
4. Usual dose: 0.3 g, which equals 0.6 ml of dilute hydrochloric acid. It is usually taken before meals.

Pancreatin (pan′kree-ah-tin)

1. Pancreatin contains lipase, protease, and amylase. These are enzymes normally found in pancreatic juice. It is used as a digestive aid in patients with pancreatic secretory deficiencies.
2. Pancreatin is prepared from the pancreas of the hog.
3. It is available in enteric-coated tablets and in granules or capsules.
4. Usual dose: 325 to 1,000 mg with meals.

Pancrelipase (pan-kre-li′pays)
(Viokase) (vy′o-kays)

1. Pancrelipase is used for the same purpose as Pancreatin. It consists of desiccated gland rather than an extract and is more active than the official preparation.
2. It is obtained from the pancreas of cattle.
3. It is available in 300-mg tablets or in powder form.

BILE AND BILE SALTS

1. Drugs that stimulate the liver to increase bile production are called choleretics. The most important are bile salts and bile acids.
2. Hydrocholeretics are drugs stimulating the production of bile of a low specific gravity. This may be desirable in conditions such as diseases of the biliary tract not associated with liver disorders.
3. Bile is secreted by the liver into the bile duct, which drains into the duodenum. It is composed of water, bile salts, bile pigments, cholesterol, lecithin, and inorganic salts.
4. Bile salts are the most important in the digestion of fats because of their hydrotropic effect. They lower the surface tension of fats and help in the emulsification of fats before digestion and absorption in the small intestine.
5. Bile acids stimulate the production of bile salts. Both of these are normally absorbed from the intestine, pass through the portal blood to the liver, are reexcreted by the liver, then pass through the bile ducts and again enter the intestine.
6. Bile and bile salts are used for patients with various hepatic disorders to aid digestion and absorption and to increase biliary drainage. They are sometimes used for patients suffering prolonged drainage of the common duct.
7. Side effects of parenteral administration of bile salts include circulatory and neuromuscular system problems, such as hypotension, bradycardia, and skeletal muscular hyperactivity.

Dehydrocholic acid (Decholin) (de'ko-lin)

1. Dehydrocholic acid (Decholin) is an oxidation product of cholic acid that comes from natural bile acids.
2. It increases bile volume without increasing total bile acid quantity and increases drainage of bile ducts. It improves lipid absorption and may be used to flush the biliary ducts to remove mucus, debris, and small obstructions and to prevent ascent of infections.
3. Usual dosage: 250 to 500 mg three times daily after meals.

DRUGS FOR OTHER GASTRIC IRRITATIONS

Simethicone (si-meth'i-koan) (Mylicon) (my'li-kon)

1. Simethicone (Mylicon) is effective for treating gastrointestinal distress caused by entrapment of gas in such conditions as air swallowing, postoperative gaseous distention, functional dyspepsia, peptic ulcer, spastic or irritable colon, and diverticulitis.
2. The defoaming action of this drug relieves the flatulence of the patient by dispersing and preventing the formation of mucus-surrounded gas pockets in the gastrointestinal tract. In the stomach and intestines it changes the surface tension of gas bubbles and enables them to coalesce. The gas is then freed and is eliminated by belching or by the passing of flatus through the rectum.
3. Usual dose: one tablet (40- and 80-mg tablets) chewed after each meal and at bedtime or as directed by the physician. Drops: 0.6 ml orally after each meal and at bedtime.
4. Another antacid containing simethicone is Di-Gel.

Gaviscon (gav'is-kon)

1. Gaviscon is an antacid with alginic acid 200 mg, aluminum hydroxide dried gel 80 mg, sodium bicarbonate 70 mg, and magnesium trisilicate 20 mg.
2. Research has shown that the symptoms of regurgitation, heartburn, gas, and other upper gastric irritations thought to result from hyperacidity rather are caused by reflux of the contents of the stomach into the lower part of the esophagus, as occurs in hiatal hernia. Gaviscon has been found to be temporarily effective for these conditions.
3. Usual dose: two to four tablets, chewed thoroughly, swallowed, then followed by half a glass of water, three times daily after meals and at bedtime, or at times according to the order of the physician. Tablets must *not* be swallowed whole.

EMETICS

Apomorphine hydrochloride (ap-o-mor'feen)

1. Apomorphine, an emetic, or agent that induces vomiting, acts by direct stimulation of the vomiting center.
2. It is given subcutaneously in a dose of 2 to 8 mg.
3. Vomiting usually occurs within 5 to 15 minutes.
4. Large doses cause depression, so they should not be administered to patients already depressed.
5. Apomorphine is available in 6-mg tablets.

Syrup of ipecac (ip'e-kak)

1. Syrup of ipecac is used to induce vomiting in cases of poisoning by orally ingested drugs and other chemicals.
2. Do not use emetics in patients deeply sedated or unconscious or in those who are convulsing or who have ingested a corrosive such as alkali (lye), strong acids, strychnine, and strong petroleum distillates (kerosene, gasoline, paint thinner, or cleaning fluid).
3. Administer 15 to 30 ml of syrup of ipecac. Follow with a large glass of water. Vomiting may not be noted for 15 to 45 minutes.

Household measures

Emesis, or vomiting, can often be induced by the following household measures:
1. One teaspoon of mustard in one glass of tepid water
2. Mild soapsuds solution, one to two glasses, in warm water
3. Large amounts of plain warm water
4. Salt water, often the most effective measure, with 1 teaspoon of salt to 1 pint of water, or larger quantities if necessary

ANTIEMETICS

Control of vomiting is important to prevent dehydration and shock. Effective treatment usually depends on removal of the cause. Causes of vomiting can vary. Some are severe pain, strong emotion, labyrinth disturbances (inner ear), increased intracranial pressure, endocrine disturbances, motion sickness, gastrointestinal pathology, the action of certain drugs, effects of anesthesia, reaction to roentgen treatments, and heart disease.

Treatment varies from the simple to the complex and includes a cup of hot tea; carbonated drinks given at room temperature, unless the patient cannot eructate; a glass of warm solution of sodium bicarbonate ($\frac{1}{4}$ to $\frac{1}{2}$ teaspoonful per glass); antacids, such as salts of bismuth, magnesium oxide, and calcium carbonate, to protect the stomach and intestines and relieve irritation and vomiting; and the administration of CNS depressants, such as the antihistamines (dimenhydrinate) and phenothiazines (chlorpromazine, prochlorperazine). For further details, see Index.

Benzquinamide hydrochloride (benz-kwin′ah-myd) (Emete-Con) (em-et′ee kon)

1. Benzquinamide is an antiemetic used to prevent nausea and vomiting associated with anesthesia and surgery.
2. Side effects encountered with benzquinamide therapy include drowsiness, dry mouth, shivering, chills, nervousness, muscle tremors, and weakness.
3. Benzquinamide is administered intramuscularly in doses of 0.5 to 1 mg/kg every 3 to 4 hours as needed. Doses of 25 mg may be administered slowly by the IV route.
4. Emete-Con is available in 50-mg vials.

Meclizine hydrochloride (mek′li-zeen) (Bonine) (bo′neen), (Antivert) (an′tee-vert)

1. Meclizine is effective in the treatment of nausea and vomiting associated with motion sickness.
2. It is a long-acting drug. One dose may be effective for about 24 hours.
3. It has few side effects, but it causes drowsiness.

4. Meclizine is not recommended for use in pregnant patients. Teratogenic effects have been noted in offspring of laboratory animals treated with this product.
5. Usual dose: 25- to 50-mg about 1 hour before traveling. It can be repeated in a few hours if necessary. Meclizine is available in 12.5-, 25-, and 50-mg tablets. The drug also is available as an elixir containing 12.5 mg/5 ml.

Trimethobenzamide hydrochloride (tri-meth-o-ben′zah-myd) (Tigan) (ti′gan)

1. Trimethobenzamide (Tigan) is a specific antinauseant, antiemetic drug used to treat nausea and vomiting caused by infections, drug administration, radiation therapy, travel sickness, postoperative procedures, labyrinthitis, Meniere's syndrome, and pregnancy.
2. This drug is believed to depress the chemoreceptor trigger zone in the medulla of the brain rather than the vomiting center directly. It has long duration of action and some sedative effect. If drowsiness occurs, patients should be cautioned against driving or operating machinery until their individual dose is determined.
3. Trimethobenzamide has not proved to be safe during early pregnancy.
4. The injectable form is for IM use only, not IV. Usual dose: 200 mg (2 ml) four times daily, or as directed by the physician. Oral form: 250-mg capsule, three to four times daily for adults. Suppository: 100 and 200 mg.

DRUGS USED AS AIDS IN DIAGNOSIS
Barium sulfate (bar′ee-um)

1. Barium sulfate is a fine, white, odorless, and tasteless powder.
2. It is insoluble in water, organic solvents, and watery solutions of acids and alkalies.
3. Its insolubility makes it safe to use. All soluble barium salts are exceedingly poisonous, but barium sulfate is not, because of its insolubility.
4. It is more impermeable (not permitting passage) to x-rays than is tissue. It shows up in x-ray films as a milky, cloudy shadow. For this reason it is used in x-ray photography of the gastrointestinal tract.
5. The patient is usually examined first with the fluoroscope. Then x-ray films are taken at intervals to determine the rate of passage of the barium sulfate through the digestive tract and to locate any tumors, ulcers, or other areas of abnormality.
6. At the conclusion of the gastrointestinal series, often called "GI series," the patient receives a cleansing enema to remove as much of the barium as possible.

Azuresin (azh-u-rez′in)
(Diagnex Blue) (dy′ag-neks)

1. Diagnex Blue is a preparation used to detect gastric anacidity (achlorhydria—lack of hydrochloric acid in the stomach) without intubation.
2. The hydrogen ions of the hydrochloric acid, if acid is present, will displace the blue dye in the resin. Some of the displaced dye is excreted in the urine within 2 hours after the administration of Diagnex Blue. The dye content of the urine is estimated. This estimate is used as a measure of the amount of acid secreted by the stomach.
3. A 2-g, single dose is administered orally, in the form of granules.
4. One pharmaceutical company produces a kit of two small packets. One packet contains two tablets to be taken with a glass of water after the first voiding in the morning. One hour later the patient is instructed to void, and this urine is discarded. The second packet contains granules that are stirred in one-fourth glass of water and given to the patient. Any remaining granules should be given with a little more water. Two hours later all urine voided is saved for laboratory examination.
5. No food or fluids may be taken until the test is completed.
6. Some type of gastric stimulant, such as caffeine or histamine phosphate, is administered about 1 hour before the administration of the drug. Directions must be followed closely in regard to the administration of the drug and the urine collection. The patient should be told that his urine will range in color from green to blue for several days after the test.

Histamine (his′tah-min)

1. Histamine, another agent used to determine gastric acidity, is a powerful stimulant of the gastric glands when injected subcutaneously or intramuscularly in doses of approximately 0.3 to 0.5 mg. Its failure to stimulate secretion of hydrochloric acid from the stomach glands is considered proof of achlorhydria.
2. Side effects include a wheal at site of injection, vertigo, headache, superficial vasodilation, larger vessel vasoconstriction, or occasional drop in blood pressure.

Histamine phosphate

1. This drug is also called histamine diphosphate or histamine acid phosphate.
2. When it is administered during an augmented histamine test, it is accompanied by a simultaneous injection of an antidote such as epinephrine to antagonize all effects of histamine, except those on gastric secretions.
3. Usual dose: 0.04 mg/kg of body weight, subcutane-

ously on the day of the test. The patient is to have nothing by mouth after midnight until the test is completed.

Betazole hydrochloride (bay′tah-zol)
(Histalog) (his′tah-log)

1. This analogue of histamine is used more frequently than histamine phosphate because it has fewer side effects.
2. The routine administration of an antihistaminic compound is not necessary and augmentation of gastric secretion is equally effective.
3. Betazole should be used with caution in patients with allergies.
4. Usual dose: 0.5 mg/kg of body weight, subcutaneously or intramuscularly.

ANTIDIARRHEICS

Diarrhea is associated with such symptoms as too rapid a passage of intestinal contents, frequent fluid stools, and gripping. Causes of diarrhea are many and varied and include bacterial or protozoan infection; certain nervous disorders; the eating of contaminated or partially decomposed food; disturbances of gastric physiology, such as the absence of hydrochloric acid or the effects of resectional surgery of the stomach; the effects of certain drugs, such as certain antibiotics; and inflammatory processes of the intestine or adjacent viscera.

Diarrhea should be brought under control, but it is important to determine the cause first, if possible. Diarrhea can cause exhaustion, dehydration, and loss of vitamins, food materials, and electrolytes.

Diarrhea drugs are selected on the basis of what is causing the diarrhea and can be grouped as follows:

1. Demulcents-protectives—***bismuth subcarbonate, bismuth subnitrate, precipitated calcium carbonate, bismuth magma, milk of bismuth***
2. Adsorbents—***kaolin, kaolin mixture with pectin (Kaopectate)***
3. Antiperistaltic agents—***diphenoxylate, loperamide***

Kaolin, light kaolin (kay′o-lin)

1. Kaolin, an adsorbent, is a drug effective in the treatment of diarrhea.
2. Usual dose: 50 to 100 g suspended in water, every 3 to 4 hours until the diarrhea is brought under control.

Kaolin mixture with pectin
(Kaopectate) (kay-o-pek′tayt)

1. Kaopectate contains kaolin and pectin.
2. It is used for its soothing effect on the gastrointestinal tract, as well as in the treatment of diarrhea. Kaopectate acts as both an adsorbent and demulcent.
3. Usual dose: 2 to 4 oz four times daily until diarrhea subsides.

Bismuth subcarbonate (biz'muth)

1. Bismuth preparations have a soothing effect on the stomach and intestines. They coat these areas and help control gastritis and diarrhea.
2. Usual dose: 1 to 4 g four times a day.

Donnagel (don'ah-gel)
Donnagel-PG

1. Donnagel contains kaolin, pectin, hyoscyamine sulfate, atropine sulfate, hyoscine hydrobromide, sodium benzoate (preservative), and alcohol.
2. Donnagel-PG contains the preceding basic Donnagel formula plus powdered opium.
3. The actions of Donnagel are adsorbent, detoxicant, demulcent, spasmolytic, and anticholinergic.
4. Donnagel is used to treat diarrhea. It also is of aid in treating enteritis, colitis, gastritis, acute gastrointestinal upsets, and nausea accompanying these conditions.
5. Donnagel preparations should be administered with caution to patients with incipient glaucoma or prostatic hypertrophy because of the effects of the belladonna alkaloids.
6. Blurring of vision, dry mouth, and difficult urination may occur in a few patients taking an increased dosage but rarely in those taking the usual dosage.
7. Dose: 1 to 2 tablespoons every 3 hours.

Camphorated opium tincture (Paregoric) is also used in the treatment of diarrhea (see Index).

Other sedative antispasmodic drugs used for diarrhea include the following:

Lomotil (lo'mo-til)

1. Lomotil (diphenoxylate hydrochloride and atropine sulfate) has come into popular use for its effect in inhibiting gastrointestinal hypermotility.
2. It is contraindicated in severe hepatic dysfunction.
3. Usual dose: 2.5 to 5 mg four times daily.

Loperamide (lo-per'ah-myd)
(Imodium) (im-o'dee-um)

1. Loperamide is a recently introduced antiperistaltic antidiarrheal drug similar to diphenoxylate (Lomotil).
2. It may be effective in the control of acute or chronic diarrhea associated with inflammatory bowel disease and excess ileostomy output.
3. This drug has some opiate-like properties, although the drug appears to be nonaddicting in recommended dosages. Naloxone is the recommended antidote for overdosages.
4. Such antidiarrheal agents as diphenoxylate (Lomotil) and loperamide (Imodium) should not be used in some forms of infectious diarrhea since they may prolong the course of the disease by slowing the elimina-

tion of the pathogenic bacteria and their metabolic products from the colon.
5. Usual adult dose: two 2-mg capsules initially, followed by one 2-mg capsule every 4 to 6 hours as needed for diarrhea.

CATHARTICS
Classification

Cathartics may be classified as laxatives or purgatives. Laxatives are cathartics that cause few movements of the bowel. The stool is formed, and there is usually no gripping. Purgatives are cathartics that produce several bowel movements. The stool is soft or liquid, and there may be gripping.

It is difficult to place cathartics in any one group, since dosage is the factor that determines the action. A small dose may have a laxative effect, but a large dose of the same cathartic may have a purgative effect.

Causes of constipation

Drugs have been used for centuries for the purpose of overcoming the problem of constipation. Today, many people believe that even occasional failure of the bowel to move should be treated with a cathartic. This frequently is not necessary. Many people are normal even though they have but one or two bowel movements per week, provided their health is good and the bowel movement is not hardened or impacted. The nurse should remember that chronic use of cathartics is habit-forming. A number of causes of constipation are cited.

1. Improper diet—too little residue, too little fluids, or not enough vitamins
2. Muscular weakness of the colon
3. Sedentary habits
4. Failure to respond to the normal defecation impulse
5. Weakness of abdominal muscles
6. Certain diseases, such as anemia or liver, stomach, and intestinal diseases
7. Drug habits, such as morphine addiction
8. Tumors of the bowel or pressure on the bowel
9. Disease conditions of the rectum and anus

Contraindications

Cathartics should not be administered, or should be administered with caution, in the following conditions:

1. Inflammation of the gastrointestinal tract, such as gastritis, appendicitis, and colitis
2. Conditions of abdominal pain that have not been diagnosed
3. Chronic and spastic constipation
4. After surgery of the stomach, bowel, and rectum
5. Anemic conditions or states of malnutrition

Indications

Cathartics are indicated under the following situations:

1. To relieve some cases of acute constipation
2. To assist in the majority of cases of drug or food poisoning or gastrointestinal problems, on the advice of a physician
3. To remove gas and feces before x-ray examination of kidneys, colon, or gallbladder
4. To help keep the stool soft in order to avoid irritation from hardened stool and to keep certain patients from straining, such as those with coronary occlusion, a heart condition
5. To control certain types of diarrhea by removing the irritating substance from the bowel
6. To relieve edema, or excessive accumulation of fluid in the tissues. Saline cathartics are usually used for relieving edema. They are sometimes used to relieve intracranial pressure caused by edema.

Advice to the nurse in the use of cathartics

It is well for nurses to remember to use great caution about giving advice to persons on the subject of cathartics. Nurses should realize that they are diagnosing and prescribing when they give such advice to patients, and this is not their responsibility. *The physician diagnoses and prescribes; the nurse carries out the physician's orders.*

Remember, too, that many conditions of so-called constipation need to have the *cause determined. The physician does this.* People are likely to take cathartics for digestive upsets or abdominal pain, and the cause of the condition may be appendicitis. *No cathartic should be taken in the presence of abdominal pain. A physician should be consulted and his advice followed.*

The nurse may teach some basic hygiene to the patient for the prevention of constipation, such as the need for adequate diet and fluids, regular exercise, and regularity in bowel habits. The nurse should remind the patient that the physician should be consulted concerning the cause of the constipation, whether a cathartic is needed, and if so, what type.

One of the most essential points to teach people is that they do not have to have a watery, profuse bowel movement each day to be normal. This is a surprise to many people. Many are quite healthy and normal with only one or two bowel movements per week.

Lubricant laxatives
Mineral oil

1. Mineral oil softens the feces and aids in the easy passage of the stool. This is important after rectal operations and hernia repair.
2. The oil is not digested. There is little absorption.
3. It is useful in chronic types of constipation.
4. Some physicians object to its use because it dissolves certain fat-soluble vitamins and bile salts and therefore inhibits their absorption.
5. In large doses the drug may cause leakage from the rectum and soiled clothing or bedding. The dose can be reduced in this case.
6. It should not be administered immediately after meals, since it may cause nausea or delay the passage of food from the stomach. A slice or two of orange eaten just after the taking of the oil will remove the oil taste from the mouth.
7. Usual dose: 15 to 30 ml between meals or at bedtime.

Agoral (ag'or-ahl)

1. Agoral is a finely homogenized, stable emulsion of mineral oil with phenolphthalein. (For discussion of phenolphthalein, see Index.)
2. The drug aids in producing a normal evacuation without cramping, gripping, or oil leakage.
3. The mineral oil acts as an intestinal lubricant. The phenolphthalein stimulates intestinal musculature and therefore increases peristalsis.
4. This drug is used to prevent straining or pain during defecation by cardiac patients, patients with hemorrhoids before and after surgery, and geriatric and obstetric patients.
5. Usual dose: $1/2$ to 1 tablespoon at night. It may be repeated in the morning if necessary.

Bulk laxatives

Constipation may be caused by eating too little food or food that leaves too little residue. Bulk-forming cathartics provide more content to the stool, making it easier to pass.

Agar (ahg'ar)

1. Agar is a dried, mucilaginous substance obtained from several varieties of seaweed.
2. When it is moistened, it swells. This forms a bulk or mass of material that makes the stool large and soft. It is then easily passed through the colon and into the rectum.
3. Usual dose: 4 to 16 g twice daily. It may be taken in hot water or soaked in hot water and added to cereal, soup, or mashed potatoes.
4. It may be emulsified with liquid petrolatum.
5. The effect of agar is not observed at once. It may take a week or two to establish regular bowel movements. The drug can then be gradually reduced in dosage until it is no longer necessary.

Plantago seed (plan-tah'go), psyllium seed (sil'ee-um)
(Siblin) (sib'lin)

1. This bulk-forming cathartic is a small brown seed ground to a powder.

2. When water is added to it, plantago seed forms an abundant amount of mucilaginous material that absorbs more water, swells, and helps to form a larger, softer stool.
3. The seeds should be soaked before using.
4. One disadvantage to the use of this drug is that even though the seeds swell, their ends remain sharp and may cause irritation of the gastrointestinal tract.
5. Usual dose: $7^1/_2$ g; two rounded teaspoons in a glass of water, followed by another glass of fluid.

Psyllium hydrophilic mucilloid with dextrose (Metamucil) (met-ah-mu′sil)

1. Metamucil is a white or cream-colored powder.
2. It contains about 50% powdered mucilaginous part of psyllium seeds and about 50% dextrose.
3. Metamucil is useful in the treatment of constipation, since it helps to form a soft, water-retaining, gelatinous residue in the lower bowel.
4. It also has a demulcent, or soothing, effect on inflamed mucosa of the intestines.
5. Metamucil should be thoroughly stirred into a full glass of water or fruit juice. The patient should drink the entire glass of fluid and Metamucil and follow it with another glass of water or fruit juice. This is important so that Metamucil can achieve its effect of causing a soft, easily passed stool.
6. Usual dose: 4 to 7 g one to three times daily. Metamucil is available in premeasured single-dose packets for oral use and in instant-mix packets for single doses. The latter are effervescent and require no stirring. Patients on a low-sodium diet should not use the effervescent form because it contains sodium.

Effersyllium Instant (ef-er-sil′ee-um)

1. Each rounded teaspoonful of Effersyllium, or individual packet, contains psyllium hydrocolloid, 3 g.
2. Effersyllium is used to relieve constipation caused by decreased intestinal motility and lack of bulk in the intestinal contents.
3. It produces a soft, lubricating bulk that promotes natural elimination.
4. As is true of other bulk-forming cathartics, Effersyllium is not a one-dose, fast-acting agent. Administration for several days may be needed to establish regularity.
5. Effersyllium contains less than 7 mg sodium per rounded teaspoonful.
6. Usual adult dose: one rounded teaspoonful, or one packet, in a glass of water one to three times a day, or as directed by the physician. Caking can be avoided by using a dry spoon and dry glass. Add water, stir, and drink immediately. Replace cap tightly and keep drug in a dry place.

Plantago ovata coating (Konsyl) (kon′sil)

1. This is a cream- to brown-colored granular powder obtained from the *Plantago ovata* (mucilaginous portion of the blond psyllium).
2. Usual dose: 5 to 10 g three times daily before meals in a glass of water or milk that must be swallowed before the mixture thickens.

Methylcellulose (meth-il-sel′u-los) (Cellothyl) (sel′o-thill), (Hydrolose) (hy′dro-los), (Methocel) (meth′o-sel), (Syncelose) (sin-se′los)

1. Cellothyl (methylcellulose) is a grayish white powder that swells in water.
2. In the intestine this solution loses water and forms a gel. This gel increases the bulk and softness of the stool.
3. Cellothyl is available in tablets or granules.
4. Usual dose: 1 to 1.5 g with plenty of water two to four times daily. Dosage is gradually reduced.

Carboxymethylcellulose sodium (kar-bok-se-meth-il-sel′u-los) (Carmethose) (kar′me-thos), (C.M.C. Cellulose Gum), (Thylose sodium) (thy′los)

1. Carboxymethylcellulose sodium is a synthetic hydrophyllic colloid gum.
2. It is similar to methylcellulose in that it forms a soft bulk in the intestine after oral ingestion.
3. This drug is insoluble in gastric juices, which is not true of methylcellulose.
4. Carboxymethylcellulose sodium is available in 225- and 500-mg tablets and in 5% solution for oral administration. The usual adult dose is 4 to 6 g daily with one or two glasses of water. Tablets should not be chewed before swallowing.

Saline cathartics

Saline cathartics are soluble salts. They are relatively nontoxic and nonabsorbable, but they do exert toxic actions if injected intravenously. If administered by mouth, they are nontoxic because they are not absorbed.

Solutions of saline cathartics remain in the intestine and are only slightly absorbed. Water is retained because of osmosis, which is the passage of a solvent through a membrane from a dilute solution into a more concentrated one. Osmosis develops because the intestine acts as a semipermeable membrane for these cathartic salts.

The volume of water in the intestine speeds the passage of stool to the colon and rectum. In the colon and rectum, defecation reflexes, or the desire to expel, are stimulated.

There must be water present in the intestines for saline cathartic action to occur. Saline cathartics cause a loss of fluid from the bowel and the general circulation. Dehydration must not be allowed to develop.

Therapeutic uses

Saline cathartics are used with certain anthelmintics and in certain cases of drug and food poisoning. If the purpose is only to empty the intestine, saline cathartics such as magnesium sulfate, sodium phosphate, magnesium citrate, or milk of magnesia are probably the most effective. Milk of magnesia is the mildest of the saline cathartics and is best suited for children. For adults, heavy magnesium oxide is usually better. The most agreeable salines to take are the effervescent preparations:

1. To treat acute constipation
2. To treat intestinal putrefaction (decomposition of organic matter, with production of gases, acids, and toxic substances)
3. To obtain a stool specimen for purposes of examination
4. To treat food poisoning and drug poisoning

Administration

Saline cathartics have a rapid action, especially if taken in the morning before breakfast. They will act on the entire intestine. Results occur in 1 to 4 hours.

Saline cathartics sometimes cause distention with gas. They should all be taken with plenty of water because the salts do not leave the stomach quickly unless they are well diluted.

Magnesium sulfate
(Epsom salt)

1. Magnesium sulfate is available in glassy crystals or white powder.
2. It has a disagreeable taste.
3. Usual dose: 10 to 30 g orally.

Magnesium hydroxide mixture
(Milk of Magnesia)

1. Magnesium hydroxide enters the stomach, reacts with hydrochloric acids secreted by the stomach glands, and forms magnesium chloride. The magnesium chloride then acts as a saline cathartic in the bowel.
2. Usual dose: 15 to 30 ml orally for cathartic action.

Magnesium citrate solution

1. The taste of magnesium citrate solution is not unpleasant, since it is carbonated and flavored.
2. Usual dose: $1/2$ to 1 bottle (6 to 12 oz) orally.

Cathartics that act by irritation
Castor oil
(Oleum ricini) (o'lee-um ri-si'nee)

1. Oleum ricini (castor oil) originates from the seeds of the castor bean, a plant that grows in India. It can be cultivated in other warm climates.
2. It slows the emptying time of the stomach, so it should be given on an empty stomach.
3. The oil changes in the intestine to glycerin and fatty acid. Both the acid and the resulting salts cause the irritant action.
4. Castor oil acts mainly on the small intestine.
5. An average dose will produce several semifluid stools within 2 to 6 hours.
6. Some patients may experience severe cramping and diarrhea.
7. The semifluid nature of the stools is caused by the rapid passage of the stool.
8. Castor oil empties the bowel completely. There is usually no bowel movement for a day or two following the dose.
9. It is excreted into the milk of nursing mothers.
10. It is very useful in dysentery and fermentative diarrhea (if given early before dehydration occurs), food or drug poisoning, cleansing of the bowel for x-ray examination, preoperative preparation of the bowel, and acute constipation.
11. It should not be used in chronic constipation or in ulcerative bowel conditions.
12. Usual dose: 15 to 60 ml. The unpleasant and nauseating taste of the natural oil may be overcome by the use of orange juice or other fruit juices or pharmaceutical mixtures to emulsify and disguise the oil.

Aromatic cascara sagrada fluidextract (kas-kar'ah sah-grah'dah)

1. Cascara sagrada comes from the bark of the *Rhamnus purshiana* tree. It grows in the Pacific Coast region.
2. Cascara sagrada is one of the more commonly used cathartics, acting in about 6 to 12 hours.
3. It is used mainly for habitual constipation, acting mainly on the large intestine.
4. It may cause gripping but is less likely to do so than some of the other irritant cathartics.
5. Usual dose: 5 ml orally.
6. Other forms of cascara sagrada are:
   a. *Cascara sagrada fluidextract.* Usual dose: 1 ml orally.
   b. *Cascara sagrada extract tablets.* Usual dose: 0.3 g (300 mg) orally.
   c. *Cascara tablets.* Usual dose: 120 to 250 mg.
7. Notice the difference in dose of cascara sagrada fluidextract and aromatic cascara sagrada fluidextract.

Aloe (al'o)

1. Aloe is the dried juice of the leaves of a plant that grows well in Africa and the West Indies.
2. Aloe is one of the most irritating types of irritant cathartics, acting mainly on the large bowel.
3. It causes marked gripping, and in large doses it may cause pelvic congestion.
4. It is the active ingredient in a number of proprietary preparations, such as **Carter's Little Pills** and **Nature's Remedy.**
5. Usual dose: 0.25 g orally.

Senna fluidextract (sen'ah)

1. Senna originates from the dried leaves of the *Cassia senna* plant.
2. It resembles cascara, although cascara is not as powerful as senna.
3. Senna will produce cathartic action in about 6 to 12 hours and will cause gripping.
4. This drug is in some proprietary remedies, such as **Gentlax, Castoria,** and **Senokot.**
5. Usual dose: 10 to 15 ml orally.

Phenolphthalein (fee-nol-thayl'ee-in)

1. Phenolphthalein is a synthetic substance similar in action to that of the irritant cathartics already mentioned.
2. It will produce cathartic action in about 8 to 12 hours, with little or no gripping.
3. Its action is on both the small and the large intestines, but especially the large intestine.
4. It is sometimes prepared in ''candy tablet'' form. Children should be cautioned that it is *not* candy; the drug should be kept out of their reach.
5. Usual dose: 60 mg orally. It is found in many proprietary medicines, including **Amlax, Ex-Lax,** and **Feen-A-Mint.**

Danthron (dan'thrahn)
(Dorbane) (dor'bayn)

1. Danthron is a synthetic product tablet that contains dihydroxyanthraquinone.
2. The active ingredient is closely related to emodin, the active principle in such vegetable-type laxatives as cascara, senna, aloe, and rhubarb.
3. It acts chiefly on the large intestine.
4. It is effective in the treatment of functional constipation of all types.
5. Usual dose: one or two tablets orally 1 hour after the evening meal.

Bisacodyl (bis-ak'o-dil)
(Dulcolax) (dul'ko-laks)

1. Bisacodyl is a laxative that acts by stimulating the colonic mucosa.
2. It has little effect on the small intestine.
3. It may be effective in the treatment of atonic, spastic, and dietary constipation. It provides satisfactory cleansing of the bowel in preparation for surgery, proctoscopy, or radiologic examination, often making the need for an enema unnecessary.
4. It is given to persons of all ages, including pregnant and lactating women, patients with severe and chronic illness, and patients with hepatitis and renal disease.
5. Bisacodyl is available in oral tablets and rectal suppositories. It causes peristalsis and soft, formed stools.
6. Usual dose: one to three tablets at bedtime or $1/2$ hour before breakfast, for action within 6 hours. It is available in 5-mg enteric-coated tablets.
7. Tablets should not be taken within 1 hour of taking antacids and should not be crushed prior to administration.

DRUGS BELONGING TO THE DETERGENT GROUP (FECAL MOISTENING AGENTS)

In the past few years there has been a new approach to the problem of chronic constipation. In many persons with constipation or bowel irregularity, the waste matter in the intestines loses water content. The intestinal waste then becomes harder and drier. The harder and drier it is, the greater is the problem of elimination. A drug that is not a laxative, dioctyl sodium sulfosuccinate, acts as a wetting agent or detergent, to moisten and soften the intestinal waste. Natural peristalsis (muscular contraction of the intestine) then produces normal elimination without an unnatural urgency. Immediate relief should not be expected. This drug should be taken for several days before full benefits are achieved. The dose can then be reduced.

This drug is an aid in functional constipation caused by hardened fecal matter and in atonic and spastic constipation. Sometimes the drug is combined with a mild laxative such as danthron (Dorbane).

Remember: Dioctyl sodium sulfosuccinate is *not* a laxative, *not* a lubricant, and *not* a bulk-producer. It acts as a *wetting* agent, moistening and softening the stool. Natural muscular contractions of the intestines then produce a normal bowel movement.

An essential part of the treatment with this drug is reeducation of the patient concerning the subject of constipation. He should be taught that a daily bowel movement is not absolutely necessary to health and that even this drug should be reduced in dose when bowel habits are restored.

Dioctyl sodium sulfosuccinate (dy-ok'til so'dee-um sul-fo-suk'si-nayt)
(Colace) (co'lase), **(Dialose)** (dy'ah-los), **(Disonate)** (di'so-nayt), **(Doss), (Doxinate)** (dok'si-nayt), **(Regutol)** (rej'u-tol)

1. Average dose for all of these preparations varies between 100 and 300 mg (tablets or capsules) per day. Dose is usually 60 to 100 mg twice a day. It can be increased to 360 mg with no untoward effects.
2. For action and uses see, the discussion of this drug.
3. Two other preparations of a similar nature are **Kasof** and **Surfak.**
4. **Peri-Colace** is another preparation that combines the stool softener Colace with casanthranol, a mild stimulant laxative. It is available in capsule and syrup.

Doxidan (dok'si-dan)

1. Doxidan is a combination of calcium bis-dioctyl sulfosuccinate, an excellent fecal softener, with danthron (Dorbane), a mild peristaltic stimulant.
2. Doxidan acts only on the lower intestine and is a safe, gentle, nonirritating laxative for the management of chronic functional constipation.
3. Usual adult dose: one to two capsules daily, taken with a glass of water.

Dialose (dy'ah-los)

1. **Dialose Plus** contains casanthranol, dioctyl sodium sulfosuccinate, and sodium carboxymethylcellulose.
2. Dialose itself is a combination of dioctyl sulfosuccinate and sodium carboxymethylcellulose. It combines the advantages of both agents: fecal softening and bulk producing.
3. Usual dose: one capsule two or three times a day, taken with a glass of water.

**The physician prescribes the medicine and treatment.
The nurse carries out the physician's orders.
Self-medication is dangerous. Consult your physician first.
There is in every medicine a possible danger.
When in doubt—ASK!**

ASSIGNMENT

Review previous lessons and questions according to the directions of your instructor.

1. What is a common personal discomfort in the hospitalized patient? What is the most effective treatment of oral discomfort? Name two commonly used mouthwashes. What is the main use of a 0.9% sodium chloride solution? What is the main use of a hydrogen peroxide solution for mouth care? What do most dentifrices contain? What is the essential requirement of a toothpowder or toothpaste? What is the purpose of stannous fluoride in dentifrices? What is the proportion of stannous fluoride and drinking water in order to prevent caries? Which toothpastes are recommended by the American Dental Association as the only toothpastes having caries-inhibiting properties?
2. What are antacids and for what purposes are they used? What are the main digestive substances secreted by the stomach? What is the function of hydrochloric acid? What are the results of oversecretion of hydrochloric acid? What is the main purpose of antacids when oversecretion of hydrochloric acid is a problem? List other uses for antacids. What is a disadvantage of long-term therapy with antacids? The most effective antacids available are combinations of what other antacids? How do all of these antacids act? Why should a combination of these compounds be used? Give examples of the severe side effects that may be caused by use of any one of these antacid compounds alone.
3. What other ingredients are found in antacid combination products? Describe the effects of simethicone. What is a possible use of alginic acid? List the drug interactions when antacids are administered with other medications. Before recommending antacid therapy, which questions should be asked of the patient and why? How long should antacids for "indigestion" be administered? If no relief is obtained during this time, what should the patient do? What are the restrictions in antacid administration for patients with edema, congestive heart failure, hypertension, renal failure, pregnancy, or salt-restricted diets? Do antacid *tablets* effectively give relief in peptic ulcer disease? Why not? What are possible results of excessive use of antacids? What problems should be considered in selection of an antacid for the patient with *acute* ulcer disease?
4. Name five commonly used antacids. See Table 18-1 and ask your instructor for several examples commonly used in your hospital.

5. Cimetidine (Tagamet) (several choices are correct)
   a. Has been on the market for many years as an effective drug to increase gastric secretion
   b. Decreases daytime and nighttime secretions of gastric acid
   c. Is effective in the treatment of stomach ulcer only
   d. Can be used safely in pregnant and nursing mothers and in children
   e. Is available in injectable and tablet form
   f. Has as an initial oral dose of 300 mg four times a day, with meals and at bedtime
   g. Is an effective drug to heal ulcers, with healing occurring within 3 to 6 months
   h. Will heal an ulcer within the first 2 weeks of treatment, but therapy should continue for 4 to 6 weeks to ensure adequate healing
   i. Should be used concomitantly with antacid therapy if oral cimetidine is used

6. What is the main use of carbenoxolone (Biogastrone)? Is it commonly used in the United States? List its adverse effects.

7. What is the medical term for insufficient secretion of hydrochloric acid in the stomach? Name three possible causes of this condition. Can this condition be found in normal people? Describe the method of mixing dilute hydrochloric acid before administration and the method of administration. What is the average dose of dilute hydrochloric acid and at what times should it be administered? Why? Name one drug available in capsule form containing hydrochloric acid for the treatment of achlorhydria. This drug is a combination of what two agents? When is it administered?

8. What does pancreatin contain and what are its purposes? Name one other drug used for the same purpose as pancreatin.

9. What is the source of bile? What is the purpose of bile and bile salts? What is the purpose of dehydrocholic acid (Decholin)?

10. Explain the defoaming action of simethicone (Mylicon). What is the usual dose? Name another antacid carminative containing simethicone.

11. What are the main uses of Gaviscon? It is an example of what type of drug? What is the usual dose? Describe the method of administration.

12. Define *emetic*.

13. Name two emetics and tell the method of administration of each. What is the purpose of inducing vomiting with the drug Syrup of ipecac? For which conditions should it *not* be used? What is the dose?

14. Name two household measures that can be used as emetics.

15. In the discussion of antiemetics, on what does effective treatment usually depend? What are causes of vomiting? List the treatments for vomiting. Name three drugs discussed as antiemetics. List the main uses, side effects, duration of action, and usual doses for these three drugs. Which drug was mentioned as useful in the treatment of Meniere's syndrome? When you named your drugs, did you use both generic and trade names?

16. Name one drug used in x-ray photography of the gastrointestinal tract, and explain the aftercare at the conclusion of the x-ray examinations.

17. Name a drug used to detect gastric anacidity and describe the method of administration. In addition to the procedure of administration of this drug, what would you consider important to tell the patient?

18. What is the purpose of histamine? What are its side effects?

19. Why is betazole (Histalog) used more frequently than histamine phosphate in diagnostic stimulation of hydrochloric acid secretion?

20. What are the causes of diarrhea? Diarrhea should be brought under control, but it is important to determine what first? What conditions can diarrhea cause? Give two examples for each of the following: demulcents-protectives, adsorbents, and antiperistaltic agents, and tell the purpose of all drugs.

21. Kaopectate can be expected to relieve diarrhea by producing which of the following effects?
   a. Carminative and sedative
   b. Adsorbent and astringent
   c. Demulcent and cathartic
   d. Adsorbent and demulcent

22. What is the action of bismuth subcarbonate and what conditions does it control?

23. What does Donnagel contain? What are the actions of Donnagel? It is used to treat what conditions? For which conditions should it be administered with caution? What is the usual dose?

24. Camphorated opium tincture (Paregoric) is used for what condition?

25. Name two other sedative antispasmodics used in the treatment of diarrhea.

26. Give the trade name for loperamide. What type of drug is it? For what conditions is it effective? It has opiate-like properties, but is it addicting in recommended dosages? What is the antidote for overdosage?

27. What is the difference between laxatives and purgatives? Explain why it is difficult to place cathartics in any one group.

28. List some causes of constipation. List contraindications for cathartics. List indications for the use of cathartics.

29. Outline the advice you as a nurse may give patients in the use of cathartics. Who is the one to give detailed specific advice to the patient regarding use of cathartics? What is an essential point to teach people in regard to frequency and type of bowel movements?

30. If a person went into the drugstore asking for a cathartic, why would a pharmacist ask whether the person has any nausea, vomiting, or abdominal pain?

31. A mother told you that her 10-year-old daughter "seems perfectly well, but she hasn't had a bowel movement in 2½ days. What kind of cathartic do you think I should give her?" Which is the one best, safest, and most helpful reply you can give her?
   a. A teaspoon of milk of magnesia is a mild cathartic and effective for the needs of children
   b. Use a glycerin suppository and see that she gets plenty of raw fruits, vegetables, and water

c. You had better see your doctor; cathartics can be dangerous if taken at the wrong time or in the wrong amount

d. A dose of castor oil should be very effective for her

32. Name two lubricant laxatives and give the dose of each. Describe the method of administration for mineral oil. If it causes leakage, what is the best procedure? For what conditions beside constipation are mineral oil and Agoral used?

33. Name four bulk laxatives. How do bulk laxatives achieve their effect? Give the correct method of mixing Metamucil and administering it to the patient. Why are fluids during administration and throughout the day important? What is the usual dose of Metamucil? Metamucil is available in effervescent form, but for which patients is this form contraindicated? Describe the method of administration and dosage of Effersyllium and methylcellulose. What is the source of carboxymethylcellulose sodium? What is the method of administration and amount of dosage for this drug? It is available in tablet form, but what precaution should be given to the patient in regard to the tablets?

34. Saline cathartics achieve their quick action by
    a. Being completely insoluble
    b. Increasing the volume of water in the intestines
    c. Decreasing the volume of water in the intestines
    d. None of these

35. Saline cathartics should best be given
    a. At bedtime
    b. Between lunch and supper
    c. Before breakfast
    d. After breakfast

36. Saline cathartics act usually in how many hours?
    a. 12 to 16
    b. 1 to 4
    c. 6 to 8
    d. 8 to 12

37. Saline cathartics are used mainly in the treatment of what conditions or for what purposes?

38. Name three commonly used saline cathartics.

39. To achieve cathartic action, saline cathartics need water present
    a. In the rectum
    b. In the stomach only
    c. In the intestines
    d. Nowhere

40. Milk of magnesia is a saline cathartic. Which of the following substances is responsible for the cathartic effect of milk of magnesia in cathartic dosage?
    a. Magnesium citrate
    b. Magnesium carbonate
    c. Magnesium hydroxide
    d. Magnesium chloride

41. Castor oil (several choices are correct)
    a. Is an example of a bulk laxative
    b. Is an example of a cathartic that acts by irritation
    c. Originates from the seeds of the castor bean
    d. Comes from the *Rhamnus purshiana* tree
    e. Is also known by its generic name, oleum ricini
    f. Acts mainly on the small intestine
    g. Causes little gripping in persons with normal bowels,

although some patients may experience severe cramping and diarrhea

h. Will produce semifluid stools in average dose

i. Is an excellent cathartic choice in chronic constipation and ulcerative bowel conditions because of the oil

j. Has as the usual dose 15 to 60 ml

k. Is very useful in dysentery and fermentative diarrhea (if given early before dehydration occurs) and in food or drug poisoning, cleansing of the bowel for x-ray examination, preoperative preparation of the bowel, and acute constipation

l. Causes one or two bowel movements a day during the next 48 hours

42. The source of cascara sagrada is
    a. The castor bean
    b. *Rhamnus purshiana* tree bark
    c. Synthetic
    d. Animal

43. Cascara sagrada acts chiefly on the large intestine, or the small intestine? For what type of constipation is it commonly used? It acts in how many hours? What is the usual dose and at what time should it be administered? Name other forms of cascara sagrada. What is the difference in dosage of cascara sagrada fluidextract and aromatic cascara sagrada fluidextract?

44. What is the source of aloe? What type of cathartic is it? It acts mainly on large intestines, or small intestines? Does it cause gripping? Name two proprietary preparations that contain aloe.

45. What is the source of senna? In how many hours does it produce action? Name three proprietary remedies that contain senna.

46. What type of cathartic is phenolphthalein? In how many hours does action occur? Its action is on small intestines, large intestines, or both small and large intestines? Phenolphthalein is sometimes prepared in "candy tablet" form. What instructions should be given to children and parents and where should the drug be kept? What is the usual dose? Name three proprietary medicines containing phenolphthalein.

47. Danthron (Dorbane) acts chiefly on the large intestine, or the small intestine? It is effective for what type of constipation? What is its usual dose?

48. Bisacodyl (Dulcolax) acts mainly on the large intestine, or small intestine? It is effective in what types of constipation? What are some of its uses? To which type of patients may bisacodyl be given? What is the usual dose? In how many hours does action occur? What drug should *not* be given within an hour of administration of bisacodyl?

49. Is dioctyl sodium sulfosuccinate a laxative? What type of drug is it? Does it bring immediate relief? It is an aid in what type of constipation? Sometimes it is combined with a mild laxative. Name one. What are the points to remember about this drug? What is an essential part of the treatment with this drug? Name several examples of dioctyl sodium sulfosuccinate. Doxidan is a combination of what two drugs? It acts on the large intestine, or small intestine? It is effective for which type of constipation? What does Dialose contain and what are its chief effects?

CHAPTER 19

Histamine, antihistamines, and drugs used for motion sickness

Histamine is derived from an amino acid called histidine. It is stored in small granules in most body tissues. Its physiologic functions are not completely known, but it is released in response to allergic reactions and tissue damage from trauma or infection.

When histamine is released in the area of tissue damage or at the site of an antigen-antibody reaction, such as pollen being inhaled into the nose of a patient allergic to that specific pollen:

1. Arterioles and capillaries in the region dilate, allowing an increased blood flow to the area, resulting in a "blush"
2. Capillaries become more permeable, resulting in the outward passage of fluid into the extracellular spaces, with formation of edema; this edema is manifested by congestion in the mucuous membranes of the patient's nose and lungs
3. Nasal, lacrimal, and bronchial secretions are released, resulting in the running nose and eyes noted in patients with allergies

When large amounts of histamine are released, blood pressure drops (hypotension) and the skin becomes flushed and edematous with severe itching (urticaria). Bronchospasm makes respiratory effort more difficult (dyspnea), changes in intracranial pressure result in severe headache, and copious quantities of gastric secretions are released.

Small doses of histamine were once used as a diagnostic aid to stimulate gastric acid secretion. Presence of gastric acid is significant in the diagnosis of certain malabsorption disorders and pernicious anemia. Because of the many adverse effects of histamine, however, betazole hydrochloride is now used.

Betazole hydrochloride (bay'tah-zol)
(Histalog) (his'tah-log)

1. Betazole is an analogue of histamine, with similar pharmacologic actions.
2. It is now used in diagnostic tests of gastric secretion instead of histamine.
3. Betazole stimulates gastric secretion equal to that of

histamine, especially during the first hour of gastric analysis. The amount of acid secreted during the second hour and later is generally greater with betazole.
4. This drug is particularly advantageous because it produces fewer side effects than histamine. Side effects include sweating, a feeling of warmth, and flushing in about 20% of the patients, and headache occurs in about 3% of the patients. Rarely observed are urticaria and syncope.
5. Betazole should be used with caution in patients with recent gastrointestinal bleeding, heart disease, or bronchial asthma.
6. Usual adult dose: 50 mg, or 0.5 mg/kg of body weight administered subcutaneously or intramuscularly.

HISTAMINE ANTAGONISTS

Histamine response can be antagonized by two types of drugs: rapidly acting epinephrine and the more slowly acting group of antihistamines.

Epinephrine is a life-saving drug in anaphylactic shock. The most serious effects of anaphylaxis, or severe acute allergic reactions, are extensive arteriolar dilation, with hypotensive shock and collapse and constriction of bronchial tubes that can lead to extreme respiratory difficulty and suffocation. Epinephrine promotes vasoconstriction and dilates the bronchial tubes, thus antagonizing the physiologic effects of massive histamine release or anaphylaxis.

Antihistamines

Antihistamines can modify and lessen the severity of the symptoms observed in the allergic patient. Antihistamines are chemical agents that act by competing with the allergy-liberated histamine for receptor sites in the patient's arterioles, capillaries, and glands. Antihistamines do not prevent histamine release, and because they act by competitive inhibition, if the histamine concentration at the receptor site exceeds the antihistamine concentration, histaminic effects will predominate. Antihistamines are therefore more effective if taken at the beginning of adverse symptomatology.

All of the antihistaminics are palliative and do not immunize the patient or protect over time from allergic reactions. Relief of various allergic symptoms is obtained only while the drug is being taken. There is apparently no cumulative action, so these drugs can be taken over a long period. Some patients requiring frequent antihistamine use find that they do not obtain the same degree of relief after several weeks or months of therapy. This is apparently because of more rapid metabolism of the chemical compound. If tolerance does develop, patients may easily switch to another antihistamine that does provide relief.

The most common side effect of many of the antihistaminic drugs is drowsiness. Persons who are working around machinery, driving a car, pouring and giving medicines, or performing other duties in which they must remain alert mentally and employ good judgment should not take these drugs while working. Most patients acquire a tolerance to this adverse effect. Reduction in dosage or a change to another antihistamine may occa-

sionally be necessary, however. The sedative properties of the antihistamines may enhance the effects of alcohol and other CNS depressants, including sedative-hypnotics, analgesics, and tranquilizers.

All antihistamines display anticholinergic side effects, particularly when higher dosages are used. Symptoms may include dry mouth, stuffy nose, blurred vision, constipation, and urinary retention. Patients with asthma, prostatic enlargement, and glaucoma should take antihistamines only under a physician's supervision.

Table 19-1 represents a list of commonly used antihistamine products, most of which are available without prescription.

Cimetidine represents another type of histamine antagonist. It is used to block histamine receptors in the stomach, reducing the secretion of gastric acid. (See Index for a more complete description of its use.)

DRUGS USED FOR MOTION SICKNESS

In addition to their histamine-blocking effects, certain antihistamines have the capability to reduce nausea and vomiting from motion sickness. Vomiting is thought to

Table 19-1. Antihistamines*

Generic name	Available form	Common brand names	Adult dosages	Maximum daily dose (mg)
Brompheniramine maleate	Injection, tablets, elixir	Bromatane, Dimetane, Dimetane-Ten	10 mg three times daily	40
Chlorpheniramine maleate	Tablets, capsules, syrup	Antagonate, Chlor-Trimeton, Trymegen	4 mg three or four times daily	40
Cyproheptadine hydrochloride	Tablets, syrup	Periactin, Cyprodine	4 mg three times daily	32
Diphenhydramine hydrochloride	Injection, capsules, tablets, syrup, elixir	Benadryl, Bendylate, Nordryl	25 to 50 mg three or four times daily	300
Doxylamine succinate	Tablets, syrup	Decapryn	12.5 to 25 mg every 4 to 6 hours	100
Pheniramine maleate	Tablets	Inhiston	20 mg every 4 hours	150
Promethazine hydrochloride†	Injection, tablets, syrup, suppository	Phenergan, Prothazine, Pentazine, Prorex	12.5 to 25 mg three or four times daily	100
Pyrilamine maleate	Tablets	Allertoc, Zem-Histine	25 to 50 mg four times daily	200
Tripelennamine	Tablets, elixir	PBZ, Pyrizine	25 to 50 mg every 4 to 6 hours	300

*Many of these antihistamines are also available in combination with decongestants and analgesics for relief of cold and flu symptoms.
†Promethazine is a phenothiazine with antihistaminic properties.

be induced by impulses from the vestibular canals in the ear, stimulating the chemoreceptive trigger zone (the ''vomiting center''). The most effective agents that block these impulses to the vomiting center are: cyclizine, dimenhydrinate, meclizine, and promethazine (see Index).

Cyclizine hydrochloride (si'kli-zeen) *(Marezine Hydrochloride)* (mar'eh-zeen)

1. This drug has been found effective in a high percentage of cases of nausea and vomiting caused by motion sickness.
2. The usual symptoms of dry mouth, drowsiness, and blurred vision seldom appear with normal dosage but may appear with large doses.
3. Cyclizine should not be administered during pregnancy because of possible harm to the fetus.
4. Usual dose: 50 mg 30 minutes before departure and 50 mg three times daily before meals. Dosage can be reduced after the initial dose. It relieves dizziness and other symptoms associated with vestibular disorders in a dosage of 50 mg three times a day.

Dimenhydrinate (dy-men-hy'dri-nayt) *(Dramamine)* (dram'ah-meen)

1. Dimenhydrinate is an effective antihistaminic drug used mainly in the treatment of nausea and vomiting from motion sickness (seasickness, train sickness, and air sickness).

2. This drug has also been used to control nausea, vomiting, and dizziness associated with such conditions as fenestration operations, radiation sickness, Meniere's disease, and postoperative nausea and vomiting. It is not as effective as promethazine.
3. It produces mild sedation and can cause drowsiness.
4. For motion sickness, its best effect is obtained by taking 50 mg orally before meals and at bedtime for the first 4 days of a sea voyage. The initial oral dose before an airplane trip is 50 mg about 30 minutes before departing. The usual IM dose is 50 mg.

Meclizine hydrochloride (mek'li-zeen) *(Antivert), (Bonine)* (bo'neen)

1. Meclizine has a mild but prolonged antihistaminic action and is effective in the prevention of motion sickness.
2. Its effects may last as long as 24 hours. It appears to affect the central nervous system and the inner ear, as do other members of this group of drugs.
3. It can cause drowsiness, dry mouth, and blurred vision, but incidence of side effects is low.
4. This drug should not be administered during pregnancy because it may possibly harm the fetus.
5. Usual adult dose: 25 to 50 mg orally once a day for the prevention of motion sickness (1 hour before departure) and for the relief of nausea and vomiting from other causes. The drug is available in tablets of 12.5 and 25 mg.

The physician prescribes the medicine and treatment.
The nurse carries out the physician's orders.
Self-medication is dangerous. Consult your physician first.
There is in every medicine a possible danger.
When in doubt—ASK!

ASSIGNMENT

Review previous lessons and questions according to the directions of your instructor.

1. What are the sources for histamine? List the action and effects of histamine. When large amounts of histamine are released, what symptoms occur? Small amounts of histamine were once used as a diagnostic aid for what purpose? Why is betazole hydrochloride now used in place of histamine?
2. What type of a drug is betazole (Histalog)? What are its main use and effects? What is its particular advantage? List the side effects and contraindications for this drug.

3. Name two histamine antagonists. Epinephrine is a lifesaving drug in anaphylactic shock. Explain the symptoms of anaphylactic shock. What effect does epinephrine have on the blood vessels and bronchial tubes in overcoming anaphylactic shock?
4. What effect do antihistamines have on the body? Do they cure the allergic condition or give immunization? What is the most common side effect of many of the antihistaminic drugs? What instructions should be given the patient in this regard? List the anticholinergic side effects of antihistamines. Name a drug that represents another type of histamine antagonist. What is its chief effect that makes it useful in the treatment of some allergy patients?

5. List the antihistamines that seem to be most effective in blocking the nausea and vomiting impulses and are of aid in treating motion sickness.

6. What is the chief use of cyclizine (Marezine)? Side effect symptoms seldom appear with normal dosage, but list the symptoms that may appear with large doses. Can cyclizine be administered safely during pregnancy? What is the usual dose and when is it administered? Is it effective in relieving dizziness and other vestibular disorders symptoms? What dosage is effective for this condition?

7. What is the main use of dimenhydrinate (Dramamine)? List its other uses. Can it cause sedation? Drowsiness? Is it as effective as promethazine? What is the usual dose and when should it be administered?

8. What is the main use of meclizine (Antivert, Bonine)? How long may its effects last? What two body sysems does it affect? List the possible side effects. Is this a safe drug to use during pregnancy? Why not? Tell the usual dose for this drug and when it should be administered?

9. Name six antihistamine drugs from Table 19-1, giving both the generic name and trade name for each drug. Your instructor will help you select six of the most commonly used drugs in your hospital for patient use at home.

10. The physician ordered a dose of meclizine (Antivert) 25 mg once a day for motion sickness. You had on hand meclizine 12.5 mg. How many tablets will you administer?

CHAPTER 20

Drugs affecting the reproductive system

DRUGS THAT STRENGTHEN UTERINE CONTRACTIONS

Ergot (er'got)

Ergot is a drug that comes from a mold on the grain rye. Its derivatives stimulate uterine contractions and aid in preventing or controlling uterine hemorrhage after childbirth.

The entire group of individual alkaloids derived from ergot can be divided into three groups: the ergotamine, the dihydroergotamine, and the ergonovine groups. All three groups increase the motor activity of the uterus. Ergonovine is the preparation of ergot most used in obstetrics. Oral doses are readily absorbed; therefore, it is more effective than the other alkaloids and is taken in smaller doses and weaker concentrations. Because of this, side effects are rare in obstetric use.

Side effects from ergonovine usually result from stimulation of the central nervous system and include symptoms such as nausea, vomiting, weakness, tremor, excitement, rapid pulse, dilated pupils, and convulsive seizures. Side effects from the ergotamine alkaloids usually produce circulatory system disturbances before they produce effects in the nervous system. These symptoms include itching, tingling, and coldness of the skin, rapid weak pulse, headache, thirst, nausea, vomiting, dizziness, diarrhea, and abdominal cramps.

Treatment of ergot poisoning includes complete withdrawal of the medication plus the use of vasodilators (nitroprusside) and sedatives.

The following two ergot preparations are used in obstetrics.

Ergonovine maleate (er-go-no'veen)
(Ergotrate Maleate) (er'go-trayt)

1. Usual dose: 0.2 to 0.4 mg orally two or three times daily for 2 to 3 days. Some physicians prescribe 0.2 mg every 4 hours for six doses starting immediately after delivery. Parenteral dose: 0.2 to 0.4 mg IM.
2. Prolonged therapy should be avoided.

Methylergonovine maleate (meth-il-er-go-no'veen)
(Methergine) (meth'er-jin)

1. Methergine is an outstanding synthetic oxytocic that stimulates uterine contractions and aids in prevention or control of hemorrhage after childbirth.
2. It should be administered at the end of the third stage of labor. Under constant obstetric supervision, it may be administered in the second stage following delivery of the anterior shoulder.
3. Methergine is said to be more intense and sustained and relatively free of vasopressor action when compared to ergonovine.
4. Caution should be used in administering this drug to patients with sepsis, hepatic or renal involvement, or obliterative vascular disease. The drug is contraindicated during pregnancy.
5. Methergine has less tendency to cause an elevation of blood pressure and is preferred for patients with threatened or definite eclampsia.
6. Usual dose: 0.2 mg orally. Parenteral dose: 0.2 mg/ml.

• • •

Ergotamine tartrate has been used for the treatment of migraine headache and for the relief of excessive itching associated with jaundice conditions (see Index).

Posterior pituitary hormone

The pituitary gland is a small, ductless gland situated in a saddle-shaped depression in the sphenoid bone at the base of the brain. It has two lobes, the anterior and the posterior. Extracts are obtained from the posterior lobe of the pituitary glands of cattle and sheep. When injected they produce the following effects: (1) stimulation of uterine muscle (oxytocic effect), (2) constriction of peripheral blood vessels (pressor effect), and (3) promotion of water reabsorption in the tubules of the kidney (antidiuretic effect).

Two major hormones that have been obtained from the gland are oxytocin and vasopressin. These are both peptides containing eight amino acids. It has proved possible to synthesize them chemically.

Vasopressin (vas-o-pres'in)
(Pitressin) (pi-tres'in)

1. Vasopressin is a purified form of the posterior pituitary hormone that possesses vasopressor and antidiuretic (ADH) activity. It is used primarily in the treatment of polyuria associated with diabetes insipidus.
2. Side effects associated with vasopressin therapy include tremor, sweating, abdominal cramps, diarrhea, urticaria, and bronchial constriction. Vasopressin should be used very cautiously in patients with cardiovascular disease. The vasopressor effects of this drug may produce hypertension, anginal pain, and possible myocardial infarction.
3. Dosage for treatment of diabetes insipidus: 5 to 10 units intramuscularly or subcutaneously two to three times daily.
4. *Vasopressin tannate (Pitressin Tannate in Oil)* may produce a duration of action of 48 to 96 hours.

Oxytocin injection, synthetic (ok-se-to'sin)
(Pitocin) (pi-to'sin), *(Syntocinon)* (sin-to'si-non),
(Uteracon) (u'ter-ah-kahn)

1. This hormone in its original form was from the posterior lobe of domestic animals. It is now available in synthetic form with fewer side effects.
2. This synthetic form of the drug has three uses:
   a. To induce active labor or to increase the force and rate of existing contractions during delivery when they are not strong enough to expel the fetus
   b. To contract uterine muscle and decrease hemorrhage after delivery of the placenta
   c. To occasionally promote milk ejection when ineffective ejection is believed to be a cause of inadequacy of breast feeding
3. Side effects and toxic effects:
   a. Constant observation is absolutely essential, including frequent blood pressure readings, accurate and periodic check of the fetal heart tones, and observation of the strength and duration of uterine contractions; prolonged contractions of the uterus cause a diminished blood flow and decreased oxygen for the fetus
   b. When used unwisely, oxytocin can cause hypertensive crisis, cerebral hemorrhage, and uterine rupture, as well as pelvic hematomas, arrhythmias, and bradycardia; arrhythmias may also occur in the fetus—fetal deaths have resulted
   c. Water intoxication may occur when large doses of oxytocin, without the addition of electrolytes, have been infused over long periods
4. It is contraindicated in fetal distress, severe toxemia, cephalopelvic disproportion, malpresentation of the fetus, predisposition to uterine rupture (from mul-

tiparas, previous cesarean section, or uterine surgery), and medical conditions such as severe cardiovascular disease.

5. Usual dosage:
   a. IV infusion dose: 1 ml (10 units) of oxytocin added to 500 or 1,000 ml of 5% dextrose or normal saline, infused at an initial rate of 1 to 2 milliunits per minute; the rate is carefully increased until an optimal uterine response is obtained (three or four effective contractions in 10 minutes)
   b. IV injection for emergency treatment of postpartum bleeding: 0.06 to 0.18 ml (0.6 to 1.8 units) of oxytocin is diluted with 3 to 5 ml of normal saline and slowly injected; effects occur in 15 to 60 seconds
   c. IM injection to control postpartum bleeding: 0.3 to 1 ml (3 to 10 units); effects appear in 3 to 7 minutes and last for 30 to 60 minutes
   d. Nasal spray is used to promote milk ejection for breast feeding: dose is 1 spray into one or both nostrils 2 to 3 minutes before nursing
   e. Buccal administration: one or more tablets are placed in the buccal space or inner cheek every 30 minutes until the desired uterine response is obtained, or a total of 15 tablets (3,000 units) have been administered over 24 hours; buccal administration is less reliable and less precise than IV administration because the rate of absorption is unpredictable

DRUGS THAT DECREASE UTERINE MOTILITY

Sometimes, the inhibition of uterine contractions is necessary, for example, when a patient begins premature labor or when uterine tone is high and contractions are unusually frequent and uncoordinated. Drugs to control such conditions include certain depressants of the central nervous system and muscle relaxants.

Large doses of opiates, barbiturates, and general anesthetics tend to decrease uterine motility. Average doses of barbiturates have little effect other than to reduce anxiety. Morphine relieves pain and lessens fear and anxiety. Meperidine relieves pain and has less effect on respiration, although the lessened effect on respiration may not occur with larger doses. Promethazine hydrochloride (Phenergan) is used in obstetrics for sedation, relief of apprehension, and increase in effect of drug such as morphine sulfate and meperidine hydrochloride, allowing a reduction in their dosage.

Unfortunately, heavy doses of narcotics, barbiturates, and anesthetics are apt to cause maternal and infant respiratory depression during labor, endangering the lives of both mother and infant and even possibly causing brain damage of the infant because of the lack of oxygen.

Magnesium sulfate

1. When magnesium sulfate is administered parenterally, it will depress all forms of muscle tissue (skeletal, smooth, and cardiac).
2. It is effective to counteract uterine tetany that may occur after large doses of oxytocin or when the myometrium is contracting abnormally.
3. Because of its depressant effect on skeletal muscle, it is used to treat preeclampsia to prevent the development of seizure activity.
4. Toxic effects are possible. Respiratory depression can occur. Fast injection of large doses can cause respiratory arrest. Never leave a patient who is receiving magnesium sulfate parenterally alone.
5. Calcium gluconate (10% solution) is usually an effective antidote, since it counteracts the effect of magnesium sulfate on muscle tissue. In addition, the patient may need artificial respiration.
6. Magnesium sulfate is administered intramuscularly and sometimes intravenously. For rapid effect an IV dose of 20 ml of a 20% solution is used followed by a continuous infusion of 2 to 3 g/hr. This drug is poorly absorbed after oral administration and may cause severe diarrhea.

A beta-adrenergic drug being used to decrease uterine motility is **isoxsuprine hydrochloride (Vasodilan).** It has potent relaxant effects on vascular and uterine smooth muscle. It is approved for use in the treatment of peripheral vascular spasm, Buerger's and Raynaud's diseases, and arteriosclerotic vascular disease. Side effects are relatively mild and include nausea, vomiting, dizziness, and occasionally, transient hypotension and tachycardia. These symptoms usually subside with a reduction in dosage. Oral dosage is 10 to 20 mg three or four times daily, and is preferred for long-term therapy over the IM route.

Terbutaline sulfate (Brethine, Bricanyl), a sympathomimetic amine, similar in chemical structure and pharmacologic action to isoproterenol and metaproterenol, is being tried for the prevention of premature uterine activity. Its main use is as a bronchodilator in the treatment of bronchial asthma and bronchospasm. Usual adult oral dose is 2.5 or 5 mg at 4- to 8-hour intervals. Dosage should not exceed 15 mg daily. It is also available for injection. Terbutaline has many side effects, such as nausea, vomiting, headache, restlessness, lethargy, drowsiness, sweating, tremors, increase in heart rate, nervousness, palpitations, dizziness, and tinnitus. These side effects, however, are rare when terbutaline is used in recommended dosages.

This drug should be used with caution in patients with hypertension, hyperthyroidism, diabetes, or cardiac disorders associated with arrhythmias. It should also be used with caution when combined with other sympathomimetic agents because of the possibility of increasing the cardiovascular side effects.

SEX HORMONES THAT AFFECT THE OVARIES

The hormones concerned with ovarian function are the anterior pituitary hormones. They are required for the normal development and function of the gonads, the ovarian hormones, and the gonadotropic hormones of placental origin.

Pituitary gonadotropic hormones

The anterior pituitary endocrine gland is made up of six or seven different types of secretory cells. These cells function independently in producing their characteristic hormones. These hormones are the adrenocorticotropic hormone (ACTH), the thyroid-stimulating hormone (TSH), the luteinizing hormone (LH), the melanocyte-stimulating hormone (MSH), the follicle-stimulating hormone (FSH), the growth hormone (GH), and prolactin (PL).

The secretion of these hormones is stimulated by hypothalamic releasing factors, also called hypophysiotropic hormones, such as ACTH-releasing factor (CRF), TSH-releasing hormone (TRH), FSH-releasing factor (FRF), LH-releasing factor (LRF), PL-inhibiting and PL-releasing factors (PIF and PRF), MSH-releasing and MSH-inhibiting factors (MRF and MIF), and GH-releasing and GH-inhibiting factors (GRF and GIF).

Several neuropharmacologic agents alter anterior pituitary secretions by acting on the production of hypothalamic releasing factors. It is thought that the neurons that secrete the releasing factors are located in the ventral hypothalamus, and that a number of neurotransmitters regulate their functional activities. Among the possible transmitters are norepinephrine, dopamine, and serotonin.

Three hormones are of interest in their effect on the ovary:

1. FSH, which stimulates the development and growth of the graafian follicle and the secretion of estrogens and initiates the monthly cycle of hormonal activity in the ovary
2. LH, which produces ovulation and promotes secretion of progesterone from the corpus luteum
3. LTH, which is a luteotropic hormone probably identical with the lactogenic hormone:
   a. Promotes the secretory activity of the corpus luteum and the formation of progesterone
   b. In the absence of LTH, the corpus luteum undergoes regressive changes and fails to make progesterone

FSH and LH both cause the graafian follicle to grow, mature, secrete estrogen, ovulate, and form the corpus luteum.

In the male, FSH acts only on the seminiferous tubules and promotes the formation of sperm cells. Interstitial cell-stimulating hormone stimulates the interstitial cells in the testes and promotes the formation of androgen.

The clinical use of the pituitary gonadotropic hormones has been limited by the lack of sufficiently refined preparations. Commercial preparations often contain other proteins and inert substances that cause painful injections and make allergic reactions possible.

Gonadotropic hormones from the placenta

Gonadotropic substances are formed by the placenta during pregnancy in the human being and in some animals. Human chorionic gonadotropic hormone (HCG) differs from pituitary gonadotropin both biologically and chemically. It produces little of the follicle-stimulating effect, mainly affecting the growth of the interstitial cells of the testes and ovaries and maintaining the secretion of luteal hormone. Its chief function seems to be to enhance and prolong the secretion of the corpus luteum during early pregnancy. It does not initiate the formation of corpus luteum. In women it prolongs the luteal phase of the menstrual cycle. In men it stimulates the interstitial cells of the testes, causing them to increase production of androgen. This in turn promotes the growth and development of accessory sex organs.

Gonadotropic hormones are used in the treatment of cryptorchidism (if no anatomic obstruction is present), of hypogonadism, and for induction of ovulation. There is considerable difference of opinion about its value. Examples of gonadotropic hormones are *Follutein, Pregnyl, Antuitrin-S,* and *A.P.L.* secules.

The gonads

The gonads are the glands of reproduction: the testes of the male and the ovaries of the female. In addition to producing sperm, the testes produce testosterone, the male sex hormone. Testosterone controls the development of the sex organs of the male and influences characteristics such as voice, hair distribution, and male body form. Other steroid hormones that produce masculinizing effects are a group called androgens.

The ovaries produce estrogen and progesterone. These are hormones that stimulate maturing of the female sex organs. They influence breast development, voice quality, and the broader pelvis of the female body form. Menstruation is established because of the hormone production of the ovaries. Estrogen is the hormone responsible for most of these changes. Progesterone is thought to be concerned mainly with body changes that favor the implantation of the fertilized ovum and continuation of pregnancy. Both hormones seem to influence mood changes and the emotional balance of the female.

Estrogens

The estrogens are responsible for the development of the sex organs at puberty and for characteristics such as growth of hair, texture of skin, and distribution of body fat.

Estrogenic substances are found in many places in both plants and animals. These substances can be found in the blood of both female and male, in testicular fluid of the male, and in feces, bile, placenta, and urine of pregnant women and mares. Some physicians believe that estrogens may cause cancer in persons who may have an inherited sensitivity to certain types of cancer. They believe that estrogens should not be given to women with a personal or family history of cancer of the reproductive system.

Estrogens relieve some symptoms of menopause, such as nervousness, "hot flashes," irritability, and emotional upsets. In menopause, there is a gradual lessening of ovarian function and therefore a gradual decrease in ovarian secretion. Estrogens aid in an attempt to restore the balance of the secretions. They are also used to relieve breast engorgement in women who do not nurse their babies and to relieve pain in postmenopausal women who have an inoperable breast cancer that has spread to the soft tissues. Estrogens are also used to relieve discomfort and pain of prostatic cancer with metastases (spreading of the growth to other tissues) and to treat senile vaginitis and pruritus vulvae (or itching of the vulva). Some are available in suppository form for these purposes. Estrogens are powerful drugs that should be taken only under medical advice.

Estrone (es'troan)
(Theelin) (thee'lin), *(Foygen)* (foi'jin)

1. Estrone is obtained from the urine of pregnant mares. It is effective in the treatment of menopause, vulval conditions, and prostatic carcinoma.
2. Usual dose for menopause: 0.2 to 1 mg intramuscularly, once or twice weekly. Large doses may cause uterine bleeding.

Ethinyl estradiol (eth'i-nil es-trah'dee-ol)
(Estinyl) (es'ti-nil), *(Feminone)* (fem'i-noan),
(Rolidiol) (ro-li'dee-ol)

1. Ethinyl estradiol is a derivative of estrone and is one of the most powerful estrogens.
2. Side effects such as headache, nausea, and vomiting may occur, as they may with other estrogens.
3. The doses vary, depending on whether the drug is administered for menopause symptoms, breast engorgement after childbirth, prostatic cancer, or breast cancer. Usual dose for menopause: 0.02 to 0.05 mg orally in tablets one to three times daily and cyclically.

4. Other estradiol preparations include **estradiol (Estrace), estradiol cypionate in oil (D-Est, Estroject-L.A.),** and **estradiol valerate in oil (Dioval, Estate, Delestrogen).**

Diethylstilbestrol (dy-eth-il-stil-bes′trol)

1. Diethylstilbestrol is a synthetic estrogenic substance that is less expensive than some other types of estrogens. It is effective in practically all the various uses of estrogens.
2. It may cause headache, nausea, and vomiting.
3. Its dose varies, depending on its purpose. Usual dose for menopause: 0.2 to 0.5 mg daily.

Estrogenic substances, conjugated
(Premarin) (pre′mah-rin), **(Estrocon)** (es′tro-kahn), **(Genisis)** (jen′i-sis), **(Kestrin)** (kes′trin), **(Menotab)** (men′o-tab)

1. These preparations have as their source the urine of pregnant mares. Action and uses are similar to those of other estrogens.
2. Usual dose for menopause: 1.25 mg daily. Larger doses are given for senile vaginitis, breast cancer, and pruritus vulvae.

Piperazine estrone sulfate (pi-per′ah-zeen)
(Ogen) (o′jin)

1. Piperazine has the same actions and uses as the naturally occurring conjugated estrogens.
2. Dosage is oral. For control of menopause symptoms: 1.5 mg. For treatment of senile vaginitis and pruritus vulvae: 1.5 to 4.5 mg.

There is much controversy today about the long-range effects of estrogens (conjugated estrogens), and questions have not been resolved. It is now recommended, however, that courses of estrogen supplementation be as short as possible.

Luteal hormones
Progesterone (pro-jest′er-own)
(Profac-O) (pro-fak′oh), **(Lipo-Lutin)** (li-po-lu′tin), **(Gesterol)** (jes′ter-ol)

1. Progesterone, secreted by the corpus luteum, inhibits the secretion of pituitary gonadotropins, thus preventing follicular maturation and ovulation. Progesterones are used primarily to treat secondary amenorrhea and functional uterine bleeding.
2. The use of progestational agents is not recommended during the first 4 months of pregnancy. Several studies indicate that there is a greater risk of congenital heart and limb defects when progestational agents are used during this time.
3. Side effects associated with administration of progesterone are rare but include nausea, vomiting, diar-

rhea, breakthrough bleeding, spotting, amenorrhea, headache, cholestatic jaundice, mental depression, and hirsutism.
4. Dosage for functional uterine bleeding: intramuscularly, 5 to 10 mg daily for six doses. Bleeding may be expected to cease within 6 days.

Fertility drugs
Menotropins (men-o-tro′pins)
(Pergonal) (per′gon-al)

1. Menotropins is a purified preparation of gonadotropic hormones extracted from the urine of postmenopausal women.
2. It is also known as human menopausal gonadotropin (HMG). It contains both luteinizing (LH) and follicle-stimulating hormones (FSH) in a 1:1 ratio.
3. Menotropins is used to promote follicular growth and maturation in women with secondary anovulation.
4. To accomplish ovulation therapy with menotropins, it must be followed by the administration of human chorionic gonadotropins (HCG).
5. Adverse side effects include diarrhea, nausea, vomiting, and fever.
   a. Mild hyperstimulation may cause ovarian enlargement, flatulence, and abdominal discomfort for a period of 1 to 3 weeks and usually requires no treatment.
   b. Severe hyperstimulation may occur about 2 weeks after therapy begins. If it does occur, it is evidenced by weight gain, hypotension, ascites, oliguria, pleural effusion, and hypercoagulability. Daily fluid intake and output, weight, hematocrit, serum and urinary electrolytes, and urinary specific gravity must be monitored.
6. Menotropins is contraindicated in patients with overt thyroid and adrenal dysfunction, abnormal vaginal bleeding of undetermined cause, ovarian cysts, pregnancy, and infertility other than secondary ovarian failure.
7. The preparation is injected intramuscularly and is administered daily for 10 days. The same dosage regimen may be repeated for two or more courses of treatment if there is evidence of ovulation but no pregnancy. Dosage can be increased thereafter if the patient tolerates treatment.
8. Monitoring of urinary estrogen permits the clinician to determine the dose and duration of treatment according to response of the patient. There is marked variability in individual response to menotropins.
9. Pregnancy occurs in 20% to 45% of patients within four to six treatment cycles. Spontaneous miscarriages occur in about 25% of the patients.
10. Daily sexual intercourse should occur from the day

before HCG is administered until ovulation occurs.

11. Patients with significant ovarian enlargement following ovulation should not have sexual intercourse because of the danger of hemoperitoneum from ruptured ovarian cysts. Ovarian rupture with intraperitoneal hemorrhage may require surgery.

12. The couple should be fully informed about possible complications from menotropins and about the frequency and potential hazards of multiple births. Incidence of multiple births in patients treated with menotropins is 17% to 53% of the cases.

Clomiphene citrate (klo'mi-feen)
(Clomid) (klo'mid)

1. Clomiphene is an agent used to increase pituitary secretion of gonadotropin with the intention of inducing ovulation.

2. The mechanism of action of clomiphene is not fully known, but it may compete with estrogen at the hypothalamic level, causing an increase in secretion of the hypothalamic releasing factor, resulting in an increase in the pituitary gonadotropins LH and FSH and, as a consequence, ovarian stimulation. Its stimulant effect on gonadotropin output in women may be a result of removal of inhibition exerted by estrogens.

3. Short-term therapies seem to be more effective than long-term therapies.

4. Side effects include nausea, breast engorgement, cyclic ovarian pain (mittelschmerz), abnormal uterine bleeding, hot flashes, ovarian enlargement with or without cyst formation, and visual abnormalities. If blurred vision or other visual abnormalities occur, the drug should be discontinued and the patient referred for an ophthalmic evaluation. Effects usually disappear when the drug is stopped.

5. Incidence of ovulation has been found in one study to be 76%, although further research is needed.

6. Pregnancy occurs in 25% to 30% of patients treated. Multiple pregnancies may occur in 5% to 10% of patients.

7. Dosage: 50 to 100 mg daily for 5 to 7 days.

OVULATORY SUPPRESSANTS—ORAL CONTRACEPTIVES

Enovid as a contraceptive was introduced in 1960. By 1965 more than 5 million American women were using oral contraceptives. Few drugs have created the interest and study as have the oral contraceptives. This is because of (1) the need for a simple method of population control in densely populated countries, (2) the interest aroused concerning the effects of these drugs on the human body when hormone levels and relationships are altered for the one purpose of preventing conception, and (3) the desire of many couples for planned parenthood.

The development of the oral contraceptives was based on the knowledge that ovulation did not occur during pregnancy and that large amounts of estrogen and progesterone were produced by the placental secretion and the continuing function of the corpus luteum.

A summary of the physiology of the menstrual cycle indicates that:

1. The hypothalamus regulates the secretion of two hormones from the anterior pituitary gland:
   a. FSH—for maturation of the ovum
   b. LH—for release of the mature ovum from the ovary
   c. The hypothalamus regulates secretions of these hormones by secreting hormones known as releasing factors

2. Ovulation is dependent on these functions.

3. Estrogen in large amounts (secreted by the maturing follicle and following ovulation, by the corpus luteum) inhibit the hypothalamic releasing factors. This inhibits FSH and LH release and blocks further ovulation.

4. Progesterone (secreted by the corpus luteum) inhibits the hypothalamic releasing factor for the luteinizing hormone. This also intereferes with ovulation.

5. Estrogen and progesterone are responsible for endometrial buildup. A decreased production of estrogen and progesterone results in endometrial sloughing and menstrual bleeding. Oral contraceptives probably act, in part, by inhibiting the secretion of gonadotropins from the pituitary gland. Other possible actions may be a direct inhibitory effect on the ovary, changes in the endometrium, or changes in tubal motility that would result in a failure of implantation of fertilized ova.

The combination of drugs rapidly transforms the early secretory stage of the endometrium to one resembling secretory exhaustion. The estrogen encourages change that inhibits ovulation, while progesterone ensures that withdrawal bleeding will be physiologic, brief, and prompt.

Naturally occurring progesterone is extremely weak or inactivated when taken orally and must be administered by injection to be effective. Therefore, steroidal compounds related to progesterone have been developed. These are called progestogens. The majority of the oral contraceptives contain a synthetic progestogen, usually **norethynodrel** or **norethindrone.**

Three methods of oral contraception are available:

1. Combination therapy **(Ovral, Norinyl, Ortho-Novum)** consists of taking tablets containing a progestogen and an estrogen; 21 (or 28) tablets are taken during each menstrual cycle. The pill is started on the first Sunday after menstruation be-

gins; the first tablet is taken whether or not menstruation has ceased. One tablet a day is taken thereafter, for 21 days. Menstruation will occur within 2 to 7 days after the last tablet has been taken. The pill is started again on the next Sunday. If using a 28-day pill pack, a new pack is started the day after completing the last one. If breakthrough bleeding occurs, the drug should be continued and the physician notified at once so the dosage or the drug may be changed. If bleeding resembles that of the menses, the drug should be stopped, with medication begun again 5 days later, beginning a new cycle. Spotting or brownish discharge is not breakthrough bleeding and eventually disappears.

If menses does not occur following completion of a medication cycle, patients should begin another medication cycle on the seventh day and not wait for menstruation to occur, since ovulation may occur within 9 or 10 days after stopping the medication. Ovulation can occur if a menstruation is delayed or missed.

Women who ovulate early or who have shortened menstrual cycles should use another method of birth control during the first medication cycle. With hormonal therapy, these women usually convert to a 28-day cycle.

The combination method of therapy is very effective; many authorities claim it to be 95% to 99% effective. Failures are often the result of missed dosage.

2. Contraceptive tablets that contain only a very low dosage level of 0.35 mg of the progestogen norethindrone or 0.075 mg of norgestrel are known as the minipill **(Nor-QD, Micronor, Ovrette).** These preparations probably exert their contraceptive action by interfering with luteal function by suppressing the secretion of gonadotropins, by interfering with the implantation of the ovum, and by reducing the penetrability of the sperm in the cervical mucus. The minipill does not prevent ovulation and is perhaps slightly less effective as a contraceptive than the contraceptives containing both estrogen and progestogen. It does have unpredictable bleeding patterns. The dose is one tablet daily without interruption.

3. The mechanism of action of diethylstilbestrol (DES) as a postcoital contraceptive is not well understood. It appears to lower the level of circulating progesterone and to inhibit implantation of the fertilized ovum in the uterus when taken within 72 hours after intercourse (preferably within 24 hours). This drug may increase tubal motility causing the ova to arrive in the uterus sooner than nor-

mal. Diethylstilbestrol should be used only as an emergency method and not as a routine method of birth control. Repeated use should be avoided.

There are many side effects: headache, nausea, vomiting, diarrhea, abdominal cramps, weight gain, dizziness, breast tenderness, increased vaginal secretions, darkening of the breast areola, rash, leg cramps, anorexia, changes in menstrual flow or spotting, thrombophlebitis, pulmonary embolism, and cerebral thrombosis. Diethylstilbestrol is contraindicated in blood-clotting disorders, impaired liver function, a history of thrombophlebitis, cancer of the breast or uterus, abnormal uterine bleeding of unknown origin, or pregnancy. All efforts must be made to determine whether a patient is pregnant before contraceptive therapy. If a patient is pregnant and has been taking diethylstilbestrol, the patient should be informed about the risk of vaginal or cervical cancer occurring in her female child. The patient should then be given the choice of deciding whether or not the pregnancy should be terminated.

The oral postcoital contraceptive dosage is 25 mg twice a day for 5 days beginning not later than 72 hours and preferably no more than 24 hours after sexual intercourse. The dose can prevent pregnancy but cannot terminate pregnancy. To be effective, the full course of treatment must be taken regardless of the nausea that commonly occurs.

It is important that yearly physical examinations be performed on patients receiving oral contraceptives. Also of vital importance is to confirm with tests and other means that the patient about to receive contraceptives is not pregnant, for reasons already cited. Patients should always inform their physician of the use of oral contraceptives regardless of the purpose of the appointment.

MALE SEX HORMONES

Testosterone propionate (tes-tos′te-roan pro′pee-oh-nayt)
(Oreton) (or′e-ton), **(Andronate)** (an′dro-nayt)

1. Testosterone is a testicular hormone useful in the treatment of climacteric in males and metastatic bone cancer in females when the primary cancer site is the breast. It is obtained synthetically or from bull testes. It may also be effective in the treatment of male hypogonadism, eunuchism, androgen deficiency, prevention of postpartum pain and breast engorgement, and palliation of breast cancer.

2. Symptoms include nausea, gastrointestinal upsets, and retention of sodium, chloride, potassium, and water, which may contribute to heart failure. Edema can often be treated with a low-salt diet and diuretics.

Patients receiving androgens should be checked frequently for hypercalcemia, appearance of edema, and acceleration of the disease being treated. Women receiving androgen therapy may experience growth of hair on the face, upper lip, and chin, deepening or masculinization of the voice, flushing, acne, regression of the breasts, enlargement of the clitoris, and loss of feminine contours. The adverse effects will disappear when therapy is discontinued.

3. Androgens are contraindicated in prostatic cancer, with serious cardiorenal dysfunction, and in pregnant women because of the possibility of masculinization of the female fetus.

4. Dosage is variable and depends on the condition being treated.

Methyltestosterone (meth-il-tes-tos'ter-own) *(Oreton M), (Metandren)* (me-tan'dren)

1. Methyltestosterone is a synthetic derivative. Its uses and action are similar to those of testosterone propionate.

2. It is available in oral, buccal, and sublingual forms. Buccal form is available in 10-mg dosage. Absorption from the buccal membranes is more effective than from the gastrointestinal tract. Avoid eating, drinking, chewing, or smoking while buccal tablet is in place. Thorough oral hygiene is important after the buccal tablet is completely absorbed.

3. Usual dose: Oral—10 mg three times daily. Buccal—5 to 20 mg daily. Sublingual—5 mg three to four times daily.

4. Doses for suppression of lactation are larger. Doses for breast cancer are 50 to 200 mg daily. In all forms of dosage the dose is individualized, adjusted, and reduced according to the needs and response of the patient, as is true of most androgens.

Testosterone, Testosterone enanthate *(Delatestryl)* (del-ah-tes'tril)

A single IM dose of testosterone enanthate provides prolonged effect for 3 to 4 weeks.

Fluoxymesterone (floo-ok-se-mes'ter-own) *(Halotestin)* (hal-o-tes'tin), *(Ora-Testryl)* (oar-ah-tes'tril)

Fluoxymesterone is several times more potent than methyltestosterone in both androgenic and anabolic activity and for palliation of breast cancer.

Deladumone-OB is a combination of an estrogen, estradiol valerate, and an androgen, testosterone enanthate. Deladumone-OB is administered in one or two doses intramuscularly to suppress lactation and prevent breast engorgement.

PREMENSTRUAL TENSION PRODUCTS

Premenstrual and menstrual tension are relatively common discomforts to the average woman. Symptoms characteristically occur 2 to 3 days before menstruation and include headache, occasional nervousness, and depression.

Most products sold without prescription for the symptomatic relief of premenstrual tension include an analgesic (aspirin or acetaminophen), an antihistamine (pyrilamine maleate), and a diuretic (caffeine, pamabrom, ammonium chloride). The antihistamine and diuretic are frequently available only in subtherapeutic doses, making the product no more effective than the less expensive analgesic alone.

Nurses are occasionally requested to recommend a product for premenstrual tension. Prior to making any recommendation, the nurse should determine whether the symptoms are normal functional menstrual discomforts consistent with previous cycles. Any irregularities concerning the frequency, volume, or consistency of the menstrual flow or any unusual pain or fluid retention should require prompt referral to a gynecologist.

The most effective agent for premenstrual tension is frequently aspirin or acetaminophen taken in oral doses of 325 to 650 mg every 4 to 6 hours. The patient should not exceed 2.6 g in 24 hours. Premenstrual edema or "puffiness" can often be controlled by avoiding food high in salt content, such as soda pop, french fries, pickles, and snacks, 3 to 4 days prior to menstruation.

The physician prescribes the medicine and treatment.
The nurse carries out the physician's orders.
Self-medication is dangerous. Consult your physician first.
There is in every medicine a possible danger.
When in doubt—ASK!

ASSIGNMENT

Review previous lessons and questions according to the direction of your instructor.

1. What is the source of ergot? What are its main effects on the uterus during labor and after childbirth? Name the three groups of individual alkaloids derived from ergot. Which one is the preparation most used in obstetrics? Why are its side effects rare? What side effects of ergonovine can occur? What is the treatment of ergot poisoning? Name two ergot preparations used in obstetrics. When should ergonovine maleate (Ergotrate Maleate) be administered and how frequently? What is the parenteral dose?

2. Methylergonovine maleate (Methergine) (several choices are correct)
   a. Lessens uterine contractions so that the mother may have much needed rest during labor
   b. Is a synthetic oxytocic
   c. Stimulates uterine contractions and aids in prevention or control of hemorrhage after childbirth
   d. Should be administered usually during the early part of the first stage of labor
   e. Should be administered at the end of the third stage of labor and under constant obstetric supervision, may be administered in the second stage following delivery of the anterior shoulder
   f. Can be administered freely and safely to patients with sepsis, hepatic or renal involvement, or obliterative vascular disease
   g. Is contraindicated during pregnancy
   h. Has less tendency to cause an elevation of blood pressure and is preferred for patients with threatened or definite eclampsia
   i. Has as a usual dose 0.2 mg orally and 0.2 mg/ml parenterally

3. Give two medical conditions for which Ergotamine tartrate has been found useful.

4. Locate the pituitary gland. Name its two lobes. From which lobe are extracts obtained? List the effects obtained from injection of these extracts. Name two hormones that have been obtained from the pituitary gland. What do these peptides contain? Is it possible to synthesize them chemically?

5. What is the source of vasopressin (Pitressin)? What action does it possess? State the main use of this drug. List the side effects of vasopressin (Pitressin). Vasopressin should be used very cautiously in patients with what medical condition? The vasopressor effects of this drug may produce what undesirable conditions? What is the duration of action of vasopressin tannate (Pitressin Tannate in Oil)?

6. What is the original source of the hormone oxytocin (Pitocin)? Name the present source of oxytocin and tell its advantage. List the three uses of the synthetic form of oxytocin. List the side and toxic effects of oxytocin. When used unwisely, what conditions may it cause? What are the contraindications of oxytocin? Explain the IV infusion dosage in detail, including the uterine response desired. What is the IM injection dosage to control postpartum bleeding?

7. When is it necessary to decrease uterine motility? List the groups of drugs that in large doses tend to decrease uterine motility. What are their disadvantages?

8. Magnesium sulfate administered parenterally will cause what effect on what types of muscle tissue? What are its main uses in its effect on the uterus? List the toxic effects of this drug. Name an effective antidote for magnesium sulfate overdosage. What other treatment for magnesium sulfate overdosage may still be necessary? What are the methods of administration for this drug? Why?

9. What are the chief effects of isoxsuprine hydrochloride (Vasodilan), and for which diseases has it been found effective? List the side effects and state how they are brought under control or eliminated. What is the preferred method of administration?

10. Terbutaline sulfate (Brethine, Bricanyl) is being tried for what uterine condition? What is its main use? List its many side effects. Are these side effects commonly or rarely seen in recommended dosages? List the medical conditions for which terbutaline sulfate should be used with caution.

11. What is the name for the hormones concerned with ovarian function? What are their functions? State the function of ACTH, TSH, LH, MSH, FSH, GH, and PL. What stimulates the secretion of these hormones? Where are the neurons that secrete the releasing factors located? Name three neurotransmitters and tell their function in regard to anterior pituitary secretions.

12. Name three hormones that are of interest in their effect on the ovary and state the function of each.

13. Why is the clinical use of the pituitary gonadotropic hormone limited? What is the source of gonadotropic substances? Human chorionic gonadotropic hormone is known by what initials? What are its effects? What is the chief function? Does it initiate the formation of corpus luteum? What effect does it have on women? On men? List the conditions for which gonadotropic hormones are used. Is their value in these conditions considered highly effective, moderately effective, or is there considerable difference of opinion concerning their effectiveness?

14. Locate and give the function of the gonads and the ovaries. What hormone do the testes produce, and what are the effects? What hormones do the ovaries produce and what are the effects?

15. State the function of the estrogens. Where are estrogenic substances found? Why do some physicians believe that estrogens should not be administered to women with a personal or family history of cancer of the reproductive system? List the symptoms and conditions that estrogens relieve. Why should estrogens be taken only under medical advice?

16. What is the source of estrone (Theelin)? It is used in the treatment of what conditions? What is the usual dose for menopause? What is the disadvantage of large doses?

17. Ethinyl estradiol (Estinyl) (more than one choice is correct)
   a. Is one of the more mild estrones
   b. Is a derivative of estrone and is one of the most powerful estrogens

c. Has side effects such as headache, nausea, and vomiting, as is true of many other estrogens

d. Rarely has the usual side effects of other estrogens

e. Has doses that vary, depending on the conditions to be treated

f. Is taken orally in tablets for menopause: 0.2 to 0.5 mg one to three times daily

18. Diethylstilbestrol (several choices are correct)

a. Is a synthetic estrogenic substance

b. Has a disadvantage in being more expensive than other types of estrogens

c. Is effective in practically all the various uses of estrogens

d. Rarely causes headache, nausea, vomiting

e. Has various doses, depending on its purpose, the usual for menopause being 0.2 to 0.5 mg daily

19. A conjugated estrogen substance (Premarin) (more than one choice is correct)

a. Has as its source the urine of pregnant mares

b. Is synthetic

c. Has action and uses similar to those of other estrogens

d. Is administered in a usual dose of 1.25 mg daily for menopause

e. Requires much smaller doses than for menopause if administered for senile vaginitis, breast cancer, or pruritus vulvae

20. Piperazine estrone sulfate (Ogen) has the same action and uses as what group of estrogens? Does the dose vary depending on the purpose? What is the dosage for menopause?

21. Since there is much controversy today about the long-range effects of estrogens (conjugated estrogens), what is the recommendation for their use?

22. What secretes progesterone and what type of hormone is it? What is its function and use? Why are progestational agents *not* recommended during the first 4 months of pregnancy? List the side effects for progesterone. What is the dosage for functional uterine bleeding and how soon will bleeding be expected to cease?

23. Menotropins (Pergonal) belongs to what group of drugs? What type of drug is it and what is its source? What is another name for it? What is its chief use? To accomplish ovulation therapy with menotropins, it must be followed by the administration of what hormone? List adverse side effects, tell how long they last, and what type of treatment is used for the side effects, if any. If hyperstimulation occurs, what symptoms develop and how are they treated? List the contraindications for menotropins. Explain the method of administration of this drug. What is the percentage of chance that pregnancy will occur and in what period of time? Spontaneous miscarriages occur in what percent of the patients? What treatment is used if a patient develops significant ovarian enlargement following ovulation? Why should the couple be fully informed about possible dangers from menotropins? What is the frequency of multiple births?

24. Clomiphene citrate (Clomid) belongs to which group of drugs? What is its use? What is the theory of its mechanism of action? Which are more effective: short-term therapies or long-term therapies? List the side effects. If blurred vision or other visual abnormalities occur, what is the method of treatment? In what percent of the patients treated does pregnancy occur? Multiple births (or pregnancies) may occur in what percent of the patients? What is the usual dosage and for how long?

25. Enovid belongs to which group of drugs? What are the reasons for the intense interest and study of oral contraceptives? The development of the oral contraceptives was based on what knowledge? Summarize in outline form the physiology of the menstrual cycle. Since naturally occurring progesterone is extremely weak or inactivated when taken orally and must be administered by injection to be effective, steroidal compounds related to progesterone have been developed and are called by what name? List the three methods of oral contraception available and describe each method, including examples of drugs. Why is it of vital importance to confirm with tests and other means that the patient about to receive contraceptives is *not* pregnant? Why are yearly physical examinations important for the patients receiving oral contraceptives?

26. Testosterone propionate (Oreton, Andronate) (several choices are correct)

a. Is a female sex hormone

b. Is a testicular hormone useful in the treatment of male climacteric

c. Is useful in the treatment of metastatic bone cancer in females when the primary cancer site is the breast

d. Originates from the corpus luteum

e. Is obtained from bull testes

f. May cause such symptoms as nausea, gastrointestinal upsets, and retention of sodium, chloride, potassium, and water, which may contribute to heart failure

g. May cause edema, which can be treated with a low-salt diet and diuretics

h. Can cause hair growth on the face, upper lip, and chin, deepening of the voice, and other masculinization symptoms in women receiving testosterone therapy

i. Can be used safely in prostatic cancer, in serious cardiorenal dysfunction, and during pregnancy

27. What is the source of methyltestosterone? Its uses and action are similar to those of what other androgen? Give two trade names for this drug. It is available in what forms for administration? What is the dosage for the buccal form and how is it administered? What instructions should be given to the patient while the buccal tablet is in place and after the buccal tablet is completely absorbed? What is the usual dose: oral, buccal, and sublingual? Doses for suppression of lactation are larger, or smaller? What are the doses for breast cancer? Are all these doses strictly adhered to?

28. How long does the effect last for testosterone enanthate (Delatestryl)?

29. Fluoxymesterone (Halotestin, Ora-testryl) is more, or less, potent than methyltestosterone for androgenic and anabolic activity and for palliation of breast cancer? Deladumone-OB is a combination of what hormones (estrogen and androgens)? What is the main use of Deladumone-OB?

30. List the symptoms of premenstrual tension and tell when they usually occur. What drugs do most premenstrual ten-

sion products contain? Do the antihistamine and the diuretic in the products make the products much more effective?

31. You were bathing your female patient, who seemed slightly tense and depressed this morning. She asked you to recommend a premenstrual product for her to take. What advice would you give her concerning her tension, menstrual irregularities, pelvic pain, or fluid retention? Why?

32. What is probably the most effective agent for premenstrual tension and in what dose? How can premenstrual edema or "puffiness" often be controlled?

33. The physician orders the patient to receive orally 2.5 mg of one of the estrogens for senile vaginitis and pruritus vulvae. The medicine bottle label strength of the tablets is 1.25 mg. How many tablets will you administer?

34. The physician orders the patient to receive orally 0.04 mg of estrogen for menopause. The bottle label strength of the tablets is 0.02 mg. How many tablets will you administer?

Drugs affecting the endocrine system

Hormones are natural chemical substances that act after they have been secreted into the bloodstream from the ductless, or endocrine glands. Some act on many other tissues and organs and in general regulate body growth, development of sex organs, and, as with the pituitary hormones, growth and function of the endocrine glands. Thyrotropic hormone from the anterior pituitary gland is necessary for normal development and function of the thyroid gland. The thyroid gland itself exerts an influence on other endocrine glands, such as the thymus, adrenals, and gonads.

THYROID GLAND

The thyroid gland is a large, reddish, ductless gland in front of and on either side of the trachea, or windpipe. It consists of two lateral lobes and a connecting isthmus and is roughly butterfly shaped. It is enclosed in a covering of areolar tissue, is made up of numerous closed follicles containing colloid matter, and is surrounded by a vascular network. This gland is one of the most richly vascularized tissues in the body; only the lungs and carotid body have a greater blood supply.

As with other endocrine glands, thyroid gland function is regulated by the hypothalamus and the anterior pituitary gland. The hypothalamus secretes thyrotropin-releasing hormone (TRH), which stimulates the anterior pituitary gland to release thyroid-stimulating hormone (TSH). TSH stimulates the thyroid gland to release its hormones triiodothyronine (T_3) and thyroxine (T_4).

The thyroid hormones regulate general body metabolism. Imbalance in thyroid hormone production may interfere with growth and maturation; carbohydrate, protein, and lipid metabolism; thermal regulation; cardiovascular function; lactation; and reproduction.

Drugs used to treat thyroid disorders are of two general classes: (1) those used to replace thyroid hormones in patients whose thyroid glandular function is inadequate to meet metabolic requirements (hypothyroidism) and (2) antithyroid agents used to suppress synthesis of thyroid hormones (hyperthyroidism). Thyroid hormone replacements available are levothyroxine (T_4), liothyronine (T_3), liotrix, thyroglobulin, and thyroid, USP. Antithyroid agents discussed are the iodides, propylthiouracil, and methimazole.

Thyroid replacement hormones
Levothyroxine (le-vo-thy-rok′sen)
(Synthroid) (sin′throyd), **(Letter)**

1. Levothyroxine (T_4) is one of the two primary hormones secreted by the thyroid gland. It is partially metabolized to liothyronine (T_3), so that therapy with levothyroxine provides physiologic replacement of both hormones.
2. It is now the drug of choice for hormone replacement in hypothyroidism.
3. Symptoms of adverse effects are tachycardia, anxiety, weight loss, abdominal cramping and diarrhea, cardiac palpitations, arrhythmias, angina pectoris, fever, and intolerance to heat.
4. Therapy may be initiated in low doses of 0.025 mg (25 μg) daily. Dosages are gradually increased over the next few weeks to an average daily maintenance dose of 0.1 to 0.2 mg (100 to 200 μg).

Liothyronine sodium (ly-o-thy′ro-neen)
(Cytomel) (sy′to-mel)

1. Liothyronine is a synthetic form of the natural thyroid hormone, triiodothyronine, (T_3).
2. Liothyronine has an onset of action more rapid than levothyroxine and is occasionally used as a thyroid hormone replacement when prompt activity is necessary.
3. Liothyronine therapy should not be used in patients with cardiovascular disease unless a rapid onset of activity is deemed essential.
4. Usual starting dose depends on the particular condition but is usually 0.025 mg (25 μg) daily. The usual maintenance dose is 0.025 to 0.075 mg (25 to 75 μg) daily.

Liotrix (ly′o-triks)
(Euthroid) (you′throyd), **(Thyrolar)** (thy′ro-lar)

1. This is a synthetic mixture of levothyroxine and liothyronine in a ratio of 4:1, respectively.
2. A few endocrinologists prefer this combination because of the standardized content of the two hormones that results in consistent laboratory test results more in agreement with the patient's clinical response.

3. Liotrix is administered orally, usually as a single dose before breakfast. The two available commercial preparations of liotrix contain different amounts of each ingredient, so patients should not be changed from one preparation to the other unless differences in potency are considered.
4. Dosage range is 0.060 to 0.180 mg (60 to 180 μg) of levothyroxine and 0.015 to 0.045 mg (15 to 45 μg) of liothyronine.

Thyroglobulin (thy-ro-glob'you-lin) *(Proloid)* (pro'loyd)

1. Thyroglobulin is obtained from a purified extract of hog thyroid.
2. It contains thyroxine and triiodothyronine. It is effective in the treatment of inadequate thyroid hormone production.
3. The potency of thyroglobulin is equal to that of thyroid, USP, but it is twice as costly.
4. Dosage should be started in small amounts and increased gradually. Oral maintenance dose for adults: 30 to 180 mg daily. Many oral strengths are available.

Thyroid, USP (thy'royd)

1. Thyroid, USP (desiccated thyroid), is derived from pig, beef, and sheep thyroid glands. Thyroid, USP is the oldest thyroid hormone replacement available and the least expensive. Because of its lack of purity, uniformity, and stability, however, it is generally not the drug of choice for the initiation of thyroid replacement therapy.
2. Usual dosage range: 60 to 180 mg daily.

Antithyroid drugs

The synthesis of the thyroid hormones and their maintenance in blood in sufficient amounts depend greatly on sufficient iodine intake through food and water. Iodine is converted to iodide and stored in the thyroid gland before reaching circulation.

Excessive formation of thyroid hormones and their escape into the circulation causes hyperthyroidism, also known as thyrotoxicosis, exophthalmic goiter, or Graves' disease. Symptoms include increased metabolic rate, increased pulse rate to perhaps 140 beats per minute, increased body temperature, restlessness, nervousness, anxiety, sweating, muscle weakness and tremors, and complaint of feeling too warm. This condition is treated with the antithyroid drugs or surgical removal of the thyroid gland.

An antithyroid drug is a chemical agent that lowers the basal metabolic rate by interfering with the formation, release, or action of the hormones made by the thyroid gland. Radioactive iodine is one of the more effective antithyroid drugs.

Radioactive iodine (^{131}I)

1. Iodine 131 is a radioactive isotope of iodine. It is the most commonly used drug for treating hyperthyroidism.
2. Iodine 131 has a half-life of 8.08 days. This means that at the end of about 8 days, 50% of its atoms have undergone disintegration. In another 8 days, 50% of the remaining amount has undergone disintegration, and so on until an inappreciable amount remains. The radioactivity of this material is therefore dissipated in a relatively short time. During the period of radioactivity, the energy liberated is in the form of beta particles and gamma rays. Since the thyroid gland actively concentrates iodine, the radioactivity is released into the thyroid gland, destroying the hyperactive tissue, with essentially no damage to other tissues in the body.
3. Radioactive iodine is therefore effective for treatment of hyperthyroidism and thyroid carcinoma and for diagnosis of thyroid function. Some physicians believe radioiodine is most effective as a therapeutic agent in older patients who are beyond the childbearing years, those with severe complicating diseases, those with recurrent hyperthyroidism after previous resection of the thyroid, those who are poor surgical risks, and those who have unusually small glands. The theoretical danger of radiation injury has caused many of these limitations.
4. Radioiodine is useful because it may be located even when present in minute amounts. Radioiodine behaves exactly as does ordinary nonradioactive iodine. Thus, an infinitesimal quantity of it can be used to trace to follow the behavior of any amount of ordinary iodine with which it is mixed. These tiny doses, called ''tracers,'' when administered to a patient, can trace all of the ordinary iodine in the patient's body, permitting the physician to trace the behavior of the radioiodine, study problems of physiology and disease of the thyroid gland, diagnose functional states of the thyroid gland, and treat certain select cases of cancer of the thyroid gland.
5. Administration of radioiodine preparations seems simple: it can be added to water and swallowed like a drink of water and has no color or taste. However, the radiation from this substance is dangerous in the same way and to the same extent as radiation from radium and roentgen rays.
   a. Exposure should be avoided or minimized as much as possible.
   b. Special precautions must be taken, since the drug can be easily spilled on yourself, the patient, his gown, his bedding, the furniture, or the floor.
   c. The contamination that results from this or from spilling the urine or excreta from the patient requires that clothing, bedding, floor, bedpan, urin-

al, bedpan disposal unit, and other surroundings be checked and measured with special monitoring instruments, such as a small, portable Geiger counter.

    d. Nurses and technicians should wear rubber gloves whenever administering radioiodine to patients and disposing of their excreta.

    e. *Be careful: avoid spills! Report any accidental contamination at once to your supervisor, head nurse, team leader, or instructor and follow directions for your hospital contamination cleanup technique.*

6. Side effects include radioactive thyroiditis, causing tenderness over the thyroid area and occurring during the first few days or few weeks after radioactive iodine therapy. Recurrence of hyperthyroidism after therapy is low but does occur and can be especially dangerous in the patient with severe heart disease. Many of the patients who receive radioactive iodine develop hypothyroidism, which requires thyroid hormone replacement therapy. Long-term follow-up is important. Radioactive iodine should not be administered to pregnant women or nursing mothers.

Propylthiouracil (pro-pil-thy-o-you'rah-sil)
(PTU, Propacil)

1. Propylthiouracil is an antithyroid agent that acts by blocking synthesis of T_3 and T_4 in the thyroid gland. Propylthiouracil does not destroy any T_3 or T_4 already produced, so there is usually a latent period of a few days to 2 weeks before symptoms improve once therapy is started. Propylthiouracil may be used for long-term treatment of hyperthyroidism or for short-term treatment prior to subtotal thyroidectomy.
2. Side effects include skin rash, drug fever, headache, leukopenia, pruritus, loss of the sense of taste, enlargement of the salivary glands and lymph nodes in the neck, paresthesias, hepatitis, and arthralgias. Agranulocytosis is a most grave complication. Symptoms such as head cold, sore throat, fever, or malaise may signal the onset of agranulocytosis, so patients should be warned to report any of these symptoms to their physician, and nurses should be alert to notice these warning symptoms and report them. Untoward reactions occur in about 3% to 5% of the cases, with agranulocytosis in about 0.5% of the cases. Close medical supervision is vital.
3. If these drugs must be administered to pregnant women, the smallest possible dose must be given, since there is danger of large doses leading to goiter in the newborn. Mothers should not nurse their babies when taking propylthiouracil, since it is excreted in the breast milk.
4. Initial adult dose: orally, 300 mg daily. Daily dosage may range up to 900 mg daily. Usual maintenance dose: 100 to 150 mg daily.

Methimazole (meth-im'ah-zoal)
(Tapazole) (tap'ah-zoal)

1. Methimazole is another antithyroid agent similar in uses and side effects to propylthiouracil.
2. It is effective for treatment of hyperthyroidism in preparation for subtotal thyroidectomy or radioactive iodine therapy.
3. Initial daily dose: 15 mg for mild hyperthyroidism, 30 to 40 mg for moderately severe hyperthyroidism, and 60 mg or more for severe cases. These amounts are administered in divided doses every 8 hours. Maintenance dose: 5 to 15 mg daily.

PITUITARY GLANDS

See Index for discussion of vasopressin injection.

Corticotropin injection (ACTH) (kor-ti-ko-tro'pin)
(Acthar) (ak'thar)

1. ACTH is the anterior pituitary adrenocorticotropic hormone that stimulates the adrenal gland to secrete cortisone.
2. It has been used in the treatment of rheumatoid arthritis, rheumatoid spondylitis, rheumatic fever, severe asthma or hay fever, drug sensitivities, contact dermatitis, many acute inflammatory conditions of the eye and skin, ulcerative colitis, and secondary adrenal cortical hypofunction. Its primary use now, however, is in diagnostic testing of adrenocortical function.
3. The following signs of overdosage should be observed for and reported to the physician: ''moon'' face (edema and swelling), acne and growth of hair on face and other body parts, and glycosuria (sugar in the urine). The physician also will monitor the blood sugar level. Additional insulin is usually needed in patients who have diabetes mellitus.
4. Usual dose for testing adrenocortical function: up to 80 units in a single or divided dose. Various diagnostic tests use doses administered intramuscularly, subcutaneously, or intravenously, depending on the test protocol.

ADRENAL GLANDS
Adrenocortical hormones—
the corticosteroids

The corticosteroids are hormones secreted by the adrenal cortex. They are divided into two categories, based on their structure and biologic activity. The mineralocorticoids (desoxycorticosterone, aldosterone) are used for maintaining water and electrolyte balance, while the glucocorticoids (cortisone, hydrocortisone, prednisone) are used to regulate carbohydrate, protein, and fat metabolism. The mineralocorticoids are also used to treat adrenal insufficiency, such as hypopituitarism and Addison's disease.

Glucocorticoids are used most frequently for their antiinflammatory and antiallergic properties. They do not cure any disease, but rather relieve the symptoms associated with tissue inflammation. Glucocorticoids are quite effective for relief of allergic manifestations, such as serum sickness, severe hay fever, status asthmaticus, and exfoliative dermatitis. In addition, they have been used for the "collagen" diseases, such as lupus erythematosus, dermatomyositis, and acute rheumatic fever, and some forms of shock.

Glucocorticoids are most commonly used, however, in the treatment of rheumatoid arthritis. Relief of arthritic symptoms is noted within a few days. Joint and muscle stiffness, muscle tenderness and weakness, joint swelling, and soreness are all considerably lessened. Appetite, weight, and energy are increased, fever is reduced, and sedimentation rates are reduced or become normal. Anatomic changes and joint deformities already existing remain unchanged. Symptoms generally return a short time after withdrawal of these drugs.

Possible side effects of the glucocorticoids include a rise in blood sugar, glycosuria, aggravation of diabetes mellitus symptoms, negative nitrogen balance, increase of white cell count, reduced resistance to some infectious diseases, delay in wound healing, peptic ulcer formation, tendency for embolic formations and thrombosis, a rounded contour of the face, hirsutism, purplish or reddish striae of the skin, retention of salt and water, restlessness, insomnia, and euphoria.

These drugs must be used with caution in patients with diabetes mellitus, congestive heart failure, hypertension, peptic ulcer, mental disturbance, and suspected or newly healed tuberculosis.

Corticosteroids are available in many different preparations, brand names, and dosage forms. See Table 21-1 for a listing of the generic names, brand names, and dosage forms available.

See Chapter 9 for a discussion of the insulins and Chapter 20 for a discussion of reproductive hormones.

Table 21-1. Corticosteroid preparations*

Generic name	Brand names	Dosage forms
Betamethasone	Celestone, Valisone, Diprosone	Tablets, syrup, injection, cream, ointment, lotion, aerosol
Cortisone	Cortone	Tablets, injection
Desoxycorticosterone	Doca, Percorten	Injection
Dexamethasone	Decadron, Dexone, Hexadrol, Solurex, Dezone	Injection, cream, ointment, aerosol
Fludrocortisone	Florinef	Tablets
Fluocinolone	Fluonid, Synalar	Ointment, cream, solution
Fluprednisolone	Alphadrol	Tablets
Flurandrenolide	Cordran	Cream, ointment, tape, solution
Hydrocortisone (cortisol)	Cortef, Hydrocortone, Solu-Cortef, others	Tablets, suspension, injection, enema, gel, cream, ointment, lotion
Meprednisone	Betapar	Tablets
Methylprednisolone	A-Methapred, Solu-Medrol, D-Med, Depo-Medrol	Tablets, injection, enema, ointment, cream, aerosol
Paramethasone	Haldrone	Tablets
Prednisolone	Hydeltrasol, Delta-Cortef, Delcort-E, Sterane, Dura-Pred, others	Tablets, injection, cream, aerosol
Prednisone	Deltasone, Fernisone, Meticorten, Ro-pred, Paracort, others	Tablets
Triamcinolone	Aristocort, Kenalog, Kenacort, Trilone, Amcort, Spencort, others	Tablets, syrup, injection, ointment, cream, lotion, gel, aerosol

*For ophthalmic preparations, see Chapter 22.

> **The physician prescribes the medicine and treatment.**
> **The nurse carries out the physician's orders.**
> **Self-medication is dangerous. Consult your physician first.**
> **There is in every medicine a possible danger.**
> **When in doubt—ASK!**

ASSIGNMENT

Review previous lessons and questions according to the directions of your instructor.

1. What are hormones and how and where in the body do they act? What is the function of thyrotropic hormone and what is its source? The thyroid gland exerts an influence on what other endocrine glands?
2. Locate and describe the thyroid gland. What regulates thyroid gland function? Explain the results of this regulation.
3. What are the two general classes of drugs used to treat thyroid disorders? List the thyroid hormone replacements available.
4. Levothyroxine (Synthroid, Letter) (more than one choice is correct)
   a. Is a hormone formerly commonly used in the treatment of hypothyroidism
   b. Is one of the two primary hormones secreted by the thyroid gland
   c. Is now the drug of choice for hormone replacement in hypothyroidism
   d. Rarely, if ever, has any symptoms of adverse effects
   e. May have such adverse effects as tachycardia, anxiety, weight loss, abdominal cramping and diarrhea, cardiac palpitations, arrhythmias, angina pectoris, fever, and intolerance to heat
   f. May be administered in large doses at beginning of treatment, such as 0.1 to 0.4 mg daily
   g. Has initial low doses of 0.025 mg daily
5. What is the source of liothyronine sodium (Cytomel)? Compare its onset of action with that of levothyroxine. Occasionally liothyronine is used as a thyroid hormone replacement for what purpose? What are the contraindications for this drug? What is the usual starting dose? What is the maintenance dose?
6. What is the source of liotrix (Thyrolar, Euthroid)? Why do some endocrinologists prefer this combination of two hormones? What is the method and time of administration of this drug? There are two available commercial preparations of liotrix. What precautions should be taken if the patient is changed from one preparation to the other? What is the dosage range of both drugs of this preparation?
7. What is the source of thyroglobulin (Proloid)? What hormones does it contain? It is used for the treatment of what condition? Compare its potency to that of thyroid. What is

thyroglobulin's disadvantage? Tell the usual dosage and the method of administration.
8. Give the source for thyroid, USP. Why is it generally *not* the drug of choice for the initiation of thyroid replacement therapy? What is the usual dosage range?
9. On what does the synthesis of the thyroid hormones and their maintenance in blood in sufficient amounts greatly depend? What happens to iodine ingested through food and water?
10. Explain the term hyperthyroidism and give three other of its names. List the symptoms of *hyper*thyroidism and make another list of the symptoms of *hypo*thyroidism. Place the second list beside the first list and compare or contrast the symptoms. Be familiar with these differences.
11. What is an antithyroid drug? Give an example of one of the more effective antithyroid drugs.
12. What is the source of Iodine 131? For what condition is it most commonly used? Describe the half-life of Iodine 131. Is the radioactivity dissipated in a relatively short time or relatively long time? What effect does the iodine and radioactivity have on the thyroid gland? Does it damage other tissues in the body?
13. List the many conditions for which radioactive iodine is effective. Tiny amounts or "tracers" have advantages when administered to the patient. Explain "tracers" and various conditions for which they may be given.
14. Explain the method of administration of radioiodine preparations. List the dangers and precautions during and after administration. List the side effects of radioactive iodine. Why is long-term follow-up important? Can radioactive iodine be administered to pregnant women or nursing mothers?
15. Propylthiouracil (PTU, Propactil) (several choices are correct)
   a. Is an excellent thyroid preparation given for treatment of hypothyroidism
   b. Is an antithyroid agent that acts by blocking synthesis of T_3 and T_4 in the thyroid gland
   c. Destroys any T_3 or T_4 already produced, so symptoms disappear within 48 hours
   d. May be used for long-term treatment of hypothyroidism
   e. May be used for long-term treatment of hyperthyroidism or for short-term treatment prior to subtotal thyroidectomy
   f. Can cause such symptoms as head cold, sore throat,

fever, or malaise, which the observant nurse knows may signal the onset of agranulocytosis, a grave complication

g. Has many side effects, which may include skin rash, drug fever, headache, leukopenia, pruritus, loss of the sense of taste, enlargement of the salivary glands and lymph nodes in the neck, paresthesias, hepatitis, and arthalgias

h. Rarely causes dangerous side effects, so minimum medical supervision is needed

i. Should be administered to pregnant women only if absolutely necessary and then in the smallest doses, since it may cause goiter in the newborn

j. Should not be administered to nursing mothers since it is excreted in the milk

16. What type of agent is methimazole (Tapazole)? It is similar in uses and side effects to what other agent? Methimazole is effective for the treatment of what conditions? What is the initial daily dose, in divided doses, and how frequently is it administered? Tell the maintenance dose.

17. What is corticotropin injection (ACTH, Acthar)? What action does it have on what gland? List the conditions it is used to treat. What is its primary use? List the signs of overdosage.

18. What are the corticosteroids? Name their two categories and give examples for each category. Tell the conditions for which each category is used.

19. What are the uses of the glucorticoids? Tell the condition for which they are most commonly used. List the symptoms relieved by the glucocorticoids in rheumatoid arthritis. What are possible side effects of the glucocorticoids? In which conditions should the glucocorticoids and the mineralocorticoids be used with caution?

20. Select from your corticosteroid preparations table eight preparations, using generic and trade names, commonly dispensed in your hospital or by physicians for patient home use. Your instructor will help you in making this list. Become familiar with these drugs.

21. A physician has initiated low doses of levothyroxine for a patient during the past 3 weeks. During the next few weeks the dosage will be gradually increased until a daily maintenance dose of 0.2 mg is reached. The physician shows you a bottle of levothyroxine 0.1 mg and wants the patient to have 0.2 mg. How many tablets will you administer?

CHAPTER 22

Drugs affecting the eye

The eyeball has three coats or layers: the protective external, or corneoscleral, coat; the nutritive middle vascular layer, called the choroid; and the light-sensitive inner layer, or retina (Fig. 22-1).

The cornea, or outermost sheath of the anterior eyeball, is transparent to allow light to enter the eye. The cornea has no blood vessels but receives its nutrition from the aqueous humor and its oxygen supply by diffusion from the air and surrounding vascular structures. There is a thin layer of epithelial cells on the external surface of the cornea that is quite resistant to infection. An abraded cornea, however, is most susceptible to infection. The cornea has sensory fibers, and any damage to the corneal epithelium will cause pain. Seriously injured corneal tissue is replaced by scar tissue that is usually not transparent. The sclera, continuous with the cornea, is nontransparent and is the eye's white portion.

The iris is a diaphragm that surrounds the pupil and gives the eye its blue, green, hazel, brown, or gray color. The sphincter muscle within the iris encircles the pupil and is innervated by the parasympathetic nervous system. Contraction of the iris sphincter muscle causes a narrowing of the pupil, or miosis. The dilator muscle, which runs radially from the pupillary margin to the iris periphery, is sympathetically innervated. Contraction of the dilator muscle and relaxation of the sphincter muscle causes dilation of the pupil, or mydriasis.

Drugs that produce miosis (miotics) act similar to acetylcholine (cholinergic agents) at receptor sites in the sphincter muscle or interfere with cholinesterase activity (cholinesterase inhibitors), prolonging the activity of acetylcholine. Drugs that produce mydriasis (mydriatics) stimulate adrenergic receptors or inhibit the action of acetylcholine. Constriction of the pupil normally occurs with light or when the eye is focusing on nearby objects. Dilation of the pupil normally occurs in dim light or when the eye is focusing on distant objects.

The lens is a transparent, gelatinous mass of fibers encased in an elastic capsule situated behind the iris. Its function is to ensure that the image on the retina is in sharp focus. It does this by changing shape (accommodation). This occurs readily in youth, but with age the lens becomes more rigid and the ability to focus close objects is lost. The *near point,* or the closest point that can be seen clearly, recedes. With age, the lens may lose its transparency and become opaque, forming a cataract. Blindness can occur unless the cataract can be treated or surgically removed.

The lens has ligaments around its edge called zonular fibers that connect with the ciliary body. Tension on the zonular fibers helps to change the shape of the lens. In the unaccommodated eye, the ciliary muscle is relaxed and the zonular fibers are taut. For near vision, the ciliary muscle fibers contract, relaxing the pull on the ligaments and allowing the lens to increase in thickness. Accommodation depends on two factors: the ability of the lens to assume a more biconvex shape when tension on the ligaments is relaxed and ciliary muscle contraction. Paralysis of the ciliary muscle is *cycloplegia.* The ciliary muscle is innervated by parasympathetic nerve fibers.

The ciliary body forms aqueous humor, which bathes and feeds the lens, posterior surface of the cornea, and iris. After it is formed, the fluid flows forward between the lens and the iris into the anterior chamber. It drains out of the eye through drainage channels located near the junction of the cornea and sclera into a meshwork that leads into the canal of Schlemm and into the venous system of the eye.

Eyelids, eyelashes, tears, and blinking all protect the eye. There are about 200 eyelashes for each eye. The eyelashes cause a blink reflex whenever a foreign body touches them, closing the lids for a few seconds to prevent the foreign body from entering the eye. Blinking, which is bilateral, occurs every few seconds during waking hours and serves to keep the corneal surface free of mucus and spreads the lacrimal fluid evenly over the cornea. Tears are secreted by lacrimal glands and contain lysozyme, a mucolytic lubrication for lid movements. They wash away foreign agents and form a thin film over the cornea, providing it with a good optical surface. Tear fluid is lost by drainage into two small ducts (the lacrimal canaliculi) at the inner corners of the eyelids and by evaporation.

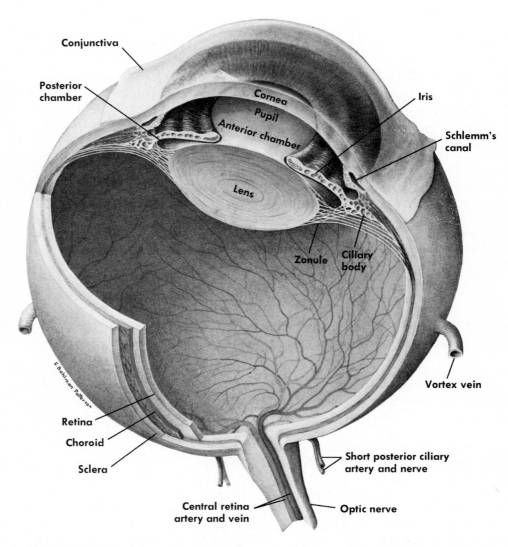

Fig. 22-1. The human eye. (From Newell, F. W.: Ophthalmology, principles and concepts, ed. 4, St. Louis, 1978, The C. V. Mosby Co.)

GLAUCOMA

Glaucoma is an eye disease characterized by abnormally elevated intraocular pressure, which may result from excessive production of aqueous humor or from diminished ocular fluid outflow. Increased pressure, if persistent and sufficiently elevated, may lead to permanent blindness. There are three major types of glaucoma: primary, secondary, and congenital. Primary includes narrow-angle, or acute congestive, glaucoma and wide-angle, or chronic, simple glaucoma. These are diagnosed by the angle of the anterior chamber where aqueous humor reabsorption takes place. Wide-angle glaucoma has an insidious onset, and its control demands long-term drug therapy. Drugs are also necessary for controlling the acute attack associated with narrow-angle glaucoma. Secondary glaucoma may result from previous eye disease or may follow a cataract extraction and may required drug therapy for an indefinite period. Congenital glaucoma requires surgical treatment.

Symptoms of chronic (open-angle) glaucoma include no symptoms in early stages, gradual loss of peripheral vision over a period of years, slow but persistent onset in older age group, and persistent elevation of intraocular pressure, as determined by serial tonometric examinations and any other examinations the ophthalmologist requires.

Cholinergic and anticholinesterase drugs are used to treat glaucoma. The selection of the drug is determined to a great extent by the requirements of the individual patient.

Cholinergic drugs

Cholinergic drugs produce strong contractions of the iris (miosis) and ciliary body musculature (accommodation). These drugs lower the intraocular pressure in patients with glaucoma by widening the filtration angle, permitting outflow of aqueous humor. Toxicity or sensitivity to these drugs may be evidenced by such symptoms as sweating, salivation, headache, abdominal discomfort, diarrhea, fall in blood pressure, and asthmatic attacks.

Acetylcholine chloride, intraocular
(Miochol) (my′o-kol)

1. Acetylcholine chloride 10% is used during cataract surgery for rapid miosis.
2. From 0.5 to 2 ml of solution is instilled into the anterior chamber of the eye after the lens has been removed in cataract surgery.
3. Since the duration of action of acetylcholine is only a few minutes, pilocarpine may be added to maintain miosis.

Carbachol (kar′bah-kol)
(Isopto-Carbachol), (Carbacel) (kar′bah-sel)

1. Carbachol produces intense and prolonged miosis because it is resistant to destruction by cholinesterase. It may be particularly useful when resistance to pilocarpine has developed.
2. The miotic action lasts 4 to 8 hours, and it is usually prescribed for use two or three times daily.
3. This drug must be combined with a wetting agent such as benzalkonium chloride for increased corneal penetration.
4. Usual dose: the ophthalmic preparation is applied topically to the conjunctiva as 0.75%, 1.5%, 2.25%, or 3.0% solution two to six times daily.

Pilocarpine (nitrate, hydrochloride) (py-lo-kar′pin)
(Isopto-Carpine, Pilocar)

1. Pilocarpine is the safest and most widely used miotic in the treatment of glaucoma.
2. Pilocarpine is also used to neutralize mydriatics used during eye examinations.
3. Usual dose: 1 to 2 drops of 0.5% to 4% solution into the eye several times daily.
4. Excess solution must be wiped away immediately to prevent the drug's flow into the lacrimal system and resulting production of systemic symptoms. (See instructions for instilling eye drops and ointment in the conclusion of this chapter.)
5. Miosis occurs within 15 minutes to 1 hour and may last 2 or 3 hours, with some effects persisting for 24 hours.

Pilocarpine ocular therapeutic system
(Ocusert Pilo-20, Ocusert Pilo-40)

A new method of delivery for ophthalmic pilocarpine consists of an ocular insert with a centrally located reservoir of drug. It is inserted into the upper or lower cul-de-sac. There has been success in using it in the management of glaucoma. The reservoir is calibrated to release either 20 or 40 μg of pilocarpine per hour, for 1 week.

Advantages of this ocular therapeutic system include the following: (1) less medication may be needed, and toxicity may be reduced; (2) more convenience is provided, which may increase patient compliance; (3) continuous, steady medication is delivered for up to 7 days, after which a replacement is necessary; (4) in younger patients with glaucoma the miosis and spasm occurring with eye drops are less prominent; and (5) better daytime control of intraocular pressure may be provided.

Some of the disadvantages of the ocular insert are: (1) conjunctival irritation, especially during initial use; (2) migration onto the cornea, which may obstruct vision and cause pain; (3) possibility of the unit falling out at night (the patient should check for this every morning);

(4) greater expense compared to other methods of therapy; (5) need for more therapy for some patients than can be given by the ocular insert, requiring frequent administration of eye drops; (6) variability in duration of action, with some inserts effective for only 2 to 4 days; (7) sudden leakage of the device; and (8) inability of some patients to learn to place the ocular insert properly.

Anticholinesterase drugs

Cholinesterase is an enzyme that destroys acetylcholine. Following are anticholinesterase agents used to reduce intraocular pressure associated with glaucoma.

1. *Demecarium bromide (Humorsol).* This agent is used in 0.125% and 0.25% ophthalmic solution; it is extremely powerful, with 1 drop producing miosis within 1 hour and ciliary muscle contraction for as long as 5 to 12 days. Excess solution must be wiped away promptly according to instructions at the conclusion of this chapter.

2. *Echothiophate iodide (Echodide, Phospholine Iodide).* This is an effective drug in the control of chronic wide-angle glaucoma, congenital glaucoma, and aphakic glaucoma; used in 0.06% to 0.125% solution. Miosis occurs within 10 to 45 minutes and may last several days to 4 weeks. Dosage should be gradually withdrawn. After reconstitution, the drug should be used within 1 month if stored at room temperature and within 6 months if refrigerated.

3. *Isoflurophate (Floropryl).* This ointment is applied to the conjunctival sac every 8 to 72 hours. A decrease in intraocular pressure should occur within a few hours. After therapy is stabilized, the ointment should be applied no more frequently than every 48 hours.

4. *Physostigmine (Eserine ointment, Isopto-Eserine solution).* This agent is used in concentrations of 0.25% and 0.5% every 4 to 6 hours; it is not to be used if the solution turns pink or brown. Conjunctivitis may occur with chronic use.

• • •

Disadvantages of cholinergic and anticholinesterase drugs include difficulty in adjusting quickly to changes in light intensity (a hazard to elderly patients, especially at night), headache, visual blurring, conjunctivitis, dermatitis, eye irritation, drainage, possible cataracts, development of tolerance and resistance, necessity of frequent instillations, nausea, fall in blood pressure, asthmatic attacks, and spasm of the wink reflex (with anticholinesterase drugs).

Some advantages of cholinergic drugs: (1) they are effective in many cases of chronic glaucoma, (2) their side effects are less severe and less frequent than those of anticholinesterase agents, (3) instillations are less frequent, and (4) they give better control over and less fluctuation in the intraocular pressure.

Two antidotes to cholinergic drugs are atropine and pralidoxime chloride (Protopam Chloride).

ANTICHOLINERGIC DRUGS

Parasympatholytic drugs cause the smooth muscle of the ciliary body and iris to relax, producing mydriasis (extreme dilation of the eye pupil) and cycloplegia (paralysis of the ciliary muscle). Ophthalmologists use these effects to examine the interior of the eye, to measure the proper strength of lenses for eyeglasses (refraction), and to put the eye at rest in inflammatory conditions of the uveal tract. Systemic absorption of large quantities of these drugs can result in serious side effects, such as inhibition of sweating, flushing, dryness of the mouth, fever, tachycardia, delirium, and coma.

Atropine sulfate (at'ro-peen)

1. Atropine sulfate is a potent cycloplegic and mydriatic agent used for refraction and pupillary dilation necessary for inflammatory conditions of the iris and uveal tract.

2. Mydriasis occurs within 30 to 40 minutes; cycloplegia occurs within a few hours. Effects may persist for 12 days or longer. During therapy patients may be unable to focus on nearby objects and will be unusually sensitive to light.

3. Side effects of dryness of mouth and tachycardia are indications for dosage reduction.

4. Atropine sulfate is contraindicated in patients with glaucoma.

5. Atropine sulfate ophthalmic solutions are available in 0.125%, 0.25%, 0.5%, 1%, 2%, 3%, and 4% concentrations. Atropine sulfate ophthalmic ointment is available in 0.5% and 1% concentrations.

Cyclopentolate hydrochloride (sy-klo-pen'to-layt) (Cyclogyl) (sy'klo-jil)

1. The greatest use of this drug is as an aid to eye examination and refraction.

2. In 0.5%, 1%, and 2% solution, it produces rapid and brief mydriasis and cycloplegia. One drop of a 1% solution or 2 drops of 0.5% solution 5 minutes apart will produce cycloplegia within 45 minutes. Although recovery usually occurs in 24 hours, 1 or 2 drops of 1% to 2% pilocarpine reduces recovery time to 3 to 6 hours in most patients.

3. Patients with darkly pigmented irises may be resistant to the effects of cyclopentolate. The 2% solution is recommended.

Homatropine hydrobromide (ho-mat′ro-pin)
(Isopto-Homatropine), (Homatrocel)
(ho-mat′ro-sel)

1. Homatropine is a moderately long-acting mydriatic and cycloplegic with uses similar to those of atropine sulfate.
2. Homatropine hydrobromide is available in 1%, 2%, and 5% solutions.

Scopolamine hydrobromide (sko-pol′ah-meen)
(Isopto-Hyoscine Hydrobromide)

1. Scopolamine in aqueous solutions of 0.2%, 0.25%, and 0.5% has actions and side effects similar to those of atropine.
2. The instillation of a 0.5% scopolamine solution causes cycloplegia within 40 minutes.

Tropicamide (tro-pik′ah-myd)
(Mydriacyl) (my-dree′ah-sil or my-dry′ah-sil)

1. This agent is a rapid-acting cycloplegic and mydriatic with a short duration of action.
2. Two drops of a 1% solution 5 minutes apart are effective within 20 to 35 minutes.
3. There is complete recovery from the cycloplegic effect in 2 to 6 hours.

ADRENERGIC DRUGS

Adrenergic agents have several uses in ophthalmology. Sympathomimetic agents cause pupil dilation, increased outflow of aqueous humor, vasoconstriction, relaxation of the ciliary muscle, and a decrease in the formation of aqueous humor. Adrenergic agents are used to treat open-angle glaucoma, to relieve congestion and hyperemia, and to produce mydriasis for ocular examination.

Epinephrine hydrochloride (ep-i-nef′rin)
(Adrenalin Chloride), (Epifrin) (e′pi-frin),
(Glaucon) (glaw′kahn), *(Epinal)* (e′pi-nahl)

1. Epinephrine ophthalmic solutions are used to treat open-angle glaucoma and conjunctivitis, to provide rapid dilation of the pupil, and to control bleeding during surgery.
2. Systemic effects from ophthalmic instillation are infrequent; however, systemic absorption may occur from drainage via the lacrimal drainage system into the nasal pharyngeal passages. Effects observed are palpitations, tachycardia, hypertension, anxiety, trembling, sweating, and cardiac arrhythmias.
3. Epinephrine is available in 0.25%, 0.5%, 1%, and 2% solutions.

Naphazoline hydrochloride (naf-az′o-leen)
(Albalon Liquifilm, Vaso-Clear, Clear Eyes, Vasocon ophthalmic)

1. Naphazoline is used as a topical ocular vasoconstrictor. It is a common ingredient in nonprescription eye drops.
2. It is available in concentrations of 0.012%, 0.02%, 0.05%, and 0.1%.

Phenylephrine hydrochloride (fen-il-ef′rin)
(Neo-Synephrine) (nee-o-si-nef′rin)

1. Phenylephrine solutions are available in four general strengths: 0.02%, 0.08%, 0.12%, and 0.15%.
   a. The weak solutions are used as decongestants to provide temporary relief of minor eye irritation caused by eye strain, hard contact lens, smoke, dust, wind, swimming, and hay fever.
   b. The 2.5% strength is commonly used for ophthalmic examination and refraction, diagnostic procedures, and prior to ophthalmic surgery.
   c. The 10% solutions are used as mydriatics and vasoconstrictors in uveal inflammation, wide-angle glaucoma, and surgery.
2. Be cautious of systemic side effects, particularly with the 10% solution.

Tetrahydrozoline hydrochloride
(tet-rah-hi-dro′zo-leen)
(Murine-2) (mur′een), *(Tetracon)* (tet′rah-kahn),
(Visine) (vi′zeen)

1. Tetrahydrozoline is a vasoconstrictor used to reduce eye irritation caused by smoke, allergens, close work, and after contact lens removal.
2. Dosage: 1 or 2 drops of the 0.05% solution in each eye two or three times daily.

Adrenergic blocking agent
Timolol maleate (tim′o-lol)
(Timoptic) (tim-op′tik)

1. Timolol is a new beta-adrenergic blocking agent that reduces normal and elevated intraocular pressure. Unlike the anticholinergic agents, there is no blurred or dim vision or night blindness, because intraocular pressure is reduced with little or no effect on pupil size or visual activity.
2. Timolol is now used to reduce intraocular pressure in patients with chronic open-angle glaucoma, in aphakic patients with glaucoma, in certain cases of secondary glaucoma, and in ocular hypertension. Onset of action occurs within 2 hours. Duration of action may last up to 24 hours.
3. Occasionally, patients will suffer systemic side effects from this beta-adrenergic blocking agent. Use with caution in patients with a history of bronchial

asthma or heart disease or in those patients already taking propranolol (Inderal) or other beta blockers.

4. Timolol is available in 0.25% and 0.5% solutions. Usual initial dose: 1 drop twice daily of the 0.25% solution.

OSMOTIC AGENTS

Osmotic agents are administered intravenously, orally, or topically to reduce intraocular pressure. These agents elevate the osmotic pressure of the plasma, which causes fluid from the extravascular spaces to be drawn into the blood. The effect on the eye is reduction of volume of intraocular fluid, which produces a decrease in intraocular pressure.

Glycerin (glis'er-in)
(Glycerol) (glis'er-ol), **(Glyrol)** (gly'rol),
(Ophthalgan) (off-thal'jin), **(Osmoglyn)**
(oz'mo-glin)

1. Glycerin is used to reduce intraocular pressure in patients with acute narrow-angle glaucoma, prior to iridectomy, and preoperatively and postoperatively in conditions such as congenital glaucoma, retinal detachment, cataract extraction, and keratoplasty, and in some secondary glaucomas. It reduces edema and improves visualization.
2. Side effects include headache, nausea, vomiting, diarrhea, and thirst. Headache is a result of cerebral dehydration and may be relieved by having the patient lie down during and after oral administration of glycerin.
3. Glycerin should be used with caution in patients with cardiac, hepatic, or renal disease; the shift in body water may cause congestive heart failure or pulmonary edema. Elderly patients may be subject to dehydration. In diabetic patients, the metabolism of the glycerin may cause hyperglycemia and glycosuria, so the diabetic patient should be observed for symptoms of acidosis.
4. Usual topical dose: 1 or 2 drops for edema of the cornea to reduce edema and improve visualization. Ophthalmic glycerin may be used in combination with miotic agents to prolong the effects of glycerin. Oral administration: 1 to 1.5 g/kg of body weight for adults and children at 5-hour intervals. Flavoring the glycerin with lemon or lime juice, pouring it over cracked ice, and having the patient sip it with a straw may lessen the nausea and vomiting.

Mannitol (man'i-tol)
(Osmitrol) (os'mi-trol)

1. Mannitol is administered intravenously to reduce intraocular pressure.
2. It is used for the same conditions and has the same side effects as glycerin. The drug can also cause disorientation, agitation, and convulsions; some fatalities have occurred after large doses.
3. Usual dose: 0.5 to 2 g/kg of body weight for adults and children. The solution should be infused slowly over 30 to 60 minutes. Maximal decrease in intraocular pressure occurs in 30 to 60 minutes and lasts about 6 to 8 hours.
4. Mannitol should be used with caution in elderly patients, patients with cardiovascular or pulmonary disease, and severely ill patients. Patients receiving mannitol should be carefully checked for vital signs, electrolyte and fluid balance, and urinary output.

Urea (your'ee-ah or your-ee'ah)
(Urevert) (your'eh-vert), **(Ureaphil)** (your'ee-ah-fil)

1. Urea is administered intravenously to reduce intraocular pressure. It is used for the same conditions as glycerin.
2. Common side effects are nausea, vomiting, headache, dehydration, and massive diuresis. Disorientation, agitation, and dizziness may occur, and pulmonary edema, convulsions, and death have occasionally been reported.
3. Usual dosage for adults: 0.5 to 2 g/kg of body weight of a 30% solution administered at a rate of 60 drops each minute. Maximal decrease in intraocular pressure occurs 1 hour after injection and lasts about 8 to 12 hours.
4. Urea is unstable in solution and must be freshly prepared for administration. It is irritating to the tissues and causes pain at the injection site. Extravasation should be prevented because tissue necrosis can occur.

ANTISEPTICS

Antiseptics prevent or lessen the possibility of infection. Antiseptic solutions are employed in ophthalmology for irrigation, dissolution of secretions, precipitation of mucus, and when specific antimicrobial agents cannot be used.

Mild silver protein
(Argyrol S.S. 20%) (ar'ji-rol)

1. Mild silver protein is an antiseptic used preoperatively in ophthalmic surgery, in eye infections, and for prevention and treatment of ophthalmia neonatorum.

Silver nitrate

1. A 1% solution of silver nitrate is used routinely as a prophylaxis against gonorrhea infection of the eye or ophthalmia neonatorum.
2. It is available in collapsible capsules that contain about 5 drops of a 1% solution.

Thimerosal ointment (thi-mer′o-sol)
(Merthiolate ophthalmic ointment) (mer-thi′o-layt)

1. Thimerosal ointment is a mercurial ointment that has mild antiseptic activity against most common bacterial and fungal pathogens.
2. It is used in conjunctivitis and for the prevention of infection following removal of foreign bodies.

ANESTHETICS

Local anesthetics (Table 22-1) may be used in such ophthalmic procedures as removal of foreign objects, tonometry, gonioscopy, suture removal, and for short corneal and conjunctival procedures. Since the "blink" reflex is temporarily eliminated, it is wise to protect the eye with a patch after procedures are completed.

ANTIBACTERIAL AGENTS

Antibacterial agents (Table 22-2) are occasionally used in the treatment of superficial infections of the eye. Prolonged or frequent intermittent use of topical antibiotics should be avoided because of the possibility of hypersensitive reactions and the development of resistant organisms, including fungi. If hypersensitivities or new infections appear during use, an ophthalmologist should be consulted immediately. (Refer to Index for a discussion of these antibiotics.)

ANTIFUNGAL AGENT

Natamycin (na-tah-my′sin)

1. Natamycin is an antifungal agent effective against a variety of yeast, including *Candida*, *Aspergillus*, and

Table 22-1. Ophthalmic anesthetics

Generic name	Brand names	Availability
Benoxinate hydrochloride	Dorsacaine	0.4% solution
Cocaine hydrochloride	Various	1% to 4% solution
Proparacaine hydrochloride	Alcaine, Ophthetic, Ophthaine	0.5% solution
Tetracaine hydrochloride	Anacel, Pontocaine Eye	0.5% solution, 0.5% ointment

Table 22-2. Ophthalmic antibiotics

Antibiotic	Brand names	Availability
Bacitracin	Baciguent Ophthalmic	Ointment
Chloramphenicol	Chloromycetin Ophthalmic, Chloroptic, Econochlor, Ophthochlor	Drops, ointment
Chlortetracycline	Aureomycin Ophthalmic	Ointment
Erythromycin	Ilotycin Ophthalmic	Ointment
Gentamicin	Garamycin Ophthalmic	Drops, ointment
Neomycin	Myciguent Ophthalmic	Ointment
Polymyxin B	Polymyxin B Sulfate, Aerosporin	Drops
Sulfacetamide	Sulamyd, Sulf-10	Drops, ointment
Tetracycline	Achromycin Ophthalmic	Drops
Combinations		
Chloramphenicol Polymyxin B	Chloromyxin Ophthalmic	Ointment
Neomycin Polymyxin B	Stratrol Ophthalmic, Polyspectrin Liquifilm Ophthalmic	Ointment, drops
Neomycin Polymyxin B Bacitracin	Neo-Polycin Ophthalmic, Mycitracin Ophthalmic, Neosporin Ophthalmic, Neotal, Pyocidin	Ointment
Neomycin Polymyxin B Gramicidin	Neo-Polycin Ophthalmic, Neosporin Ophthalmic	Drops

Fusarium. It is effective in the treatment of fungal blepharitis, conjunctivitis, and keratitis caused by susceptible organisms.

2. If little or no improvement is noted after 7 to 10 days of treatment, resistance to the antifungal agent may have developed. Topical administration does not appear to result in systemic effects.

3. Initial dose in fungal keratitis: 1 drop instilled in the conjunctival sac every 1 to 2 hours.

ANTIVIRAL AGENT

Idoxuridine (i-doks-ur′i-deen)
(Dendrid) (den′drid), *(Stoxil)* (stok′sil), *(Herplex Liquifilm)* (her′pleks)

1. Idoxuridine is used in the treatment of herpes simplex keratitis. Idoxuridine blocks viral reproduction by alteration of normal DNA synthesis.

2. Side effects are minimal but may include irritation, pain, pruritus, inflammation, and edema of the eyes or eyelids. Do not exceed the recommended frequency and duration of administration.

3. Do not use boric-acid eye solutions during the course of therapy since it may cause further irritation.

4. Idoxuridine is available in a 0.1% solution and a 0.5% ointment.

STEROIDS

Corticosteroid therapy is indicated for allergic reactions of the eye and other acute, noninfectious inflammatory conditions of the conjunctiva, sclera, cornea, and anterior uveal tract. Corticosteroid therapy must not be used in bacterial, fungal, or viral infections of the eye because corticosteroids decrease defense mechanisms and reduce resistance to pathologic organisms. This therapy should be used for a limited time only, and the eye should be checked frequently for an increase in intraocular pressure. Prolonged ocular steroid therapy may cause glaucoma and cataracts.

The following are some corticosteroids available for topical ophthalmic use as solutions, suspension, or ointments: *cortisone acetate, dexamethasone, fluorometholone, hydrocortisone, medrysone,* and *prednisolone.*

INSTRUCTIONS FOR INSTILLING EYE DROPS AND OINTMENT

1. Place the patient's head on a suitable support, such as a firm pillow, and direct his face toward the ceiling.

2. Instruct the patient to fix his gaze on a point above his head.

3. With clean fingertips, apply gentle traction to the lid bases at the bony rim of the orbit; do not apply pressure to the eyeball.

4. Approach the eye from below with the dropper or the ointment tube, outside the patient's field of vision; do not touch the eye with the dropper or the tube.

5. Release the dose; drops should not fall more than 1 inch before striking the eye.

6. Apply gentle pressure inward and downward against the bones of the nose for about 2 minutes to the lacrimal canaliculi at the inner corner of the eyelids. This prevents the eye medication from entering the nasal cavity and being absorbed through the nasal cavity's highly vascular mucosa. Many eye medications are very powerful; take care to prevent their systemic absorption.

**The physician prescribes the medicine and treatment.
The nurse carries out the physician's orders.
Self-medication is dangerous. Consult your physician first.
There is in every medicine a possible danger.
When in doubt—ASK!**

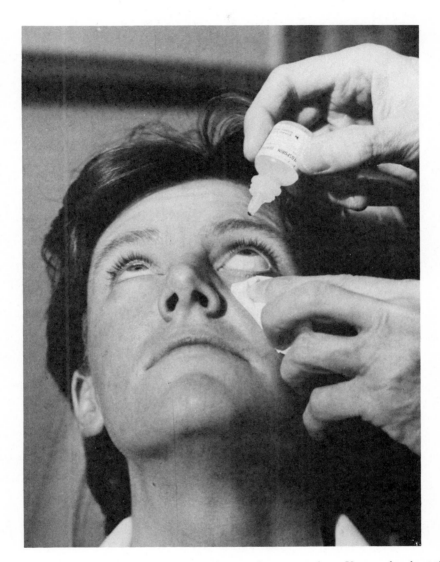

Fig. 22-2. The patient should tilt her face upward to receive an eye drop. Use an absorbent tissue to prevent excess drops and tears from flowing down the patient's face. (From Saunders, W. H., and others: Nursing care in eye, ear, nose, and throat disorders, ed. 4, St. Louis, 1979, The C. V. Mosby Co.)

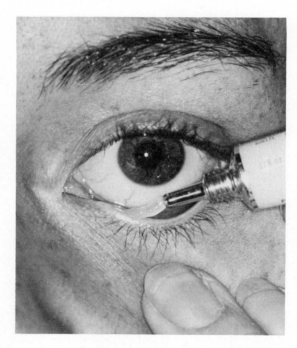

Fig. 22-3. To instill ointment, pull down the lower eyelid as the patient looks upward. Squeeze the ointment into the lower conjunctival sac. Avoid touching the tube to the eye or lid. (From Saunders, W. H., and others: Nursing care in eye, ear, nose, and throat disorders, ed. 4, St. Louis, 1979, The C. V. Mosby Co.)

ASSIGNMENT

Review previous lessons and questions according to the directions of your instructor.

1. Name the three coats or layers of the eyeball. Describe and tell the function of the cornea, the sclera, and the iris.
2. What is the effect of contraction of the iris sphincter muscle? What is the effect of relaxation of the sphincter muscle? Define *miosis* and *mydriasis*.
3. Explain the action of drugs that produce miosis (miotics) and mydriasis (mydriatics).
4. Locate, describe, and give the function of the lens. What is its function and how does it achieve its function? What is meant by the terms accommodation, near point, and cataract? How is the shape of the lens changed? Accommodation depends on what two factors? Define *cycloplegia*.
5. Explain the function of the ciliary body. What is the function of aqueous humor? Once it is formed, where does it flow? Locate these drainage channels. Once the aqueous humor has drained into the drainage channels and into a meshwork, where else does it drain?
6. What is the function of the eyelids, eyelashes, tears, and blinking? About how many eyelashes are there for each eye? Explain the function of the eyelashes and blinking in greater detail. Tears are secreted by what glands and contain a mucolytic lubrication called by what name and with what function? How is tear fluid lost?
7. Define glaucoma and tell the possible results of increased pressure that is persistent and sufficiently elevated. Name the three major types of glaucoma and explain the meaning of each type. What is a possible cause of secondary glaucoma and what is the treatment? What is the treatment for congenital glaucoma? List the general symptoms of glaucoma.
8. Name two groups of drugs used in the treatment of glaucoma. Explain the actions and effects of the cholinergic drugs. List toxic or sensitivity symptoms of the cholinergics.
9. What is the intraocular use of acetylcholine chloride (Miochol), and where is it instilled? What is its duration of action? What drug may be added to maintain miosis?
10. Describe the action and effect of carbachol (Carbacel), and tell its possible particular use. How long does its miotic action last and how often per day is it usually prescribed? For increased corneal penetration with what drug must carbachol be combined? What is the usual dose of carbachol and the method of application?
11. Pilocarpine (nitrate, hydrochloride) (several choices are correct)
    a. Is the safest and most widely used miotic in the treatment of glaucoma
    b. Has wide use but is powerful and must be used with caution and with adequate supervision only
    c. Is also used to neutralize mydriatics used during eye examinations
    d. Gives a miotic effect within 2 to 6 minutes, which lasts usually 15 to 30 minutes
    e. Has a usual dose of 1 to 2 drops of 0.5% to 4% solution into the eye several times daily

    f. Must have the excess solution wiped away immediately after administration to prevent the drug's flow into the lacrimal system with resulting production of systemic symptoms
    g. Is so safe that no precautions have to be taken after its administration
    h. Has a miotic action that occurs within 15 minutes to 1 hour and may last 2 or 3 hours, with some effects possibly persisting for 24 hours
12. Explain the new method of ocular insert of pilocarpine (Ocusert Pilo-20, Ocusert Pilo-40) and list its advantages and disadvantages.
13. What is cholinesterase and what effect does it have on acetylcholine? Name four anticholinesterase agents used to reduce intraocular pressure in glaucoma, tell the method of administration of each, and list any precautions each drug may have.
14. What are the disadvantages to cholinergic and anticholinesterase drugs? What are some advantages of cholinergic drugs?
15. Name two antidotes to cholinergic drugs.
16. List the actions and effects on which part of the eye for anticholinergic drugs. What do ophthalmologists use these effects for? What are the results of systemic absorption of large quantities of these drugs?
17. Atropine sulfate (several choices are correct)
    a. Is a potent cycloplegic and mydriatic agent used for refraction and pupillary contraction
    b. Is a potent cycloplegic and mydriatic agent used for refraction and pupillary dilation
    c. Has a mydriatic effect occurring within 30 to 40 minutes and a cycloplegic effect occurring within a few hours; effects persist for 12 days or longer
    d. May cause patients to be unable to focus on nearby objects and to be unusually sensitive to light
    e. May cause patients to be unable to focus on distant objects and to be completely insensitive to light
    f. Has side effects of dryness of mouth and tachycardia, which are indications for dosage reduction
    g. Is a specific drug to use for glaucoma patients
    h. Is contraindicated for glaucoma patients
    i. Has several ophthalmic solution dosages available, such as 0.125%, 0.25%, 0.5%, 1%, 2%, 3%, and 4%
18. What is the greatest use of cyclopentolate (Cyclogyl)? What is a usual dose? How soon will it produce cycloplegia? How long does its effect last and what drug may reduce its recovery time?
19. What type of drug is homatropine for ophthalmic use? Its uses are similar to what other drug?
20. What ophthalmic effects does scopolamine have? Its effects are similar to what other drug? How soon does its cycloplegic effect occur?
21. What type of ophthalmic drug is tropicamide (Mydriacyl)? What is its duration of action? What dosage causes its effects in what period of time? When does recovery occur?
22. What are the uses of adrenergic drugs in ophthalmology?
23. What are the uses of epinephrine ophthalmic solutions?
24. Systemic effects from ophthalmic instillation of epinephrine are infrequent but can occur. What may cause their

occurrence, and what are these effects? What are ophthalmic dosages of epinephrine?

25. What is the ophthalmic use of naphazoline? It is a common ingredient in what type of eye drops?

26. What are the uses of phenylephrine (Neo-Synephrine) in weak solutions? What are the uses of phenylephrine in 2.5% and in 10% solutions? Why is it necessary to be cautious of systemic side effects, particularly with the 10% solution?

27. What type of drug is tetrahydrozoline (Murine-2, Tetracon, Visine)? What are its uses? Tell the usual dose and how often it is administered.

28. Timolol (Timoptic) is what type of drug, and what is its effect? Unlike the anticholinergic agents, is there blurred or dim vision or night blindness with use of Timolol? Why not? What are the uses of Timolol? When does onset of action occur, and what is the duration of action? Does Timolol have occasional systemic side effects? In what conditions should Timolol be used with caution? What is the usual initial dose?

29. What are the methods of administration of the osmotic agents? Tell the ophthalmic uses of the osmotic agents. How is their effect obtained?

30. Glycerin (Glycerol) is an example of what group of ophthalmic agents? What are its uses and effects and for what ophthalmic medical conditions? List the side effects of glycerin. List the conditions in which glycerin should be used with caution. What is the usual dose, topical and oral? How may the oral dose be administered to help prevent nausea and vomiting?

31. What is the method of administration of mannitol (Osmitrol), and what is its main ophthalmic use? It is used for the same conditions and has the same side effects as what other osmotic agent? List additional conditions that may occur after large doses. What is the usual dose, and what is the method and length of administration? When does maximal decrease in intraocular pressure occur, and how long does it last? Mannitol should be used with caution in what conditions? Patients receiving mannitol should be carefully checked for what signs and symptoms?

32. What is the method of administration of urea for ophthalmic purposes, and what is its ophthalmic use? List the common side effects of urea. Describe the usual dosage and method of administration. When does maximal decrease in intraocular pressure occur, and how long does the effect last? Why must urea be freshly prepared for administration? What effect does urea have on the injection site? Why is it important to prevent extravasation?

33. What is the effect of antiseptic eye preparations? What are the various uses of antiseptics in eye treatment? Name three ophthalmic antiseptics and tell the main uses of each. What strength of silver nitrate is used in the eyes of the newborn, and for what purpose?

34. List the conditions for which local anesthetics may be used in ophthalmic procedures.

35. Select from Table 22-1 four drugs often used in eye treatment, including brand names. Your instructor will help you to select drugs often used in your hospital or by your ophthalmologist.

36. Antibacterial agents have their place in the treatment of superficial infections of the eye, but what is the disadvantage for prolonged or frequent intermittent use?

37. Give an example of one antifungal ophthalmic agent and tell its main use.

38. Give an example of one antiviral ophthalmic agent and tell its main use. List the side effects. What eye solution should be avoided during therapy with idoxuridine and why?

39. Select from Table 22-2 ten antibiotics often used for ophthalmic purposes, including trade names. Your instructor will help you to select antibiotics commonly used in your hospital or by your ophthalmologist.

40. What are the indications for use of corticosteroid therapy in eye treatment? Why must corticosteroid therapy *not* be used in bacterial, fungal, or viral eye infections? Why should corticosteroid therapy be used for a limited time only? Why should the eye be checked frequently during corticosteroid therapy? What are complications of prolonged ocular steroid therapy? Name six corticosteroids available for topical ophthalmic use as solutions, suspensions, or ointments.

41. In class your instructor demonstrated instructions for instilling eye drops, with you demonstrating these instructions with one of your classmates acting as patient. Outline the instructions given to you several times until you are familiar with them.

42. The physician orders for a patient 0.0006 g of a drug in tablet form, orally. The medicine bottle label strength of each tablet in the bottle is 0.3 mg. How many tablets will you administer? *Remember:* This is a conversion problem. Convert your grams to milligrams. Then try converting from milligrams to grams, using the same problem. (See Index for Conversion.)

CHAPTER 23

Antimicrobial agents

Antimicrobial agents are chemicals that eliminate living microorganisms pathogenic to the patient. Antimicrobial agents may be of chemical origin, such as the sulfonamides, or may be derived from other living organisms. Those derived from other living microorganisms are called *antibiotics;* for example, penicillin was first derived from the mold *Penicillium notatum.* Most antibiotics used today are harvested from large colonies of microorganisms, purified, and chemically modified into semisynthetic antimicrobial agents. The chemical modification makes the antibiotic more effective against certain pathogenic organisms.

The selection of the antimicrobial agent must be based on the sensitivity of the pathogen and the possible toxicity to the patient. If at all possible, the infecting organisms should be isolated and identified. Culture and sensitivity tests should be completed; the antimicrobial therapy is then started based on the sensitivity results and the clinical judgment of the physician.

Side effects common to all antimicrobial agents include (1) allergy, (2) direct tissue damage, and (3) superinfection.

Allergy. The severity of allergic reaction ranges from a mild rash to fatal anaphylaxis. Allergic reactions may develop within 30 minutes of administration (anaphylaxis, laryngeal edema, shock, dyspnea, or skin reactions) or may occur several days after discontinuance of therapy (skin rashes or fever). All patients must be questioned for previous allergic reactions, and allergy-prone patients must be observed closely. When a patient says he is allergic to medications, ask him to describe the symptoms of the reaction. Nausea, vomiting, or diarrhea are not symptoms of allergy. It is important not to label a patient allergic to a particular medication without adequate documentation. The medication that a patient claims he is allergic to may be a lifesaving drug for him.

Direct tissue damage. All drugs have at least the potential for causing damage to tissues of certain organs. Examples include kidney damage by the aminoglycosides and penicillins and liver damage by isoniazid. Fortunatley, these adverse effects are rare. The physician will order certain laboratory tests during antimicrobial treatment to help monitor the patient's therapy. Patients with preexisting diseases, such as renal failure or hepatitis, will require lower doses to prevent toxicity.

Common side effects of antimicrobial agents taken orally include nausea, vomiting, and diarrhea. These effects are often dose-related and result from changes in normal bacterial flora in the bowel, from irritation, and from superinfection. Symptoms resolve within a few days and rarely require discontinuation of therapy.

Superinfection. Antimicrobial agents may induce overgrowths by resistant bacterial strains or fungal organisms. Superinfections occur most frequently with the use of broad-spectrum antibiotics and with agents causing diminished host resistance, such as corticosteroids and antineoplastic agents. Stomatitis, glossitis, itching, and vulvovaginitis are often caued by candidal species of fungi. Viral infections may also develop, especially on the lips (cold sores) and oral mucosa (canker sores).

AMINOGLYCOSIDES

1. The aminoglycoside antibiotics are used primarily against gram-negative microorganisms that cause urinary tract infections, meningitis, wound infections, and life-threatening septicemias. They are a mainstay in the treatment of hospital-acquired gram-negative infections.

2. Allergic reactions to the aminoglycosides are not common; however, they may be quite serious should they occur. Ask patients about any allergies prior to the administration of any medication. Discontinue therapy if the patient develops a rash, fever, or itching skin.

3. Two serious reactions may occur with the aminoglycosides: ototoxicity, manifested by dizziness, tinnitus, and deafness; and nephrotoxicity, manifested by protein and blood in the urine, particularly in patients receiving high dosages or medications for longer than 10 days. If any of these symptoms should occur, report them immediately. Continue to observe patients for ototoxicity or nephrotoxicity after therapy has been discontinued. These adverse effects may appear several days later.

4. See Table 23-1 for aminoglycoside products available and dosage ranges.

207

Table 23-1. The aminoglycosides

Generic name	Brand names	Availability	Dosage range
Amikacin	Amikin	0.1-, 0.5- and 1-g vials	IM, IV: 15 mg/kg/24 hr
Gentamicin	Garamycin	20- and 80-mg vials	IM, IV: Up to 240 mg/24 hr
Kanamycin	Kantrex, Klebcil	75- and 500-mg vials	IM, IV: 15 mg/kg/24 hr
Neomycin	Mycifradin	500-mg vial	IM: 15 mg/kg/24 hr
Streptomycin	Streptomycin Sulfate	1- and 5-gm vials	IM: 1 to 4 g/24 hr
Tobramycin	Nebcin	20- and 80-mg vials	IM, IV: Up to 5 mg/kg/24 hr

Table 23-2. The cephalosporins

Generic name	Brand names	Availability	Dosage range
Cefadroxil	Duricef	500-mg capsules	po: 1 g twice daily
Cefamandole	Mandol	0.5-, 1-, and 2-g vials	IM, IV: 0.5 to 1 g/4 to 8 hr; do not exceed 2 g/4 hr
Cefazolin	Ancef, Kefzol	0.25-, 0.5-, and 1-g vials	IM, IV: 250 to 500 mg/8 hr up to 6 to 12 g/24 hr
Cefoxitin	Mefoxin	1- and 2-g vials	IM, IV: 1 to 2 g/6 to 8 hr
Cephalexin	Keflex	250- and 500-mg capsules 1-g tablets 125 and 250 mg/5 ml suspension 100 mg/1 ml drops	po: 1 to 4 g daily in divided doses
Cephalothin	Keflin	1-, 2-, and 4-g vials	IM, IV: 500 mg to 1 g/4 to 6 hr; do not exceed 2 g/4 hr
Cephapirin	Cefadyl	1-, 2-, and 4-g vials	IM, IV: 500 mg to 1 g/4 to 6 hr
Cephradine	Anspor, Velosef	0.25-, 0.5-, 1-, and 2-g vials 250-, 500-mg capsules 125 and 250 mg/5 ml suspension	IM, IV: 2 to 4 g/24 hr in four divided doses po: 250 to 500 mg four times daily

CEPHALOSPORINS

1. The cephalosporins are chemically related to the penicillins and have a similar mechanism of activity. The cephalosporins may be used as alternatives when patients are allergic to the penicillins.
2. Some patients allergic to the penicillins are also allergic to the cephalosporins. You must always ask the patient whether he is allergic to any medications. Allergy may develop during therapy; discontinue if the patient develops a rash, fever, or itching skin.
3. The cephalosporins are used for certain pneumonias, urinary tract infections, septicemias, and osteomyelitis.
4. Side effects with the cephalosporins are usually minor. Nausea, vomiting, and diarrhea are most common.
5. A false positive reaction for glucose in the urine may occur with Clinitest tablets, but not with Tes-Tape or Diastix.
6. See Table 23-2 for products available and dosage ranges.

PENICILLINS

1. The penicillins were the first true antibiotics to be grown and used against pathogenic bacteria in human beings. They are still one of the most widely used classes of antibiotics today.
2. The penicillins act by interfering with the synthesis of bacterial cell walls. They are therefore most effective against bacteria that multiply rapidly. They do not hinder growth of human cells, because human cells have protective membranes but no cell wall.
3. Penicillin G is the naturally occurring parent compound of this class of antibiotics. Semisynthetic compounds are made from modification of the penicillin G molecule to alter the spectrum of activity, enhance oral absorption, and reduce enzyme resistance by pathogenic microorganisms.
4. The penicillins are used to treat middle ear infections (otitis media), pneumonia, meningitis, urinary tract infections, syphilis, gonorrhea, and as a prophylactic antibiotic for patients with rheumatic fever.
5. Before any penicillin therapy is started, you must ask the patient about any allergy to medications. Patients most susceptible to penicillin allergy are those who already have a history of hives, asthma, hay fever, or allergies to other drugs. Allergy may develop during therapy; discontinue if the patient develops a rash, fever, or itching skin.
6. See Table 23-3 for the different penicillin derivatives available, common brand names, and recommended dosage ranges.

Table 23-3. The penicillins

Generic name	Brand names	Availability	Dosage range
Amoxicillin	Amoxil, Trimox, Larotid, Wymox, Polymox	250- and 500-mg capsules 125 and 250 mg/5 ml suspension	po: 250 to 500 mg/8 hr
Ampicillin	Amcill, Polycillin, A-cillin, Omnipen, Principen, Pensyn, Totacillin	0.125-, 0.25-, 0.5-, 1-, and 2-g vials 125-, 250-, and 500-mg capsules 125 and 500 mg/5 ml suspension	IM, IV: 0.5 to 1 g/4 to 6 hr po: 250 to 500 mg/6 hr
Carbenicillin	Geopen, Pyopen	1-, 2-, 5-, 10-g vials	IM: Do not exceed 2 g/injection site IV: Up to 40 g/24 hr
Cloxacillin	Tegopen, Cloxapen	250- and 500-mg capsules 125 mg/5 ml suspension	po: 250 to 500 mg/6 hr
Dicloxacillin	Dynapen, Dynacill, Pathocil, Veracillin	125-, 250-, and 500-mg capsules 62.5 mg/5 ml suspension	po: 125 to 500 mg/6 hr
Methicillin	Azapen, Celbenin, Staphcillin	1-, 2-, 4-, 6-g vials	IM, IV: 1 g/4 to 6 hr
Nafcillin	Nafcil, Unipen	0.5-, 1-, 2-g vials 250- and 500-mg tablets 250 mg/5 ml suspension	IM, IV: 0.5 to 1 g/4 to 6 hr po: 250 to 500 mg/6 hr
Oxacillin	Bactocill, Prostaphlin	0.5-, 1-, 2-, 4-g vials 250- and 500-mg capsules 250 mg/5 ml suspension	IM, IV: 0.5 to 1 g/4 to 6 hr po: 250 to 500 mg/4 to 6 hr
Penicillin G, potassium or sodium	Pfizerpen, K-Cillin-500, Pentids	Vials of 0.2-, 0.5-, 1-, 5-, and 10-million units Capsules of 1-, 2-, 2.5-, 4-, 5-, and 800,000 units	po: 400,000 to 1.6 million units IM, IV: 600,000 to 30 million units daily
Penicillin V potassium	V-Cillin K, Betapen VK, Pen-Vee-K, Veetids	125-, 250-, and 500-mg tablets 125 and 250 mg/5 ml suspension	po: 250 to 500 mg/6 hr
Ticarcillin	Ticar	1-, 3-, and 6-g vials	IM: Do not exceed 2 g/injection site IV: Up to 18 g/24 hr

SULFONAMIDES

1. The sulfonamides are not true antibiotics because they are not synthesized by microorganisms; however, they are highly effective antibacterial agents used to treat urinary tract infections and otitis media.
2. Sulfonamides act by inhibiting bacterial biosynthesis of folic acid, which eventually results in bacterial cell death. Human cells do not synthesize folic acid so are not affected.
3. Allergic reactions may occur with sulfonamides. Ask patients about any allergies prior to the administration of any medication. Allergy may develop during therapy; discontinue if the patient develops a rash, fever, or itching skin.
4. Sulfonamides have many side effects, the most common of which are nausea and diarrhea. Rashes may represent more serious underlying disorders; report them immediately. Patients receiving sulfonamides longer than 14 days should have routine red and white cell counts with differential completed.
5. A false positive reaction for glucose in the urine may occur with Clinitest tablets, but not with Tes-Tape or Diastix.
6. Patients should be encouraged to drink 8-oz glasses

of water several times daily while ingesting sulfonamides. Crystals may form in the urinary tract if the patient becomes too dehydrated.
7. See Table 23-4 for the different sulfonamide derivatives available, common brand names, and recommended dosages.

TETRACYCLINES

1. The tetracyclines are a class of antibiotics that are effective against both gram-negative and gram-positive bacteria. They act by inhibiting protein synthesis by bacterial cells; they are particularly effective against rickettsial and mycoplasmic infections. The tetracyclines are often used for patients allergic to the penicillins for the treatment of certain venereal diseases, urinary tract infections, upper respiratory tract infections, pneumonia, and meningitis.
2. Before any tetracycline therapy is initiated, you must ask the patient about any allergy to medications. Patients most susceptible to allergic reactions are those who already have a history of hives, asthma, hay fever, or allergies to other drugs. Allergy may develop during therapy; discontinue if the patient develops a rash, fever, or itching skin.

Table 23-4. The sulfonamides

Generic name	Brand names	Availability	Dosage range
Sulfacytine	Renoquid	250-mg tablets	po: initial dose is 500 mg, then 250 mg four times daily
Sulfadiazine	Microsulfon Sulfadiazine	300-, 500-mg tablets	po: initial dose is 2 to 4 g, maintenance dose is 4 to 8 g/24 hr in divided doses
Sulfamerazine	Sulfamerazine	Powder	po: initial dose is 3 to 4 g, maintenance dose is 1 g/6 to 8 hr
Sulfamethizole	Thiosulfil, Bursul, Proklar, Unisul	0.25-, .5-, 1-g tablets 250 and 500 mg/5 ml suspension	po: 0.5 to 1 g three to four times daily
Sulfamethoxazole	Gantanol	0.5-, 1-g tablets 500 mg/5 ml suspension	po: initial dose is 2 g, then 1 g/12 hr
Sulfasalazine	Azulfidine, S.A.S.-500, Sulcolon	500-mg tablets	po: initial therapy is 3 to 4 g daily in divided doses, maintenance dose is 2 g daily
Sulfisoxazole	Gantrisin, Sulfalar, J-Sul, Rosoxol	500-mg tablets 500 mg/5 ml syrup 400 mg/ml vial	po, IM, IV: initial dose is 2 to 4 g, maintenance dose is 4 to 8 g/24 hr divided into 3 to 6 doses
Triple Sulfas	Neotrizine, Sulfose, Trisem	Tablets Suspension	po: initial dose is 2 to 4 g, followed by 2 to 4 g/24 hr divided into 3 to 6 hr

Table 23-5. The tetracyclines

Generic name	Brand names	Availability	Dosage range
Chlortetracy-cline	Aureomycin	250- and 500-mg vials	IV: 250 to 500 mg/12 hr po: 250 to 500 mg/6 hr
Demeclocy-cline	Declomycin	150-mg capsules 75-, 150-, and 300-mg tablets 75 mg/5 ml syrup	po: 150 mg four times daily or 300 mg two times daily
Doxycycline	Vibramycin, Doxychel	100- and 200-mg vials 50- and 100-mg capsules 25 and 50 mg/5 ml syrup	IV: 100 to 200 mg one or two times daily po: 200 mg on day 1, then 100 mg divided in two doses
Methacycline	Rondomycin	150- and 300-mg capsules 75 mg/5 ml syrup	po: 150 mg four times daily or 300 mg two times daily
Minocycline	Minocin, Vectrin	100-mg vial 50- and 100-mg capsules 50 mg/5 ml syrup	po, IV: 200 mg, followed by 100 mg/12 hr
Oxytetracycline	Terramycin, Oxlopar, Tetramine	100-, 250-, and 500-mg vials 125- and 250-mg capsules 125 mg/5 ml syrup	IM: 250 mg/24 hr or 100 mg/8 hr IV: 250 to 500 mg/12 hr; po: 250 to 500 mg four times daily
Tetracycline	Achromycin, Tetracyn, Pan-mycin, Robitet, Sumycin	100-, 250-, and 500-mg vials 100-, 250-, and 500-mg capsules and tablets 125 mg/5 ml syrup	IM: 250 to 800 mg/24 hr IV: 250 to 500 mg/12 hr po: 250 to 500 mg four times daily

3. Patients should be cautioned to avoid bright sunlight when taking tetracyclines. A severe sunburn may develop in a short time.

4. Tetracyclines should not be used during the age of tooth development (the last half of pregnancy, infancy, and childhood to 8 years of age). Permanent staining of the teeth (yellow, gray, or brown) may result. Tetracyclines are secreted in milk of lactating women. Infant nourishment by formula is recommended during the course of the mother's tetracycline therapy.

5. Oral tetracyclines should be administered 1 hour before or 2 hours after the ingestion of iron, milk, food, and antacids. These products inhibit the absorption of tetracycline.

6. A false positive reaction for glucose in the urine may occur between parenteral tetracycline and Clinitest tablets, but not between tetracycline and Tes-Tape or Diastix.

7. See Table 23-5 for the different tetracycline derivatives available, common brand names, and recommended dosage ranges.

OTHER ANTIBIOTICS

Chloramphenicol (klo-ram-fen'i-kol) (Chloromycetin) (klo-ro-my-se'tin)

1. Chloramphenicol is an antibiotic that acts by inhibiting bacterial protein synthesis. It is particularly effective in treating rickettsial infections, meningitis, and typhoid fever. It must not be used in the treatment of trivial infections or when it is not indicated, such as in colds, influenza, throat infections, or as a prophylactic agent to prevent bacterial infection.

2. Serious and possibly fatal bone marrow suppression may occur after therapy is initiated with chloramphenicol. Early signs include sore throat, a feeling of fatigue, elevated temperature, and small petechial hemorrhages and bruises on the skin. If patients report any of these symptoms, report them to your supervisor immediately.

3. Allergies may occur with chloramphenicol. You must ask the patient about any allergy to medications prior to administering this antibiotic. Allergy may develop during therapy; discontinue if the patient develops a rash, fever, or itching skin.

4. Chloramphenicol may cause a false positive reaction when determining glucose content in the urine by the Clinitest method. Tes-Tape or Diastix may be used instead to test for the presence of glucose.

5. Usual adult doses: between 50 and 100 mg/kg/day in divided doses at 6-hour intervals. Chloramphenicol is available in 50- and 250-mg capsules, 150-mg/5 ml suspension, and 100- and 500-mg ampules for IV injection. IM administration is not recommended.

Clindamycin (klin-dah-my'sin) (Cleocin) (klee-o'sin)

1. Clindamycin is an antibiotic that acts by inhibiting protein synthesis. It is useful against infections caused by gram-negative aerobic organisms as well a variety of gram-positive and gram-negative anaerobes.

2. Severe diarrhea may develop from the use of clindamycin. If diarrhea consisting of more than 5 stools per day develops, the physician should be notified. The use of Lomotil, loperamide, or paregoric may prolong or worsen the condition. Large doses of kaolin-pectin (Kaopectate) may be effective in diminishing the diarrhea.

3. Before any clindamycin therapy is started, you must ask the patient about any allergy to medications. Patients most susceptible to clindamycin allergy are those who already have a history of hives, asthma, hay fever, or allergies to drugs.

4. Adult dosages: from 600 to 2,700 mg daily in 2 to 4 divided doses. Clindamycin may be administered by oral, IM, or IV routes. It is available in 75- and 150 mg capsules, 75 mg/5 ml suspensions, and 300- and 600-mg ampules for injection.

Erythromycin (e-rith-ro-my'sin) (Erythrocin) (e-rith'ro-sin), (E-Mycin)

1. Erythromycin may be used as an alternative antibiotic for those patients allergic to penicillin. It acts by inhibition of protein synthesis and is effective in treating respiratory tract infections, meningitis, syphilis, and gonorrhea and may be used in prophylaxis against rheumatic fever.

2. Before erythromycin therapy is initiated, the nurse must first ask the patient whether he is allergic to any medications. Allergy may develop during therapy; discontinue if the patient develops a rash, fever, or itching skin.

3. The most common side effects of oral erythromycin products are epigastric distress, with possible nausea and vomiting.

4. Adult dosage: 15 to 20 mg/kg/day administered in divided doses every 6 hours. Erythromycin is available in 125-, 200-, 250-, and 500-mg tablets; 125, 200, and 400 mg/5 ml suspension; 125 mg/2.5 ml drops; and 250- and 500-mg vials for IV injection. IM injection is quite painful and generally is not recommended.

Spectinomycin (spek-ti-no-my'sin) (Trobicin) (tro'bi-sin)

1. Spectinomycin is used specifically for the treatment of gonorrhea in both males and females. It has a particular advantage: most bacterial strains of gonorrhea

respond to one administration of the recommended dosage.

2. It is used as an alternative to penicillin for gonorrhea only. It is not effective against syphilis.
3. The dosage for both males and females is 2 g. An IM injection into the upper outer quadrant of the gluteal muscle using a 20-gauge needle is recommended. Spectinomycin is available in 2- and 4-g vials for injection.

ANTIFUNGAL AGENTS
Clotrimazole (klo-trim′ah-zoal)
(Lotrimin) (lo′tri-min)

1. Clotrimazole inhibits the growth of both dermatophytes and yeasts.
2. It is effective in treating skin infections caused by species of fungi that burrow into superficial skin layers to cause athlete's foot (tinea pedis), ringworm of the groin (tinea cruris), and ringworm of the body (tinea corporis). It is also effective against *Candida albicans,* the yeast-like fungus that causes an inflammation of the corners of the mouth (perlèche), and candidal vulvitis. Vaginal tablets (Gyne-Lotrimin) are available for treating vaginal fungal infections.
3. The topically applied products are applied twice daily for up to 4 weeks. Treatment may be repeated if necessary. Topical strength: 1% cream or solution.

Griseofulvin (gris-ee-o-ful′vin)
(Fulvicin) (ful′vi-sin), *(Grifulvin)* (gri-vul′vin)

1. Griseofulvin is a fungistatic antibiotic used to treat ringworm of the scalp, body, nails, and feet, although response to treatment is sometimes slow in the nails and feet.
2. After griseofulvin is absorbed, it is incorporated into the keratin of the nails, skin, and hair in therapeutic amounts. The infecting fungus is not killed, but its growth into new cells is prevented. Once the cells are shed or removed, they are replaced by new cells free from the infection.
3. Infrequent side effects that may occur include nausea, headache, diarrhea, skin rash, and epigastric distress. The possible occurrence of leukopenia necessitates periodic blood examinations.
4. Griseofulvin is not recommended for infections that will respond readily to topical antifungal agents.
5. Usual dose: 1 g daily in divided doses. This drug is available in 250- and 500-mg tablets for oral administration. Administer with meals for improved absorption.

Nystatin (nis′tah-tin)
(Mycostatin) (my-ko-stat′in)

1. Nystatin is an antifungal agent used in the treatment of candidal infections of the skin, mouth, vulvovag-inal mucosa, and intestinal tract. Nystatin acts by damaging the permeability of the fungal cell membrane.
2. Allergy to nystatin is quite rare, although patients may develop rashes from the preservatives in the topical preparations.
3. When treating topical candidal infections, with moist lesions, such as on skin folds or on feet, the powder is recommended. The affected areas should be kept dry and exposed to air if possible. Proper hygiene must also be maintained to prevent reinfection.
4. Nystatin is available as 500,000-unit oral tablets; 100,000-unit vaginal tablets; 100,000-units/ml oral suspension; and as cream, ointment, and topical powder.

TUBERCULOSIS MEDICINES
Ethambutol (e-tham′bu-tol)
(Myambutol) (my-am′bu-tol)

1. Ethambutol inhibits tuberculosis bacterial growth by altering RNA synthesis and phosphate metabolism. Ethambutol must be used in combination with other antitubercular agents to prevent the development of resistant organisms.
2. Some patients receiving ethambutol develop blurred vision and possible green color blindness. These adverse effects disappear within a few weeks after therapy is discontinued.
3. Other side effects include nausea, vomiting, mental confusion, disorientation, and hallucinations.
4. Nurses must emphasize to patients the need for continuing therapy as prescribed. Discontinuation of therapy may result in drug resistance, reversal of clinical improvement, and increased susceptibility of family members to tuberculosis.
5. Ethambutol is available in 100- and 400-mg tablets. Dosage range: 15 to 25 mg/kg as a single dose every 24 hours.

Isoniazid (i-so-ny′ah-zid)
(INH), (Hyzyd) (hy′zid), *(Nydrazid)* (ny′dra-zid)

1. Isoniazid is used for the treatment of tuberculosis, but its mechanism of action is not known. It should be used in combination with other antitubercular agents for therapy of active disease.
2. Tingling and numbness of the hands and feet, nausea, vomiting, dizziness, and ataxia are relatively common side effects of isoniazid and are dose-related.
3. Pyridoxine (vitamin B_6), 25 to 50 mg daily, is recommended to prevent peripheral neuropathies.
4. Isoniazid may produce a false positive reaction for glucose in the urine with Clinitest tablets, but not with Tes-Tape or Diastix.
5. Nurses must emphasize to patients the need for continuing therapy as prescribed. Discontinuation of

therapy may result in drug resistance, reversal of clinical improvement, and increased susceptibility of family members to tuberculosis.

6. Usual adult dose: 300 mg orally daily. Isoniazid is available in 50-, 100-, and 300-mg tablets, 100 mg/ml vials, and powder.

Rifampin (rif'am-pin)
(Rifadin) (rif'ah-din)

1. Rifampin is used in combination with other agents against tuberculosis. It acts against enzymes within the bacterial cell that are required to produce DNA.
2. Patients should be told that rifampin may tinge the urine, feces, saliva, sputum, sweat, and tears a red-orange color. No pathologic damage is caused by this

color change, and it will disappear when the medication is discontinued.

3. When female patients are taking rifampin, they should be counseled to use birth control methods other than oral contraceptives. Rifampin apparently interferes with the contraceptive activity of birth control pills.
4. Nurses must emphasize to patients the importance of continuing therapy as prescribed. Discontinuation of therapy may result in drug resistance, reversal of clinical improvement, and increased susceptibility of family members to tuberculosis.
5. Usual adult dose: 600 mg daily, either 1 hour before or 2 hours after meals. Rifampin is available in 300-mg capsules.

The physician prescribes the medicine and treatment.
The nurse carries out the physician's orders.
Self-medication is dangerous. Consult your physician first.
There is in every medicine a possible danger.
When in doubt—ASK!

ASSIGNMENT

Review previous lessons and questions according to the directions of your instructor.

1. Define antimicrobial agents and tell the origins of antimicrobial agents. What are antimicrobial agents derived from other living microorganisms called? What was the original source of penicillin? Explain the source and processing of most antibiotics used today. What is the purpose of the chemical modification?
2. What is the basis for selection of an antimicrobial agent? What points must be considered in this selection?
3. List three groups of side effects common to all antimicrobial agents. Completely explain each group. Are nausea, vomiting, or diarrhea symptoms of allergy? Are these symptoms common side effects of antimicrobial agents? What is often a cause of these symptoms? Do they disappear? Do they usually require discontinuation of therapy?
4. The aminoglycosides (several choices are correct)
   a. Are used primarily against gram-positive microorganisms
   b. Are used primarily against gram-negative microorganisms that cause urinary tract infections, meningitis, wound infections, and life-threatening septicemias
   c. Can be considered a mainstay in the treatment of hospital-acquired gram-negative infections
   d. Have a high rate of severe allergic reactions
   e. Rarely give any allergic reactions, so it is not necessary

to ask the patient about any allergies before administration of this antibiotic
   f. Rarely cause any serious reaction
   g. May cause ototoxicity or nephrotoxicity, particularly if the antibiotic is administered in high dosages or for longer than 10 days
   h. May cause such symptoms as ototoxicity or nephrotoxicity, which usually disappear quickly and are of little consequence, so they do not need to be reported to the physician or head nurse
   i. Sometimes cause such symptoms as ototoxicity or nephrotoxicity, which always appear only during administration of the drug
5. Give four examples of the aminoglycosides, using both the generic and brand name for each example (see Table 23-1).
6. The cephalosporins may be used as an alternate to which group of antibiotics? Name the medical conditions the cephalosporins are used to treat. Are side effects major or minor problems? Name three common side effects of cephalosporins. Are allergic reactions possible? What question must you ask the patient before administering this, or any, antibiotic? What is the name of the preferred test for glucose in the urine during therapy with this drug? Why?
7. Name five cephalosporins in common use. Your instructor will help you in this selection. Use both generic and brand names for each selection (see Table 23-2).
8. What is the name of the group of antibiotics that were the

first true antibiotics to be grown and used against pathogenic bacteria in human beings?

9. How do penicillins act? This makes them effective against what bacterial process? What is the name of the naturally occurring parent compound of the penicillin group? What are the uses of penicillin? What question must you ask the patient before starting penicillin therapy? What type of patient is apt to be most susceptible to penicillin? With the aid of your instructor, select from Table 23-3 six of the most commonly used penicillins, using both generic and brand names for each selection. Your instructor will tell you which dosage selections you should remember.

10. Are the sulfonamides true antibiotics? If not, why not? What are the main uses of sulfonamides? How do sulfonamides act? Do they have many side effects? Which are the most common side effects? Should rashes be ignored or reported? Why? What laboratory tests are essential for the patient receiving sulfonamides longer than 14 days? Which test for glucose in the urine is preferred for the diabetic patient receiving sulfonamides? Why? Why should the patient receiving sulfonamides be encouraged to drink several 8-oz glasses of water daily during sulfonamide therapy and probably several days after discontinuance of this therapy? With the aid of your instructor, select from Table 23-4 five of the most commonly used sulfonamides, using both generic and brand names in your selection of each drug. Your instructor will tell you which dosage selections you should remember.

11. The tetracyclines (several choices are correct)
    a. Are effective against both gram-negative and gram-positive organisms and against rickettsial and mycoplasmic infections
    b. Act by inhibiting protein synthesis by bacterial cells
    c. Can rarely be used as a substitute for patients allergic to penicillins for the treatment of certain venereal diseases, urinary tract infections, upper respiratory infections, pneumonia, and meningitis
    d. So rarely cause any allergic reactions that it is not necessary to ask the patient about any allergy to medications
    e. May cause a severe sunburn to the patient, so bright sunlight should be avoided during its administration
    f. Should not be used during the last half of pregnancy, infancy, and childhood to 8 years of age, since permanent staining of the teeth may result
    g. Are not secreted in milk of lactating women, so it is safe to continue nursing while taking tetracyclines
    h. Should be administered 1 hour before or 2 hours after the ingestion of iron, milk, food, and antacids, since these products inhibit the absorption of tetracycline
    i. May cause a false positive reaction for glucose in the urine if Tes-Tape is used

12. With the aid of your instructor, select from Table 23-5 four of the most commonly used tetracyclines, using both generic and brand names in your selectioin of each drug. Your instructor will tell you which dosage selections you should remember.

13. How does chloramphenicol act? For which conditions is it particularly effective? Should it be used for trivial infections, colds, influenza, and sore throat? Why not? What serious and possible fatal bone marrow suppression may occur with the use of this drug? What are early signs of this possibility, and what should be your action? What question must you ask the patient before administration of this drug? Which test is preferred when determining glucose content in the urine for the diabetic patient receiving chloramphenicol? Why? What is the usual adult dose of chloramphenicol?

14. How does clindamycin act? For which infections is it useful? What is a serious side effect of this drug? Is the use of Lomotil, loperamide, or paregoric helpful in overcoming this serious side effect? Why not? What drug may be effective in overcoming diarrhea caused by this drug? What question should you ask the patient before administration of clindamycin?

15. Erythromycin may be used as an alternative antibiotic for those patients allergic to what other antibiotic? How does it act? Name the medical conditions for which it is used. What question must you ask the patient before administration of this or any antibiotic? Can allergic symptoms develop during erythromycin therapy? What symptoms would advise discontinuance of this drug? List some common side effects of erythromycin. What is the adult dose?

16. Name four additional antibiotics discussed and tell the main uses of each. What type of antibiotic are griseofulvin and nystatin? Does griseofulvin kill the fungus? What is its action? How does nystatin achieve its effect?

17. To which group of antimicrobial agents does ethambutol belong? Why must ethambutol be used in combination with other antitubercular agents? List all the side effects of this drug. Why must the need to continue therapy with this drug be explained to the patient? What is the dosage range of this drug?

18. What is the one use of isoniazid? Should it be used in combination with other antitubercular agents? Why? List the side effects of this drug. What drug is recommended for daily administration while the patient is receiving isoniazid? Why? Which test should be used for glucose in the urine? Why? Why must nurses emphasize to patients the need for continuing therapy with isoniazid? What is the usual adult dose?

19. How is rifampin used against tuberculosis? How does it act? What color may it tinge the urine, feces, saliva, sputum, sweat, and tears? Should patients by taught this? Is there any pathologic damage caused by this color change? What advice should be given to female patients before they take rifampin concerning oral contraceptives? Why? Why must nurses emphasize to patients the importance of continuing therapy? What is the usual adult dose of rifampin?

20. The physician ordered an oral, 500-mg dose of sulfisoxazole (Gantrisin) to be administered to his patient. What dose in *grams* would you be administering if you gave the 500-mg tablet? (See Index for converting milligrams to grams.)

21. The physician ordered an oral, 250-mg dose of oxytetracycline (Terramycin) to be administered to his patient. You have on hand 125-mg capsules. How many capsules will you administer?

CHAPTER 24

Vitamins, minerals, and electrolytes

Vitamins, by definition, are a group of chemicals needed in the human diet for metabolism. The absence of these substances results in malnutrition and specific deficiency diseases. Vitamins are not sources of energy, but they are indispensable for normal functions and the maintenance of health. Most vitamins are not synthesized by the body and must be applied by adequate nutrition. The Food and Nutrition Board of the National Academy of Sciences–National Research Council has been charged with the responsibility of evaluating the vitamin and nutritional requirements of the American populace. This board periodically publishes a brochure that contains a set of "recommended dietary allowances" (RDA) (see Table 24-1). These have replaced the minimum daily requirement (MDR). The RDA is just what it indicates—a recommended allowance of nutritional needs in essentially healthy adults in the United States under current standards of living. The board emphasizes that it is not a minimum requirement. The RDA is calculated to allow the differences resulting from individual variation and is estimated to exceed the requirements of most individuals, thereby ensuring that the needs of nearly everyone are met. The RDA is not designed to meet vitamin requirements of patients with chronic illness or to consider vitamins lost in cooking.

Those who need vitamin supplementation are patients with (1) inadequate food intake as a result of dieting, chronically poor appetite, alcoholism, or food restriction for religious beliefs or for the control of other diseases; (2) poor absorption, resulting from chronic diarrhea, long-term use of antibiotics, or gastrointestinal surgery; and (3) increased nutritional needs, such as during pregnancy and lactation, growth, and frequent periods of hard physical activity.

Vitamin A

1. Vitamin A is essential to promote normal growth and development of bones and teeth, to maintain the health of epithelial body tissues, and to aid in maintaining normal vision and preventing night blindness. The use of vitamin A has also been proposed for the treatment of acne, for enhancement of wound healing, and for prevention of infection. Clinical studies have not supported these uses, however.

2. The carotene of plants supplies the provitamin from which the body tissues prepare vitamin A. Animal fats, such as those found in milk, eggs, butter, fish, and liver, are also sources of the carotenoids, which are originally derived from plants and then stored in the animal tissues.

3. Efficient absorption of vitamin A is depedent on fat absorption and on the presence of adequate bile salts in the intestine. Obstructive jaundice, malabsorption syndrome, and the presence of mineral oil in the intestines may diminish vitamin A absorption.

4. Hypervitaminosis A is now being reported more frequently because of consumer interest in health food supplementation. Prolonged daily dosages over 25,000 IU should be under close medical supervision. Fatigue, malaise, and lethargy, followed by nausea, throbbing headaches, insomnia, brittle nails, loss of body hair, and rough, scaly skin, are all signs of chronic vitamin A toxicity.

5. Vitamin A is available in various concentrations in the form of tablets, capsules, lozenges, drops, and parenteral injection. Many brands are available.

6. Vitamin A deficiency may be treated orally with 100,000 IU daily for 3 days, followed by 50,000 IU daily for 2 weeks.

Vitamin B₁ (thiamine) (thy′ah-min)

1. Thiamine is a coenzyme necessary for carbohydrate metabolism. Natural sources include the hull of rice, fresh peas and beans, beef, and pork.

2. Thiamine deficiency results in beriberi, a disease that affects the nervous and cardiovascular systems. Beriberi is commonly seen in regions where the diet consists primarily of polished rice.

3. Signs of thiamine deficiency become evident within 2 to 3 weeks after thiamine ingestion is stopped. In the Western world this is most commonly seen in the alcoholic who is nutritionally deficient.

4. Usual adult dose, for treatment of beriberi: 10 to 20 mg intramuscularly three times daily for 2 weeks.

Table 24-1. United States recommended dietary allowances*

	Unit	Infants (0-12 mo.)	Children under 4 yrs.	Adults and children 4 or more yrs.	Pregnant or lactating women
Vitamin A	μg retinol equivalents	400-420	400	500-1000	1000-1400
Vitamin D	μg	10	10	5-10	10-15
Vitamin E	mg α-tocopherol equivalents	3-4	5	6-10	10-11
Vitamin C	mg	35	45	45-60	80-100
Folacin	μg	30-45	100	200-400	500-800
Thiamine (B_1)	mg	0.3-0.5	0.7	0.9-1.5	1.4-1.6
Riboflavin (B_2)	mg	0.4-0.6	0.8	1.0-1.7	1.6-1.8
Niacin	mg niacin equivalents	6-8	9	11-19	15-20
Vitamin B_6	mg	0.3-0.6	0.9	1.3-2.2	2.5-2.6
Vitamin B_{12}	μg	0.5-1.5	2	2.5-3.0	4
Biotin	μg	35-50	65	85-200	—
Pantothenic acid	mg	2-3	3	3-7	—
Calcium	mg	360-540	800	800-1200	1200-1600
Phosphorus	mg	250-360	800	800-1200	1200-1600
Iodine	μg	40-50	70	90-150	175-200
Iron	mg	10-15	15	10-18	†
Magnesium	mg	50-70	150	200-400	450
Copper	mg	0.5-1.0	1.0-1.5	1.5-3.0	—
Zinc	mg	3-5	10	10-15	20-25

*Modified from Recommended dietary allowances, ed. 9, Washington, D.C., 1980, National Academy of Sciences–National Research Council.
†Use of 30 to 60 mg of supplemental iron is recommended.

Vitamin B₂ (riboflavin) (ri-bo-fla'vin)

1. Vitamin B_2 is an essential coenzyme necessary for cell growth. The body's need for riboflavin is increased during periods of increased cell growth, such as during pregnancy. Natural source of vitamin B_2 are eggs, meat, milk, fish, and liver.
2. Vitamin B_2 deficiency is manifested by sore throat, cheilosis, angular stomatitis, and later, generalized dermatitis. Deficiency is rarely seen outside the nutritionally deficient alcoholic population.
3. Usual therapeutic dose: orally, 10 mg daily. Larger doses are occasionally used but do not provide additional benefit. Excess riboflavin is excreted in the urine, imparting a bright yellow color to it. Vitamin B_2 is also available for IM injection.

Vitamin B₆ (pyridoxine) (peer-i-dok'seen)

1. Vitamin B_6 acts as a coenzyme in the metabolism of fat, carbohydrate, and protein. Vitamin B_6 deficiency results in seizure activity in infants and in dermatitis, peripheral neuropathy, diminished mental function, and oral sores in adults. It is often difficult to distinguish between niacin, riboflavin, and pyridoxine deficiencies.
2. Several drugs inhibit the action of vitamin B_6. Patients receiving isoniazid, cycloserine (antitubercular drugs), hydralazine, or penicillamine should be observed for vitamin B_6 deficiency. Patients requiring isoniazid or cycloserine are routinely placed on vitamin B_6 therapy as well.
3. Vitamin B_6 may antagonize the pharmacologic activity of levodopa, an antiparkinsonian agent. Patients treated with levodopa should avoid supplemental vitamins that contain more than 5 mg of vitamin B_6 in the daily dose.
4. Vitamin B_6 dietary deficiency is treated orally with 10 to 20 mg daily for 3 weeks. Follow-up treatment is recommended daily for several weeks with an oral multivitamin containing 2 to 5 mg of vitamin B_6. Patients should correct poor dietary habits and adhere to an adequate, well-balanced diet. Patients receiving isoniazid therapy should also receive 50 mg of vitamin B_6 daily. Vitamin B_6 is available as tablets, capsules, and in solution for parenteral injection.

Vitamin B₁₂ (cyanocobalamin) (sy-ah-no-ko-bal'ah-min)

1. Vitamin B_{12} is essential for growth, cell reproduction, hematopoiesis, and myelin synthesis. It is also necessary for the incorporation of folic acid into cells. Meat protein is the primary source of vitamin B_{12}.
2. Pernicious anemia develops if there is a deficiency of vitamin B_{12}. Deficiencies secondary to malabsorption induced by regional enteritis, celiac disease, idiopathic steatorrhea, or surgical removal of portions of the stomach and small intestine are most common.

Occasionally, pernicious anemia will develop in a patient on a vegetarian diet.
3. Deficiencies are manifested by numbness of the hands and feet, poor muscular coordination, mental confusion, agitation, and possible psychosis.
4. Those deficiencies developing from inadequate nutrition may be treated orally, with 10 to 15 μg daily. Those patients with intestinal malabsorption are treated intramuscularly with 30 μg daily for 5 to 10 days, followed by 100 to 200 μg monthly.

Vitamin C (ascorbic acid) (as-kor'bik)

1. Vitamin C is an essential vitamin in human beings; however, its exact biologic actions are not fully documented. It does play a role in the chemical reactions necessary for cellular respiration and is necessary for the formation and the maintenance of intercellular ground substance and collagen.
2. Deficiency of vitamin C results in scurvy, a disease that causes degenerative changes in capillaries, bone, and connective tissue. Scurvy can be prevented by 50 mg of vitamin C daily, a quantity readily attained in a normal diet containing fresh fruits and vegetables. It is therefore seen only in cases of inappropriate nutrition. Infants fed artificial formulas without vitamin supplementation may also develop scurvy.
3. Vitamin C has been recommended for the prevention and treatment of the common cold. After reviewing the literature available, the Department of Drugs of the American Medical Association has concluded that little evidence exists to support the use of vitamin C against the common cold.
4. Vitamin C is routinely used as a urinary acidifier for patients taking methenamine compounds. The acid environment created converts methenamine to formaldehyde, a germicidal agent useful in preventing recurrent urinary tract infections. This urinary acidification causes a greater reabsorption of aspirin from the renal tubules back into circulation and will cause greater urinary excretion of basic drugs, such as the tricyclic antidepressants, quinidine, the amphetamines, and the aminoglycosides.
5. Usual therapeutic dose for treatment of scurvy: 100 mg or more daily. Urinary acidification requires at least 500 mg four times daily. The pH of the urine should be checked several times daily to determine if the vitamin C dose is adequate. Optimal pH for methenamine-formaldehyde activity is 4.5 to 5.0.

Vitamin D

1. Vitamin D is a collective name for a series of compounds required by the body for the functional use of calcium, phosphorus, and magnesium. The primary source for most vitamin D is sunlight. Vitamin D is synthesized from sterols in the skin when irradiated with sunlight. If sunlight exposure is not adequate, vitamin D must be supplemented in the diet.
2. Food sources of vitamin D are fish liver oils and irradiated yeast. Most milk products and cereals are fortified with vitamin D. A deficiency of vitamin D results in rickets, osteomalacia, or tetany. Vitamin D deficiency is quite rare in the general population, but patients with malabsorption syndromes, short bowel syndromes, renal disease, or hypoparathyroidism are quite susceptible to this deficiency.
3. The optimum daily dose must be carefully determined for each patient when a true deficiency exists. Excess vitamin D may result in hypercalcemia, cardiac arrhythmias, and further renal failure. Patients should avoid taking mineral oil while ingesting therapeutic doses of vitamin D, since mineral oil may diminish the absorption of this group of compounds.

Vitamin E

1. Vitamin E is another vitamin that is essential for normal metabolic activity but whose exact mechanisms of action have eluded investigators. The absolute daily requirement has not been established. Natural sources of vitamin E are nuts and cereal and vegetable oils, especially safflower oil.
2. Vitamin E deficiency develops in infants fed with commercial formulas low in vitamin E and in patients with malabsorption diseases secondary to sprue, cystic fibrosis, pancreatitis, and biliary cirrhosis.
3. Therapeutic dosage for both infants and adults: 100 IU daily for several weeks. Vitamin E preparations are available in drops, chewable tablets, capsules, elixir, and parenteral dosage forms.
4. If vitamin E is prescribed for an infant, it should not be taken at the same time as any prescribed iron supplements, since they apparently inhibit absorption of vitamin E.

Folic acid

1. Folic acid is a vitamin required for protein synthesis and production of red blood cells. It is present in the normal diet from fresh fruits and vegetables, yeast, and liver.
2. Folic acid deficiency readily occurs from improper diet. Early symptoms include sore mouth, diarrhea, irritability, and mental confusion. Examination of the red blood cells will frequently indicate that a megaloblastic anemia has also developed.
3. Folic acid absorption and utilization can be impaired by several drugs. Patients taking phenytoin, trimethoprim, oral contraceptives, methotrexate, and pyrimethamine on a long-term or recurrent basis should be monitored periodically for folic acid deficiency.

4. The symptoms of a megaloblastic anemia from folic acid deficiency are quite similar to a pernicious anemia induced by vitamin B_{12} deficiency. Attempted correction of a pernicious anemia with folic acid will result in further damage to the central nervous system as a result of the vitamin B_{12} deficiency. If a vitamin deficiency is suspected, the patient must not attempt to treat the deficiency with over-the-counter vitamins.

5. Usual dose for treatment of a folic acid deficiency: orally, 1 mg daily. Doses above 1 mg daily are excreted in the urine and are unnecessary.

Niacin (ny'ah-sin) (nicotinic acid) (ni-ko-ti'nik)

1. Niacin is a constituent of two primary enzymes necessary for the transfer of electrons in chemical reactions within the cell. A deficiency of niacin results in pellagra, a disease manifested by peripheral neuropathies, diarrhea, dementia, and dermatitis (the ''3 Ds'' of niacin deficiency). Foods rich in niacin are beef, cow's milk, and whole eggs.

2. Niacin has also been used to lower serum lipid concentrations and as a vasodilator in patients with vascular disease. The dosages required for therapeutic response are usually associated with serious adverse effects, such as cholestatic jaundice, hyperuricemia, and gastritis.

3. Niacin deficiency is treated orally with 300 to 500 mg daily in divided doses, taken with meals to reduce gastritis. Available dosage forms of niacin are tablets, capsules, timed-released capsules, an elixir, and a solution for parenteral injection.

Vitamin K

Vitamin K is discussed elsewhere in the text (see Index).

MULTIPLE VITAMINS

Multiple vitamins contain several vitamins and minerals in one tablet, capsule, or liquid preparation. They are used for patients with dietary deficiencies, multiple vitamin deficiencies, or impaired gastrointestinal absorption or for patients who have increased metabolic needs, such as pregnant or lactating patients. A multiple vitamin supplement should be selected based on the number of vitamins in the product and whether they provide the RDA. There are many multiple vitamin products available, with a wide range in cost. Asking your pharmacist for a recommendation and then comparing ingredients and prices is a good way to find a suitable product. A word of caution, however—never try to diagnose or treat a vitamin deficiency without your physician's advice.

MINERALS AND ELECTROLYTES

Minerals are elements occurring in nature that are essential constituents of all living cells. They are excreted daily from the body and must be replaced by ingestion of food and water. Requirements are greater for growing children, pregnant women, and patients with certain pathologic conditions. The Food and Nutrition Board of the National Academy of Sciences–National Research Council has also published a list of recommended dietary allowances for certain minerals (see Table 24-1). As with vitamins, the RDAs for minerals are based on the nutritional needs of essentially healthy adults in the United States under current standards of living and are not designed to meet the requirements of patients with chronic illness. There are no RDAs for such minerals as sodium, chlorine, fluorine, manganese, sulfur, or potassium; nutritional requirements for these elements are highly dependent on a particular patient's medical condition and must be monitored closely by the physician. Minerals discussed in this chapter are copper, iron, and zinc, although many other minerals, such as selenium, manganese, magnesium, and cobalt, are also essential.

Many minerals serve a dual role as electrolytes. The body fluid consists mainly of water and dissolved minerals that are capable of an electrical activity when ionized. These substances are termed electrolytes because they give off electrical charges, some positive and others negative. They establish an electrical balance when correctly distributed in the circulating fluid. Electrical currents generated are also essential for such standard activities of the body as conduction of nerve impulses, beating of the heart, absorption of food from the gastrointestinal tract, and muscular contraction.

Body fluid is distributed into two compartments: (1) the internal cell (cellular) and (2) the area surrounding the cell (extracellular), in a ratio of 3:1. The exchange of water, electrolytes, and other dissolved chemicals between these areas is a continual body process influenced by the electrical potential between cells and their environment. This ratio of fluids and electrolytes must be maintained for the body to function normally. Certain organs in the body monitor this exchange, such as kidneys, endocrine glands, and lungs. When any of these organs break down, the physician must intervene.

The primary electrolytes and their symbols are potassium (K), sodium (Na), calcium (Ca), and chloride (Cl).

Calcium

1. Calcium is a primary constituent of bones and teeth and is essential for muscle contractions, nerve conduction, and blood coagulation.

2. Calcium supplements are often required in pregnancy and lactation, long-term treatment with corticosteroids, hypoparathyroidism, and certain malabsorption syndromes. It is also used for immediate cardiac stimulation, but it must be used with extreme caution in patients also receiving digitalis glycosides such as digoxin or digitoxin.

3. Commonly used products for calcium administration are calcium chloride, calcium lactate, calcium gluconate, calcium glubionate, and calcium phosphate.

Copper

1. Copper is a constituent of all human tissues. The highest concentrations occur in the brain, kidneys, heart, liver, and pancreas. It is essential for the synthesis of hemoglobin and is a component of several enzyme systems.
2. The only deficiencies that develop are in patients who are fed entirely by IV parenteral nutrition. Supplementation of the IV fluid with trace minerals is mandatory for adequate metablism.

Iron

1. Iron is essential for hemoglobin formation and for many chemical reactions in living tissues.
2. The most common way of losing iron from the body to such an extent that anemia develops is by blood loss. This could be the sudden blood loss of an acute large hemorrhage or the gradual loss that might occur from hemorrhoids, a silent ulcer, or a tumor of the gastrointestinal tract. The major problem, apart from replacing the iron, is to find the source of blood loss.
3. Iron preparations have irritant properties that may cause nausea, vomiting, constipation, diarrhea, and abdominal distress. They should be administered after meals to prevent some of these symptoms.
4. Oral preparations of iron will usually cause the stool to be dull black; patients should be informed of this.
5. Iron preparations include:
   a. **Ferrous sulfate (Feosol).** Ferrous sulfate is one of the most common, least expensive iron preparations available.
   b. **Ferrous gluconate (Fergon).** Ferrous gluconate is occasionally recommended for patients who cannot tolerate ferrous sulfate.
   c. **Iron dextran injection (Imferon).**
      (1) Imferon is available in 2- and 5-ml ampules in a 10-ml vial for deep IM injection into the gluteal muscles. Do not use the 10-ml ampule for IV use.
      (2) The subcutaneous tissue should be pushed aside before insertion of the needle to prevent leakage along the tract of the needle. (This is often called the Z, or zigzag, technique.) A fresh needle placed on the syringe just before injection helps to assure that no drops from the needle penetrate the skin during injection and often prevents skin discoloration and soreness at the needle site. Adequate student and graduate nurse supervision for the first few injections of this drug prevents many of the administration problems.
      (3) Initial dose: usually 50 mg the first day. This may be increased gradually thereafter until amounts up to 250 mg may be administered daily or every 2 days until blood studies show the desired response has been obtained.

Potassium

1. Potassium is the principal intracellular electrolyte of most body tissues. Potassium is essential for contraction of cardiac, skeletal, and smooth muscle, for nerve conduction, and for normal renal function.
2. Potassium depletion may develop slowly from excess excretion by diuretics, long-term use of corticosteroids, diabetic ketoacidosis, hyperaldosteronism, severe diarrhea, or inadequate replacement by maintenance IV fluid therapy.
3. Potassium may be replaced orally or intravenously.
   a. Oral therapy is used to replace potassium lost by the use of thiazide diuretics, corticosteroids, or testosterone. Diluted liquid preparations taken with food are most effective in reducing gastric irritation that may accompany oral potassium therapy. A few oral potassium chloride products are **Kay Ciel, Kaon,** and **Klorvess.**
   b. Intravenous therapy is used to replace acute losses from severe diarrhea or in those patients who do not have an adequate oral intake, such as postsurgical patients. Potassium chloride is usually used for parenteral therapy, although potassium phosphate may also be used in certain clinical situations.
4. Dosages for potassium therapy will be dependent on each patient's requirements. It is essential that the patient understand the need for adherence to the prescribed therapy and to report to the physician any discomfort that may develop while undergoing potassium therapy.

Sodium and Chloride

1. Sodium and chloride are the principal electrolytes of the extracellular fluid. They are essential for the maintenance of fluids between the intracellular and extracellular compartments of the body.
2. Historically, sodium chloride (saline) solutions have been named in terms of "normality."
   a. Normal saline is 0.9% sodium chloride. It is approximately equal to the sodium concentration of blood. It is used to restore both water and sodium chloride losses.
   b. Half-normal saline ($\frac{1}{2}$ normal) is 0.45% sodium chloride. This solution provides fluid replacement when fluid losses exceed sodium chloride losses.
   c. Quarter-normal saline ($\frac{1}{4}$ normal) contains 0.2% sodium chloride. This solution is most commonly used for maintenance fluid therapy and to prevent

excessive losses of water, sodium, and chloride when oral intake is inadequate to meet metabolic needs.

Zinc

1. Zinc is an essential element in metabolism. It participates in several vital enzyme systems, is necessary for wound healing, and is present with insulin in the pancreas.
2. Zinc supplementation is most important for patients with inadequate diet, with chronic, nonhealing wounds, and with wounds from major trauma or surgery.
3. Therapeutic zinc replacements should be administered with meals in divided doses rather than once daily since zinc is an irritant and may cause nausea and vomiting.
4. Zinc sulfate supplements are available in tablet, capsule, and parenteral forms.

**The physician prescribes the medicine and treatment.
The nurse carries out the physician's orders.
Self-medication is dangerous. Consult your physician first.
There is in every medicine a possible danger.
When in doubt—ASK!**

ASSIGNMENT

Review previous lessons and questions according to the direction of your instructor.

1. Define the term vitamin.
2. What conditions occur as a result of vitamin absence?
3. What is the function of the Food and Nutrition Board of the National Academy of Sciences in relation to vitamins?
4. What is meant by the abbreviations RDA and MDR?
5. Which conditions require vitamin supplementation?
6. Why is vitamin A essential? The carotenoids from which vitamin A is obtained are found in what foods? What conditions may diminish vitamin A absorption? List the symptoms that may occur with prolonged daily overdosage of vitamin A.
7. What is another term for vitamin B_1? What is thiamine? List the natural sources of vitamin B_1 (thiamine). What is the result of thiamine deficiency? Where is the condition commonly seen and why?
8. What is vitamin B_2 (riboflavin)? At what times are the body's needs of vitamin B_2 increased? List the natural sources of vitamin B_2. What are the symptoms of vitamin B_2 deficiency? What is the usual therapeutic dose? What changes will excess riboflavin cause in the urine? Should this be explained to the patient?
9. How does vitamin B_6 (pyridoxine) act? What conditions develop as a result of vitamin B_6 deficiency? Name the drugs that may inhibit the action of vitamin B_6. What effect does vitamin B_6 have on levodopa, a drug used for Parkinson's disease? In addition to the administration of vitamin B_6, what other therapy is essential to overcome vitamin B_6 deficiencies? Is this true for all other vitamin deficiencies?
10. For what conditions is vitamin B_{12} essential? What is the primary source of vitamin B_{12}? What condition develops if there is a deficiency of vitamin B_{12}? List the deficiency symptoms for this vitamin.
11. For what conditions in the human body does vitamin C (ascorbic acid) play a role? What disease is the result of vitamin C deficiency? What food sources will prevent or overcome this disease? What is the danger of feeding infants artificial formulas without vitamin supplementation? What is the conclusion of the Department of Drugs of the American Medical Association in regard to the use of vitamin C to lessen or prevent colds? Explain the routine use of vitamin C with methenamine compounds. What does the urinary acidification cause when vitamin C is administered with such drugs as aspirin, tricyclic antidepressants, quinidine, and the amphetamines? What is the usual dose of vitamin C for treatment of scurvy? What is the dose for urinary acidification? How often should the pH of the urine be checked, and for what reason?
12. What is vitamin D? What is the primary source of vitamin D? If sunlight exposure is not adequate, what is the appropriate therapy? List the food sources of vitamin D. What medical conditions are a result of vitamin D deficiency? What medical conditions may result from excess vitamin D dosage? What drug is contraindicated for the patient taking vitamin D, and why?
13. Vitamin E is essential for what body condition? List the natural sources of vitamin E. In what medical conditions may vitamin E deficiency develop? If vitamin E is pre-

scribed for an infant, it should not be taken at the same time as what other drug? Why?

14. What effects does folic acid have on the body? List its natural sources. What is a common cause of folic acid deficiency? List the symptoms of folic acid deficiency. List the drugs taken on a long-term or recurrent basis that may cause folic acid deficiency. What are the symptoms of megaloblastic anemia from folic acid deficiency?

15. Define niacin (nicotinic acid). List the symptoms that may develop as a result of niacin deficiency. List the food sources of niacin. What other uses are there for niacin? What complications may occur with therapeutic dosages of niacin? Why is it taken with meals?

16. What is the main use of vitamin K? (See Index).

17. In your selection of a multiple vitamin preparation at the pharmacy, what three cautions should you follow?

18. Define minerals and tell how they are excreted and replaced by the body. What board publishes a list of recommended dietary allowances (RDA) for certain minerals? Explain on what the recommendations of this Board are based. List seven minerals considered essential for nutrition. Many minerals serve a dual role as electrolytes. Explain the process of electrolytes. List the primary electrolytes, including the symbol for each.

19. Why is calcium essential for the body? For what conditions are calcium supplements necessary? What is its immediate cardiac effect? It must be used with extreme caution in patients receiving which other drugs? List four commonly used products for calcium administration.

20. The highest concentrations of copper are found where in the body? Copper is essential for what purposes in the body? In what condition will the only deficiencies develop? How can this deficiency be prevented?

21. Why is iron essential in the human body? What is the most common way of losing iron from the body? What conditions could cause this blood loss? Apart from replacing the iron, what is the major problem in this blood loss? What symptoms may iron preparations cause, and how can some of these symptoms be controlled or prevented? What is the appearance of the stool from oral iron preparations? Should patients be informed of this? Name three iron preparations. Explain the precautions in injecting iron dextran injection (Imferon). May the student or graduate nurses administer their first few iron dextran injections without supervision, especially if they have administered several subq and IM injections?

22. Where is potassium, the electrolyte, found in the body? For what is it essential? List the conditions which may cause potassium depletion. How is oral therapy used to replace potassium lost by the use of thiazide diuretics, corticosteroids, or testosterone? Name four oral potassium products. For what conditions IV therapy with potassium used? Why is it essential that the patient understand the need for adherence to potassium therapy?

23. Sodium and chloride are the principal electrolytes of what part of the body system? For what are they essential? What percent sodium chloride is normal saline? What in the body does it approximate? What are its uses? Name two other saline solutions, tell their approximation to normal, and tell the main use of each.

24. Zinc is an essential element in _____. It participates in several _____, is necessary for _____, and is present with _____. Zinc supplementation is most important for what medical conditions? Why should zinc be administered with meals in divided doses?

CHAPTER 25

Antiseptics and disinfectants

Antiseptics (bacteriostatics) are substances that inhibit the growth of microorganisms. Disinfectants (germicides) are substances that destroy microorganisms. A disinfectant can be an antiseptic if it is in a weak enough solution, but an antiseptic cannot be a disinfectant. The disinfectant (germicidal) effectiveness of a solution depends on the strength of the solution, the temperature of the solution, the degree of ionization (mechanism of action), and the length of time the solution has been in contact with the infected material or tissue.

THE ALCOHOLS

1. As a chemical group, the alcohols possess many desirable features of a disinfectant. They are bactericidal, are relatively inexpensive, have a cleansing action, and readily evaporate.
2. Alcohols apparently act by destroying proteins within microorganisms.
3. Alcohols are used most frequently to prepare the skin prior to venipuncture, subq and IM injection, and ear or finger pricks for blood samples. They are also effective for swabbing down flat surfaces and cleaning thermometers. Alcohols are not very effective on rough surfaces or surfaces contaminated with blood or pus. They are also not effective against bacterial spores.
4. Products:
   a. **Ethyl alcohol.** This is most effective in concentrations of 50% to 70%.
   b. **Isopropyl alcohol.** Commonly known as "rubbing alcohol," it is most effective in 70% to 75% concentrations. Isopropyl alcohol is also used to remove oils or fats from the skin.

THE CHLORINE COMPOUNDS

1. Chlorine is a greenish yellow gas that is very irritating and has a characteristic odor. It does not exist in the free state in nature. Numerous chlorine compounds may be used as disinfectants, however, because chlorine is liberated. Very small amounts (1 part of chlorine in 1 million parts of water) will destroy most bacteria in a few minutes.
2. Although the chlorine compounds have been studied

extensively, their mechanism of action is unknown.
3. Products:
   a. **Halazone.** Halazone is used as a disinfectant for contaminated water, especially water contaminated with *Escherichia coli* and typhoid fever. Two 4-mg tablets added to a liter of water will destroy bacteria in 30 to 60 minutes.
   b. **Sodium hypochlorite (modified Dakin's solution, Clorox).** The hypochlorites are the oldest and most widely used chlorine compounds for disinfection. They are used as deodorizers and sanitizers for restaurants, food processing plants, dairies, sewage plants, and in swimming pools and drinking water. A 0.5% solution of sodium hypochlorite may be used to disinfect walls, furniture, and floors.

THE IODINES

1. Iodine and iodine compounds have been used as antiseptics since the late 1800s. Iodines act by destroying protein, thus killing bacteria, fungi, viruses, yeast, and protozoa.
2. Iodine and compounds that release iodine have a variety of uses. These solutions may be used to sterilize instruments, disinfect small wounds and skin abrasions, prepare skin preoperatively, and disinfect drinking water as an emergency measure.
3. Disadvantages of the iodines include allergic reactions and staining of clothing and skin.
4. Products:
   a. **Iodine tincture.** This preparation contains 2% iodine and 2.4% sodium iodide in 46% ethyl alcohol. It is used most frequently as a disinfectant for cuts and abrasions.
   b. **Iodine solution.** This contains the same concentrations of iodine and sodium iodide found in iodine tincture, but they are dissolved in sterile water. It is less irritating to the skin but stains more readily and dries more slowly.
5. The *iodophors* are complex combinations of iodine and a carrier that slowly release free iodine when diluted with water.
   a. **Povidone-iodine solution (Betadine, PVP, Iso-**

dine). This iodophor is a complex of iodine and polyvinylpyrrolidone that is water soluble. The complex breaks down on contact with the skin or mucous membranes, and free iodine is slowly released. This combination provides the disinfectant properties of iodine and the antibacterial properties of povidone. It is routinely used in most hospitals as a presurgical disinfectant for both the patient and the surgical team members. It is available as a soap, an aerosol, an ointment, an antiseptic gauze pad, and a solution. It does not stain as do other iodine compounds.

THE MERCURIALS

1. Although the mercurials have been used as antiseptics since the turn of the century, they are far from ideal germicides. They irritate the tissues, penetrate poorly, and may be toxic to the patient if absorbed internally.
2. The mercurials do have a distinct advantage over other disinfectants because they penetrate and kill spores. Their mechanism of action appears to be that of enzyme inhibition. The mercurials are now used primarily as antiseptics against common skin bacterial and fungal pathogens.
3. Products:
   a. **Ammoniated mercury ointment.** Ammoniated mercury is used in ointments of 2% to 10% concentrations as antiseptics in parasitic skin diseases, such as impetigo.
   b. **Thimerosal (Merthiolate).** Thimerosal is still frequently used as a household first-aid product for minor cuts and abrasions. It is available as an aerosol, cream, ointment, solution, and tincture.

THE PHENOLS

1. The phenolic compounds have been the most extensively used disinfectants and antiseptics. For many years they were the standard against which all other disinfectants were compared. The phenols act through inhibition of key enzyme systems and destruction of cell walls.
2. Phenol is also used in soothing lotions and ointments because it penetrates the skin and anesthetizes local nerve endings.
3. The use of phenols has declined over the past 2 decades because of better product development. These improved products are less irritating to tissues and more effective against bacterial spores and viruses than the phenols.
4. Phenolic derivatives still in use:
   a. **Hexachlorophene (pHisoHex, WescoHex, Septisol).** Hexachlorophene is a white powder added to water, soaps, and detergents. It is frequently used

as a presurgical scrub and as an antibacterial agent in certain dermatologic conditions. Cumulative antibacterial action develops with frequent use. Hexachlorophene is less effective in the presence of alcohol, blood, or other organic debris. Hexachlorophene should not be used on a regular basis for newborn infants. On continued use, infants absorb hexachlorophene, which may cause neurologic tissue damage. Rinse thoroughly after use.
   b. **Phenol.** The parent compound to this class of disinfectants, phenol may be used in a 5% solution to disinfect clothing, bed linen, instruments, sinks, and floors. It does not stain metal, paint, wood, or fabrics. It will redden and burn skin with prolonged application.

THE QUATERNARY AMMONIUM COMPOUNDS

1. The quaternary ammonium compounds were once a very popular class of disinfectants used in medicine. They have been employed as all-purpose antiseptics for application to skin, tissue, and mucous membranes and as disinfectants for surgical, industrial, and laboratory instruments. There are several shortcomings, however, that now limit the use of these agents to areas where complete sterility is not necessary.
2. Disadvantages include deactivation by soaps, alcohol, and tissue debris, slow disinfectant action compared with other agents available, occasional allergic responses with chronic use in diaper washes and deodorants, and lack of sufficient activity against certain types of bacteria that may be pathogenic.
3. Products available:
   a. **Benzalkonium chloride (Zephiran, Spensomide)** and **benzethonium chloride.** These are common ingredients in creams, dusting powders, and solutions for topical use.
   b. **Cetylpyridinium Chloride.** This is a constituent in **Cēpacol** and **Scope** mouthwashes. It may also be used for the treatment of superficial infections of the mouth and throat.
   c. **Methylbenzethonium chloride (Diaparene).** This compound is used as a diaper rinse to kill bacteria that may induce diaper rash.

MISCELLANEOUS ANTISEPTICS AND DISINFECTANTS

1. **Boric acid.** In concentrations of 1% to 4%, boric acid is a commonly used ingredient in eyewashes, mouthwashes, douches, dusting powders, and topical anti-infective and hemorrhoidal products. It inhibits bacterial growth but does not kill many forms of bacteria. Boric acid toxicity may develop if used for prolonged

periods or if used on large areas of abraded skin or wounds.

2. *Chlorhexidine (Hibiclens).* This is a disinfectant used as a presurgical hand scrub and a wound cleanser. It is also used as a preservative for pharmaceutical preparations. Do not use in eyes or ears; if it should enter eyes or ears, rinse thoroughly with water.

3. *Gentian violet.* This dye kills gram-positive organisms and many fungi. It is used in concentrations of 1:1,000 to 1:5,000. It has the disadvantages of staining and a narrow spectrum of activity.

4. *Hydrogen peroxide.* Diluted hydrogen peroxide decomposes to water and oxygen on contact with skin. Its germicidal action is weak, but because of its effervescent action, it is commonly used as a cleansing agent for draining wounds, sockets after tooth extraction, and ear canals. It is usually diluted with 1 to 4 parts of water. It deteriorates and must be kept in a cool, dark place in dark bottles with tight caps.

**The physician prescribes the medicine and treatment.
The nurse carries out the physician's orders.
Self-medication is dangerous. Consult your physician first.
There is in every medicine a possible danger.
When in doubt—ASK!**

ASSIGNMENT

Review previous lessons and questions according to the directions of your instructor.

1. Explain the difference between disinfectant and antiseptic. What is a germicide? What factor is necessary for efficient action of a disinfectant (germicide?)

2. List the desirable features for alcohols as disinfectants. What is the action of the alcohols? What are some of the common uses of the alcohols? List the conditions and excretions from the body for which the alcohols are *not* very effective. Are they effective against bacterial spores? Name two alcohol products. In what concentrations is ethyl alcohol most effective? What are the uses of isopropyl alcohol, and in what concentrations is it most effective?

3. Describe the chlorine compounds. Why may numerous chlorine compounds be used as disinfectants? About what amount of chlorine in what amount of water will destroy most bacteria in a few minutes? Name two chlorine products and describe the uses of each.

4. When were iodine and iodine compounds first used as antiseptics? What is their action, and which microorganisms do they kill? List the uses of iodine and iodine compounds. What are the disadvantages of the iodines? Name two iodine products and describe the uses of each product.

5. Describe the iodophors. Name one example and give its uses. What is the advantage of the combinations of iodine and polyvinylpyrrolidone? Tell the forms in which povidone-iodine solution is available.

6. When were the mercurials first used as antiseptics? Are they ideal germicides? Why not? What is a definite advantage the mercurials have over other disinfectants? What appears to be the mechanism of action of the mercurials? What is the primary use today of the mercurials? Name two mercurial products and tell the common uses of each. What is the strength of ammoniated mercury ointment? List the forms of availability for thimerosal (Merthiolate).

7. For many years the phenols were the most extensively used disinfectants and antiseptics and were the standard against which all other disinfectants were compared. Why has the use of phenols declined over the past 2 decades? What is the purpose of their use in soothing lotions and ointments? Name two phenolic derivatives still in use, including their names, and tell the uses of each. Should hexachlorophene be used on a regular basis for newborn infants? Why not?

8. The quaternary ammonium compounds were once a very popular class of disinfectants. What are the common uses of these compounds? List the disadvantages of the quaternary ammonium compounds. List four products available in these compounds, including generic and brand names for each product, common uses, and the different forms in which each is a constituent. Which one is a constituent in Cēpacol (a mouthwash used in many hospitals) and Scope? Which one is known by many young mothers as Diaparene?

9. Name four miscellaneous antiseptics and disinfectants and tell the common uses of each. What is the strength of boric acid used in eyewashes, mouthwashes, douches, dusting powders, and topical antiinfective and hemorrhoidal products? What is its action? If during a presurgical hand scrub you accidentally got some chlorhexidine (Hibiclens) in your eye, what would you do? What are the disadvantages of gentian violet? The staining from gentian violet is most difficult to remove from both linen and skin. What precautions would you take during its application to the patient's skin? Since the germicidal action of hydrogen peroxide is weak, why is it commonly used as a cleansing agent for draining wounds, sockets after tooth extraction, and ear canals? What group of organisms has it been used to control or eradicate, aerobes or anaerobes? Why? (See Index for aerobes and anaerobes.)

CHAPTER 26

Drugs affecting the skin and mucous membranes

The skin is the largest organ of the body. Absorption from the skin is poor and uncertain. The outermost layer is composed of flat cells containing keratin, a substance that waterproofs the skin and prevents the absorption of water and other substances. Absorption is affected by the presence of sweat pores and sebaceous glands. Drugs that cannot penetrate the horny first skin layer are sometimes absorbed by way of the sebaceous glands. Absorption is increased if the skin is macerated (softened by soaking) either by water or by perspiration, is raw or denuded, or is thin. Drugs may be excreted by the skin in small amounts. Arsenic, copper, silver, mercury, bromides, borates, salicylates, phenol, methylene blue, and phenolphthalein can be deposited in the skin and sweat glands, which may explain the skin eruption observed at times after their use. Many other drugs can also cause skin eruption.

Complete instructions for application of the following drugs will be given by the physician, instructor, supervisor, head nurse, or team leader. The drugs are, therefore, merely listed according to their main effect.

SOOTHING AGENTS

Calamine lotion
Glycerin, glycerol
Lanolin (hydrous wool fat)
Petrolatum (petroleum jelly); light liquid petrolatum
Rose water ointment
Theobroma oil (cocoa butter)
White ointment
Yellow ointment
Zinc oxide ointment
Zinc stearate

ANTIBACTERIAL AGENTS

Nitrofurazone (Furacin)

Antibiotics

Bacitracin (Baciguent)
Chloramphenicol (Chloromycetin)
Chlortetracycline (Aureomycin)

Erythromycin (Ilotycin)
Gentamicin (Garamycin)
Neomycin sulfate (Myciguent)
(There are also many antiinfective combination products containing bacitracin, neomycin, gramicidin, and polymyxin B.)

ANTIFUNGAL AGENTS

Acrisorcin (Akrinol)
Amphotericin B (Fungizone)
Benzoic and salicylic acid ointment (Whitfield's Ointment)
Clotrimazole (Lotrimin)
Haloprogin (Halotex)
Iodochlorhydroxyquin (Clioquinol)
Methylrosaniline chloride (gentian violet)
Miconazole (Micatin)
Nystatin (Mycostatin)
Potassium permanganate solution, 1:1000 to 1:10,000
Triacetin (Enzactin)
Undecylenic acid (Desenex, Cruex, Caldesene)

AGENTS THAT DESTROY SCABIES (ANTIPRURITICS, ANTIPARASITICS)

Crotamiton (Eurax)
Gamma benzene hexachloride, lindane (Kwell, Gamene)

AGENTS THAT DESTROY LICE (PEDICULICIDES)

A-200 Pyrinate
Blue Gel
Cuprex
RID
TISIT
Triple X
Vonce

BURN PREPARATIONS

Mafenide (Sulfamylon)
Nitrofurazone (Furacin, Furazyme)
Silver nitrate, 0.5%
Silver sulfadiazine (Silvadene)

225

ACNE PREPARATIONS

Benzoyl Peroxide, 4% to 10% (Benoxyl, Epi-Clear Antiseptic, Persa-Gel)

Sulfur Compounds (Xerac, Postacne, Transact, Bensulfoid)

Tetracycline hydrochloride (Topicycline)

Tretinoin, retinoic acid (Retin-A)

CORTICOSTEROID AGENTS

Corticosteroid agents should be used only when indicated because of possible side effects (see Index). These topical preparations are effective because of their antiinflammatory, antipruritic action.

Betamethasone benzoate (Benisone Gel and Cream)
Desonide (Tridesilon)
Dexamethasone (Aeroseb-D)
Flumethasone pivalate (Locorten)
Fluocinolone acetonide (Fluonid, Synalar)
Fluocinonide (Lidex)
Flurandrenolide (Cordran)
Halcinonide (Halog)
Hydrocortisone (Cort-Dome)
Triamcinolone (Kenalog, Aristocort)

The physician prescribes the medicine and treatment.
The nurse carries out the physician's orders.
Self-medication is dangerous. Consult your physician first.
There is in every medicine a possible danger.
When in doubt—ASK!

ASSIGNMENT

Review previous lessons and questions according to the direction of your instructor.

1. What is the largest organ of the body?
2. What factors cause an increase in absorption of drugs through the skin?
3. Name three common soothing agents.
4. Name one antibacterial agent.
5. Of the many antibiotics used for skin disease, name four used most commonly. (Your instructor will aid you in this selection.)
6. Of the many antifungal agents, select five used most commonly for fungus skin diseases. (Your instructor will aid you in this selection.)
7. Name two agents used to destroy scabies. Include generic and trade names.
8. Name four agents used most commonly to destroy lice. (Your instructor will aid you in this selection.)
9. Name four burn preparations.
10. List four acne preparations. Give one trade name for each preparation.
11. Can corticosteroid agents be used freely, frequently, and without medical supervision for treating skin diseases? Why not? (See Index).
12. Name five of the most commonly used corticosteroid preparations for the treatment of skin diseases. Give generic and trade name for each preparation. (Your instructor will aid you in this selection.)

CHAPTER 27

Antineoplastic drugs

Malignant diseases represent a significant cause of death. Chemical agents have become increasingly important in the treatment of cancer and related disorders. The drugs discussed here are placed in a separate chapter because they all have the same aim: the pharmacologic eradication or control of malignant tumors. The various groups of drugs presented in this chapter act in different ways, just as the individual types of tumors may represent different disorders. At present there is no known drug that cures malignant disease. True cures of malignant tumors are the result of early surgery and irradiation, and they occur in only a small percentage of the cases. Chemotherapeutic agents provide an adjunct to surgery by attempting to kill malignant cells that may have been released during surgery. These drugs may also be quite successful in slowing the growth of metastatic tumors and providing an improved quality of life to the patient, although not actually providing a cure.

Malignant tumors are those made up of cells that grow rapidly and without normal controls or restraints. These tumors invade, growing into surrounding tissues and destroying them by pressure or by taking over their supply of nutrients and oxygen. Malignant tumors may also metastasize. They send off daughter cells by way of the bloodstream or lymphatic stream or by the serous fluids in the body cavities to form new colonies of tumor. In general such cells are as fatal as the tumors unless both are totally removed from the body by surgery or irradiation.

The cause of malignant growths is unknown at present, although constant study and research is directed to this area. Since the cause is not known, there can be no rationally based pharmacologic treatment. The useful chemical agents have been obtained chiefly by screening many different kinds of compounds. The compounds used today are not highly selective in manner of treatment—they are not able to destroy malignant tissue alone; healthy cells or tissue may also be injured. These drugs are comparatively toxic—many would not ordinarily be considered safe enough for use, but the disease makes the situation desperate and allows little alternative in treatment.

One of the most serious toxic effects of the antimalig-

nant drugs is the depression of bone marrow. Rigid precautions must be observed continuously to prevent the development of infection in the patient who has leukopenia or depression of bone marrow. The patient needs constant protection from all attendants and other people who harbor microorganisms, and everything that comes in contact with the patient must be absolutely clean.

Antineoplastic drugs damage normal cells, too. Since none have been discovered that are free of toxic effects or selective, these drugs are used for short periods in small doses, with frequent intermissions in the dosage schedule. A favorable response to treatment is usually the result of cancer cells being more sensitive to the drug than normal cells. The normal cells most often affected are those that are rapidly produced, such as blood cells and gastrointestinal epithelium.

Great expenditures of time, money, and effort are being directed toward the development of drugs that would effectively destroy cancer cells without affecting vital cells or metabolic processes, but such drugs are not yet available. Meanwhile, the search for drugs to eradicate cancer, which ranks today as the second major destroyer of human life, goes on.

A number of antineoplastic drugs are used in the treatment of malignancies that affect the blood and blood-forming tissues. The neoplastic processes in which "cure," or more correctly, long-term remission, can be achieved are in certain types of Hodgkin's disease, lymphocytic leukemia, gestational choriocarcinoma, Burkitt's lymphoma, Wilms' tumor, Ewing's sarcoma, childhood acute lymphocytic leukemia, embryonal carcinoma of the testicle, retinoblastoma, and rhabdomyosarcoma.

LEUKEMIA

Leukemia affects the bone marrow, lymph nodes, and spleen. It reduces the production of erythrocytes and thrombocytes, which aids in causing anemia and hemorrhagic tendencies.

A characteristic of leukemia is an excessive production of white blood cells of abnormal type. The type of white cell that predominates in the blood determines the type of leukemia.

227

In myelogenous leukemia the white cell most often found is a granulocyte or a typical cell preceding it. Lymphatic leukemia is characterized by a large number of lymphocytes. Both myelogenous and lymphatic leukemia may be acute or chronic.

The white blood cells found in the blood of a patient with acute leukemia are immature, whereas more fully matured white blood cells are found in the blood of a chronic leukemia patient. While the number of white blood cells may be excessive, they give little protection against infection.

LYMPHOMA

Lymphomas are tumors that invade the lymph nodes, causing enlargement of the nodes, the liver, and the spleen. Characteristic problems include fever, itching, hemorrhagic tendencies, anemia, and thrombocytopenia. Radiation therapy is the treatment of choice, although nitrogen mustards and related compounds are considered valuable as helpful additions to treatment.

In lymphosarcoma the lymphocytes multiply in excess numbers and involve the lymph nodes, lymphoid tissue of other organs, and spleen. Almost any part of the body can be invaded. Hodgkin's disease involves lymph nodes as well as nonnodal tissues, but it involves reticulum cells rather than lymphocytes. These diseases are usually fatal within a few years or less.

POLYCYTHEMIA VERA

Polycythemia vera is characterized by an excessive production of erythrocytes. Increased numbers of thrombocytes and leukocytes are also frequently observed.

EXAMPLES OF ANTINEOPLASTIC DRUGS

The antineoplastic drugs can be divided into several large groups: alkylating agents, antimetabolites, radioisotopes, and miscellaneous agents.

Details regarding dosage and drug administration will be omitted, since these functions are generally performed by physicians and may vary depending on the type of cancer being treated.

Alkylating agents

The mechanism by which alkylating agents cause cellular injury is not completely known. Perhaps they act as anticancer agents by reacting with essential molecules in the cells of the tumor, such as nucleic acids. Rapidly reproducing cells are sensitive to the alkylating agents. This means that many of these compounds are also toxic to the gastrointestinal tract and bone marrow. Alkylating agents inhibit cell division in any cell-cycle phase. This inhibits multiplication of malignant cells as well as certain normal cells.

Mechlorethamine hydrochloride (Nitrogen mustard) (me-klor-eth'ah-meen) *(Mustargen Hydrochloride)* (mus'tar-jen)

1. Mechlorethamine is an analogue of sulfur mustard gas used in World War I. In some respects its action on body cells is similar to that of radiation.
2. Mechlorethamine is used in the treatment of lymphosarcoma, Hodgkin's disease, bronchogenic carcinoma, and mycosis fungoides.
3. Nitrogen mustard often gives marked relief of such symptoms as fever, lack of appetite, weakness, itching, and pain. In addition, it reduces the size of the liver and spleen. Remissions may vary from a few weeks to several months.
4. This is a drug of choice for hospitalized patients in need of prompt treatment. It is most effective when the disease has become generalized or the patient cannot take radiation therapy.
5. Side effects may include thrombophlebitis or thrombosis (from the effect of the drug on veins), sloughing of tissues around needle site caused by leakage of solution, severe nausea, vomiting, decreased formation of blood cells, granulocytopenia, lymphopenia, thrombocytopenia, agranulocytosis, anemia, and gastrointestinal and gonadal injury. Mechlorethamine can produce severe tissue damage when it comes in contact with eyes, skin, or respiratory tract. Toxic effects are directly proportional to dosage, so careful calculation of dosage is essential.
6. Nausea and vomiting may be prevented by administering the drug late in the day and sedating the patient for the night.
7. Additional treatment with this drug is not resumed until there is satisfactory recovery in the bone marrow. Additional treatment generally does not produce the responses as satisfactorily as did the initial treatment.
8. *Mechlorethamine hydrochloride* for injection is administered intravenously, after special dissolving, by injecting the solution into the tubing of an IV infusion. Dosage is calculated on the basis of body weight.

Other alkylating agents

1. *Busulfan* (byou-sul'fan) *(Myleran)* (mil'er-an). The cytotoxic action is restricted chiefly to the cells of the bone marrow. Busulfan gives remissions to 90% of chronic granulocytic leukemia.
2. *Carmustine* (kar-mus'teen) *(BiCNU).* Carmustine is used alone or in combination with other agents in the treatment of certain brain tumors, multiple myeloma, Hodgkin's disease, and other lymphomas.
3. *Chlorambucil* (klo-ram'byou-sil) *(Leukeran)*

(loo'ker-an). Chlorambucil is a derivative of nitrogen mustard, and its actions and uses are similar to those of mechlorethamine hydrochloride. In recommended doses it is the slowest-acting and least toxic nitrogen mustard in use and is well tolerated, with few side effects. Large doses or prolonged administration will cause nausea, vomiting, and anorexia and may cause severe depression of the bone marrow. Weekly blood counts are necessary. The drug is effective in the palliative treatment of lymphomas, chronic lymphocytic leukemia, reticulum cell sarcoma, and some forms of Hodgkin's disease.

4. *Cyclophosphamide* (sy-klo-fos'fah-myd) *(Cytoxan)* (sy-tok'san). This agent was developed in a search for greater selective toxicity and is similar in its antineoplastic activity to mechlorethamine hydrochloride. It is used for treatment of lymphoma, lymphosarcoma, leukemias, Hodgkin's disease, multiple myeloma, malignancy of the ovary, breast, and lung, and mycosis fungoides. In the treatment of Burkitt's lymphoma complete remissions of more than 5 years have occurred when this drug is used in conjunction with other agents. Cyclophosphamide can produce severe bone marrow depression. Nausea and vomiting are not as violent as with mechlorethamine but are more prolonged. Alopecia and hemorrhagic cystitis are common, and hepatotoxicity can occur. Sterility commonly follows administration of this drug.

5. *Lomustine* (lo-mus'teen) *CCNU (Cee NU).* Lomustine is used as secondary therapy in the treatment of certain brain tumors and Hodgkin's disease.

6. *Melphalan* (mel'fah-lan) *(Alkeran)* (al'ke-ran). Melphalan is used to treat multiple myeloma, bringing improvement to 70% to 80% of the patients for 6 months to 2 years.

7. *Thiotepa* (thy-o-te'pah). This alkylating agent is particularly useful for therapy of cancer of the urinary bladder, breast, and ovaries. It is not effective for acute leukemia. It has a slow onset of action, and immediate side effects of nausea and vomiting are minimal.

8. *Uracil mustard* (your'ah-sil). Uracil mustard is used in the treatment of chronic lymphocytic leukemia, lymphomas, Hodgkin's disease, and sometimes other malignancies such as ovarian cancer. It may cause loss of hair in addition to the usual side effects.

Antimetabolites

Antimetabolite agents include the folic acid antagonists (methotrexate), purine antagonists (mercaptopurine), and pyrimidine antagonists (fluorouracil).

Folic acid is a vitamin that acts as a catalytic agent in the synthesis of nucleic acid. Nucleic acid is an essential component of cellular protein. For this activity folic acid is converted to a biologically more active form called folinic acid. Folic acid antagonists block the formation of folinic acid from folic acid. Cells are not prevented from going into cell division, but the normal mitotic progress is arrested. Cells that proliferate rapidly, such as white blood cells in the leukemia patient, are markedly affected.

Folic acid antagonists are used primarily in treating acute leukemia of childhood. They are less effective in the treatment of adult leukemia and have limited success in the treatment of solid tumors.

Remissions bring relief from pain in bones, improved appetite, a feeling of well-being, increased strength, disappearance of fever, and reduction in the size of enlarged organs such as the liver, spleen, and lymph nodes. Laboratory studies of the blood indicate an approach to normal during the remission period.

The first clinically useful folic acid antagonist was aminopterin. This drug is not available in the United States. Methotrexate is used in its place.

Methotrexate (meth-o-trek'sayt)

1. Methotrexate is a folic acid antagonist used chiefly in the treatment of acute leukemia in children. It has been used to treat a rare type of cancer in women, choriocarcinoma, in which the tumor is composed of cells of fetal origin.

2. This drug may be accompanied by the administration of folinic acid, or leucovorin. This acts as an antidote to lessen the toxicity of the methotrexate.

3. Side effects and toxic effects are similar to those already discussed: depression of the bone marrow, marked leukopenia, thrombocytopenia, anemia, nausea, vomiting, and diarrhea.

Other antimetabolites

1. *Azathioprine* (a-zah-thy'o-preen) *(Imuran)* (im'u-ran). This drug is a derivative of mercaptopurine and is an immunosuppressive agent used in the treatment of rejection reactions, systemic lupus erythematosus, idiopathic thrombocytopenic purpura, and autoimmune hemolytic anemia.

2. *Cytarabine* (sy-tar'ah-been) *(Cytosar)* (sy'toe-sar). Cytarabine is used for the induction of remission in acute granulocytic leukemia of adults and secondarily for other acute leukemias of adults and children.

3. *Fluorouracil* (floo-o-ur'ah-sil) *(5-FU).* Fluorouracil causes remissions in nonresectable carcinoma of the rectum, sigmoid, and colon and in advanced breast and ovarian cancer. It brings relief from pain and permits the patient to become ambulatory. Remissions in gastrointestinal cancer may last 6 months to 4

years. Many side effects may occur that may cause withdrawal of the drug: lip and mouth ulceration, severe diarrhea, leukopenia, loss of scalp hair, anorexia, nausea, and vomiting.

4. *Mercaptopurine* (mer-kap-to-pu′reen) *(6-Mercaptopurine Purinethol)* (pu′reen-thol). This is used chiefly in the treatment of acute leukemia in children. It causes remissions varying from a few weeks to several months.

5. *Thioguanine* (thy-o-guah′neen) *(2-amino-6-mercaptopurine).* Thioguanine is used to treat chronic myelocytic leukemia and acute leukemia. It gives greater remissions in children than in adults and is used chiefly after administration of busulfan or mercaptopurine has developed resistance or toxicity. It should be used with caution in patients with impairment of the liver.

Hormones

The cortical hormones made by the adrenal gland and the adrenocorticotropic hormone (ACTH) are known to slow the growth of cells, especially the young, actively growing and multiplying cells. How this action is achieved is not known.

Prednisone and prednisolone are most frequently used in the treatment of lymphomas and leukemia. Their action is somewhat similar to that of cortisone. They do have the advantage of causing less retention of fluid and salt than hydrocortisone does. These hormones also are used in the treatment of Hodgkin's disease, multiple myeloma, lymphosarcoma, and chronic lymphatic leukemia.

Temporary remissions are achieved in a fairly good percentage of children with acute leukemia. Remissions are not so marked or sustained in adults. Some physicians use hormones in treating complications of lymphoma and chronic lymphatic leukemia rather than the disease itself, feeling that true remissions rarely occur with the use of hormones and that toxic effects of the hormones may be too dangerous.

Side effects from these drugs may be a serious problem and are difficult to treat. (For details on these side effects see Index.) Prolonged use of the drug may make restriction of sodium and administration of potassium chloride necessary to maintain electrolyte balance. Abrupt withdrawal of the drug should be avoided to prevent a hypoadrenal state.

Hormones for the treatment of cancer of the breast include androgens, such as testosterone propionate and fluoxymesterone. If the patient is well past menopause, such estrogens as diethylstilbestrol are sometimes administered. In women still menstruating, estrogens may increase the growth and metastasis of cancer.

Prostate gland cancer in the male is treated with an estrogen such as diethylstilbestrol or by a combination of an orchiectomy, or excision of both testicles, and administration of an estrogen.

A good percentage of the patients with breast or prostate cancer show subjective improvement. They feel better, have less pain, and their appetite improves. Some patients receive these benefits for a number of years, although the malignant process may have changed very little.

Radioactive isotopes

The radiations produced by radioactive isotopes are commonly spoken of as alpha, beta, and gamma rays, and more correctly as alpha and beta particles and gamma rays. Alpha and beta rays penetrate poorly into tissues; gamma rays are highly penetrating. All radioactive isotopes are a possible hazard to the patient and to all persons who handle the preparations. The cytotoxic action of these preparations is the result of their ability to ionize molecules in a cell by injecting electrons. Tissues vary in sensitivity to ionizing radiations. Cells with a short life and a high rate of reproduction are especially vulnerable to these radiations. Cells of the body that are particularly affected include the germinal cells of the ovaries and testes, bone marrow, lymphocytes, and the epithelial cells of the gastrointestinal tract. This explains some of the symptoms of radiation sickness: nausea, vomiting, diarrhea, weakness, and reduction of cells in the circulating blood. Death can result from depression of the bone marrow, infection, or hemorrhage.

Radioactive isotopes occasionally used in medicine are sodium radiophosphate, radiogold colloid, and sodium radioiodide.

Radioactive sodium phosphate ^{32}P

1. Large doses of radioactive sodium phosphate may result in severe depression of bone marrow. Cells from which red blood cells develop, as well as other cellular elements, are also depressed. This helps control excessive formation of white blood cells and thrombocytes and decreases the size of an enlarged liver or spleen.

2. Remissions usually last for several months to a year or more; they last longer than after the use of radiation therapy or other drugs.

3. This radioactive isotope has been used extensively in the treatment of polycythemia vera. It is also used to treat chronic myelogenous and chronic lymphatic leukemia. It does not benefit acute leukemia patients.

4. This drug is excreted in the urine. This necessitates the careful disposal of the urine according to hospital rules, the wearing of rubber gloves in disposal technique, and the cleansing of urinals and bedpans.

5. Side and toxic effects are similar to those for x-ray

irradiations. Radiation sickness does not usually occur, but serious depression of the bone marrow may. Leukopenia, anemia, and thrombocytopenia are the chief untoward effects. Frequent blood examinations are necessary to discover developing states of toxicity. This isotope produces fewer complications than several other effective agents and is relatively inexpensive.

6. *Sodium phosphate ^{32}P solution (^{32}P, Phosphotope).* This is administered intravenously or orally in aqueous solution. It is supplied in glass containers. Great care must be taken in handling the material to prevent radiation burns from contact with the skin.

7. Dosage is expressed in millicuries (mc) and is usually measured and administered by physicians, registered nurses, or pharmacist. Dose is individualized according to needs and responses of patient.

Gold ^{198}Au solution, Aureotope

1. The main use of this agent is in the treatment of recurrent pleural effusion and ascites associated with metastatic malignancy.

2. It does not cure the malignancy but does reduce the accumulation of fluid and thus adds to the comfort of the patient.

3. It is administered by injection into the pleural cavity or peritoneal cavity.

4. Mild radiation sickness may occur after 3 to 4 days, and a decrease in the number of white blood cells may be found.

5. This drug is a greater hazard to nursing personnel than ^{32}P because ^{198}Au emits the penetrating gamma rays and ^{32}P emits only beta rays.

Sodium iodide ^{131}I solution

1. This solution is used for palliative therapy of thyroid cancer and hyperthyroidism.

2. This substance, which is colorless and tasteless, can be added to water and given to the patient to swallow.

3. Radioactive iodine is absorbed rapidly from the stomach. Most of the dose is in the blood within the first hour.

4. Since radioiodine can be taken by mouth and is collected and concentrated by the thyroid tissue, a much greater degree of irradiation can be obtained than from radium or roentgen rays. There is a possibility of damage to normal tissue, especially the skin, when large doses of radium or roentgen rays are used.

5. The tiny doses administered, called ''tracers,'' have become useful in studying problems of physiology and disease of the thyroid gland, diagnosing functional states of this gland, and treating certain cases

of hyperthyroidism and cancer of the thyroid gland.

6. It is useful in medicine because it may be located, because of its radioactivity, even when present in very small amounts. During the period of activity the energy liberated is in the form of beta particles and gamma rays.

7. Some physicians believe that this agent is more useful and effective as a therapeutic agent when used in patients over 50 years of age and in those with very small glands, severe complicating diseases, or recurrent hyperthyroidism after resection of the thyroid.

8. Radioiodine treatments of patients with toxic goiter have been encouraging, but the possible danger of radiation injury has limited the treatment to patients beyond the child-bearing period and to patients who are poor surgical risks.

9. Cancerous tissue of the thyroid gland demonstrates a variable degree of capacity to collect iodine, depending on the degree of function of the tissue in the tumor. Thus, the possibility of treating cancer of the thyroid gland with radioiodine is perhaps somewhat limited. Metastasis from a malignant tumor of the thyroid gland sometimes can be traced with the use of the Geiger-Mueller counter and radioactive iodine. In some cases prolonged treatment with radioiodine may arrest widespread metastatic lesions.

10. Side and toxic effects are dangerous, since radiation from the substance is just as hazardous as that from radium and roentgen rays. Special precautions must be taken to prevent the spilling of the drug on persons or property. Rubber gloves should be worn during administration of this substance and in handling the disposal of the gloves and of the patient's excreta. Surroundings of patients receiving this substance should be checked with special monitoring instruments such as a small portable Geiger counter.

11. The hospital's routine care for such special patients, with emphasis on avoiding the problems of contamination just discussed, should be strictly followed for the safety of the nurse, patient, other patients, hospital personnel, and visitors.

Antibiotics and miscellaneous agents
Dactinomycin (dak-tin-o-my'sin), *(Actinomycin D)* (ak-ti-no-my'sin)
(Cosmegen) (kos'me-jen)

1. Dactinomycin is one of the actinomycins produced by a species of *Streptomyces*. The exact mechanism of its action is unknown. It probably inhibits cellular activity and cell reproduction. It also inhibits the normal rapidly proliferating cells of the body. It is used

for Wilms' tumor, rhabdomyosarcoma, and carcinoma of the uterus and testes.

2. Dactinomycin can be used alone or in combination with surgery or radiation.
3. Side and toxic effects include nausea, vomiting, oral ulcerations, skin eruptions, diarrhea, bone marrow depression with platelet depression, extravasation, or the discharge of blood or other substances into the tissues. The last may cause severe local reactions. These effects are observed after several days of treatment.
4. This agent is given intravenously for 5 days and can be repeated if toxic symptoms do not develop. Single smaller doses once a week for 3 weeks have been used.

Doxorubicin (dok-so-ru'bi-sin)
(Adriamycin) (ay-dree-ah-my'sin)

1. Doxorubicin has proved effective in treating such hematologic malignancies as acute lymphocytic leukemia, malignant lymphomas including Hodgkin's disease, and especially sarcomas, a class of solid tumors not usually responsive to cancer chemotherapy.
2. Doxorubicin has had some success in treating ovarian, prostate, bladder, testicular, and thyroid cancers.
3. Remissions of several years have occurred in some cases of sarcoma.
4. Symptoms of toxicity include bone marrow depression, liver impairment, loss of hair, red color to the urine (the latter during the first 2 days after injection), burning in the mouth or mouth ulceration, redness of the tongue, nausea, vomiting, diarrhea, and myocardial damage.
5. One injection is administered every 3 weeks, followed by close monitoring of white blood cells and platelet levels for early detection of bone marrow depression, and liver function tests.
6. Care must be taken during IV administration to prevent extravasating, because it can cause severe cellulitis, blistering, and local tissue necrosis. The drug is best administered by injection into the tubing of a freely running IV infusion of saline-dextrose solution.

Mitomycin C (mi-to-my'sin)
(Mutamycin) (mew-tah-my'sin)

1. The chief use of mitomycin is in advanced cases of metastatic malignancies that have been treated either surgically or by radiation and are now resistant to other kinds of chemotherapy.
2. For cancer of the stomach, pancreas, colon, and rectum, the response rate to this drug is approximately 10%. Mitomycin has sometimes produced regression

for a short time in advanced adenocarcinoma of the breast, malignant melanoma, and squamous cell carcinomas of the lungs, head, and neck.

3. Mitomycin is highly toxic. Symptoms include bone marrow toxicity, alterations in coagulation and bleeding times, thrombocytopenia, leukopenia, irreversible bone marrow depression, fever, nausea, vomiting, diarrhea, and headache.
4. There is daily administration of the drug for 5 days, 2 days without the drug, and then 5 days of daily administration. The course can be repeated in 2 or 3 weeks if no bone marrow toxicity occurs. Care must be taken during IV administration of the drug (preferably through IV tubing) to prevent pain, necrosis, and sloughing that may require skin grafts.
5. Treatment is terminated whenever platelets or white cells fall below certain levels to prevent the blood changes and bone marrow depression already cited.

Mithramycin (mith-rah-my'sin)
(Mithracin) (mith'rah-sin)

1. Mithramycin is a toxic antibiotic. It acts in a manner similar to that of actinomycin D.
2. It is used in the treatment of hypercalcemia that may result from bone metastasis and in the treatment of testicular tumors.

Bleomycin (ble-o-my'sin)
(Blenoxane) (blen-ok'sayn)

1. Bleomycin is a product of a *Streptomyces*.
2. It is toxic but is said to have good results in the treatment of squamous cell carcinomas, Hodgkin's disease, and non-Hodgkin's lymphomas.

Other miscellaneous antineoplastic agents

1. **Mitotane** (mi'toe-tayn) **(Lysodren)** (ly'so-dren). Mitotane is used in the treatment of inoperable adrenal cortical carcinoma, acting by adrenal suppression. Side effects include adrenal suppression, drowsiness, lethargy, dizziness and vertigo, nausea, vomiting, and diarrhea. Infrequent side effects include blurred vision, hemorrhagic cystitis, orthostatic hypotension, generalized aching, and hyperpyrexia. Dosage is administered orally and should be given daily and continued as long as clinical benefits are noted.
2. **Procarbazine hydrochloride** (pro-kar'bah-zeen) **(Matulane)** (ma'tu-layn). Procarbazine is a hydrazine derivative. It is cytoxic and has many toxic effects, but has some effectiveness in the treatment of Hodgkin's disease and may have some effect in the treatment of bronchogenic carcinoma.
3. **Vinblastine sulfate** (vin-blas'teen) **(Velban)** (vel'ban). Velban is useful as a supplement or alternative

in treatment of Hodgkin's disease, choriocarcinoma, or breast cancer when resistance to methotrexate and other drugs has occurred.

4. *Vincristine sulfate* (vin-cris'teen) *(Oncovin)* (on'ko-vin). Vincristine is a drug chemically related to vinblastine. It is used chiefly to treat acute leukemias of childhood and childhood neoplasms. It is also used to treat Hodgkin's disease and lymphosarcoma. Remissions occur in 50% to 60% of the cases; if combined with corticosteroids, they occur in 85% of the cases. Use of this drug is limited because of its neurotoxicity, which includes possible permanent neural damage, such as loss of deep tendon reflexes and ataxia.

Nursing care measures for patients receiving antineoplastic therapy

1. One of the most vitally important nursing measures is to provide emotional support to patients. They have a destructive disease, and the drug therapy for this is both physically and psychologically distressing.
   a. Assure the patient that the symptoms arising from drug therapy will subside; nausea and vomiting will disappear, and hair will regrow within a few months after drug therapy is discontinued.
   b. Prepare patients receiving antineoplastic drugs for the symptoms that usually occur. Such preparation will lessen both the physical and psychologic stress.
2. Strict adherence to hospital regulations regarding spe-

cial care of patients receiving radioactive materials is vital to prevent spread or contamination from these radioactive materials and maintain the safety of patients, nurses, and other personnel.

3. Patients receiving antineoplastic therapy have lowered resistance and are prone to infections as a result of the depression of antibody formation and red and white cell production. Medical asepsis must be strictly enforced when caring for these patients. Protective isolation may also be necessary.
4. Observe patients closely for bleeding tendencies, such as ecchymosis or purpura and bleeding gums.
5. Avoid physical trauma to the patients, such as bruising or undue pressure on body parts, since this may further increase bleeding into body tissues.
6. Observation of patients for neural involvement is very important. Watch for signs of paresthesia (numbness or tingling sensations), loss of reflexes, ataxia, and mental depression. As for all symptoms, these should be recorded and reported.
7. Give patients with stomatitis a highly nutritious, bland, and nonirritating diet. Foods with a high content of acid, such as tomatoes, fresh fruits, highly seasoned foods, and raw vegetables, should be avoided.
8. Frequent checks on the patient's blood examinations and liver tests will help you plan your nursing care and your work with the dietitian concerning the diet of the patient.

The physician prescribes the medicine and treatment.
The nurse carries out the physician's orders.
Self-medication is dangerous. Consult your physician first.
There is in every medicine a possible danger.
When in doubt—ASK!

ASSIGNMENT

Review previous lessons and questions according to the directions of your instructor.

1. As far as we know today, is there any drug that cures malignant disease?
2. How can true cures of malignant tumors be accomplished at this time?
3. What is the difference between a malignant growth and a benign one?
4. Is the cause of malignant growths known, or unknown, at present?

5. What is a serious toxic effect of the antimalignant drugs? How is the patient protected in an effort to prevent this serious side effect?
6. Do antineoplastic drugs damage normal cells as well as malignant ones? Which normal cells are most often affected?
7. Do any antineoplastic drugs effect a total cure of malignant processes? Have any antineoplastic drugs been discovered at the present time to be free of toxic effects?
8. List the types of neoplastic processes in which "cure," or more correctly, long-term remission, can be achieved.
9. What areas of the body are affected by leukemia? What is

a characteristic of leukemia? What determines the type of leukemia? Describe the two types of leukemia discussed in your chapter. Describe the white cells found in the blood of a patient with acute leukemia. Are the white cells increased or decreased, and do they give normal, or little, protection against infection?

10. Describe the malignant medical disease lymphoma.

11. Define polycythemia vera.

12. Give four examples of the antineoplastic drug groups.

13. Name two nitrogen mustard drugs and list the symptoms that they may relieve. List the side effects for these drugs. How may nausea and vomiting during nitrogen mustard therapy be lessened or prevented? The nitrogen mustard drugs are examples of what antineoplastic drug group?

14. Name five additional antineoplastic drugs of the alkylating agents group. (Your instructor will help you select the ones most commonly used.) For each drug you selected, list the symptoms observed during drug therapy and the types of cancer it is used to treat.

15. Name the three drugs included in the antimetabolites group. What age group and type of cancer do each treat?

16. What type of antimetabolite is methotrexate? What is its primary use? Which drug may be administered with methotrexate? What is its purpose? List the side effects and toxic effects of methotrexate.

17. Name four other antimetabolites, giving both generic and trade names. Tell the main uses of each drug. What are the side effects of fluorouracil? How long do remissions last for each of the drugs you selected?

18. For many of the drugs discussed, weekly blood counts and bone marrow examinations frequently are essential. Why is this? What results might indicate a temporary or permanent withdrawal of the drug?

19. Name two hormone drugs and tell for which malignancies each is commonly used. List some of the more serious side effects possible from use of hormones. Which hormones are used for the treatment of cancer of the breast? If the patient is well past menopause, which hormone may be used for breast cancer treatment? What effect may the administration of estrogens cause in a menstruating female? What hormone is used to treat prostate gland cancer in the male? What results occur in a considerable percentage of the patients with breast or prostate cancer? Is a cure obtained?

20. What symptoms are apt to occur with the use of radioactive isotopes in the treatment of cancer? What can cause death? Name three radioactive isotopes frequently used in the treatment of malignancies.

21. Outline the precautions and nursing care in administration of sodium iodide to the thyroid cancer patient.

22. Name three of the antibiotics or miscellaneous agents. Give the main uses and side effects for each drug selected.

23. Name four miscellaneous antineoplastic agents and tell the main uses and side effects for each drug selected.

24. Explain several important points in the nursing care for patients on antineoplastic therapy.

25. What is meant by giving emotional support to the adult, child, or child's parents when the patient is receiving, or about to receive, antineoplastic therapy? How can you provide such emotional support?

CHAPTER 28

Serums and vaccines

There are two kinds of immunity: natural and acquired. *Natural immunity* is endowed at birth and is retained for life. Microorganisms that live within a parent organism such as a human being are harmless to that organism because it has natural defense mechanisms to ward off infection from that microorganism.

Acquired immunity may be *active* or *passive*. Active acquired immunity results when the parent organism develops antibodies against the invading antigens, or microorganisms. Active immunity may be induced by artificial means, such as by injection of antigens. Examples of antigens include a suspension of living microorganisms such as the vaccinia virus or a suspension of dead microorganisms such as typhoid vaccine. The antigen may be a soluble toxin produced by bacteria, such as diphtheria toxin, or an extract of the bodies of bacteria, such as tuberculosis vaccine.

Passive acquired immunity can be obtained in two ways: (1) an individual may be given the serum of an animal that has been actively immunized by injections with the specific organisms or toxins of a particular disease or diseases or (2) an individual may be given an injection of the serum of an immune person. This serum is rich in antibodies developed to protect the organism against the specific disease antigen. Passive is used to describe this type of acquired immunity because the body plays no active part in the preparation of antibodies. The body does not produce antibodies to resist infection as it does in active immunity. As the blood is renewed, the acquired antibodies are lost, so the individual must be reimmunized periodically to maintain protection against that specific microorganism.

AGENTS CONTAINING ANTIBODIES
Immune serums

An immune serum is the serum of a human being or animal that has specific antibodies in the bloodstream. The immune serum is transferred into the circulation of the patient and contains specific antibodies that act on disease microorganisms, providing passive acquired immunity.

Naturally produced human serums are preparations obtained from the serum of patients who have recovered from a disease and still have the immune bodies in their blood serum. Examples of naturally produced human serums follow.

Hepatitis B immune globulin (human) (H-Big)

1. Hepatitis B immune globulin contains a high titer of antibody to hepatitis B antigen.
2. It is used for patients who have had direct exposure to blood or mucous membrane secretions of patients infected with the hepatitis B antigen.
3. Recommended dose: 0.06 ml/kg, as soon as possible after exposure (up to 7 days) and repeated 28 to 30 days after exposure.

Immune serum globulin (human) (Gammagee) (gam'ah-jee), (Immu-G), (Gammar) (gam'ar)

1. Immune serum globulin is a sterile solution of globulins that contains those antibodies normally present in adult human blood. Each lot of the preparation is derived from an original plasma or serum pool. This pool represents serum collected from at least 1,000 individual patients.
2. It is useful for prevention or modification (weakening of the toxicity of microorganisms or viruses) of measles and for prevention of rubella (German measles), poliomyelitis, and infectious hepatitis.
3. The injection of the proper dose of serum immune globulin into pregnant women soon after exposure to rubella may modify or prevent the disease. It is unlikely that this treatment is able to prevent rubella virus infection in the fetus.
4. Dosage varies. It is administered intramuscularly.

Pertussis immune globulin (human) (Hypertussis) (hy-per-tus'is)

1. This is the liquid or dried serum of blood obtained from donors who have recovered from pertussis (whooping cough).
2. The donors must have been without active clinical symptoms of the disease for 7 or more days before giving blood.

3. Usual dose: intramuscularly, 1.25 ml for 3 to 5 doses or 3 to 6.75 ml as a single dose. Efficacy has never been proved in active cases.

Rabies immune globulin (human) (Hyperab)

1. This immune globulin is used in combination with rabies vaccine of duck origin to provide passive protection to those patients who have been exposed to rabies. Rabies immune globulin provides protective coverage to the patient during the 2 weeks or longer that it takes for the rabies vaccine to develop antibodies to the rabies exposure.
2. Rabies immune globulin must not be administered in repeated doses once vaccine treatment has been initiated. Repeating the immune globulin may interfere with antibody production initiated by the vaccine.
3. Recommended dose: intramuscularly, 20 IU/kg at the time of the first vaccine dose.

RH$_0$ (D) immune globulin (human) (RhoGAM, Gamulin Rh)

1. This globulin is used to prevent the formation of active antibodies in the Rh$_0$ (D) negative individual who has received Rh positive blood as a result of delivering an Rh$_0$ (D) positive infant or as a result of a transfusion accident.
2. With an injection of this antibody to the mother after delivery or to the recipient of a transfusion accident, the person's antibody response to the foreign Rh$_0$ (D) cells is suppressed. This protects the patient from red blood cell destruction resulting from the transfusion reaction.
3. Rh$_0$ immune globulin is to be administered *only* to the recipient in a transfusion accident or the postpartum mother or postmiscarriage woman. It must not be administered to the infant.
4. This serum must not be administered to:
   a. An Rh$_0$ (D) positive individual
   b. An Rh$_0$ (D) negative patient who has inadvertently received an Rh$_0$ (D) positive blood transfusion within 3 months of delivery
   c. A patient previously immunized to the Rh$_0$ (D) blood factor
5. Side effects include fever, muscular aches, lethargy, and jaundice.
6. Dosage must be individualized to the patient and is dependent on the amount of Rh$_0$ positive blood received.

Antitoxins

These antitoxic serums are formed in the bodies of animals that have been injected with a specific toxin. The animal forms antibodies to that toxin and is then bled, with the serum separated from the blood. The serum is purified to remove inactive substances and to concentrate the antibodies.

The purpose of the antitoxins is to produce passive immunity in certain diseases. Animals most often used for the artificial production of immune serums are horses and rabbits.

One inoculation with the animal product may sensitize a patient to the blood components of that species. Future inoculations of products from the same animal source may cause serum sickness or an anaphylactoid shock condition in which severe sudden shock symptoms occur and prompt treatment is necessary to save the patient's life.

Tests for sensitivity to horse serum or other suspected antigens should be made on patients before injection of antitoxins to prevent possibilities of serum sickness and anaphylactic shock. The antitoxin should be withheld if a reaction characterized by a red, swollen area develops around the site of the intradermal test injection.

Diphtheria antitoxin

1. Diphtheria antitoxin is a sterile solution of antitoxic substances obtained from the blood serum or the plasma of a healthy animal that has been immunized against diphtheria toxin.
2. It gives a passive immunity to the individual who has been exposed to diphtheria or to a patient ill with diphtheria.
3. Usual prophylactic dose: 1,000 to 5,000 units. Usual therapeutic dose: 20,000 units, although it may vary from 10,000 to 100,000 units. It is administered intramuscularly and intravenously.

Tetanus antitoxin (Equine) (ek'win)

1. Tetanus antitoxin is prepared from the horse in much the same way as diphtheria antitoxin. The animal in this case, however, has been immunized against tetanus toxin.
2. Usual therapeutic dose: 50,000 to 100,000 units, intravenously or intramuscularly. Usual prophylactic dose: 1,500 to 5,000 units, subcutaneously or intramuscularly.

ANTIGENIC AGENTS USED TO PRODUCE ACTIVE IMMUNITY: VACCINES
Definition and important points about vaccines

1. Vaccines are suspensions of either attenuated or killed microorganisms.
2. They are administered for the prevention or treatment of infectious diseases.
3. The viruses for vaccines are usually grown in living tissue, such as chick embryos.
4. This type of vaccine is absolutely contraindicated in

persons with a history of hypersensitivity to eggs, chicken, or chicken feathers.

5. Vaccines do not give immediate protection. An interval of days or even several weeks passes between inoculation and production of antibodies.

6. If there is danger of immediate infection and a serum is available, a prophylactic dose of serum is first administered to give immediate protection. It is followed later by the vaccine injection to give prolonged immunity.

Cholera vaccine

1. This is a sterile suspension of killed cholera vibrios *(Vibrio comma)* in isotonic sodium chloride solution or other suitable diluent.

2. Cholera vaccine contains 8 billion killed cholera organisms in each milliliter of suspension at the time of manufacture.

3. Usual dose: subcutaneously, 0.5 ml, followed by another dose of 1 ml after 7 to 10 days, making a total of 2 injections. The 0.5-ml dose may be repeated every 6 months if necessary.

Influenza virus vaccine, Trivalent; (Fluogen) (floo-o'jen), (Fluax) (floo'aks)

1. This vaccine is a suspension of recommended, contemporary, inactivated influenza viruses cultivated in chick embryos. Its content will change annually based on viruses expected to be prevalent.

2. Influenza virus vaccine is used prophylactically to produce active immunization against influenza.

3. Maximum amount of antibody formation occurs during the second week after vaccination. The titer remains constant for about a month; thereafter there is a gradual decline.

4. Dosage and frequency of injection will vary annually based on the viral antigens present.

5. This vaccine should not be administered to individuals sensitive to derivatives of chick or egg protein.

Measles (rubeola) virus vaccine, live attenuated (Attenuvax) (ah-ten'u-vaks), (M-Vac)

1. The measles virus is grown in chick embryo tissue culture. Live, attenuated virus vaccine is prepared from this culture.

2. Since the vaccine is lyophilized, or dried, it must be reconstituted with the diluent before use.

3. After a single dose the vaccine induces an active form of immunity that lasts at least 4 years.

4. A mild, or sometimes fairly severe, febrile response follows the vaccination.

5. Measles virus, live attenuated, is available in an injectable suspension of 0.5 ml. This is administered subcutaneously in the upper arm.

6. The live vaccine should not be administered to pa-

tients who are pregnant, who suffer from severe or debilitating illnesses, whose resistance may be lowered by irradiation, toxic antineoplastic drugs, or steroids, or who may be allergic to some of the constituents of the vaccine preparation, such as egg proteins or the neomycin in the preparation.

German measles (rubella) virus vaccine (Meruvax II) (mer'u-vaks)

1. Attenuated strains of rubella virus, grown in human cell culture, are injected subcutaneously.

2. This produces a mild, systemic infection, perhaps followed by long-term immunity to the natural infection.

3. Children tolerate the vaccine well. Fever and arthralgia (pain in a joint) commonly occur in adults.

4. Rubella vaccine must not be administered to pregnant women because the vaccine strain may infect the fetus.

5. Some physicians prefer to administer rubella vaccine only to prepubertal girls. If administered to seronegative adolescent girls and women, it must be ascertained that pregnancy will not occur for 3 months after immunization.

6. Do not administer to patients allergic to neomycin.

Measles, mumps, and rubella virus vaccine, live (M-M-R II)

1. This product allows simultaneous immunization against measles, mumps, and rubella in children from 15 months of age to puberty in 1 subq injection.

2. Do not administer to patients allergic to chicken feathers, eggs, or neomycin.

3. The lyophilized powder should be stored at 2° to 8° C and protected from light. Reconstitute only with the diluent provided and use as soon as possible after dissolution. Dosage is the contents of one reconstituted vial. Store the reconstituted vaccine in a dark place at 2° to 8° C and discard if not used within 8 hours.

Mumps virus vaccine, live, attenuated (Mumpsvax)

1. This vaccine is a preparation of live organisms of the Jeryl Lynn (B level) strain of mumps virus that has been grown in chick embryo tissue culture.

2. Refrigeration is necessary at 2° to 8° C. The vaccine must be used within 8 hours after its reconstitution. Unused portions must be discarded. The vaccine should be protected from bright light and sunlight. Color may be red, pink, or yellow.

3. Duration of immunity is not yet determined, but study indicates that good protection exists for 1 to 2 years after vaccination and probably lasts up to 10 years.

4. This vaccine is not recommended for use in children under 1 year of age or in pregnant women.

5. Inject the entire contents of vial subcutaneously into the upper arm. Antibodies develop in about 28 days.

6. Serious reactions are rare, but fever, redness, and soreness at the injection site may occur. Do not administer to patients allergic to chickens or neomycin.

Pneumococcal vaccine, polyvalent (Pneumovax)

1. Polyvalent pneumococcal vaccine contains the capsular coats (antigenic substance) of fourteen of the most prevalent types of pathologic pneumococcal bacteria.

2. Immunization against pneumonia and bacteremia is suggested in patients who have an increased risk of pneumococcal infection, such as those with chronic heart disease, lung disease, renal disease, or diabetes mellitus.

3. Patients should not be immunized during the time of an active infection. Most patients will note redness and swelling at the site of injection, and an occasional patient may develop a fever.

4. At this time, it is recommended that patients not be revaccinated more than every 3 years.

5. The vaccine should be stored at 2° to 8° C. Normal dosage: 0.5 ml, administered subcutaneously or intramuscularly.

Live oral poliovirus vaccine, trivalent (TOPV) (Orimune, Trivalent)

1. Dr. Albert Sabin introduced attenuated live virus strains 1, 2, and 3 vaccines.

2. This vaccine can be cultured in renal tissue cells of monkeys.

3. Strains 1, 2, and 3 represent the three separate monovalent vaccines for the prevention of poliomyelitis caused by types 1, 2, or 3 of the poliovirus.

4. The U.S. Public Health Service now recommends TOPV as the vaccine of choice for primary immunization of children in the United States.

5. This vaccine is preferred over the Salk vaccine because it provides longer lasting immunity, produces an immune response similar to that induced by natural poliovirus infection, and is easier to administer.

6. This liquid vaccine is for oral administration only, not for injection. Normal dose: 0.5 ml of vaccine, diluted with distilled water, simple syrup, or milk. It may also be absorbed on bread, cake, or cube sugar for administration.

7. Three doses of the trivalent vaccine are administered; the first two doses 8 weeks apart and the third dose 8 to 12 months after the second dose.

8. Oral poliovirus vaccine is stored in the frozen state.

When thawed for use, it is stored at refrigeration temperatures up to 8° C. When thawed, it must be used within 30 days. Once opened, vials must be kept refrigerated and used within 7 days.

Rabies vaccine (duck embryo) dried, killed virus (DEV)

1. Rabies vaccine is a sterile freeze-dried suspension of killed rabies virus prepared from duck embryo.

2. Caution should be used in administering vaccine to persons with a history of allergy, especially to duck or chicken eggs or proteins. Local redness and soreness are common. Patients often complain of headache, listlessness, numbness of hands or feet, and photophobia.

3. Rabies vaccine is injected subcutaneously for 14 to 21 days. One milliliter of the reconstituted suspension of killed virus vaccine is administered subcutaneously daily at different sites.

4. Rabies vaccine injections are painful and dangerous, but the mortality rate of rabies is very high—almost 100%.

Smallpox vaccine

1. This vaccine, the first of all vaccines prepared, consists of a glycerinated suspension of *Vaccinia* viruses that were grown in healthy vaccinated animals of the bovine family.

2. Failure of vaccination is often caused by inactive virus and indicates that the vaccination should be repeated.

3. Usual dose: the contents of one container, administered by multiple puncture of the skin. It should cause no bleeding or pain if properly administered. Patients must not scratch the pustules that develop; secondary infection may develop.

4. In 1971, the U.S. Public Health Service, with the support of the Committee of Infectious Diseases of the American Academy of Pediatrics, recommended discontinuation of routine smallpox vaccination, because the dangers of vaccination now exceed the risk of contracting the disease. Deaths and encephalitis have occurred from smallpox vaccine. The last recorded case of smallpox in the United States occurred in 1949 by importation. Smallpox vaccination is recommended for international travel to specified countries and for health personnel considered to be at risk. Persons with chronic dermatitis or eczema should not be vaccinated.

Tuberculosis vaccine; BCG vaccine (Bacillus Calmette-Guérin Vaccine)

1. This vaccine is a freeze-dried preparation of the culture of an attenuated strain of the bovine tubercle bacillus.

2. It is used only in individuals who are negative in their reaction to the tuberculin skin test.

3. Conversion of negative tuberculin-tested subjects to positive reactors after vaccination is usually presumptive evidence that immunity has developed similar to that following a naturally resisted or healed primary sensitizing infection.

4. Physicians may choose either to use the vaccine to reduce the risk of clinical disease or to not use the vaccine and give the tuberculin skin test for early diagnosis and as a guide to the patient's symptoms.

5. Tuberculosis vaccine is usually administered by intradermal injection: 0.1 ml (equivalent to 0.2 mg) is injected with a tuberculin syringe and a 26-gauge needle as superficially as possible so that a wheal of 8 to 10 mm occurs.

Typhoid vaccine

1. This is a sterile suspension of killed *Salmonella typhosa* in physiologic saline solution or other suitable diluent.

2. Usual dose: 0.5 ml, subcutaneously, administered two times at an interval of 4 or more weeks.

3. Routine immunization is not required. It is recommended for travelers to countries where typhoid is endemic, for persons exposed to a typhoid carrier, and for those in a community where there is an outbreak of typhoid fever.

Typhus vaccine

1. This vaccine is a sterile suspension of the killed rickettsial organism of strains of epidemic typhus rickettsiae cultured in chick embryos.

2. Usual dose: 1 ml, subcutaneously, to be repeated once after at least a 4-week interval. Booster injections are necessary every 6 to 12 months.

Yellow fever vaccine

1. Yellow fever vaccine is an attenuated strain of the living virus. It is prepared by culturing the microorganism in the chick embryo.

2. It is dried from the frozen state. The powder is rehydrated immediately before use.

3. Usual dose: 0.5 ml, administered subcutaneously.

4. A single dose provides protection for at least 6 years.

5. All rehydrated vaccine and containers which remain unused after 1 hour must be sterilized and discarded.

TOXOIDS

A toxoid is a toxin that is chemically modified to be nontoxic but still antigenic. The agent generally used for the detoxification of toxins is formaldehyde. Toxoids are available in the plain form and as adsorbed and precipitated preparations. Aluminum hydroxide and aluminum phosphate are used to provide an adsorption surface for the adsorbed products, and alum is used for the precipitated products. The adsorbed and precipitated products are absorbed more slowly by the circulating and tissue fluids of the body and are excreted more slowly; thus, they provide higher immunizing titers than does plain toxoid.

Diphtheria toxoid, adsorbed (pediatric)

1. This adsorbed diphtheria toxoid is a sterile suspension of diphtheria toxoid adsorbed by the addition of aluminum hydroxide.

2. It is recommended for active immunization of infants and children under 6 years of age.

3. Usual dose: for active immunization, 0.5 ml intramuscularly, 2 injections 6 to 8 weeks apart. A third reinforcing dose is administered approximately 12 months later.

Tetanus toxoid, fluid

1. This toxoid is a sterile solution of the products of growth of *Clostridium tetani*. The products of this growth are so modified by formaldehyde that it has lost the ability to cause serious toxicity but still has the power to induce active immunity.

2. Usual dose: 0.5 or 1 ml, subcutaneously or intramuscularly, according to label directions. The dose is repeated three times at intervals of 4 to 8 weeks. A fourth dose of 0.5 ml should be administered 6 to 12 months after the third injection.

Tetanus toxoid, adsorbed

1. Adsorbed tetanus toxoid is precipitated or adsorbed by the addition of alum, aluminum phosphate, or aluminum hydroxide.

2. Usual dose: for active immunization, 2 injections of 0.5 ml at intervals of 4 to 8 weeks, intramuscularly. A third dose should be administered 6 to 12 months after the second injection.

3. To maintain adequate protection for the actively immunized person, booster doses should be repeated every 10 years.

Diphtheria and tetanus toxoids, adsorbed (DT)

1. This is a sterile suspension prepared by mixing the desired quantities of the adsorbed forms of diphtheria and tetanus toxoids.

2. Usual dose: 2 injections of 0.5 ml, as directed on the label 4 to 8 weeks apart. A third reinforcing dose is administered 6 to 12 months later.

3. This combination is used for adults for whom the triple vaccine (including pertussis) is not recommended.

Diphtheria and tetanus toxoids and pertussis vaccine, adsorbed (DPT)

1. This is a sterile mixture of diphtheria toxoid, tetanus toxoid, and pertussis vaccine adsorbed on alum, aluminum hydroxide, or aluminum phosphate.
2. DPT is recommended for active immunization of infants and children under 6 years of age.
3. Primary immunization: a complete immunizing treatment for children 6 weeks to 3 months of age or older consists of three 0.5-ml doses injected intramuscularly, each 4 to 8 weeks apart, with a reinforcing dose approximately 1 year after the third injection. A booster dose should be administered when the child is 3 to 6 years of age. For boosters thereafter, use the recommended dose of diphtheria and tetanus toxoids, adsorbed (for adult use) every 10 years.

AGENTS FOR CUTANEOUS IMMUNITY TESTS
Mumps skin test antigen

1. This skin test is most commonly used in patients to determine whether skin sensitivity exists. The antigen is a suspension of killed mumps virus prepared from virus cultured in chicken embryo.
2. Those known to be sensitive to chicken, chicken eggs, or chicken feathers should not be tested.
3. Dose: 0.1 ml of antigen, injected intradermally. An area of erythema, 1.5 cm or more in diameter, indicates sensitivity to the virus and probable immunity. If the reaction is negative, it indicates susceptibility to infection.

Purified protein derivative of tuberculin (PPD) (Aplisol)

1. This is a sterile soluble purified product of the growth of the *Mycobacterium tuberculosis*.
2. It is prepared in a special liquid medium free from protein.
3. Its chief use is as a diagnostic aid in determining exposure to *Mycobacterium tuberculosis*.
4. Usual dose: 5 TU (0.1 ml) intradermally.
5. If the patient has been infected with tuberculosis at some time, an area of redness develops, usually with a papule at the point of application of the tuberculin.
6. A reaction indicates that the patient has at some time been infected with tuberculosis but not necessarily that he has clinical tuberculosis.

ALLERGENS

Allergy is a condition of hypersensitivity to certain antigens. Antigens are usually proteins, such as the proteins present in the hair or skin of animals, the feathers of fowl, the pollen of plants, or the proteins of food, serum, or bacteria. Persons who come in contact with the proteins to which they are unusually sensitive develop such symptoms as coryza, sneezing, headache, fever, hives, and asthmatic attacks.

Allergens are extracts prepared from the proteins of various substances and are used to determine the susceptibility of the patient to proteins and to prevent and relieve the conditions caused by his hypersensitivity.

Susceptibility is tested by intradermal injection of the allergen. If the patient is sensitive to that particular protein, an elevated red spot or urticarial wheal results.

Prevention and treatment of allergy

Once the identity of the particular protein causing the allergy symptoms has been discovered, attacks may be prevented or ameliorated by removing the causative factor, such as eliminating contact with dogs and cats, removing hair mattress or feather pillows, or removing offending food from the diet.

The patient with hay fever may have to be immunized against the specific pollens causing the attack. This process is called desensitization. It consists of a series of 10 or more injections of dilute solutions of the particular offending pollen or pollens in graduated strengths, administered at intervals of about 5 days. The treatment should be started early enough so that the maximum dose is reached by the time the first attack of the disease is expected; this dose is repeated once a week during the pollen season. Immunity lasts about a year. In some cases of asthma and urticaria, the patient may be desensitized to the specific proteins causing their symptoms. Individuals vary as to dosage and the frequency and length of time for injections, depending on their response to treatment.

Antihistaminic drugs are commonly used today in the treatment of allergic symptoms. (For a discussion of antihistaminic drugs, see Index.) Cortisone, hydrocortisone, and related compounds provide symptomatic relief of allergic manifestations, but should not be used for minor allergic conditions such as hay fever because of their serious side effects.

> **The physician prescribes the medicine and treatment.**
> **The nurse carries out the physician's orders.**
> **Self-medication is dangerous. Consult your physician first.**
> **There is in every medicine a possible danger.**
> **When in doubt—ASK!**

ASSIGNMENT

Review previous lessons and questions according to the directions of your instructor.

1. Name two kinds of immunity and explain each.
2. Why is the term passive is used to describe passive acquired immunity?
3. What is an immune serum? What are naturally produced human serums?
4. Explain the uses of immune serum globulin (human).
5. How is rabies immune globulin (human) used, and for how long does it provide protective coverage?
6. What is the use of $RH_0(D)$ immune globulin (human)? Learn well the uses of this serum in obstetrical patients. When must this *not* be administered?
7. How are antitoxins prepared? What is the purpose of antitoxins? Explain anaphylactic shock. What is the purpose of tests for sensitivity to horse serum or other suspected antigens?
8. What is the purpose of diphtheria antitoxin, and what type of immunity does it give?
9. What is the source of tetanus antitoxin, and what type of immunity does it give?
10. Define vaccines and list the important points about them.
11. List all the vaccines discussed and select from this list the vaccines you think should be administered to people of your community.
12. Study the types of measles and measles-mumps vaccines discussed. Do you think a measles vaccine is important statewide and nationwide?
13. Why does the U.S. Public Health Service recommend Sabin vaccine (live oral poliovirus vaccine, trivalent; TOPV)?
14. What is rabies vaccine (duck embryo) dried, killed virus (DEV)? What cautions should be used before administering this vaccine? What symptoms often occur? How long does the subq injectable treatment last? Are rabies vaccine injections painful and dangerous? If so, why is the vaccine given?
15. When did the U.S. Public Health Service and the Committee of Infectious Diseases of the American Academy of Pediatrics recommend discontinuance of routine smallpox vaccination? Why? When is smallpox vaccination recommended?
16. For what conditions is typhoid vaccine recommended?
17. What is tuberculosis vaccine (BCG vaccine)? What is its use? If the physician decides not to use the vaccine, what else may be used and what is its purpose? How is tuberculosis vaccine usually administered?
18. What is a toxoid? List five toxoids. What type of immunization do they give?
19. Name three cutaneous immunity tests and tell the purpose of each.
20. Define allergy and name some of the symptoms an allergic person may develop. What are allergens? Discuss the prevention and treatment of allergy. What group of drugs are commonly used today in the treatment of allergic symptoms?

CHAPTER 29

Miscellaneous agents

Allopurinol (al-o-pu′rin-ol)
(Zyloprim) (zy′lo-prim)

1. Allopurinol is an entirely new approach to the treatment of gout. It blocks the terminal steps in uric acid formation by inhibiting xanthine oxidase.
2. This drug can be used for the treatment of either primary or secondary gout.
3. Allopurinol should not be used during pregnancy, by nursing mothers, or in most diseases of children.
4. Side effects are nausea, vomiting, headache, diarrhea, drowsiness, and a metallic taste. Toxic effects include liver damage, fever, skin rash, and leukopenia. The drug should be stopped when skin rash occurs, or in the opinion of the physician, at the occurrence of any other toxic symptoms.
5. Allopurinol may have some advantages over the uricosuric drugs; gouty nephropathy and the formation of urate stones are less likely with allopurinol, because the drug reduces the amount of uric acid produced.
6. Usual adult dose: 200 to 400 mg daily. Larger doses have been used. Fluid intake should be sufficient to maintain a daily urinary output of 2 liters.

Bromocriptine mesylate (bro-mo-krip′teen)
(Parlodel) (par′lo-del)

1. Bromocriptine is a new agent available for the short-term treatment of amenorrhea or galactorrhea associated with hyperprolactinemia. It is a nonhormonal, nonestrogenic agent that inhibits the secretion of prolactin. It should not be used in patients with normal prolactin levels or in the management of infertility.
2. Adverse effects are fairly common with bromocriptine therapy. Side effects include nausea, headache, dizziness, fatigue, abdominal cramps, constipation, and diarrhea. These adverse effects are usually mild and do not warrant the discontinuation of therapy.
3. Bromocriptine therapy may increase fertility. Contraceptive measures are encouraged (except oral contraceptives), since fetal effects are not known. If pregnancy should occur, discontinue therapy immediately.
4. Usual dosage: 2.5 mg two to three times daily, with meals. Duration of therapy should not exceed 6 months. Bromocriptine is available in 2.5-mg tablets.

Clofibrate (klo-fi′brayt)
(Atromid S) (a′tro-mid)

1. Clofibrate is an agent used to lower serum triglyceride levels. Its mechanism of action is unknown.
2. Common early side effects are nausea, vomiting, abdominal cramping, and diarrhea. These symptoms are usually mild and diminish with continued therapy. Administering with meals will help reduce stomach upset.
3. Clofibrate interacts with warfarin to increase the anticoagulant effects of warfarin. The dose of warfarin should be started at half the normal dose and then adjusted based on patient response.
4. Clofibrate may also interact with chlorpropamide to cause hypoglycemia. This interaction may be prevented by reducing the chlorpropamide dosage.
5. Normal adult dosage: 2 g daily in two to four doses. Clofibrate is available in 500-mg capsules.

Colchicine (kol′chi-sin)

1. Colchicine is an alkaloid obtained from the seeds and bulbous root of the *Colchicum autumnale*, or meadow saffron.
2. Extracts of the plant have been used for hundreds of years to prevent or relieve acute attacks of gout. Colchicine interrupts the cycle of urate crystal deposition in the tissues that results in an acute attack of gout. It does not affect the amount of uric acid in the blood or urine, so it is not uricosuric.
3. Side effects and toxic effects include, after prolonged use, agranulocytosis, aplastic anemia, and peripheral neuritis. In acute poisoning from the drug, abdominal pain, nausea, vomiting, diarrhea, and blood in the urine may occur. Severe abdominal cramps, rapid weak pulse, slow respirations, and shock have occurred.

242

4. It is available in 0.5-, 0.6-, and 1-mg tablets for oral administration. An initial dose of 1 mg is usually followed by 0.5 mg every 1 or 2 hours until pain is relieved or until symptoms of nausea, vomiting, or abdominal pain appear. The earlier the dose, the more effective the relief.

Disulfiram (di-sul′fi-ram)
(Antabuse) (an′tah-byous)

1. Disulfiram produces a sensitivity to alcohol that results in a very unpleasant response when the patient ingests even small amounts of alcohol. It is used in alcohol rehabilitation programs for chronic alcoholic patients who want to maintain a state of sobriety. It should not be considered a cure for alcoholism and should be used only in conjunction with other rehabilitative therapy.
2. The disulfiram-alcohol reaction is manifested by nausea, severe vomiting, sweating, throbbing headache, dizziness, blurred vision, and confusion.
3. Disulfiram may interact with several other drugs.
   a. Phenytoin: disulfiram inhibits the metabolism of phenytoin, which may result in phenytoin intoxication.
   b. Warfarin: the dosage of warfarin may need to be reduced since disulfiram may prolong prothrombin time.
   c. Isoniazid: patients taking isoniazid should be observed for the appearance of unsteady gait or marked changes in behavior; discontinue disulfiram if such signs appear.
4. Patients under disulfiram treatment should carry an identification card, stating that they are receiving disulfiram, describing the symptoms of the disulfiram-alcohol reaction, and indicating the physician or institution to be contacted.
5. Side effects of disulfiram include mild drowsiness, fatigability, impotence, headache, and dermatitis.
6. Initial adult dose: 500 mg daily for 1 to 2 weeks. The average maintenance dose is 250 mg daily, with a range of 125 to 500 mg. Disulfiram is available in 250- and 500-mg tablets.

Lactulose (lak′tu-los)
(Cephulac) (sef′u-lak), *(Duphalac)* (du′fah-lak)

1. Lactulose is used to treat portal-systemic (hepatic) encephalopathy and hepatic coma by reducing blood ammonia levels. Lactulose acts by acidifying the colon, thus preventing the absorption of ammonia, which is implicated in cause of hepatic encephalopathy and coma.
2. Side effects cause gaseous distention with flatulence, belching, abdominal cramps, and diarrhea. Dosage

reduction will often control many of these adverse effects.
3. Lactulose contains galactose and lactose. It should not be used in patients who require a low-galactose diet and should be used with caution in diabetic patients.
4. Lactulose is available as a syrup. Usual initial dose: 30 to 45 ml, three or four times daily. Dosage may be adjusted every other day to produce two or three soft stools daily.

Probenecid (pro-ben′e-sid)
(Benemid) (ben′ah-mid)

1. Probenecid is another drug used to treat mild attacks of gout and chronic gouty arthritis. It is not effective in acute attacks of gout and is not an analgesic.
2. This drug promotes renal excretion of a number of substances, including uric acid. It inhibits the reabsorption of urate in the kidney, which results in reduction of uric acid in the blood. This uricosuric action helps to prevent or to retard joint changes often seen in chronic gout.
3. Precipitation of urates in the kidney can be prevented by keeping the urine alkaline.
4. When administered with penicillin, it raises and prolongs plasma concentrations, maintaining high levels of the antibiotic in the blood.
5. Salicylates should be avoided during probenecid administration because of their antagonistic effect.
6. A high fluid intake is recommended during administration of this drug to produce increased volume of urine to minimize the formation of uric acid stones and the possibility of hematuria.
7. Side effects and toxic effects may include nausea, constipation, skin rash, liver necrosis, blood dyscrasias, and hypertensive reaction. Probenecid is generally well tolerated, and side effects are rare.
8. Usual dosage: 0.5 to 2 g daily in divided doses, orally, administered frequently with sodium bicarbonate to maintain alkalinity of urine.

Probucol (pro′bu-kol)
(Lorelco) (lor-el′ko)

1. Probucol is used to lower serum cholesterol levels. It has a variable effect on serum triglyceride levels. The mechanism of action is unknown, and therapy should be instituted only after dietary therapy has failed to reduce elevated cholesterol levels.
2. Diarrhea, flatulence, nausea, vomiting, and foul-smelling sweat occasionally occur when therapy is first initiated. These side effects usually diminish with continued use.
3. Usual adult dose: 500 mg twice daily, with meals. Probucol is available as 250-mg tablets.

ASSIGNMENT

Review previous lessons and questions according to the directions of your instructor.

1. For what medical condition is allopurinol (Zyloprim) used? What is its action? For which type of gout can allopurinol be used? Can it be used during pregnancy, in nursing mothers, or in most diseases of children? List the side effects of this drug. List the toxic effects. For what toxic effects should the treatment with allopurinol be stopped? What may be possible advantages of allopurinol over the uricosuric drugs? Does allopurinol increase or decrease the amount of uric acid produced by the body? Should fluids be increased during allopurinol therapy, and if so, to what extent?

2. What is the name of an agent available for short-term treatment of amenorrhea or galactorrhea associated with hyperprolactinemia? What type of an agent is it, and what does it inhibit? Is it indicated, or contraindicated, in patients with normal prolactin levels or in the management of infertility? List the adverse effects. Are they usually severe or mild? What effect does bromocriptine (Parlodel) have on fertility? Are contraceptive measures, except oral contraceptives, encouraged? If pregnancy occurs during bromocriptine therapy, what is the best procedure? What is the usual dose of this drug, and what is the period of treatment?

3. What is the use of clofibrate (Atromid S)? List the common side effects. Are these side effects usually mild or severe, and do they lessen with continued therapy? When is the best time to administer clofibrate to control or prevent stomach upsets? What is the interaction of clofibrate with warfarin? Explain the dose of warfarin while the patient is receiving clofibrate therapy. What is the interaction of clofibrate with chlorpropamide, and how may this interaction be prevented? What is the normal adult dosage of clofibrate? It is available in capsules of what strength?

4. Describe the source of colchicine. What is the chief use of this drug? What is the action of colchicine? Does it affect the amount of uric acid in the blood or urine? Is it, then, a uricosuric, or not a uricosuric? List the side effects of colchicine. What symptoms may occur in acute poisoning from this drug? What dose strengths are available? What is an initial dose? Explain the dosage strength and frequency

of administration that follow the initial dose. What is the advantage of early therapy with colchicine?

5. What is the effect of disulfiram (Antabuse)? What is the use of disulfiram? Is it a cure for alcoholism? How is it used for alcoholism? What are the reactions or symptoms when the patient undergoing rehabiliative therapy with complete alcohol withdrawal takes even a small amount of alcohol? Discuss the interaction of disulfiram with phenytoin, warfarin, and isoniazid. Why should patients under disulfiram treatment carry an identification card that states that they are receiving disulfiram, lists the symptoms of disulfiram-alcohol reaction, and indicates the physician or institution to be contacted? List the side effects of disulfiram. Tell the initial adult dose and the average maintenance dose.

6. Lactulose (Cephulac, Duphalac) is used to treat what medical conditions? How does it act? List its side effects. How can these side effects often be controlled? What does lactulose contain? When should it *not* be used? Lactulose is available in what form? What is the usual initial dose? What effect is produced by adjusting the dose every other day?

7. What is the use of probenecid (Benemid)? Is it effective in acute attacks of gout? How does this drug act? Does probenecid have uricosuric action? How can precipitation of urates in the kidney be prevented? What is the interaction of probenecid with penicillin? Why should salicylates be avoided during probenecid administration? Why is a high fluid intake recommended during administration of probenecid? List the side effects. Are they rare? Is probenecid generally well tolerated? What is the usual dosage? With what drug should it be administered and why?

8. What is the use of probucol (Lorelco)? Should dietary therapy be tried first? List the side effects. Do they usually diminish with continued use of this drug? What is the usual adult dose?

9. The physician ordered an initial dose of 1 mg of colchicine for a patient. You had available a bottle of cochicine in strength of 0.5 mg. How many tablets will you administer?

10. It is the patient's second week of treatment with probenecid (Benemid) for gout. The physician ordered 500 mg twice daily. What dose would you be administering in *grams* if you gave 500 mg? (See Index for conversion.)

Glossary

absorbent Medicine or substance that absorbs liquids or other secretion products; a substance that takes in, or picks up, such as a blotter that absorbs ink.

   pathologic The absorption into the blood of any bodily excretion or morbid product, such as the bile or pus.

acceleration Quickening, as of the pulse rate or respiration.

accommodation Adjustment, especially that of the eye for various distances.

   absolute The accommodation of either eye separately.

   binocular The convergence of the two eyes so as to bring the image of the object seen on each retina.

acetylation Introduction of an acetyl group into an organic molecule.

acetylcholine Acetic acid ester of choline chloride, normally present in many parts of the body and having many important physiologic functions. For example, in the central nervous system it is for the purpose of transmission of nerve impulses. It is used subcutaneously and intravenously to relax peripheral blood vessels.

acetylcholinesterase An esterase in the blood that hydrolyzes any excess of acetylcholine, splitting it into acetic acid and choline.

achlorhydria Absence of hydrochloric acid from the gastric secretions.

acidosis Condition of lessened alkalinity in the body, caused by formation of excess amounts of acid or by lessened amounts of base.

acne Any inflammatory disease of the sebaceous glands, especially acne vulgaris, or common acne. It is chronic and commonly occurs on the chest, back, and face.

acromegaly Enlargement of the bony structure characterized by gigantism and caused by a tumor of the pituitary gland with increased secretion from the gland.

Addison's disease Disease characterized by a bronze-like pigmentation of the skin, severe prostration, progressive anemia, low blood pressure, diarrhea, and digestive disturbances. This condition is caused by lack of function of the adrenal (suprarenal) glands located on top of each kidney and by initial tuberculous infiltration (the last in less than half of the cases today). It is treated with cortisone or hydrocortisone and other hormones and a high-carbohydrate, high-protein diet.

adrenal cortex Outer layer of adrenal gland that manufactures specific hormones.

adrenal gland Gland of internal secretion situated on top of the kidney; also called the suprarenal gland.

adrenalectomy Removal of adrenal bodies.

adrenergic Activated or transmitted by epinephrine (adrenalin); a term applied to that form of autonomic nerves that acts by setting free acetylcholine from their nerve terminations.

adsorbent Substance that acts by gathering up another substance on its surface in a condensed layer.

aerobe A microorganism that can live and grow in the presence of free oxygen.

afferent Carrying, for example, of blood or impulses from the periphery to the center.

aggravate To make worse or to irritate.

aggregation Crowding or clustering together.

agranulocytopenia See *agranulocytosis.*

agranulocytosis Complete or nearly complete absence of the granular leukocytes (granulocytes) from the bone marrow and blood; also called agranulocytopenia.

albumin Protein found in nearly every animal and in many vegetable tissues and characterized by being soluble in water and coagulable by heat. It contains carbon, hydrogen, nitrogen, oxygen, and sulfur.

   albumin A A certain constituent of the blood serum, reduced in amount in cancer patients but increased in cancer cells.

   acetosoluble A form of albumin soluble in acetic acid; sometimes found in urine.

albuminuria The presence of albumin in the urine, indicating either a simple mixture of albuminous matters, such as blood, with the urine or a morbid state of the kidneys that is permitting albumin to pass from the blood.

alkalosis Excessive alkalinity of the body fluids; increased alkali reserve in the blood and other body tissues.

allergy Unusual reaction to a substance that in similar amounts is harmless to most persons.

alopecia Baldness, deficiency of hair, natural or abnormal.

amebiasis State of being infected with amebae.

amenorrhea Absence or abnormal stopping of menstrual flow.

amide Any compound derived from ammonia by substituting an acid radical for hydrogen.

amine Class of compounds derived from ammonia.

amino acids Organic acids in which one or more hydrogen atoms have been replaced by the amino group NH_2. The amino acids are the building blocks of the protein molecule and the end product of protein digestion.

anabolism, anabolic To build up; any constructive process by which simple substances are converted by living cells into more complex compounds; constructive metabolism and assimilation.

anaerobe Any microorganism having the power to live without either air or free oxygen.

analeptic Restorative medicine or agent. Central nervous system stimulants used to antagonize depressant drugs are called analeptics; they restore consciousness and mental alertness.

analgesic Medication to relieve pain, such as aspirin or morphine.

analogue Part or organ having the same function as another, but of a different structure.

analogy Resemblance in structure caused by similarity of function.

anaphylaxis Unusual or exaggerated reaction of an organism or individual to foreign proteins or other substances. These reactions are immediate, shock-like, and frequently fatal within minutes. They include symptoms such as apprehension, burning, prickling sensations, generalized urticaria or hives, edema, choking sensation, cyanosis, wheezing, cough, incontinence, shock, fever, dilation of pupils, loss of consciousness, and convulsions. Reaction to penicillin is an example. Emergency drugs should always be available whenever injections are administered.

androgen Male sex hormones.

anemia Insufficient blood cells or iron.

anesthetic Drug causing a temporary loss of sensation.

angina pectoris Severe, cramp-like pain of the chest, caused by insufficient circulation and characterized by spasms of the muscles of the coronary arteries surrounding and entering the heart.

angioneurotic edema Giant hives characterized by large wheals or pinkish elevations similar to hives on the skin, with marked itching, nausea, fever, and malaise; generally caused by sensitivity to a food or foods.

anhydrase An enzyme that catalyzes anhydration.
  carbonic An enzyme that catalyzes the release of carbon dioxide from the blood in the tissues and the lungs.

anion Ion carrying a negative charge. They include all the nonmetals, the acid radicals, and the hydroxyl ion.

anomalies *(anomaly)* Marked deviations from the normal standard.

anorexia Lack or loss of appetite for food.

anthelmintic Agent to destroy worms.

anthrax Carbuncle or other infection caused by the anthrax bacillus.
  malignant A fatal infectious disease of cattle and sheep caused by anthrax bacillus and characterized by formation of hard edema or ulcers at the point of inoculation and by collapse symptoms. It may occur in humans.

anti Against.

antibiotic Against life.

antibiotics Medications used to kill living microorganisms that cause infection.

antibodies Substances in the body that react with a specific antigen. They may be present under apparently normal conditions but develop anew in response to the introduction of specific antigen into the tissues or blood. Antibodies include, among others, agglutinins, antienzymes, and antitoxins.

anticoagulant Substance used to prevent blood clotting.

antiemetic Arresting or preventing emesis or vomiting, relieving nausea.

antigen Any substance that will lead to the development of antibodies.

antihistamine Agent given to neutralize histamine produced by the body.

antipyretic Relieving fever; cooling.

antiseptic Drug that tends to prevent or lessen the activity of infection by slowing the growth of microorganisms.

antispasmodic Agent used in relieving muscular contractions, spasms, and convulsions.

antitoxin Serum used to lessen the effects of the toxins or poisons produced by bacteria.

antitussive Relieving or preventing cough.

anuria, anuresis Absolute suppression of urinary secretion.

apical pulse Heartbeat taken with a stethoscope, the bell or disc of the stethoscope being placed over the apex or pointed extremity of the heart.

aplastic anemia Rare condition in which the bone marrow cells cease to produce leukocytes in sufficient amounts to compensate for their destruction.

apnea The transient cessation of breathing that follows forced respiration; asphyxia.

apoplexy Stroke or paralysis caused by rupture of a blood vessel.

apothecary Druggist or pharmacist.

appendicitis Inflammation of the appendix.

appetite Hunger, natural longing, or desire, especially for food.

aqueous humor Fluid filling the anterior and posterior chambers of the eye in front of the lens.

arrhythmia Any variation from the normal rhythm of the heartbeat; irregularities. Some various forms of arrhythmias include sinus arrhythmia, extrasystole, heart block, auricular fibrillation, auricular flutter, and paroxysmal tachycardia.

arteriole Any minute arterial branch.

arteriosclerosis Scarring or hardening of the arteries that results from disease of the arterial walls.
  obliterans Proliferation of the intima, or innermost of the three coats of the artery, causing complete obliteration or closing of the lumen of the artery.

arthralgia Neuralgia or pain in a joint.

arthritis Rheumatism characterized by symptoms such as pain, swelling, inflammation, and stiffness of joints.

ascites Accumulation of serous fluid in the peritoneal cavity; dropsy of the abdominal cavity; painless swelling of the abdomen that gives a dull sound on percussion. Causes include local inflammation of the peritoneum and obstruction of the venous circulation by disease of the heart, kidney, or liver.

asphyxia Suffocation or a deficiency of oxygen in the blood.
  neonatorum Suffocation in the newborn.

asthma Disease of the bronchi, with difficulty and shortness of breath; often caused by allergies.

asystole Imperfect or incomplete systole; inability of the heart to perform a complete systole.

ataxia Failure of muscular coordination; irregularity of muscular action.

atelectasis Partial collapse of the lung; imperfect expansion of the lung in the newborn.

atherosclerosis Form of arteriosclerosis with marked degenerative changes and fatty degeneration of the connective tissue of the arterial walls.

athetosis A derangement marked by constant recurring series of slow, vermicular movements of the hands and feet, occurring chiefly in children and resulting principally from a brain lesion.

athlete's foot Ringworm of the feet; fungous infection.

atonic Characterized by lack of normal tone, for example, lack of muscle tone.

atrioventricular heart block A blocking at the atrioventricular or auriculoventricular junction (the auricles and ventricles beat independently of each other).

atrium See **auricle.**

atrophy Change or degeneration in a part.

attenuation Act or process of thinning or weakening, especially the weakening of the toxicity of a virus or a microorganism by repeated inoculation and successive culture, adding an agent such as formaldehyde.

auricle Atrium of the heart; chamber at the apex of the heart on either side above the ventricle; divided into right and left auricle or atrium.

autoimmunization Immunization effected by processes within the body.

autonomic Self-governing; independent in function.

azotemia The presence of urea or other nitrogenous bodies in the blood.

> *chloropenic* Condition characterized by deficiency of sodium chloride, fixation of chlorine in the tissues, and azoturia (excess urea and other nitrogenous bodies in the urine).

bacteriostasis Condition in which bacteria are prevented from growing and spreading. *Bacteriostatic* is more general in its meaning than *antiseptic*.

beriberi An endemic form of polyneuritis prevalent chiefly in Japan, India, China, the Philippines, and the Malay peninsula and often fatal. Characteristic symptoms: spasmodic rigidity of the lower limbs, with muscular atrophy, paralysis, anemia, and neuralgic pains. The disease is thought to result from an almost exclusive diet of overmilled or highly polished rice or other carbohydrate food, which is deficient in the accessory food factor known as antineuritic vitamin.

bilateral Having two sides or pertaining to two sides.

biliary colic Spasm of the gallbladder, hepatic ducts, common bile duct, and cystic duct.

belpharitis Inflammation of the eyelids.

blood pressure Pressure of the blood on the wall of the arteries, dependent on the energy of the heart action, the elasticity of the walls of the arteries, the resistance in the capillaries, and the volume and the viscosity of the blood.

> *basic* That pressure exerted on the blood by the contractile walls independent of the additional pressure caused by the systolic contraction of the heart.

> *diastolic* The lowest arterial pressure at any one time during the cardiac cycle. It results from the recoil of the elastic walls of the aorta and arteries and the pressure this recoil exerts on the blood. It is known as the resting pressure that is being constantly exerted by the aorta and arteries and which the left ventricle must overcome before blood can be ejected into the aorta. This pressure represents the constant minimal load that the arteries must bear at all times.

> *pulse pressure* The difference between systolic and diastolic pressures. Pulse pressure is an important indication of cardiac output and peripheral resistance shown by the width of pulse pressure. A wide pulse pressure is a normal finding if there is bradycardia, and a narrow pulse pressure is normal if there is tachycardia. In hemorrhage, systolic level may fall, but the diastolic level tends to rise. The result is a narrow pulse pressure indicating decreased cardiac output. A pulse pressure as low as 20 mm Hg or as high as 50 mm Hg is pathologic.

> *systolic* The highest arterial pressure at any one time during the cardiac cycle. It is a combination of the ejection of blood from the ventricles during systole and the blood pushing aginst the elastic walls of the aorta and arteries. It is also known as the active or working pressure. Normal range is about 110 to 140 mm Hg.

blood sugar A simple sugar normally found in the blood.

bolus A rounded mass; a mass of food ready to be swallowed or a mass passing along the intestines. In pharmacy, a rounded mass larger than a pill.

botulism A type of food poisoning caused by a toxin produced by *Clostridium (Bacillus) botulinum* in improperly canned or preserved foods and characterized by vomiting, abdominal pain, difficulty of vision, nervous symptoms of central origin, disturbances of secretion, motor disturbances, dryness of the mouth and pharynx, dyspepsia, barking cough, mydriasis, paralytic drooping of the eyelid, and prolapse of other parts or organs. It requires immediate medical attention; death can often occur without treatment.

Bowman's capsule Globular dilation that forms the beginning of a uriniferous tubule within the kidney. Each nephron begins as a Bowman's capsule.

bradycardia Abnormal slowness of the heartbeat, as evidenced by slowing of the pulse rate to 60 or less.

bronchial asthma Disease of the bronchi with difficulty and shortness of breath.

bronchiectasis Dilation of the bronchi or of a bronchus, marked by foul breath, paroxysmal coughing, and expectoration of mucopurulent matter.

bronchogenic Originating in a bronchus.

bronchoscopy Examination of the bronchi through a tracheal wound or through an instrument called a bronchoscope.

bronchus Tube-like structure leading to the lung; located between trachea, or windpipe, and lung. There is a left and a right bronchus (bronchi).

brucellosis The disease produced by *Brucella*, a bacteria; undulant fever characterized by wave-like changes in fever.

buccal Pertaining to the cheek. In drug administration the mucous-membrane side of the inner cheek.

Buerger's disease Chronic inflammation of the arteries of the extremities with eventual thrombus or clot formation and blocking or occlusion of the blood vessel and gangrene.

buffer Any substance in a fluid that tends to lessen the change in hydrogen ion concentration (reaction), which otherwise would be produced by adding acids or alkalis; any substance that decreases or prevents the reaction that a chemotherapeutic agent would produce if administered alone; the action produced by a buffer.

BUN A laboratory blood: blood urea nitrogen.

Burkitt's lymphoma A rapidly progressive lymphatic tumor that occurs most commonly in the jaw, abdominal cavity, and meninges. Spontaneous regressions have been observed, and many patients are highly responsive to chemotherapy.

bursitis Inflammation of the bursae, or small sacs of tissue, some of which are found in the shoulder and knee.

caduceus Emblem of the medical profession; a wand with wings at the top and two serpents twisted around it.

calcinosis Condition marked by the disposition of calcium salts in nodules under the skin and in the muscles, tendons, nerves, and connective tissue.

Candida, candidal A genus of yeast-like fungi of the family Cryptococcaceae, various species of which have been isolated from pulmonary lesions in man.

Candida albicans A yeast-like fungus that causes an inflammation of the corners of the mouth.

Candida vulva Inflammation of the vulva or external part of the organs of generation in the female, caused by a yeast-like fungus *Candida vulva*.

capillary One of the microscopic blood vessels connecting arteries and veins.

carcinoma Malignant tumor or cancer; new growth made up of epithelial cells that tend to infiltrate and metastasize.

cardiac insufficiency Inability of the heart to perform its function properly.

cardiogenic shock Shock resulting from diminution of cardiac output in heart disease.

cardiospasm Spasm of the cardiac sphincter of the stomach.

carminative Medicine that expels gas from the stomach and intestines.

carotene Yellow pigment found in carrots, sweet potatoes, other vegetables, milk fat, body fat, and egg yolk. It may be converted in the body into vitamin A.

carotenoid Marked by a yellow color resembling that produced by carotene.

catabolism Destructive metabolism; passage of tissue material from a higher to a lower plane of complexity or specialization.

cataract An opacity of the crystalline eye lens or of its capsule.

catecholamines Dopamine, norepinephrine, and epinephrine synthesized, stored, and metabolized in the brain and affecting the central nervous system slightly and the autonomic nervous system to a greater degree.

cation Element or elements of an electrolyte that appears at the negative pole or cathode. Cations include all metals and hydrogen.

cationic See cation.

causalgia, causalgic Neuralgia characterized by intense local sensation, as of burning pain.

celiac disease Childhood form of sprue characterized by im-paired absorption of fats, perhaps glucose, and with such symptoms as diarrhea (with bulky, pale, frothy, foul-smelling stools), weight loss, vitamin deficiencies, anemia, infantilism, tetany, rickets, and sometimes dwarfism. The disease responds to the elimination of wheat gluten from the diet, administration of oral iron for hypochromic anemia, and vitamin B_{12} for macrocytic anemia. Diet in celiac disease should be high calorie, high protein, low fat, and gluten free.

cellulitis Inflammation of the cellular tissue, especially purulent inflammation of the loose subcutaneous tissue.

cerebellum That division of the brain behind the cerebrum and above the pons and fourth ventricle; it is concerned with the coordination of movements.

cerebrum Main portion of the brain occupying the upper part of the cranium and consisting of two equal portions called hemispheres, which are united at the bottom by a mass of white matter called the corpus callosum. The cerebrum is the organ of associative memory, reasoning, and judgment.

cervix Lower, neck-line portion of the uterus.

cheilitis Inflammation of the lip.

chemoreceptor Receptor adapted for excitation by chemical substances, such as olfactory and gustatory receptors; a supposed group of atoms in cell protoplasm having the ability to fix chemicals in the same way as bacterial poisons are fixed.

chemotherapeutic agent Agent of chemical nature used in the treatment of disease.

chilblains Inflammation and swelling of the toes, feet, or fingers caused by cold.

cholestatic Resulting from stoppage of bile flow.

cholesterol Fat-like, pearly substance crystallizing in the form of leaflets or plates and found in all animal fats and oils, in bile, blood, brain tissue, milk, egg yolk, kidneys, and suprarenal bodies. It constitutes a large part of the most frequently occurring gallstones and appears in atheroma of the arteries.

cholinergic Stimulated, activated, or transmitted by choline (acetylcholine); term applied to nerve fibers whose activity is transmitted by acetylcholine; drugs that cause effects in the body similar to those produced by acetylcholine.

cholinesterase Enzyme that hydrolyzes or destroys acetylcholine.

chorea (St. Vitus' dance) Convulsive nervous disease with involuntary and irregular jerking movements and attended with irritability, depression, and mental impairment; it occurs in early age, more commonly in girls than boys, and may be hereditary.

choriocarcinoma Carcinoma (cancer) developed from the chorionic epithelium.

chorion The outermost envelope of the growing zygote or fertilized ovum that serves as a protective and nutritive covering.

cicatric, cicatrix A scar; the mark left by a sore or wound.

ciliary Pertaining to or resembling the eyelashes.

cirrhosis Disease of the liver marked by thickening, atrophy, degeneration, and a granular yellow appearance to the organ caused by coloring from bile pigments.

climacteric Time in life when the body undergoes marked changes and the reproductive organs no longer fully function; menopause.

clitoris A small, elongated, erectile body or organ of the female, situation at the anterior angle of the vulva and homologous with the penis in the male.

clonus Spasm in which there is alternate rigidity and relaxation in rapid succession.

   foot A series of convulsive movements of the ankle, induced by suddenly pushing up the foot while the leg is extended.

   toe Rhythmic contractions of the great toe, induced by suddenly extending the first phalanx.

   wrist Spasmodic contractions of the hand muscles, induced by forcibly bending the hand backward.

Clostridium Genus of Bacillaceae that are anaerobic or microaerophilic and that form clostridial spore forms.

   Clostridium oedematiens Strictly anaerobic organism isolated from war wounds in about 40% of the cases. It is gram-positive and forms large subterminal spores.

   Clostridium septicum (Clostridium oedematis maligni) Moderately large, motile, gram-positive, rod-shaped organism with rounded ends and oval subterminal spores; infectious for humans only through wounds.

coagulant Agent causing blood or fluid to clot.

coalesce The fusing or blending of parts.

coarctation A straightening or pressing together; a condition of stricture or contraction; for example, of the aorta, with usually severe narrowing of the vessel lumen.

coenzyme A noncolloidal substance that combines with an inactive enzyme to produce activation of the enzyme.

colectomy Excision of a portion of the colon.

colitis Inflammation of the colon.

colloid Glutinous or resembling glue; a state in which the matter is distributed through some form of dispersing medium.

   emulsion The dispersing medium is usually water, and the disperse phase consists of highly complex organic substances such as starch or glue, which absorb much water, swell, and become uniformly distributed throughout the dispersion medium.

   suspension The disperse or distributing phase consists of particles of any insoluble substance such as metal, and the medium may be gaseous, liquid, or solid.

colostomy The formation of a permanent artificial opening (artificial anus) into the colon.

conduction Transfer of sound waves, heat, nerve influences, or electricity.

conductivity Capacity of a body to conduct a current.

congestive heart failure Result of the inability of the heart to expel sufficient blood for the metabolic demands of the body. Most common causes are hypertension, coronary atherosclerosis, and rheumatic heart disease. Less common causes include chronic pulmonary disease, congenital heart disease, syphilitic aortic insufficiency, calcific aortic stenosis, and bacterial endocarditis.

conjunctiva Mucous membrane lining the inner surface of the eyelids and covering the forepart of the eyeball.

conjunctivitis Inflammation of the mucous membrane conjunctiva. See *conjunctiva*.

constipation Infrequency or difficulty in movements of the bowels.

constriction A constricted part or place, a narrowing.

contract To decrease in size, as muscle tissue.

contractility Capacity for becoming short in response to a suitable stimulus.

cornea Transparent membrane forming the anterior or front part of the outer layer of the eyeball.

coronary occlusion The formation of a clot in a branch of the coronary arteries, which supply blood to the heart muscle, resulting in obstruction of the artery and infarction of the area of the heart supplied by the occluded vessel. Also called cardiac infarction and coronary thrombosis.

cortex Outer part of a gland or structure, such as the rind or bark.

craniotomy Operation on the cranium.

creatine Crystallizable nitrogenous principle, or methyl-guanidine-acetic acid, derived from the juice of muscular tissue; therapeutically, a cardiac, muscular, and digestive tonic.

creatinine Basic substance called creatine anhydride, procurable from creatine and from urine.

cretinism A chronic condition, congenital or developed before puberty, characterized by arrested physical and mental development, with dystrophy of the bones and soft parts. It is regarded as a form of myxedema and is probably caused by deficient thyroid activity.

cryptorchidism Undescended testicle.

crystalluria Formation of crystals in the urine or in the kidneys.

curie Standard unit for measuring the amount of radium emanation. The word curie comes from the discoverer of radium, Marie Sklodowska Curie, a Polish chemist in Paris, who lived 1867-1934.

Cushing's disease Disease caused by overgrowth of the basophil cells of the anterior lobe of the pituitary gland and marked by rapidly developing obesity of the face, neck, and trunk, decreased sexual activity, abnormal growth of hair, abdominal pain, weakness, and sometimes supraclavicular fat pads, striae, and acne.

cutaneous Pertaining to the skin.

cyanosis Blueness of skin, lips, and often fingernails resulting from cardiac malformations causing insufficient oxygenation of the blood.

cycloplegia Paralysis of the ciliary muscle of the eye.

cystic fibrosis An infant and childhood disease probably inherited, with pancreatic pathology and digestive and respiratory difficulties. Respiratory failure is most frequently the eventual cause of death. Characteristic symptoms are changes in the activity of the exocrine glands, including sweat (with a salty taste to the skin), salivary, and mucus-producing glands; the newborn manifest meconium ileus, with thick meconium obstructing the lower digestive tract, resulting in the need for emergency surgery. Other infant and childhood symptoms include bulky, offensive stools, protruding abdomen, spindly arms and legs, emaciation of the buttocks, and growth retardation. Foodstuffs, especially proteins and fats, are poorly digested and assimilated; pancreatic digestive enzymes are reduced or absent. Digestive problems improve with additional pancreatic enzymes in the diet. Blocking of the bronchioles, which results from extremely thick and tenacious secretions of the mucus-producing glands of the bronchi, are serious problems, causing cough, wheezing, respiratory obstruction, emphysema, and frequently infection. The lungs are usually defenseless against microbes. In severe, chronic cases of the disease, patients manifest heart problems, a barrel-like, deformed chest, cyanosis, and clubbing of fingers and toes.

cystitis Inflammation of the bladder.

cystoscopy Examination of the bladder with an instrument called a cystoscope.

cytotoxic Having the action of a cytotoxin.

cytotoxin Toxin or antibody that has a specific toxic action on cells of special organs.

debilitated, debility Lack or loss of strength.

decrease To lessen or diminish.

defecation The discharge of fecal matter from the bowel.

degradation Reduction of a chemical compound to one less complex, as by splitting off one or more groups.

dehydration Removal of water from a substance or compound; also removal of water from the body; restriction of the water intake.

delirium tremens Condition marked by great excitement with anxiety and mental distress; caused by overuse of alcoholic drinks and characterized by hallucinations.

dementia Insanity characterized by loss or serious impairment of intellect, will, and memory.

demulcent substance Soothing preparation.

deodorant Medicine or substance that covers up, absorbs, or destroys objectionable odors.

depolarization Process or act of neutralizing polarity.

depressor Agent that causes a slowing-up action when applied to nerves and muscles.

derivative Agent that withdraws blood from the seat of a disease; anything that is obtained from another.

dermatitis Inflammation of the skin. Contact dermatitis is caused by contact with an irritating substance followed by an allergic response such as skin reddening, rash, itching, and scaling.

dermatomyositis An inflammatory disease of the voluntary muscles accompanied by characteristic skin lesions. It is attended by violent pains, swellings in the muscles, inflammation of the skin, and edema. Also called multiple myositis.

dermatophyte A plant growth, or species of plant, parasitic on the skin.

dermatoses Skin diseases.

detergent Cleansing agent.

diabetes insipidus Chronic disease, usually of young male adults, characterized by great thirst and the passage of a large amount of urine with no excess of sugar. Huge appetite, loss of strength, and emaciation are often noted. Causes include a deficiency of pitressin secretion from the posterior pituitary gland, impaired function of the supraoptic pathways regulating water metabolism, and, rarely, unresponsiveness of the kidney to pitressin.

diabetes mellitus Metabolic disorder marked by inability of the body to store or utilize carbohydrate.

diaphoresis, diaphoretic Profuse perspiration.

diarrhea Loose, watery bowel movements.

diastolic blood pressure See *blood pressure.*

diffuse Process of becoming widely spread, as through a membrane or fluid.

dilate To enlarge or stretch beyond normal measurements.

diplopia The seeing of single objects as double or two.

disinfectant An agent that destroys disease-producing substances or organisms.

disk (disc) A circular or rounded flat plate or organ.

choked An inflamed and edematous optic disk, resulting from increased intracranial pressure. Called also papilledema.

interarticular An interarticular fibrocartilage.

intervertebral A layer of fibrocartilage between adjacent vertebrae.

distal Remote, farthest from the center, origin, or head; opposed to proximal.

diuresis Increased secretion of urine.

diuretic Drug that increases the flow of urine.

diverticulitis Inflammation of a diverticulum.

diverticulum Sac or pouch protruding from the wall of a tube or hollow organ, for example, from the intestine.

dosage Determination of the amount of medication to be administered to a patient, depending on the patient's weight and age.

ductless Having no excretory duct, as in ductless glands.

duodenum Portion of the small intestine leading from the stomach.

dyscrasias Abnormal composition of the blood.

dysentery Infection of the bowel characterized by inflammation, discharge of liquid and bloody stools, and pain, especially during discharge.

dysmenorrhea Painful menstruation.

dysphoria Disquiet; restlessness; feeling of ill-being; malaise.

dyspnea Difficult or labored breathing.

ecchymosis A discharge or escape of blood; a discoloration of the skin caused by discharge or extravasation of blood.

eclampsia Toxic or poisonous condition usually observed during the last 3 months of pregnancy and characterized by edema or fluid in the tissues, rapid weight gain from the edema, increase in blood pressure, albumin in urine, headache, possible convulsions, and other symptoms.

ectopic Out of the normal place.

edema Increase of tissue fluid in the tissue space; often noticed in the face, hands, fingers, abdomen, ankles, and feet.

efferent Carrying blood or secretion away from a part; carrying impulses away from a nerve center.

effusion Escape of fluid into a part or tissue.

pleural Presence of fluid in the pleural space or area occupied by the lungs.

electrocardiogram Graphic tracing of the heart action produced by electrocardiography.

electrocardiography Recording of the electric currents in the heart through leads placed on various parts of the body.

electroencephalogram Recording made of the electric currents developed in the cortex by brain activity.

electrolytes Solution that is a conductor of electricity; acids and salts are common electrolytes.

embolism Condition of plugging of an artery or vein by a clot or obstruction that has been brought to its place by the blood current.

embolus Clot or other plug brought by the blood current from a distant vessel and forced into a smaller one, obstructing the circulation.

embryoma A tumor containing embryonic elements or those derived from a rudimentary retained twin parasite.

emetic Substance that causes vomiting, such as mustard and water or the drug apomorphine.

emphysema Presence of air in the alveolar (air sac) tissue of the lungs; distention of the alveoli with air. A few symptoms are exertional dyspnea, prolonged expiratory phase, wheezing, productive cough with difficulty in clearing the bronchi, barrel chest, overuse of accessory muscles of respiration, overaerated lung fields, and flattened diaphragm (only last two indicated in x-rays).

endocarditis Inflammation of the endocardium or epithelial lining membrane of the heart.

    bacterial Endocarditis caused by bacterial infection developing as a complication of some infectious disease.

endometriosis Presence of endometrial tissue in abnormal situations.

    internal Occurring in the wall of the uterus or fallopian tube.

    external Occurring on the external surface of the uterus, in the ovary, bladder, or intestine, or extraperitoneally.

    vesicae Endometriosis involving the bladder.

endometrium Mucous membrane lining of the uterus.

endoscopy Inspection of any cavity of the body, such as the bladder, by means of an endoscope.

endotracheal intubation Insertion of a tube into the larynx through the glottis or into the trachea for the introduction of air; often used during anesthesia to introduce an anesthetic and to keep a proper airway; also used in diphtheria and edema of the glottis to aid breathing.

enhance, enhancing Increasing.

enteric coating Type of coating for tablets and capsules to prevent dissolving until medication reaches intestines, thus preventing stomach juices from destroying certain drugs.

enteritis Inflammation of the intestine, chiefly the small intestine.

enterocolitis Inflammation of the small and the large intestines.

enzymatic Relating to enzyme.

enzyme A chemical ferment formed by living cells. Enzymes are complex organic chemical compounds capable of producing by catalytic action the transformation of some other compound or compounds.

eosinophil Structure, cell, or histologic element readily stained by eosins; particularly an eosinophilic leukocyte or white cell.

eosins Rose-colored stains or dye, the potassium and sodium salts of tetrabromofluorescein. Several other red coal-tar dyes are also called eosins.

epidemic Disease that affects a large group of people in a certain locality at about the same time.

epidermophytosis Fungous infection of the skin.

epigastric Pertaining to epigastrium.

epigastrium The upper middle portion of the abdomen over or in front of the stomach.

epilepsy Nervous system disease with convulsive seizures.

    grand mal Epilepsy in which there are severe convulsions and loss of consciousness, or coma; also called *haut mal.*

    jacksonian A form of epilepsy marked by localized spasm, mainly limited to one side and often to one group of muscles.

    petit mal epilepsy Epilepsy with no decided period of unconsciousness and no obvious spasm or only a slight one.

epistaxis Nosebleed; hemorrhage from the nose.

epithelium Covering of the skin and mucous membranes consisting wholly of cells of varying form and arrangement. The four principal varieties, named according to the shape of the cells, are modified, specialized, columnar, and squamous.

eructate The act of belching; casting up wind from the stomach.

erythema Morbid redness of the skin of many varieties caused by congestion of the capillaries; rose rash.

erythroblastosis fetalis A disease of early infancy showing marked disturbance in the formation of blood.

erythrocytes Red blood corpuscles, circular biconcave disks containing hemoglobin, that carry the oxygen of the blood. Normal red blood cell count (RBC) is $4^1/_2$ to 5 million/cu ml of blood.

erythrocytosis Increase in the number of red blood corpuscles in the circulation.

eschar A slough produced by burning or by a corrosive application.

esophagitis Inflammation of the esophagus or gullet, which is a musculomembranous canal extending from the pharynx to the stomach.

esterase An enzyme that splits esters.

estrogen Generic term for many compounds having estrogenic activity; producing effects similar to estrin; a female sex hormone.

eunuch Man or boy deprived of the testes or external genital organs.

eunuchism Condition of a castrated male.

eunuchoidism A defective state of the testicles or of the testicular secretion, with impaired sexual power and eunuch-like symptoms.

euphoria Bodily comfort; well-being; absence of pain or distress.

Ewing's tumor (endothelial myeloma) A form of bone sarcoma that usually involves widening the shaft of long bones by spreading the lamellae apart.

exacerbation Increase in the severity of any symptoms or disease.

excitation Act of irritation or stimulation; a condition of being excited.

excreta Waste matter discharged from the body, particularly fecal matter.

exfoliative dermatitis Inflammation of the skin characterized by a falling off of scales or skin layers and resembling pityriasis rubra, a skin disease.

exophthalmic, exophthalmos Protruding of the eyeballs, sometimes caused by pressure of a goiter on the vessels in the neck leading to the face.

expectorant Medication used to increase secretion and aid in expelling mucus from the respiratory tract or to modify such secretions.

extravasation Discharge or escape, as of blood, from a vessel into the tissues.

fenestration The act of perforating, or the condition of being perforated with openings.

fibrillation Condition in which the groups of muscle fibers of the heart do not contract in unison, causing a rapid and irregular pulse.

fibrin Whitish, insoluble protein formed from fibrigen by the action of thrombin (fibrin ferment), as in the clotting of blood. Fibrin forms the essential portion of the blood clot.

fibrinogen Soluble protein in the blood plasma that is converted into fibrin by the action of thrombin (fibrin ferment), thus producing clotting of the blood.

fibromyositis Inflammation of fibromuscular tissue.

fibrositis Inflammation of muscle fibers.

fimbriae Fringe-like, finger-like tissue projections at the ends of the fallopian tubes of the female reproductive system.

fissure

abnormal Cleft-shaped sore.

normal Groove or cleft, such as one of the fissures of the brain.

flatulence Distention of the stomach or intestines with air or gases.

flexion The act of bending or condition of being bent.

follicle A very small excretory or secretory sac or gland.

graafian Any one of the small spherical vesicular sacs embedded in the cortex of the ovary, each of which contains an egg cell, or ovum. Each follicle contains a liquid supplied with the hormone folliculin, or estrin.

frostbite Condition produced by the freezing of a part, such as fingers, toes, or feet.

fulminant, fulminating Sudden; severe; coming on suddenly with intense severity.

fungus Plant organism characterized chiefly by the absence of chlorophyll.

galactorrhea Excessive or spontaneous secretion of milk.

gallbladder Muscular sac that contains bile; located under the right lobe of the liver.

ganglia Plural of ganglion; any collection or mass or nerve cells that serves as a center of nervous influence.

gangrene Necrosis of tissue combined with invasion by saprophytic organisms.

gastrectomy Removal of the stomach or a portion of it.

gastritis Inflammation of the stomach.

gastroenteritis Inflammation of the stomach and the intestines.

gastrointestinal Pertaining to the stomach and the intestines.

genetic Congenital or inherited.

geriatrics That branch of medicine that treats the diseases of old age.

gestation Pregnancy; gravidity.

glaucoma A disease of the eye marked by intense intraocular pressure, resulting in hardness of the eye, atrophy of the retina, cupping of the optic disk, and blindness.

globulin Protein substance similar to albumin; examples include cell globulin, fibrinogen, lactoglobulin, and serum globulin.

glomerulonephritis Inflammation of the glomeruli of the kidney.

glomerulus Tuft or cluster; a coil of blood vessels projecting into the expanded end or capsule of each of the uriniferous tubules (channels for the passage of urine).

glossitis Inflammation of the tongue.

gluteus, gluteal Muscles of the buttock commonly used as sites for intramuscular injection of medications.

glycosuria Sugar in the urine.

goiter Enlargement of the thyroid gland, located in the neck.

exophthalmic Enlargement of the thyroid gland, with such symptoms as rapid pulse, sweating, nervousness, muscular tremors, psychic disturbance, emaciation, and increased basal metabolism.

gonads Sex glands; testes in the male, ovaries in the female.

gonioscope A kind of ophthalmoscope for examining the angle of the anterior chamber of the eye and for demonstrating ocular motility and rotation.

gonioscopy An examination of the eye with a gonioscope. See *gonioscope.*

gonorrhea Venereal disease of the mucous membrane of the genitalia; can affect the mucous membrane of the eyes.

gout A metabolic disease in which purine substances are deposited in the body, with excess uric acid in the blood, chalky deposits in the cartilages of body joints, and acute arthritis. Characteristic symptoms are acute pain, tenderness, and swelling in body joints, such as in the large toe, ankle, instep, knee, and elbow; elevation of uric acid in the blood; and formation of uric-acid or urate deposits in the cartilage of various parts of the body. These tophi (''chalk stone'' or calcareous matter) increase in size and are most often seen along the edge of the ear.

graafian follicle See *follicle, graafian.*

gram-negative Bacteria or tissues that lose the stain or become decolorized by alcohol in Gram's method of staining.

gram-positive Bacteria or tissues that retain the stain in Gram's method of staining.

granulocytes Cells containing granules.

granulocytopenia Abnormal reduction of granulocytes or white blood cells in the blood. See *agranulocytosis.*

Graves' disease See *goiter, exophthalmic.*

gravid Pregnant; with child; containing a fetus.

gripes, gripping Severe and often spasmodic pain in the bowel.

hallucination A sense perception not founded on an objective reality.

hay fever Acute seasonal disease usually caused by an allergy to pollen with characteristic symptoms similar to those of a cold.

heart failure Failure of the heart to work as a pump; characteristic symptoms are fluid in the lungs, ankles, and abdomen.

hemagglutinin Substance that causes agglutination or clumping of red blood corpuscles.

hematocrit Centrifuge for separating corpuscles from plasma or serum of blood.

hematoma Tumor containing effused (spread out, profuse) blood.

hematopoietic Pertaining to or concerned with the formation of blood.

hematuria Discharge of bloody urine.

hemiplegia Loss of function and movement of one side of the body with paralysis.

hemodialysis Installation of an arterial-venal shunt that is connected to the dialyzing machine; the blood is pumped through the dialyzing fluid with a partially porous (semipermeable) plastic membrane to protect the cells. Dialysis is usually performed three times a week for 8 hours each time, but this may vary. It is extremely expensive but lifesaving in chronic renal failure (chronic uremia).

hemoglobin Iron content of the red blood cell.

hemoglobinuria The presence of hemoglobin in the urine resulting from destruction of the blood corpuscles in the vessels or in the urinary passages.

hemolysis Separation of the hemoglobin from the corpuscles and its appearance in the fluid in which the corpuscles are suspended. A few common causes include hemolysins, chemicals, freezing, heating, and placing in distilled water.

hemolytic Causing hemolysis.

hemoperitoneum The presence of extravasated (discharged or escaped) blood into the peritoneal cavity.

hemophilia Congenital condition characterized by delayed clotting of the blood and consequent difficulty in checking hemorrhage; inherited by males through the mother as an x-linked recessive trait.

hemorrhage Massive loss of blood from the body.

hemorrhoids Varicose veins or dilated blood vessels in the anal area.

hemostatic Checking the flow of blood; an agent that arrests the flow of blood.

Henle's loop A U-shaped turn in a uriniferous tubule of the kidney.

hepar Liver.

hepatic Referring to hepar or liver.

hepatitis Infectious inflammation of the liver; a viral infection transmitted by the intestinal-oral route and characterized by symptoms such as anorexia, malaise, nausea, vomiting, fever, enlarged tender liver, jaundice, normal to low white blood cell count, and abnormal hepatocellular liver function tests. The virus is present in the feces and blood during prodromal and acute phases and often in asymptomatic carriers; it may persist for long periods without symptoms after the acute phase. Incubation period is 2 to 6 weeks.

hepatotoxicity Poisoning or toxins destructive to liver cells and originating in the liver.

herpes simplex Skin disease marked by the formation of one or more vesicles on the border of the lip, eye, external nares, or mucous surface of the genitals.

Hg Symbol for mercury; abbreviation for hemoglobin.

hiatus hernia, or **hiatal hernia** Protrusion of any structure through the esophageal hiatus of the diaphragm.

hirsutism Abnormal hairiness, especially in women.

histamine Substance found in the body and in nearly all plant tissues wherever protein is broken down or there is tissue damage.

Hodgkin's disease Characterized by an infectious granulomatous condition (inflammatory enlargement) involving particularly the lymphadenoid tissues of the body. Eosinophils, fibroblasts, giant cells, and frequently *Corynebacterium* organisms, which may be causative agents of the disease, may be found. The glandular enlargement begins at the side of the neck and then extends to the axillary, inguinal, and mediastinal glands and spleen. There is usually a relapsing fever. The disease is called by many names. A few are infectious granuloma, malignant granuloma, malignant lymphoma, lymphadenoma, and lymphosarcoma.

homologous Of similar structure or situation, but not necessarily of similar function.

hormone Chemical product manufactured by some tissue, such as a gland, which is carried by the blood and acts as a messenger to control other tissues, for example, by stimulation or depression, by control of growth sex characteristics, or by effects on the heartbeat.

hydrocholeretics Drugs stimulating the production of bile of a low specific gravity.

hydrogen ion concentration Acidic concentration of hydrogen ions that were formed and given their acid character by acid; has a vital effect on all life processes.

hydrolization, hydrolysis Decomposition resulting from the incorporation of water. The two resulting products divide the water, the hydroxyl group being attached to one and the hydrogen atom to the other.

hydrolyze To subject to hydrolysis.

hydrostatic Pertaining to the pressure exerted by liquids and on liquids; medically, stagnation of fluids.

hydrotropic Chemotropism produced by water; tendency of cells to turn or move in a certain direction under the influence of chemical stimuli.

hyper- A prefix indicating above, beyond, or excessive.

hyperacidity Excessive degree of acidity, often in the stomach.

hyperadrenalism Abnormally increased activity of adrenal gland secretion.

hypercalcemia Abnormally high calcium content in the blood.

hyperchlorhydria Excessive secretion of hydrochloric acid by stomach cells.

hypercholesterolemia Excess of cholesterol in the blood.

hyperflexia, hyperflexion Forcible overflexion or bending of a limb.

hyperglycemia Excess sugar in the blood.

hyperkalemia Abnormally high potassium content in the blood.

hyperoxemia Excessive acidity of the blood.

hyperoxia High oxygen tension in the blood.

hyperplasia Abnormal multiplication or increase in the number of normal cells in normal arrangement in a tissue.

hyperprolactinemia Elevated blood levels of prolactin, the pituitary hormone that causes lactation.

hyperpyrexia A high degree of fever.

hypertension Abnormally high tension, especially high blood pressure.

   benign Essential hypertension that exists for years without producing any symptoms; fluctuating type. Elevation of blood pressure tends to return to normal with rest or sedation.

essential, primary High blood pressure without previous inflammatory disease of the kidney or urinary tract or any other known cause. A systolic pressure above 150 mm Hg and a diastolic pressure of 100 mm Hg is abnormal at all ages. The upper limit for normal blood pressure, as established by insurance companies, is 140/90 mm Hg.

malignant Essential hypertension with an acute, stormy onset, development of neuroretinitis, a progressive course, a sustained elevation of blood pressure, and a poor prognosis.

secondary Elevation of the blood pressure for which the cause is known, such as endocrine, cardiovascular, renal, or neural origin.

hypertensive encephalopathy A complex of cerebral symptoms, including headache, convulsions, and coma, occurring in the course of glomerulonephritis.

hyperthyroid Abnormal condition caused by overactivity of the thyroid gland.

hypertonic Excessive tone, tension, or activity

hypertrophic, hypertrophy Morbid enlargement or overgrowth or an organ or part.

hypertrophic gastritis Enlargement and inflammation of the stomach.

hyperuricemia Excess of uric acid in the blood.

hyperventilation Abnormally prolonged and deep breathing.

hypnotic Any agent that will produce sleep.

hypo- A prefix denoting a lack or deficiency; also a position under or beneath.

hypocalcemia Reduction of blood calcium below normal.

hypochloremic Pertaining to or characterized by lowered chloride content of the blood.

hypochlorhydria Too small a proportion of hydrochloric acid in the gastric juice.

hypodermic Any method that employs the use of a needle and syringe to place medication under the skin.

hypogenitalism Eunuchoid condition caused by defect of the internal secretion of the testicle or the ovary.

hypoglycemia Deficiency of sugar in the blood.

hypogonadism Decrease of the internal secretion of the gonads; eunuchoidism.

hypokalemia Abnormally low potassium content of blood.

hyponatremia Deficiency of sodium in the blood.

hypoparathyroidism Insufficiency of the parathyroid hormone secretion.

hypopituitarism Condition caused by pathologically diminished activity of the hypophysis or pituitary body and marked by excessive deposits of fat and persistence or acquisition of adolescent characteristics.

hypotassemia Deficiency of potassium in the blood.

hypotension Diminished tension, lowered blood pressure.

hypothalamus The ventral subdivision of the diencephalon or forebrain.

hypothermia Abnormally low temperature.

hypothyroidism Underactivity of the thyroid gland in the neck.

hypoventilation Decrease of the air in the lungs below the normal amount.

hypoxia (hypoxemia) Lack of oxygen and deficient oxygenation of the blood.

idiopathic Morbid state of spontaneous origin; neither sympathetic nor traumatic.

idiosyncrasy Peculiar susceptibility to some drug protein or other substance; exaggerated reaction to drugs.

ileitis Inflammation of the ileus, part of the small intestine.

ileostomy The making of an artificial opening into the ileum.

ileum The distal portion of the small intestine, extending from the jejunum to the cecum.

immunization Method of preventing a first or a second attack of a certain disease.

impacted Driven firmly in, closely lodged.

impermeable Not permitting a passage, as for fluid.

impetigo Low-grade skin infection with small pustules.

incipient Beginning to exist; coming into existence.

increase To enlarge, to grow.

infantilism Condition in which the characters of childhood persist in adult life; marked by mental retardation, underdevelopment of the sexual organs, and often dwarfism.

infarct Area of coagulation necrosis in a tissue caused by local anemia resulting from obstruction of circulation to the area.

inhibits Lessens, decreases.

innervation Distribution or supply of nerves to a part; supply of nervous energy or of nerve stimulus sent to a part.

inoculation Topical or subcutaneous (under the skin) application of bacteria into a human being to produce a mild form of a disease for the purpose of creating an immunity to future attacks.

inotropic To turn or influence; affecting the force or energy of muscular contractions.

negative Weakening the force of muscular action.

positive Increasing the strength of muscular contraction.

in situ In the natural or normal place.

insomnia Inability to sleep.

insulin Hormone drug used in the treatment of diabetes mellitus; extract of the islands of Langerhans of the pancreas.

intestines The small and the large bowels.

intracranial Within the cranium or skull or brain pan.

intramuscular Into or within the muscle.

intraocular Into or within the eye.

intravenous Into or within the vein.

intrinsic Situated on the inside; situated entirely within or pertaining exclusively to a part.

inulin Polysaccharide found in Inula, Dahlia, and other plants that yield levulose on hydrolysis; also a concentration of resinoid from elecampane root; an aromatic and tonic expectorant.

involution A rolling or turning inward; the return of the uterus to its normal size after childbirth; a retrograde change; the reverse of evolution; involutional, pertaining to, due to, or occurring in involution.

senile the shriveling of an organ in aged people.

ion Atom or a group of atoms having a charge of positive (cation) or negative (anion) electricity.

ionization Dissociation of a substance in solution into its constituent ions.

ionize To separate into ions.

iris Circular pigmented membrane behind the cornea of the eye, perforated by the pupil; made up of circular muscular fibers surrounding the pupil and a band of radiating fibers by which the pupil is dilated.

irradiation Treatment by roentgen rays or other forms of radioactivity.

ischemia Local and temporary deficiency of blood, caused chiefly by contraction of a blood vessel.

isotonic Having a uniform tension. Isotonic solutions are those that have the same osmotic pressure.

isotonic salt solution Solution having the same amount of salt substance as the blood (approximately 0.9% sodium chloride).

isotope Either of two substances chemically identical but with differing atomic weights.

isthmus A narrow strip of tissue or a narrow passage connecting two larger parts; of the thyroid, the band or strip of tissue that connects the lobes of the thyroid gland.

jaundice (icterus) Condition characterized by the presence of bilirubin, a red bile pigment, and deposition of the bile pigment in the skin and mucous membranes, with resulting yellow appearance of the skin and yellow whites of the eyes. It may be caused by obstruction in the biliary system, blockage from a stone that obstructs the passage of bile from the liver to the intestines, or impairment of the liver itself, which produces the bile to aid in the digestion of fats.

juxta Situated near or in the region of, such as juxtaglomerular—near or in the region of a glomerulus.

keratitis Inflammation of the cornea of the eye.

ketoacidosis A condition of metabolism in which abnormal quantities of acetone bodies are present in the body.

kilogram Unit of weight equal to 1,000 g or 2.2 pounds avoirdupois (the ordinary system of weights in the United States).

labyrinthitis Inflammation of the labyrinth or the intercommunicating cavities or canals of the internal ear: cochlea, vestibule, and canals.

laceration Mangled or torn skin or tissue.

lacrimal canaliculi Tear channels or canals of the eye.

lactation The secretion of milk; the period of the secretion of milk; suckling.

laity The nonprofessional portion of the people.

laryngeal Pertaining to the larynx.

laryngitis Inflammation of the larynx.

larynx Musculocartilaginous, box-like structure, lined with mucous membrane, situated at the top of the trachea and below the root of the tongue and the hyoid bone; located in the midline of the neck. It is the organ of the voice, or voice box.

lateral Pertaining to a side.

laxative Drug having the property of overcoming constipation.

lecithin A monoaminomonophosphatide containing fatty acids and found in animal tissues, especially nerve tissue, semen, yolk of egg, and in smaller amount in bile and blood. Lecithins are said to have the therapeutic properties of phosphorus and have been given in rickets, dyspepsia, neurasthenia, diabetes, anemia, and tuberculosis; lecithins also are said to be antivenomous.

lens A transparent gelatinous mass of fibers situated behind the iris and pupil of the eye and having the function of giving the image on the retina a sharp focus and of converging or scattering the rays of light.

leprosy Chronic infectious disease caused by a specific microbe (Hansen's bacillus) and marked by a very gradual onset, malaise, headache, formation of nodules, ulcerations, and deformities, and loss of sensation in affected parts; often called Hansen's disease.

lethargy Condition of drowsiness of mental origin.

leukemia Often fatal disease with a marked increase in the number of leukocytes in the blood, with enlargement and proliferation of the lymphoid tissue of the spleen, bone marrow, and lymphatic glands. A few characteristic symptoms include progressive anemia, internal hemorrhage, and increasing exhaustion.

leukocyte Any colorless, ameboid cell mass, such as a white blood corpuscle, pus corpuscle, lymph corpuscle, or wandering connective tissue cell, consisting of a colorless granular mass of protoplasm having ameboid movements and varying in size. Normal white blood cell count (WBC) is 5,000 to 10,000/cu ml of blood.

leukocytosis Increase in the number of leukocytes in the blood, generally caused by the presence of infection.

leukopenia Reduction in the number of leukocytes in the blood to 5,000/cu ml of blood or less.

lipids Any one of a group of substances that include the fats and the esters having corresponding properties. The American usage of the term includes fatty acids and soaps, neutral fats, waxes, sterols, and phosphatides. Lipids have a greasy feel.

liver Largest gland of the body, located in the right upper part of the abdomen. It has many functions, including formation and secretion of bile to aid in fat digestion, storage of sugar in the form of glycogen, formation of vitamin A from carotene, and storage of vitamins A and D_2. As a drug it is produced in many forms and has lifesaving properties for many types of anemia.

local Limited to, or pertaining to, one part or spot.

lumen Transverse section of the clear space within a tube; an opening.

lupus erythematosus Chronic, nontuberculous disease of the skin marked by disk-like patches with raised reddish edges and depressed centers and covered with scales or crusts that fall off, leaving off-white scars.

lymphangitis Inflammation of a lymphatic vessel or vessels.

lymphatic system System of vessels carrying lymph (a transparent, slightly yellow liquid, alkaline in reaction) to parts of the body.

lymphocyte Variety of white blood corpuscle with a single nucleus and increased cytoplasm. These corpuscles arise in the reticular tissue of the lymph glands and lymph nodes.

lymphocytic Pertaining to lymphocytes.

lymphoma Any tumor made up of lymphoid tissue.

lymphopenia Decrease in the proportion of lymphocytes in the blood.

lymphosarcoma Malignant neoplasm arising in lymphatic tissue from proliferation of atypical lymphocytes.

lysozyme A mucolytic lubrication for eyelid movements.

macrocytic Condition referring to abnormally large erythrocytes, or red blood corpuscles.

malabsorption Disorder of normal nutritive absorption; disordered anabolism.

malaise Feeling of ill-being; not feeling well.

malignant Virulent; tending to go from bad to worse; progressive.

manic-depressive Insanity in which mania and melancholia alternate.

meconium The fecal matter of the newborn; it consists of a green, sticky substance containing mucus, bile, and epithelial threads.

medulla oblongata Cone of nervous tissue continuous above with the pons of the brain and below with the spinal cord, lying ventral to the cerebellum and forming the floor of the fourth ventricle, with its back; continuation of the spinal cord within the cranium.

megaloblast An erythroblast or primitive red blood corpuscle of large size found in the blood of pernicious anemia.

Meniere's syndrome Disease or inflammatory process and congestion of the semicircular canals in the inner ear with symptoms such as pallor, vertigo, nausea, lack of balance, and several ear and eye disturbances.

meninges The three membranes that envelop the brain and spinal cord, including the dura, the pia, and the arachnoid.

meningitis Inflammation of the meninges of the brain.

menopause Cessation of menstruation; often called "the change of life."

menorrhagia Abnormally profuse menstruation.

menstruation Monthly bloody discharge from the uterus.

mesial Situated in the middle; median; toward the middle line of the body or toward the center line of the dental arch.

metabolism Tissue change; the sum of all the physical and chemical processes by which living organized substance is produced and maintained; the transformation by which energy is made available for the uses of the organism.

metastasis The moving or spreading of infection or cell growth from one area to another.

metorrhagia Profuse bleeding from the uterus at times other than during the menstrual period.

microcurie One-millionth of a curie.

microgram One-millionth part of a gram.

migraine Periodic headache, usually on one side, with such severe symptoms as nausea, vomiting, and light sensitivity.

millicurie One-thousandth of a curie, which is a unit of radiation energy.

milliequivalent One-thousandth of an equivalent combining weight of an atom or ion; an equivalent combining weight, as the weight of an element (in grams) that will combine with 1.008 g of hydrogen.

miosis Excessive contraction of the pupil of the eye.

miotic, myotic Drug that causes the pupil to contract, such as morphine, nicotine, physostigmine, and pilocarpine.

mittelschmerz Intermenstrual pain occurring about halfway through the menstrual cycle, generally during ovulation.

molecule Very small mass of matter; a gathering together or clumping of atoms.

motion sickness Nausea, dizziness, and often vomiting caused by motion of the body when riding in a ship, airplane, automobile, or train.

multipara A woman who has borne several children.

multiple myeloma Tumor composed of cells of the type normally found in the bone marrow; a primary malignant tumor of bone marrow marked by circumscribed or diffuse, tumorlike hyperplasia (abnormal multiplication or increase in number of normal cells in normal arrangement in a tissue) of the bone marrow. It is usually associated with anemia and with Bence Jones protein in the urine. Neuralgic pains and painful swellings on the ribs and skull, occur, along with spontaneous fractures.

multiple sclerosis Nervous system disease characterized by scarring of brain and spinal cord that occurs in scattered patches. Patient shows progressive weakness, paralysis, muscle contraction, and muscle cramps. The cause is unknown, and the treatment limited.

multisynaptic See *synapse*.

myalgia Pain in a muscle or muscles.

myasthenia gravis Disease characterized by an abnormal weakness of muscles.

mycosis fungoides Fatal fungous skin disease marked by the development of firm, reddish tumors on the scalp, face, and chest that are painful and have a tendency to spread and ulcerate. The disease may last several years.

mydriasis Extreme or morbid dilation of the pupil of the eye.

mydriatic Drug that dilates the pupil of the eye, such as atropine, homatropine, cocaine, phenacaine, hyoscyamine, and ephedrine.

myelin The fat-like substance forming a sheath around the medullated (myelinated) nerve fibers.

myocardium Heart muscle; myocardial infarct; a blockage or clot in the heart muscle.

myoma Any tumor made up of muscular elements; if they are striated, it is a rhabdomyoma, if not, it is a leiomyoma.

myositis Inflammation of muscle.

myxedema Hypothyroid condition causing an edema of tissues, loss of hair, and physical and mental sluggishness in adults.

narcotic Drug that produces sleep or stupor and relieves pain.

nausea Inclination to vomit.

necrosis Death of a circumscribed portion of tissue.

neoplasm Any new and abnormal formation, such as a tumor.

nephritis Inflammation of the kidney.

nephrons Multifunctional units; the renal unit consists of Bowman's capsule, the globular upper end of the tubule, and the tubule, which is concerned with kidney circulation.

nephropathy Disease of the kidneys.

nephrosis Degenerative changes in the kidney without inflammation.

nephrotoxic Toxic or destructive to the kidneys.

neuralgia Nerve pain.

neuritis Inflammation of a nerve, or nerves, with pain.

neuroblasts Any embryonic cell that develops into a nerve cell or neuron; an immature nerve cell.

neuroblastomas Malignant tumors of the nervous system composed chiefly of neuroblasts.

neurogenic Forming nervous tissue, or stimulating nervous energy; originating in the nervous system.

nocturnal Pertaining to, occurring at, or active at night.

node Swelling or protuberance.

    auriculoventricular Remnant of primitive fibers found in all mammalian hearts at the base of the intraauricular septum (separation or partition) and forming the beginning of the bundle of His.

normotensive Characterized by blood pressure within the normal range.

nucleic acid Acid obtained from nuclein, a decomposition product of nucleoprotein.

occlusion Act of closure or state of being closed.

occlusive Effecting a complete occlusion or closure.

occult Obscure, difficult to be observed, hidden.

Ocusert A method of administration of eye drops over a continuous, extended period.

oliguria Deficient secretion of urine.

ophthalmic Pertaining to the eye.

optic Of or pertaining to the eye.

orthopnea Inability to breathe except when sitting up.

orthostatic hypotension Blood pressure lower than normal when the individual is standing or in upright position.

osmosis Passage of pure solvent (liquid used to dissolve) from the lesser to the greater concentration when two solutions are separated by a membrane that selectively prevents the passage of solute (dissolved substance) molecules but that is permeable to the solvent.

osteoarthritis Inflammation of a bony union or joint; it is not as crippling and causes less inflammation than rheumatoid arthritis.

osteomalacia An adult disease marked by increasing softness of the bones so that they become flexible and brittle and attended by rheumatic pains, weakness, and exhaustion, with the patient dying eventually from exhaustion.

osteomyelitis Inflammation of the bone marrow, or bone, or medullary cavity of bone.

osteoporosis Abnormal porousness or loss of density of bone by enlargement of its canals or the formation of abnormal spaces; softening of bone.

otitis media Inflammation of the middle ear.

ototoxicity Poisonous or deleterious to the organs of hearing and balance.

ovary Female sex organ in which ova, or eggs, develop and mature.

palliative Alleviating medicine or treatment offering relief or reducing the severity of pain but not curing the cause.

palpitation Unduly rapid action of the heart felt by the patient.

pancreas Gland of the endocrine system lying behind the stomach and containing the islands of Langerhans, which produce insulin, an internal secretion that reduces the blood and urinary sugar to normal. The pancreas also produces enzymes to aid in the digestion of proteins, carbohydrates, and fats.

pancreatitis Inflammation of the pancreas marked by abdominal pain, pain around the umbilicus or navel, abdominal distention, nausea, and vomiting.

papilla Any small, nipple-shaped elevation.

    optic The optic disk, a round white disk in the fundus oculi medial to the posterior pole of the eyes; corresponds to the entrance of the optic nerve and retinal blood vessels.

papilledema Edema of the optic papilla; a choked disk; optic neuritis caused by intracranial pressure and without inflammatory manifestations.

paralytic ileus Paralysis of the muscular coats of the ileum, a part of the small intestine characterized by possible obstruction of intestinal contents, continuous abdominal pain, distention, vomiting, severe constipation, peritonitis, minimal abdominal tenderness, decreased or absent bowel sounds, history of surgery, and x-ray evidence of gas and fluid in the bowel.

parasympathetic nervous system Part of the autonomic nervous system, including certain nerves whose fibers start from the midbrain, hindbrain, and sacral parts of the spinal cord.

parasympathomimetic drugs Drugs that cause effects in the body similar to those produced by acetylcholine; cholinergic drugs.

parathyroid gland Four small glands, two of which are found on the surface of each lateral lobe of the thyroid. These glands secrete a hormone that regulates calcium-phosphorus metabolism.

parenteral, parenterally Subcutaneous, intramuscular, or intravenous method of administration; treatment by injection.

paresthesia An abnormal sensation, such as burning or prickling.

Parkinson's disease Disease marked by slowing and weakness of voluntary movement, muscular rigidity, and tremor; also known as palsy and paralysis agitans.

paroxysm Sudden recurrence or intensification of symptoms.

patent Wide open.

pathogen Any disease-producing microorganism or material.

pathology The branch of medicine that treats the essential nature of disease, especially the structural and the functional changes caused by disease.

pediculicide Destroying lice; Pediculin is a proprietary remedy for killing lice.

pellagra Endemic skin and spinal disease occurring in southern Europe and southern and central parts of the United States; thought to be caused by deficiency of vitamins B_2 or G, which are found in lean meat, milk, yeast, and other foods. Characteristic symptoms include recurring reddening of the body surface followed by falling off of the skin in layers, along with weakness, debility, digestive disturbances, spinal pain, convulsions, melancholia, and idiocy.

pentagastrin A synthetic peptide that stimulates gastric acid without producing the undesirable side effects of histamine.

peptic ulcer Stomach ulcer.

peptide A compound formed by the union of two or more amino acids. When two amino acids unite, the result is a dipeptide, three form a tripeptide, and more than three form a polypeptide.

perfusion Pouring through or into.

peripheral, periphery Outward part or surface.

blood vessels Blood vessels near the skin or surface of the body.

neuropathy Any disease affecting peripheral nerves.

resistance Ratio of pressure to flow. It is not constant along vessels because of the plastic nature of blood. Resistance is influenced by pressure, viscosity, and vessel lumen size.

peristalsis Worm-like contraction of the muscle tissue of the intestines or certain other organs.

peritoneal cavity Space between the visceral and parietal peritoneums.

peritoneum Serous membrane that lines the abdominal walls and invests the contained viscera; holds viscera in place.

parietal Membrane that lines the abdominal walls, pelvic walls, and undersurface of the diaphragm.

visceral Membrane reflected at various places over the viscera, forming a complete covering for the stomach, spleen, liver, and many parts of the small and the large intestines.

perlèche Inflammation of the corners of the mouth caused by a yeast-like fungus, *Candida albicans.*

permeability Property or state of being permeable; may be traversed or passed through.

pernicious anemia Chronic disease characterized by a progressive decrease in the number of red corpuscles.

petechiae, petechia Small spots formed by the escape of blood into a part or tissue, as seen in typhus or purpura. See *purpura.*

pH The symbol commonly used in expressing hydrogen ion concentration.

phagocyte Any cell that ingests microorganisms or other cells and substances. The ingested material is often, but not always, digested within the phagocyte. Phagocytes are either fixed, such as endothelial cells, or free, such as leukocytes. The two forms of leukocytes that are phagocytic are the large lymphocyte (macrophage) and the polymorphonuclear leukocyte (microphage). *Polymorphonuclear* means many-shaped nucleus.

pharyngitis Inflammation of the pharynx.

pharynx Tube-shaped passage or musculomembranous sac between the mouth and nares and the esophagus. It is continuous below with the esophagus and above it communicates with the larynx, mouth, nasal passages, and eustachian tubes. It is a passage for both air and food.

pheochromocytoma Tumor of the kidney or adrenal gland consisting of chromaffin cells, which secrete epinephrine.

phlebitis Inflammation of a vein, marked by infiltration of the coats of the vein and the formation of a thrombus of coagulated blood.

phobia Any persistent insane dread or fear.

phosphatide, phosphotidate Phospholipid from which choline or colamine has been split off.

phospholipid Lipin containing phosphorus that yields fatty acids and glycerin on hydrolysis. Lecithin is the best-known example.

photophobia Abnormal sensitivity to or intolerance of light.

pituitary gland (or **body**) Small, bean-shaped body located in a depression of the sphenoid bone in the skull. It is divided into anterior and posterior lobes, each of which gives off several hormones.

placenta Any cake-like mass; the round, flat organ about 1 inch thick and 7 inches in diameter within the uterus that establishes communication between the mother and child by means of the umbilical cord.

platelets Oval disks without hemoglobin found in the blood; they are essential for clotting. Platelets, or thrombocytes, may be manufactured in the red bone marrow. There is wide variance in platelet count, but normal count may be 250,000 to 500,000/cu ml of blood.

pleura The serous membrane that invests the lungs, lines the thorax, and is reflected on the diaphragm. There are two pleurae, right and left, entirely shut off from each other. The pleura is moistened with a serous secretion that eases the movements of the lungs in the chest.

pleural effusion A second stage inflammation of the pleura in which exudation of copious amounts of serum occurs. The inflamed surfaces of the pleura may become united by adhesions, which are usually permanent. Symptoms include a "stitch" in the side, and a chill followed by a fever, a dry cough, and pain during breathing. As effusion occurs, there is an onset of dyspnea and a lessening of pain. The patient lies on the affected side.

pleurisy A disease marked by inflammation of the pleura, with exudation into its cavity and on its surface.

polarity Fact or condition of having poles; exhibition of opposite effects at two extremities.

polycythemia vera A disease lasting many years and marked by a persistent increase in the red blood corpuscles (polycythemia), resulting from excessive formation of erythroblasts by the bone marrow and characterized by increased viscosity of the blood, enlargement of the spleen, and cyanotic appearance of the patient.

polymer Any member of a series of substances concerned with, derived from, or pertaining to several pigments.

polymorphonuclear Having nuclei of many forms or shapes, as in certain leukocytes.

polysaccharides Group of carbohydrates that contain more than three molecules of simple carbohydrates combined with each other. They comprise dextrins, starches, glycogens, cellulose, gums, inulin, and pectose.

polyuria Excessive secretion and discharge of urine containing increased amounts of solid constituents.

postpartum Period occurring after delivery or childbirth.

potency Power, strength, as of medicines.

potential Existing and ready for action but not yet active.

precordial Pertaining to the precordium, the region over the heart or stomach; the epigastrium and lower part of the thorax.

precursor Something that precedes or goes before.

prognosis Forecast as to the probable result of a disease attack; the prospect of recovery from a disease gained through the nature and the symptoms of the case.

proliferation, proliferating Reproduction or multiplication of similar forms, especially of cells and morbid cysts.

prostaglandin A series of chemicals that have pressor, vasodilator, and stimulant effects on the intestinal and uterine muscles.

prostate A gland in the male that surrounds the neck of the bladder and the urethra. It consists of a median lobe and two lateral lobes and is made up of glandular matter, the ducts that empty into the prostatic portion of the urethra, and the muscular fibers that encircle the urethra.

prostatectomy Surgical removal of the prostate or a part of it.

prostatic hypertrophy An enlargement of the prostate gland.

protein Any one of a group of nitrogenized compounds, similar to each other, widely distributed in the animal and vegetable kingdoms, and forming the characteristic constituents of the tissues and fluids of the animal body. They are essentially combinations of a-amino acids and their derivatives.

proteinuria The presence of protein in the urine.

prothrombin Fibrin factor in blood plasma that is supposed to be a precursor of thrombin; also called thrombogen and thrombinogen.

proximal Nearer to or on the side toward the body; opposed to distal.

pruritus Intense itching; a symptom of many skin and other diseases.

psoriasis Chronic inflammatory skin disease marked by the formation of scaly red patches on the surface of the body.

psychomotor Pertaining to or causing voluntary movements.

psychoneurosis Borderline disorder of the mind that is not a true insanity, such as hysteria and neurasthenia.

psychosis Disease or disorder of the mind.

pulmonary embolism Blood clot or foreign material that travels through the circulation and finally lodges in a blood vessel of the lungs.

pulmonary wedge pressure A Swan-Ganz catheter or a special, pliable, multiple-lumen, balloon-tipped catheter is inserted by a highly skilled physician under sterile technique into the subclavian, jugular, or femoral vein and on through the vena cava, the right atrium, and the right ventricle to the pulmonary artery. The large or major lumen of the catheter terminates at the catheter tip and measures pulmonary artery pressure. The small lumen terminates in a latex balloon that can be inflated to surround, but not occlude, the tip of the catheter. When the balloon is inflated and wedged against the pulmonary artery, it continuously measures pulmonary pressure and transmits the measurements to an oscilloscope at the bedside. This procedure is used in congestive heart failure, in myocardial infarction, in measuring left heart pressures and function, and in many other conditions. It is a lifesaving procedure.

pulse pressure See *blood pressure.*

pulvule Proprietary capsule containing a dose of a powdered drug.

pupil Opening in the center of the iris of the eye for the passage of light rays to the retina.

purgative Strong medication administered by mouth to produce bowel evacuation or several movements of the bowels.

purpura Disease characterized by the formation of purple patches on the skin and mucous membranes, caused by the escape of blood into a part or tissue.

purulent Consisting of or containing pus.

pyelitis Inflammation of the pelvis of the kidney; it may be caused by a renal stone, extension of inflammation from the bladder, or stagnation of urine. Symptoms include pain and tenderness in the loins, irritability of the bladder, remittent fever, blood or purulent urine, diarrhea, vomiting, and peculiar pain on flexion of the thigh.

pyelonephritis Inflammation of the kidney and its pelvis.

pyloric spasm Contraction of the pylorus or pyloric sphincter caused by muscle spasm; this will not allow the pylorus to relax and the stomach to empty.

pylorus Gate to the outlet of the stomach; a ring-like band of muscle tissue between the opening of the stomach and the duodenum, or the first part of small intestine.

pyrogen A fever-producing substance.

pyrogenic Inducing fever, also caused by or resulting from fever.

rabies (or hydrophobia, fear of water) Filtrable infectious disease of certain animals, especially dogs, wolves, and squirrels; communicated to man by direct inoculation from the bite of the infected animal—the virus is in the saliva. Incubation period is 1 to 6 months. Symptoms include malaise, depression of spirits, swelling of lymphatics in the region of the wound, choking, spasmodic breathing, and increasing tetanic muscle spasms, especially of respiratory and swallowing muscles, which are increased by attempts to drink water or even by the sight of water. Fever, mental derangement, vomiting, profuse secretion of a sticky saliva, and albuminuria also occur. Disease is almost 100% fatal within 2 to 5 days after onset of symptoms unless rabies vaccine is administered within a short period after the bite occurs.

Raynaud's disease Disease characterized by disturbances in circulation in the blood vessels of the extremities, with the possibility of gangrene and amputation of a limb.

reflux A backward or return flow.

refractory Not readily yielding to treatment.

regurgitation The casting up of undigested food; a backward flowing of the blood through the left atrioventricular opening resulting from imperfect closure of the mitral valve.

remission Period during which symptoms of a disease are abated or lessened in severity.

renal Pertaining to the kidney.

resection Excision of a part of an organ; excision of the ends of bones and other structures forming a joint.

reticulin Albuminoid substance from the connective fibers of reticular tissue; a net-like tissue.

reticulocyte Young red blood cell showing a reticulum or protoplasmic network construction under vital staining.

retina, retinal The innermost tunic (coat, membrane) and perceptive structure of the eye, formed by the expansion of the optic nerve and covering the back part of the eye as far as the ora serrata (the zigzag anterior edge of the retina); often called the nerve of the sense of sight.

retinoblastoma A tumor arising from retinal germ cells.

retinopathy Disease of the retina of the eye.

rhabdomyoma A tumor (myoma) composed of striated muscular fibers.

rhabdomyosarcoma A combined sarcoma and rhabdomyoma.

rheumatic fever Inflammatory joint disease that usually occurs following a streptococcal infection and that is characterized by fever, malaise, joint inflammation and swelling, and transitory pain in the joints. It is usually recurrent and may damage the heart valves.

rheumatic heart disease Chronic disease of the heart valve or valves caused by rheumatic fever.

rheumatoid arthritis Type of arthritis marked by joint pain, swelling of joints, fever, malaise, and crippling of joints.

rhinitis Inflammation of the mucous membrane of the nose; a cold.

rhinorrhea Free discharge of a thin nasal mucus.

rickets Softness of bones in childhood caused by lack of calcium salts, which results in a slowing of the bone-hardening process; lack of vitamin D is a contributing cause.

rickettsiae (Howard Taylor Ricketts' organism) group of bacteria-like microorganisms that may be transmitted to humans by lice or other parasites. Some diseases caused by rickettsiae include Brill's disease (a form of typhus fever), endemic typhus fever, epidemic typhus fever, and Rocky Mountain spotted fever.

ringworm Parasitic fungus causing a contagious skin disease marked by ring-shaped colored patches; usually on the scalp but can appear on other parts of the body.

roentgen The international unit of roentgen radiation.

roentgen rays Electromagnetic vibrations of waves of very short wave lengths, set in motion when electrons, moving at high velocity, impinge on certain substances, especially the heavy metals. They are able to penetrate most substances, to affect a photographic plate, to bring about chemical reactions, and to produce changes in living matter. They are used in taking photographs of the human body (roentgenograms) or in visualizing portions of the body (fluoroscopy). They reveal foreign bodies in the human body such as calculi (stones) and bullets, as well as fractures of the bone and the functions of such organs as the heart, stomach, and intestines. They are also used in treating various diseases, such as lupus, cancer, and eczema. Also called x-rays.

rubella German measles; an acute eruption rash and febrile disease not unlike measles. After an incubation period of 1 to 3 weeks, the disease begins with slight fever and catarrhal symptoms, sore throat, pains in the limbs, and the eruption of red papules similar to those appearing in measles but lighter in color, not arranged in crescentic masses, and disappearing without peeling or skin flaking within a week.

rubeola A viral disease or measles, characterized by fever, coryza, cough, conjunctivitis, photophobia, and Koplik's spots; the latter usually appear about 2 days before the rash and last 4 days as tiny ''table-salt crystals'' on the dull-red mucous membranes of the inner aspects of the cheeks and often on the inner conjunctival folds and vaginal mucous membranes. Exposure occurs 14 days before the rash. The rash is brick-red, irregular, and maculopapular, with onset 4 days after initial symptoms, appearing on the face first, then on the chest, the extremities, and the back. The rash begins fading on the third day in the order that it appeared. Slight desquamation (peeling and flaking of skin) also occurs.

sacroiliac Referring to the sacrum and the ilium bones of the pelvis.

salivation Process of secreting saliva from the salivary glands in the mouth.

salpinx Fallopian or eustachian tube.

saphenous Veins in the legs.
   magna The longest vein in the body, extending from the dorsum of the foot to just below the inguinal ligament, where it opens into the femoral vein.
   parva Continues the marginal vein from behind the malleolus (ankle joint) and passes up the back of the leg to the knee joint, where it opens into the popliteal vein.

scabies Communicable skin disease caused by the itch mite and attended with intense itching.

schizoid Resembling schizophrenia; reclusive, unsocial, introspective type of personality.

schizophrenia Dementia praecox; adolescent insanity; the term includes a large range of mental disorders that occur early in life and are marked by melancholia, self-absorption, reclusive, unsocial, introspective, withdrawn type of personality, and general mental weakness.

sciatica Inflammation of the sciatic nerve, usually a neuritis. Symptoms include abnormal burning, prickling sensation (paresthesia) of the thigh and leg, tenderness along the course of the nerve, pain that is usually constant, and sometimes a wasting of the calf muscles. It may recur.

sciatic nerve Long nerve with many branches originating in the sacral plexus (a network or tangle of nerves) and distributing through the skin of muscles in thigh, leg, and foot.

sclera The tough, white supporting tunic of the eyeball, covering it entirely except for the segment covered by the cornea; continuous with the cornea; nontransparent; the white portion of the eye.

scurvy Nutritional disease caused by dietetic errors, marked by weakness, anemia, spongy gums, tendency to mucocutaneous hemorrhage, and hardening of the muscles of the calves and legs. Treatment consists of eating fresh potatoes, scurvy grass, onions, lime juice, other citrus fruits such as oranges and lemons, and vitamin C.

sebaceous gland Any gland secreting sebaceous matter (sebum, or a greasy, lubricating substance); chiefly situated in the corium, or true skin.

sedative Quieting or calming type of drug.

serum Watery fluid of the body, especially the fluid left after removal of solid materials of the blood.

SGOT A laboratory blood test: serum glutamic-oxaloacetic transaminase.

smallpox Infectious viral disease marked by a rash that passes through several successive stages.

somatic Pertaining to the body tissues, as opposed to reproductive tissues and as distinguished from the psyche.

sperm Mature male cells found in the semen or testicular secretion.

sphincter Ring-like muscle that closes a natural orifice, for example, the pyloric sphincter or the anal sphincter.

spinal cord Cord-like structure contained in the spinal canal and extending from the foramen magnum to the second lumbar vertebra. It is a center for reflex activity and also functions in the transmission of impulses to and from the higher centers in the brain.

splenic flexure syndrome Discomfort originating from the bend of the colon at the junction of the transverse and descending portions.

spondylitis Inflammation of one or more vertebrae.

sprue Chronic disease of disturbed small intestine function characterized by impaired absorption, particularly of fats, and motor abnormalities. Symptoms include bulky, pale, frothy, foul-smelling, greasy stools; weight loss; vitamin deficiencies; impaired intestinal absorption of glucose, vitamins, and fat; large amounts of free fatty acids and soaps in the stool; sore mouth and raw-looking tongue; gastrointestinal catarrh with periodic diarrhea; and change in liver size. The anemia is treated with oral iron for hypochromic anemia and vitamin B_{12} for macrocytic anemia. Therapeutic diet should be high-calorie, high-protein, low-fat, and gluten-free. Sprue occurs mostly in hot countries and is known as tropical sprue. Nontropical sprue is also called intestinal infantilism. See *celiac disease* and *infantilism*.

sputum Substance sent forth from the bronchial tubes and the mouth containing saliva, mucus, and sometimes pus; phlegm.

squamous cell A flat, scale-like epithelial cell.

stasis Stoppage of the flow of blood in any part of the body.

status asthmaticus State or condition of asthma.

status epilepticus A series of rapidly repeated epileptic convulsions with no periods of consciousness.

steatorrhea Presence of excess fat in the stools.

    idiopathic Intestinal infantilism.

stenosis Narrowing or stricture of a duct or canal.

sterol A monohydroxy alcohol of high molecular weight; one of a class of compounds widely distributed in nature, which, because their solubilities are similar to those of fats, have been classified with the lipins. Cholesterol is the best-known member of the group.

stimulant Type of drug that increases activity and hastens action in the body.

stomatitis Inflammation of the mouth.

stratum A layer or set of layers, as in the epidermis, or outermost and nonvascular layer of the skin.

Stria (striae atrophicae) Streak or line on the skin. Many of these are often seen on the abdomen of pregnant women or after childbirth, first as reddish streaks, gradually fading to white. They are permanent and are caused by atrophy or stretching of the skin.

stricture The abnormal narrowing of a canal, duct, or passage, either from cicatric contraction or the deposit of abnormal tissue.

stye Inflammation of an oil gland of the eyelid.

subaortic Situated below the aorta or the main blood vessel trunk from which the entire systemic arterial system proceeds.

subcapsular cataract Opacity or cloudiness situated beneath the anterior or posterior capsule of the eye lens.

subcutaneous Beneath the skin or in the tissues.

sublingual Beneath the tongue.

substrate A substratum, or lower stratum; the term is applied to the substance on which a ferment or enzyme acts.

supraclavicular Situated above the clavicle, or collar bone.

sympathectomy Surgical removal of a part of a sympathetic nerve, especially the superior cervical sympathetic ganglion.

sympathetic nervous system Part of the autonomic nervous system; also known as the vegetative or visceral nervous system because the organs controlled by it function unconsciously.

sympathomimetic Resembling the effects produced by disturbance of the sympathetic nervous system. Sympathomimetic drugs relieve the symptoms.

symptom Any disorder of function, appearance, or sensation that the patient experiences.

synapse Anatomic relation of one nerve cell to another; the point of contact between processes of two adjacent neurons, forming the place where a nervous impulse is transmitted from one neuron to another; also called synaptic junction.

syndrome Set of symptoms that occur together.

synovial fluid Fluid secreted by the synovial membrane and contained in joint cavities.

synovitis Inflammation of the synovial membrane, or the covering around joints.

synthesis The artificial building up of a chemical compound by the union of its elements.

syphilis A contagious venereal disease leading to many structural and cutaneous lesions, resulting from a microorganism, the *spirochete pallida*, or *Treponema pallidum*. It is generally propagated by direct venereal contact or by inheritance. Its primary site is a hard or true chancre, whence it extends by means of the lymphatics to the skin, mucosa, and nearly all the tissues of the body, even to the bones and periosteum (the tough, fibrous membrane surrounding bone).

systolic blood pressure See *blood pressure*.

tachycardia Excessive rapidity in the action of the heart, with usually a pulse rate greater than 130 beats per minute.

tachyphylaxis Rapid immunization from the effects of toxic doses of an extract by previous injection of small doses.

tapeworm Flat, tape-like, segmented parasite sometimes found in the intestines of man.

tenacious Holding fast, thick, sticky, adhesive; for example, mucus and sputum.

tenosynovitis Tendon inflammation.

teratogenic Tending to produce fetal monstrosity.

testes Male gonads; organ in reproduction.

tetanus (lockjaw) Acute infectious disease caused by a toxin related by the *Clostridium tetani* (tetanus bacillus) and characterized by more or less persistent tonic spasm of some of the voluntary muscles. Continuous spasm or steady contraction of a muscle without distinct twitching can occur. Spasm can cause locking of the jaw muscles so jaws cannot open, hence its common name.

tetany Nervous affection characterized by muscle twitching, cramps, muscle pains, and convulsions.

thalamus Mass of gray matter at the base of the brain projecting into and bounding the third ventricle.

thrombin The hypothetical fibrin ferment of the blood; the enzyme, present in clotted but not in circulating blood, that converts fibrinogen into fibrin; also called thrombase, fibrin ferment, and fibrinogen.

thromboangiitis obliterans Form of gangrene attributed to a thromboangiitis occurring generally in the larger arteries and veins of the leg, although it may appear in the upper extremity. Also called Buerger's disease and presenile spontaneous gangrene.

thrombocytes Blood platelets.

thrombocytopenia Decrease in the number of blood platelets; same as thrombopenia.

thrombocytopenic purpura Severe form of purpura, with copious hemorrhages from the mucous membranes, marked lessening of the number of blood platelets, marked loss of nuclear substance of blood platelets, and severe constitutional symptoms.

thrombophlebitis Inflammation of a vein or veins resulting from an infection or clot.

thromboplastin Substance existing in the tissue that causes clotting of the blood.

thrombosis Formation or development of a thrombus or clot in a blood vessel and remaining at its point of formation.

thyroid gland Gland of internal secretion found in the neck.

thyrotoxicosis Severe condition resulting from abnormal increase of thyroid activity.

tinea corporis Ringworm of the body.

cruris Ringworm of the groin.

pedis Ringworm of the feet, or athlete's foot.

tinnitus Ringing or singing sound heard in the ears; also a clicking sound in the ear heard in chronic catarrhal otitis media or inflammation of the middle ear.

titer Quantity of a substance required to produce a reaction with a given amount of another substance.

agglutination The highest dilution of a serum that causes clumping of bacteria.

colon The smallest amount of a certain substance that indicates the presence of the colon bacillus under standard conditions.

tone In the circulatory system, the factor responsible for a small blood vessel being stiffer or showing more resistance to stretching than a larger vessel, even though the wall material of both small and large vessels possesses exactly the same mechanical properties.

tonometry The measurement of tension, especially intraocular tension.

topical Pertaining to a particular spot; local; medicine for local application, for example, eye drops.

torticollis Wryneck; a contracted state of the cervical or neck muscles producing twisting of the neck and an unnatural position of the head.

trachea Windpipe; the cartilaginous and membranous tube descending from the larynx to the bronchi.

tracheitis Inflammation of the trachea.

tracheostomy Operative formation of an opening into the trachea (windpipe) through the neck and insertion of a trachea tube to aid breathing.

transient Temporary, passing through or over.

trauma Wound or injury.

trifacial neuralgia Pain in the fifth cranial nerve, a nerve of the face. Pain is very severe, shooting, stabbing, searing, or burning in the area of one or more branches of the nerve. Attack frequency varies from many times a day to several times a month or year. Also known as trigeminal neuralgia or tic douloureux.

trigonum vesicae Triangular area of the interior of the bladder between the opening of the ureters and the orifice of the urethra. Called also trigone of bladder and vesical trigone.

trophic Of or pertaining to nutrition.

tuberculosis Infectious disease caused by the tubercle bacillus and marked by presence of tubercles in the affected tissues; most common site is in the lungs.

typhoid fever Contagious disease marked by fever, diarrhea that is sometimes bloody, and malaise. The typhoid bacillus enters the body with food such as milk, watery vegetables such as lettuce, and drinking water.

typhus fever Rickettsial infectious disease characterized by symptoms such as petechial eruptions, high temperature, chills, backache, headache, and great prostration. See *rickettsia*.

urate Any salt or uric acid. Urates, especially that of sodium, are constituents of urine, blood, and tophi or calcerous concretions (a stone or mass containing lime or calcium).

urea White, crystallizable substance, a double amide or compound of carbonic acid, from the urine, blood, and lymph. It is the chief nitrogenous constituent of the urine and is the final product of the decomposition of proteins in the body. It is the form under which the nitrogen of the body is given off. It is thought to be formed in the liver out of amino acids and other compounds of ammonia.

uremia Toxic condition from abnormal urinary constituents in the blood.

ureter The fibromuscular tube that conveys urine from the kidney to the bladder.

ureterosigmoidostomy The operation of implanting the ureter into the sigmoid flexure.

urethra Canal leading from the bladder to the exterior of the body.

uric acid Crystallizable acid, trioxypurine, from the urine of humans and animals, being one of the products of nuclein metabolism. It forms a large portion of certain calculi, or stones, and in the blood causes morbid symptoms, such as those of gout.

uricosuric drugs Drugs administered to relieve pain in gout and increase elimination of uric acid.

urinary retention Retention of urine in the bladder, often caused by a temporary loss of muscle function.

urolithiasis The formation of urinary calculi or stones; also the diseased condition associated with the presence of urinary calculi or stones.

urologic Pertaining to the urine and urinary tract; the term now includes the male and female genitourinary tract.

uropathy Any pathologic change in the urinary tract.

urticaria Hives.

uterus The womb, or organ for containing and nourishing the infant before birth.

vaccination Inoculation with a vaccine as a disease preventive.

vaccine Substance derived from the growth of bacteria and used to confer immunity against certain diseases.

vaccinia Cowpox; a disease of cattle regarded as a form of smallpox. When given to a person via vaccination, it confers a greater or lesser degree of immunity against smallpox.

vagus nerve Tenth cranial nerve, which originates in an area on the floor of the fourth ventricle, extends by small cords from the side of the medulla oblongata, and distributes to larynx, lungs, heart, esophagus, stomach, and most of the abdominal viscera. *Vagus* is a Latin word meaning "wandering." Also called pneumogastric nerve.

varicella Chickenpox; an acute contagious disease, principally of young children, marked by slight fever and an eruption of macular vesicles appearing in crops and sometimes followed by scarring.

vascular Pertaining to or full of vessels, often blood vessels.

vasoconstriction Construction or decrease in size of blood vessels.

vasodilation Dilation or enlargement of the blood vessels.

ventricle Two lower cavities or chambers of the heart; there are right and left ventricles.

venule A minute vein.

vermicular Worm-like in shape or appearance.

vertigo Dizziness, giddiness; disorder of the equilibrating sense marked by a swimming in the head; a sense of instability and of apparent rotary movement of the body or of other objects.

Vincent's infection (trench mouth) Inflammation caused by mixed organisms. It was commonly seen among soldiers in the trenches, hence its name. It can involve the throat, stomach, and intestines and is communicable. Also called Vincent's angina.

viscera Internal organs, especially those of the cavities of the chest and abdomen.

viscosity Quality of being sticky or gummy.

vulva The external part of the organs of generation of the female, including the labia majora, the labia minora, mons veneris, clitoris, perineum, and vestibulum vaginae.

vulvovaginitis Inflammation of the vulva and vagina, or of the vulvovaginal glands.

wheal A white or pinkish elevation or ridge on the skin, as in urticaria or after the stroke of a whip.

whiplash Inflammation and muscle spasm of the neck and upper back muscles often caused by violent movement during heavy exercise or automobile accidents; often occurs as the result of a sudden backward and forward whipping movement of the neck.

Wilms' tumor A tumor containing embryonic elements; embryoma of the kidney.

Wilson's disease (progressive lenticular disease or **hepatolenticular disease)** Rare disease characterized by bilateral degeneration of the corpus striatum (a subcortical mass of gray and white matter in front of the thalamus in each cerebral hemisphere) and cirrhosis of the liver with symptoms such as tremor, spastic contractures, increasing weakness and emaciation, and psychic disturbance. Also called dermatitis exfoliativa.

Appendix

FIRST-AID ACTIONS AGAINST POISONING*

Emergency telephone numbers:

Physician _____

Hospital _____

Pharmacy _____

Poison Center _____

Fire Department _____

Police _____

Emergency medical services _____

To treat poisoning until medical treatment can be obtained

1. Call a poison center, physician, or hospital immediately. If possible, begin first-aid treatment while another person calls.
2. Loosen tight clothing and be sure that airway is clear; reposition or remove dentures.
3. Apply artificial ventilation if patient's breathing has stopped. Keep airway open if unconscious.
4. Keep patient warm with blankets but do not overheat.
5. Do not give alcoholic or carbonated beverages or any drugs.
6. Stop visible bleeding if possible.
7. Save and give to physician whatever caused the poisoning, such as remaining medicine, plant material, or a household agent, plus its container and label.

For inhaled poisons (smoke, chemical, or gas fumes)

1. Do not attempt rescue alone. Use "buddy system" and lifeline.
2. Stay close to ground or crawl to rescue patient from gas, fumes, or smoke.
3. Do not enter superheated areas unless you are wearing an independent air supply.
4. Move patient to fresh air immediately.
5. If patient is not breathing, start artificial ventilation promptly. Do not stop until patient is breathing well or help arrives.

*Revised from, 1971, American Medical Association, Council on Drugs.

264

For swallowed poisons

If a petroleum distillate product is swallowed, such as furniture polish, gasoline, lighter fluid, or kerosene, immediately call a poison center, physician, or the emergency room of a hospital for first-aid instructions.

Do not induce vomiting if:

1. Patient is unconscious
2. Patient is having convulsions
3. Patient has pain or burning sensation in mouth or throat
4. Patient has swallowed a corrosive poison

If patient can swallow and if poison is:

- An acid or acid-like corrosive
    Sodium acid sulfate (toilet bowl cleaner)
    Acids (sulfuric, nitric, oxalic, hydrochloric, phosphoric)
    Silver nitrate (caustic or styptic pencils)
    Calcium hypochlorite (chlorine bleach)
- An alkali corrosive
    Sodium or potassium hydroxide (lye, drain, cleaner)
    Sodium carbonate (washing soda)
    Ammonia water
    Sodium perborate (bleaching powder)
    Dishwashing machine detergent

1. Give milk or water if patient is conscious, alert, and can swallow. Suggested dose: for patients 1 to 5 years old—1 to 2 cups (250 to 500 ml); for patients 5 years and older—2 to 3 cups (500 to 750 ml).
2. Do not use activated charcoal (see p. 266).

If poison is a noncorrosive substance:

1. Give water—1 to 2 cups (250 to 500 ml).
2. If physician tells you to induce vomiting, use 2 tbsp (30 ml) of ipecac syrup (see p. 265), if available. (Ask physician if this is a prescription item in your state.) For children, use half of the adult amount. Follow with at least 1 cup (8 oz or 250 ml) of water.
3. If patient does not vomit within 20 to 30 minutes, repeat dose. If vomiting still does not occur after

repeating dose, take patient to hospital emergency department or physician.

4. If you do not have ipecac syrup, try inducing vomiting by placing your finger or handle of spoon at back of patient's throat.
5. When vomiting begins, have patient stand or sit up and lean forward. This prevents vomitus from entering the lungs.
6. Save vomitus and give to physician for examination. Physician may tell you to administer activated charcoal (if available) *after vomiting occurs*.

For eye injury caused by chemical agents

A delay of only seconds may greatly increase extent of injury.

1. Forcibly hold patient's eyelids open and immediately rinse his eyes and face with a gentle stream of warm, running water from the tap or a pitcher for at least 15 minutes; then take victim to the emergency department of a hospital or an ophthalmologist.
2. Do not use eye cup.
3. Remove contact lenses when present, if you know how. If not, gently slide lenses onto white of patient's eye using his eyelids.
4. Do not use eye drops, drugs, or ointments. They may increase extent of injury.

For bites and stings (spider, scorpion, snake, marine life, or bee)

1. Identify source of bite. In snakebite, identify type of snake.
2. Make patient lie down and immobilize limb as soon as possible.
3. For snakebite, flush with water and apply a constricting band between bite and heart *only* when bite occurs on extremity. Band should depress skin only slightly. Pulse in vessels below band should not disappear, nor should band produce throbbing sensation. You should be able to slip your finger under band when in place. *Do not apply ice or ice pack to snakebites.*
4. For bee stings, remove stinger carefully with flicking motion of thumb and finger. *Do not use tweezers.* Soothing skin lotion may be applied to skin. If severe allergic reactions results, such as difficult breathing or extensive swelling at site of sting, patient must have medical attention at once.
5. Use ice or ice packs at sites of all bites except snakebites.
6. Transport patient to physician or hospital immediately. Do not let him walk.
7. Since black widow and brown recluse spider bites require medical treatment, transport patient to a hospital immediately.

Note: Human bites are dangerous. If skin is broken, wash with soap and water and call a physician.

For skin injury (plant poisoning)

1. Drench patient's skin with plenty of running water from shower, hose, or faucet.
2. Immediately cut away contaminated clothing and remove jewelry.
3. Wash patient's skin with soap and water to reduce extent of poison absorption and injury. Repeat several times.
4. Cover injured area with loosely applied, clean cloth.
5. Do not apply ointments, greases (including butter or margarine), powders, or drugs to affected area and do not administer drugs of any kind unless recommended by a physician.
6. See a physician if blisters appear on skin.

AGENTS TO TREAT POISONING
Ipecac syrup (ip'e-kak)

1. The source of ipecac is the dried roots of the *ipecacuanha* or *acuminata* plants native to Central and South America.
2. It has a long history of use as a medicinal agent by the Indians of South America. It was introduced in Europe as a treatment for dysentery. The chief use of ipecac in the United States today is as an emetic to induce vomiting in cases of ingested noncorrosive poisons.
3. Ipecac probably acts both centrally and locally. It directly stimulates the vomiting center and has an irritant effect on gastric mucosa.
4. Usual dose for adults: 15 to 30 ml, followed by 200 to 300 ml of water, fruit juice, or milk or as much fluid as the patient can drink. Dose for children over 1 year of age: 15 ml preceded by 200 ml of water. Vomiting usually occurs in 15 to 30 minutes. The dose may be repeated once after 20 minutes if the first dose is not effective. If vomiting does not occur within 30 minutes, gastric lavage should be performed, since ipecac is a cardiotoxic if absorbed and may cause conduction disturbances, myocarditis, or atrial fibrillation.
5. Before giving a dose of ipecac to cause vomiting in poisoning, *call physician, poison control center, or hospital emergency room at once for advice*.
6. Some physicians recommend that ipecac syrup be kept in every home, especially where there are children. *Keep it in a safe place completely out of reach of children.*
7. *Do not use ipecac* if any of the following have been ingested: such corrosives as alkalies (lye) and strong acids, strychnine, and petroleum distillates, such as gasoline, coal oil, fuel oil, kerosene, cleaning fluid, or paint thinner.

8. *Ipecac syrup should not be confused with ipecac fluid extract,* which is fourteen times more concentrated and has caused a number of deaths.

Activated charcoal (Medicinal charcoal and active carbon)
(Charcodote) (char'ko-dote)

1. Activated charcoal is a fine, black, tasteless, odorless, and nongritty powder.
2. A charcoal may be activated by treating it at high temperatures with steam and carbon dioxide, or with such dehydrating substances as sulfuric acid, zinc chloride, phosphoric acid, or a combination of these.
3. To activate the charcoal for medicinal purposes, it must be thoroughly washed to remove inorganic matter. The surface area of 1 ml of finely divided charcoal is estimated to be 1,000 sq m.
4. Activated charcoal absorbs a large variety of substances, both simple and complex. It is used as an adjunct in the treatment of oral poisonings caused by ingestion of heavy metals, strychnine, phenol, mercuric chloride, atropine, oxalic acid, phenolphthalein, poison mushrooms, aspirin, and most drugs.
5. It is not effective for poisoning caused by cyanide, ethanol, methanol, ferrous sulfate, caustic alkalies, or mineral acids.
6. For emergency treatment of adults or children: 5 to 50 g of the powder mixed with tap water to the consistency of thick soup; this is taken orally or passed through a lavage tube. Some emergency centers use a dose of 50 g; the dose may be as high as 100 g. The dose should be five to ten times the estimated weight of the ingested substance. Palatability can be improved by adding a small amount of a flavoring agent, such as cherry, concentrated fruit juice, or chocolate powder.
7. Tablets or capsules of charcoal should not be used for treatment of poisoning, because they are less effective than the powder. Ice cream or sherbet should not be used to add flavor or appease the child because these substances decrease the absorptive capacity of the charcoal.
8. If ipecac syrup is to be used to induce vomiting, the emetic should be given before administering activated charcoal because the charcoal will absorb the syrup. The charcoal mixture should be removed from the stomach shortly afterward by inducing vomiting with ipecac syrup or apomorphine or through the gastric tube.

Heavy metal antagonists
Dimercaprol (dy-mer-kap'rol), BAL

1. BAL was developed during World War II as an antidote for lewisite, a blister gas containing arsenic. BAL comes from this blister gas and is an abbreviation for "British anti-lewisite."
2. It was first used to decontaminate the eyes of persons who had been in contact with the gas, but later it was found to be of value in the treatment of various forms of arsenic poisoning.
3. Arsenic compounds produce their toxic effects by combining with the sulfhydryl groups of enzymes. These enzymes are necessary for normal metabolism. The result is serious interference with the processes of oxidation and reduction in the tissues. BAL forms a stable combination with the arsenic and hastens its excretion from the body.
4. BAL also has been found useful in the treatment of gold and mercury poisoning. Treatment should be begun as soon as possible for effective results.
5. Side effects for doses of 300 mg may include symptoms such as nausea and vomiting, a burning sensation of the mouth, throat, and eyes, headache, muscular aching and tingling in the extremities, and a constricting sensation in the chest.
6. Dosage: 2.5 to 5 mg/kg of body weight, intramuscularly, every 4 hours the first 2 days, reduced to 2 injections on the third day, and then daily for the next 5 days. Dosage can be reduced for mild cases and may sometimes be increased for mercury poisoning.

Calcium disodium edetate
(Calcium Disodium Versenate, Calcium EDTA)

1. This antidote is most useful in the treatment of lead poisoning. It combines with the heavy metal in the body and encourages its renal excretion.
2. Renal damage may occur if more than the recommended dosage is used. Symptoms of acute lead poisoning, especially cerebral symptoms, may be aggravated at the beginning of treatment. In this case, dosage may be reduced.
3. This drug should *not* be confused with the trisodium salt of ethylenediamine tetraacetic acid, the administration of which would be very dangerous.
4. The drug is usually administered by slow IV infusion; 1 g is added to 250 or 500 ml of 5% dextrose in water or to isotonic saline. Infusions may be administered twice a day for 3 to 5 days. Dosage for children should be kept below 1 g/30 pounds of body weight.
5. The drug may be administered intramuscularly, but a local anesthetic may have to be added to the solution to decrease pain at the site of injection. Patients with mild cases of lead poisoning may take the drug orally in tablets; usual dose for adults: 4 g daily.

Penicillamine (pen-i-sil-am'een)
(Cuprimine) (koo'pri-meen)

1. This heavy metal antagonist is used to treat poisoning caused by copper and to remove copper from the body in Wilson's disease.
2. Rashes, blood dyscrasias, and possible renal damage may occur infrequently following use of penicillamine.
3. Usual dosage: orally, 250 mg four times a day.

Deferoxamine mesylate (di-fer-oks'ah-meen me'si-layt)
(Desferal) (des'fer-al)

1. Desferal binds iron and promotes its excretion, so it is useful in the treatment of iron poisoning and in diseases such as hemochromatosis or chronic accumulation of iron in the body.
2. It is well tolerated and adverse effects are uncommon. Pruritus or mild rash may occur. Rapid IV injection may cause tachycardia, erythema, hypotension, and urticaria. Tissue irritation and pain may occur at the injection site. In long-term therapy, symptoms such as allergic reactions, blurred vision, fever, diarrhea, and leg cramps may occur. Cataracts may develop after prolonged deferoxamine therapy, but not after short-term therapy.
3. Desferal can increase blood coagulability and lower blood sugar and serum calcium, so frequent blood studies should be done.
4. This drug is contraindicated in patients with severe renal impairment.
5. Usual initial dose for adults and children: 1.0 g, followed by two 0.5-g doses at 4-hour intervals. Further doses of 0.5 g may be administered every 4 to 12 hours, depending on the clinical response. Total dosage should not exceed 6 g in 24 hours.
6. Intramuscular injection is the preferred route of administration for all patients not in shock. Intravenous dose should be administered by slow infusion at a rate not exceeding 15 mg/kg/hr. Intravenous route should be used only when the patient is in shock. Subcutaneous route should not be used, since tissue irritation and damage may occur. Desferal is available in vials of 500 mg of lyophilized powder. The powder is easily dissolved by adding 2 ml of sterile water for injection.

An organophosphate insecticide antidote
Pralidoxime chloride (pral-i-doks'eem)
(Protopam) (pro'to-pam)

1. Protopam is a cholinesterase reactivator used as an antidote for poisoning by organophosphate insecticides. These insecticides inactivate cholinesterase in the body. Breaking down the binding between the organophosphate compound and cholinesterase, pralidoxime liberates the cholinesterase so it can destroy accumulated acetylcholine.
2. This drug is used to reverse respiratory muscle paralysis. It is, however, relatively ineffective on the respiratory center, so atropine must be administered concomitantly to relieve respiratory depression from accumulated acetylcholine at this site. Pralidoxime is most effective if administered immediately after poisoning.
3. Pralidoxime may cause blurred vision, nausea, dizziness, diplopia, tachycardia, muscle weakness, hyperventilation, and increased blood pressure.
4. Pralidoxime may be administered intravenously in a dosage of 1 g in 100 ml of sodium chloride solution and infused over 15 to 30 minutes or injected at a rate not exceeding 200 mg a minute. The dose may be repeated in 1 hour. Dose for children: intravenously, 250 to 500 mg or 20 to 40 mg/kg/g of body weight. The drug may be administered orally in the absence of gastrointestinal symptoms in a dosage of 1 to 3 g every 3 to 5 hours. The dosage may and should be reduced in patients with renal insufficiency.

SOME SPECIFIC POISONS, SYMPTOMS, AND EMERGENCY TREATMENT*

Poison	Symptoms	Treatment
Acids (such as hydrochloric or nitric)	Parts in contact with acid are first white, later colored (brown or yellow) Pain in throat, esophagus, and stomach; dysphagia, diarrhea, shock, circulatory collapse Death may result from asphyxia from edema of glottis	Avoid stomach tube, emesis, and solutions of carbonate, such as sodium bicarbonate Give milk of magnesia, aluminum hydroxide, plenty of milk or water with egg white Copious amounts of water Keep patient warm and quiet Corticosteroids to reduce fibrosis and possibility of esophageal stricture
Arsenic (found in weed killers, insecticides, sheepdip rodenticides, and so on)	Rapidity of onset of symptoms related to whether or not poison is taken with food Odor of garlic on breath and stools Faintness, nausea, difficulty in swallowing, extreme thirst, severe vomiting, gastric pain, "rice water" stools, oliguria, albuminuria, cold, clammy skin Collapse and death	Induce emesis with ipecac syrup Give 0.5 to 10 g of activated charcoal in a glass of water followed by repeated lavage with warm or weak sodium bicarbonate solution or by an emetic (warm water) repeated until vomiting occurs Intravenous fluids Sedation, analgesics Dimercaprol (BAL) is the antidote of choice Keep patient warm

Bromides	*Acute poisoning*
	   Deep stupor
	   Ataxia
	   Extreme muscular weakness
	   Collapse
	 Chronic poisoning (bromism)
	   Bromide acne is seen on face, chest, and back
	   Salty taste in mouth
	   Foul breath
	   Gastrointestinal disturbance
	   Mental depression
	   Faulty memory
	   Pronounced apathy
	   Ataxia—slurred speech
	   Muscular weakness
	   Malnutrition
	   Anemia
		Stop the drug
		 Large doses of physiologic salt solutions are given to hasten excretion of drug
		 As a rule, symptoms of bromism rapidly abate if drug is withdrawn
		 Diuretics are given to hasten excretion of the drug
		 For acute ingestion, induce emesis with ipecac syrup
		 Hemodialysis

Carbon monoxide (present in coal gas, illuminating gas, exhaust gas from motor cars, and so on)	Symptoms vary with concentration of carbon monoxide in blood Headache, dizziness, impaired hearing and vision, drowsiness, confusion, loss of consciousness Slow respiration, rapid pulse Coma, cherry-red or dusky lips and nails	Remove patient to fresh air; artificial respiration; high concentration of oxygen preferably under positive pressure Bed rest for 48 hours Keep patient warm

*From Bergersen, B. S.: Pharmacology in nursing, ed. 14, St. Louis, 1979, The C. V. Mosby Co. Some pharmacologists do not recommend the use of large doses of salt and water and physiologic salt solution in the treatment of poisoning, since overdosage of salt may cause kidney damage, loss of kidney function, and possible death. This is true for children also. Deaths have occurred from overdosage of salt in treatment of poison, both in home and in hospital situations. Strong salt solutions also may cause severe brain and central nervous system damage, blood vessel damage, coma, and death. Syrup of Ipecac, 20 ml, and large amounts of water, if possible, have been recommended by some authorities to replace salt solutions to induce emesis for poisoning, except for cases involving acids, alkalis, hydrocarbon poisoning, or in states of unconsciousness or coma. Fluid extract of Ipecac *should not be confused* with Syrup of Ipecac. The fluid extract form is approximately fourteen times as concentrated as is the syrup and has caused death. *The fluid extract form should be avoided under all circumstances.*

Poison	Symptoms	Treatment
Carbon tetrachloride (found in some dry-cleaning fluids and in some home fire extinguishers)	*When inhaled:* headache, nausea, vomiting, diarrhea, jaundice, oliguria, albuminuria, dark-colored urine *When swallowed:* headache, nausea, vomiting, sometimes blood in vomitus, abdominal pain, disturbance of hearing and vision, jaundice, profuse diarrhea, albuminuria, anuria	Remove patient from poisoned atmosphere; administer oxygen or oxygen with carbon dioxide Emetics, such as ipecac syrup, to produce repeated vomiting if lavage not available; if possible, lavage followed by saline cathartic High-protein, high-carbohydrate, high-calcium diet General supportive measures
Chlorophenothane (dichlorodiphenyl-trichloroethane, or D.D.T.)	Headache, nausea, vomiting, diarrhea, paresthesias of lips and tongue, numbness of extremities, malaise, sore throat Coarse tremor, convulsions, respiratory failure	Induce vomiting or use gastric lavage if convulsions do not threaten Give saline cathartic, force fluids, give strong tea or coffee Avoid fats, fat solvents, and epinephrine Wash contaminated skin areas with soap and water
Cyanides	An odor of oil of bitter almonds on breath; headache, rapid breathing, dyspnea, palpitation of heart, feeling of tightness in chest, cyanosis, convulsions Death may come within few minutes	Prompt treatment sometimes successful Immediate removal of poison by an emetic (ipecac syrup, or apomorphine) or lavage Amyl nitrite (several pearls broken into gauze and given by inhalation), followed by 1% sodium nitrite intravenously slowly, in 10-ml doses, to a total of 50 ml in an hour, and this followed by slow intravenous administration of sodium thiosulfate (50 ml. of a 25% solution) Oxygen, artificial respiration, and blood transfusion may be indicated
Fluoride (found in insecticides)	Nausea, vomiting, abdominal pain, diarrhea, muscle weakness, difficult swallowing, facial paralysis, inability to speak, convulsions at times, respiratory failure and circulatory collapse	Give emetic containing soluble calcium salts (calcium lactate or gluconate) or use plenty of warm water and follow with plenty of milk Preferable to lavage promptly with 1% calcium chloride to inactivate fluoride General supportive measures Calcium gluconate 10% intravenously if tetany occurs
Hydrocarbons or **Petroleum distillates** (present in kerosene, gasoline, naphtha, cleaning fluids, paint thinner)	Symptoms of intoxication similar to those of alcohol; burning sensation in mouth, esophagus, and stomach Vomiting, dizziness, tremor, muscle cramps, confusion, fever Cold, clammy skin, weak pulse, thirst, unconsciousness, coma Pulmonary symptoms: cough, cyanosis, bloody sputum rales Death from respiratory failure	Emetics and lavage usually avoided unless large amounts swallowed; saline cathartics after small amounts taken Some authorities recommend large doses of mineral oil for severe poisoning, followed by lavage with 1% or 2% sodium bicarbonate solution General supportive measures Avoid epinephrine
Iodine	Brown-stained lips, tongue, and mouth, which are painful Odor of iodine in vomitus Intense thirst, fainting attacks, giddiness, vomiting, burning, abdominal pain, diarrhea, shock	Give plenty of water promptly, with starch or flour or mashed potatoes Gastric lavage if possible with thin, cooked suspension of starch or 5% sodium thiosulfite solution Give drinks of milk or white of egg, with water

Poison	Symptoms	Treatment
Lye (a severe caustic)	Severe burning pain in mouth, throat, and stomach Strong soapy taste in mouth Early violent vomiting with mucus and blood in vomitus Mucous membranes become white and swollen; lips and tongue swell; throat may become constricted Respirations difficult Skin cold and clammy Pulse rapid Violent purging Great anxiety	Emetics and lavage frequently not recommended Give large amounts of water containing weak acids, lemon, vinegar, lime juice, and so on; later give demulcents, white of egg, gruel, olive oil or salad oil Analgesics, parenteral fluids Corticosteroids
Mercury and its compounds	Burning sensation of throat Nausea and vomiting (vomitus blue if antiseptic tablets of bichloride used) Sense of constriction in throat and esophagus Ashen-gray color of mucous membranes that have been in contact with poison Bloody, profuse diarrhea, with shreds of mucous membrane in stool and vomitus Shock, albuminuria, and hematuria During acute phase, pain and prostration; late, progressive uremia	Give 0.5 to 10 g of activated charcoal in a glass of water and then lavage with 5% sodium formaldehyde sulfoxylate solution followed by sodium bicarbonate solution If not feasible, give emetic of ipecac syrup Give milk and egg white in water Dimercaprol indicated as specific antidote Parenteral fluids Keep patient warm Recovery depends on dose taken, amount of absorption, and amount of kidney damage
Nicotine (Black Leaf 40 contains about 40% nicotine sulfate)	Burning sensation in mouth and throat, increased flow of saliva, abdominal pain, vomiting, diarrhea, headache, sweating, confusion, weakness, dilation of pupils, faintness, death from respiratory paralysis	Activated charcoal, 10 to 30 g in a glass of water; lavage with 0.5% tannic acid or 1:5000 potassium permanganate Ipecac syrup Artificial respiration Wash contaminated skin with cold water Atropine for parasympathetic overstimulation
Organophosphorus insecticides (Parathion, Malathion, TEPP, HEPT, etc.)	Headache, dizziness, diarrhea, blurred vision, abdominal pain, dyspnea, chest pain, sweating, salivation, tearing Cyanosis, respiratory failure Collapse	Removal of secretions, maintenance of patent airway Decontaminate patient with soapy water or tincture of green soap Oxygen, artificial respiration to combat shock Atropinization is mandatory as soon as cyanosis has been relieved Adults: 2 to 4 mg atropine intravenously; repeat at 5- to 10-minute intervals until signs of atropine toxicity appear (dry flushed skin, tachycardia, mydriasis) Children: 0.5 to 1 mg intravenously or intramuscularly every 10 to 15 minutes Mild degree of atropinization should be maintained for 48 hours Pralidoxime (Protopam) Gastric lavage if poison ingested Close supervision for 48 to 72 hours

Poison	Symptoms	Treatment
Paris green (copper arsenite and copper acetate)	Vomiting of green material followed by gastric and abdominal pain; diarrhea with dark and sometimes bloody stools; metallic taste; neuromuscular weakness Thirst, oliguria, anuria Cold, clammy skin Coma, convulsions, death	Potassium ferrocyanide, gr 10 in water as soon as possible (forms an insoluble salt of copper), followed by lavage with sodium bicarbonate solution or emetic until stomach cleansed Demulcents (milk, egg white in water, gelatin) Supportive measures
Phenolic compounds (carbolic acid, cresol, Lysol, creosote)	Corrosion of mucous membranes that have come in contact with poison Severe pain, vomiting, bloody diarrhea, headache, dizziness Cold, clammy skin Oliguria, hematuria, unconsciousness, slow respiration, respiratory failure Urine dark and turns very dark on exposure to air	Of utmost importance to remove poison before absorption, prompt lavage with olive oil (a good solvent); leave some oil in stomach after lavage; give egg white and milk for demulcent effect Parenteral fluids, oxygen, carbon dioxide, analgesics Other supportive measures Phenol on skin can be removed with 50% solution of alcohol, followed by thorough rinsinig with water, or wash external burns with olive oil or castor oil
Quaternary ammonium compounds (such as Zephiran)	Burning pain in the mouth and throat, nausea and vomiting, apprehension and restlessness; muscle weakness, collapse, coma, sometimes convulsions	Induce vomiting or use gastric lavage if it can be done promptly; mild soap solution will serve as antidote or unabsorbed portions Give cathartic
Strychnine (symptoms occur within 15 or 20 minutes after drug has been taken)	Feeling of stiffness in muscles of face and neck Twitching of face and limbs Violent convulsions of whole body at intervals varying from a few minutes to an hour "Risus sardonicus" Opisthotonos Death may result from asphyxia caused by spasm of respiratory muscles or during period of relaxation from respiratory paralysis	Administer diazepam If diazepam is not available, barbiturates, chloroform, paraldehyde, or amobarbital are recommended Gastric lavage may be done with solutions of potassium permanganate, 1:1000, or 2% tannic acid After convulsions have been checked, chloral hydrate or phenobarbital may be needed to prevent convulsions from returning During treatment patient should be in cool, quiet room and protected from sudden noise, jarring or change of any kind that might precipitate another seizure

The physician prescribes the medicine and treatment.
The nurse carries out the physician's orders.
Self-medication is dangerous. Consult your physician first.
There is in every medicine a possible danger.
When in doubt—ASK!

References

General references

American Hospital Formulary Service, Washington, D.C., 1979, American Society of Hospital Pharmacists.

American Medical Association: Drug evaluations, eds. 4 and 5, Acton, Mass., 1978, 1979, Publishing Sciences Group, Inc.

American Pharmaceutical Association: Handbook of nonprescription drugs, ed. 6, Washington, D.C., 1979, American Pharmaceutical Association.

Bergersen, B. S.: Pharmacology in nursing, ed. 14, St. Louis, 1979, The C. V. Mosby Co.

Falconer, M. W., and others: The drug, the nurse, the patient, ed. 6, Philadelphia, 1978, W. B. Saunders Co.

Goodman, L. S., and Gilman, A., editors: The pharmacological basis of therapeutics, ed. 5, New York, 1975, The Macmillan Co.

Goth, A.: Medical pharmacology, ed. 9, St. Louis, 1978, The C. V. Mosby Co.

Kastrup, E. K., and Boyd, J. R.: Facts and comparisons, St. Louis, 1979, Facts and Comparisons, Inc.

Meyers, F. J., Jawetz, E., adn Goldfien, A.: Review of medical pharmacology, ed. 6, Los Altos, Calif., 1978, Lange Medical Publications.

Modell, W., editor: Drugs of choice, 1978-1979, St. Louis, 1978, The C. V. Mosby Co.

Pharmacopoeia internationalis, supplement to the U.S. Pharmacopoeia, ed. 2, Geneva, 1971, World Health Organization.

Physicians' desk reference, ed. 34, Oradell, N.J., 1980, Medical Economics Co.

Ryan, S. A., and Clayton, B. D.: Handbook of practical pharmacology, ed. 1, St. Louis, 1980, The C. V. Mosby Co.

The national formulary, supplement to the U.S. Pharmacopeia, Easton, Pa., 1975, The Mack Publishing Co.

Unlisted drugs, various monthly publications, New York, 1979, Special Libraries Association.

U.S. pharmacopeia, ed. 19, Easton, Pa., 1975, The Mack Publishing Co.

United States dispensatory and physicians' pharmacology, ed. 27, Philadelphia, 1973, J. B. Lippincott Co.

Chapter 1

Goodman, L. S., and Gilman, A., editors: The pharmacological basis of therapeutics, ed. 5, New York, 1975, The Macmillan Co.

Goth, A.: Medical pharmacology, ed. 9, St. Louis, 1978, The C. V. Mosby Co.

Chapter 2

American Hospital Formulary Service, Washington, D.C., 1979, American Society of Hospital Pharmacists.

American Pharmaceutical Association: Evaluations of drug interactions, ed. 2, Washington, D.C., 1976, American Pharmaceutical Association.

American Pharmaceutical Association: Handbook of nonprescription drugs, ed. 6, Washington, D.C., 1979, American Pharmaceutical Association.

Billups, N. F.: American drug index, ed. 23, Philadelphia, 1979, J. B. Lippincott Co.

Hansten, P. D.: Drug interactions, ed. 4, Philadelphia, 1979, Lea & Febiger.

Hoover, J. E., editor: Remington's pharmaceutical sciences, ed. 15, Easton, Pa., 1975, Mack Publishing Co.

Medical letter, New Rochelle, N.Y., 1979, The Medical Letter, Inc.

Modell, W., editor: Drugs of choice 1978-1979, St. Louis, 1978, The C. V. Mosby Co.

Physician's desk reference, ed. 34, Oradell, N.J., 1980, Medical Economics Co.

USAN and the USP dictionary of drug names, Rockville, Md., 1978, United States Pharmacopeial Convention, Inc.

United States pharmacopeia, ed. 20, Rockville, Md., 1980, United States Pharmacopeial Convention, Inc.

Wade, A.: Martindale—the extra pharmacopoeia, ed. 27, London, 1977, The Pharmaceutical Press.

Chapter 3

Hoover, J. E., editor: Remington's pharmaceutical sciences, ed. 15, Easton, Pa., 1975, The Mack Publishing Co.

Chapter 4

Featherstone, R.: A guide to molecular pharmacology toxicology, New York, 1973, Marcel Dekker.

Goodman, L., and Gilman, A., editors: The pharmacologic basis of therapeutics, ed. 5, New York, 1975, The Macmillan Co.

Hartshorne, E.: Handbook of drug interaction, Cincinnati, Ohio, 1970, Donald Francke.

La Du, B. N.: Fundamentals of drug metabolism and drug disposition, Baltimore, 1971, The Williams & Wilkins Co.

Levine, R.: Pharmacology: drug actions and reactions, Boston, 1974, Little, Brown and Co.

Saunders, L.: The absorption and distribution of drugs, London, 1974, Bailliere, Tindall Publishers.

Tearell, T.: Pharmacology and pharmacokinetics: proceedings of an international conference, New York, 1974.

Zimmerman, A.: Drugs and the cell cycle, New York, 1973, Academic Press, Inc.

Chapter 6

Hart, L.: The arithmetic of dosages and solutions—a programmed presentation, ed. 4, St. Louis, 1977, The C. V. Mosby Co.

Jessee, R., and McHenry, R.: Self-teaching tests in arithmetic for nurses, ed. 9, St. Louis, 1975, The C. V. Mosby Co.

Saxton, D., Ercolano, N., and Walter, J.: Programmed instruction in arithmetic, dosages, and solutions, ed. 4, St. Louis, 1977, The C. V. Mosby Co.

Vervoren, T., and Oppeneer, J.: Workbook of solutions and dosage of drugs: including arithmetic, ed. 11, St. Louis, 1980, The C. V. Mosby Co.

Chapter 7

Dison, N.: Clinical nursing techniques, ed. 4, St. Louis, 1979, The C. V. Mosby Co.

Johns, M.: Pharmacodynamics and patient care, St. Louis, 1974, The C. V. Mosby Co.

Loebl, S., Spratto, G., and Wit, A.: The nurse's drug handbook, New York, 1977, John Wiley & Sons, Inc.

Roberts, F.: Review of pediatric nursing, St. Louis, 1974, The C. V. Mosby Co.

Shields, E.: Introduction to drug therapy for older adults, 1975.

Chapter 8

Bergersen, B. S.: Pharmacology in nursing, ed. 14, St. Louis, 1979, The C. V. Mosby Co.

Gahart, B.: Intravenous medications: a handbook for nurses and other allied personnel, ed. 2, St. Louis, 1977, The C. V. Mosby Co.

Newton, D., and Newton, M.: Route, site, and technique: three key decisions in giving parenteral medication, Nursing 79 9(7):18-25, 1979.

Chapter 9

Bergersen, B. S.: Pharmacology in nursing, ed. 14, St. Louis, 1979, The C. V. Mosby Co.

Koda-Kimble, M. A., Katcher, B., and Young, L.: Applied therapeutics for clinical pharmacists, ed. 2, San Francisco, 1978, Applied Therapeutics, Inc.

Ryan, S. A., and Clayton, B. D.: Handbook of practical pharmacology, ed. 2, St. Louis, 1980, The C. V. Mosby Co.

Chapter 10

American Hospital Formulary Service, Washington, D.C., 1979, American Society of Hospital Pharmacists.

American Medical Association: Drug evaluations, eds. 4 and 5, Acton, Mass., 1978, 1979, Publishing Sciences Group, Inc.

Bergersen, B. S.: Pharmacology in nursing, ed. 14, St. Louis, 1979, The C. V. Mosby Co.

Brown-Skeers, V.: How the nurse practitioner manages the rheumatoid arthritis patient; agents used in rheumatoid arthritis; a basic pyramid of RA treatment, Nursing 79 9(6):26-37, 1979.

Drug Data: Lopressor, Am. J. Nurs. **79**(3):509, 1979.

Drug Data: Stadol, Am. J. Nurs. **79**(6):1129, 1979.

Drug data: What's new in drugs: butorphanol tartrate, R.N. **42**(3):107, 1979.

Falconer, M. W., and others: The drug, the nurse, the patient, ed. 6, Philadelphia, 1978, W. B. Saunders Co.

Goodman, L. S., and Gilman, A., editors: The pharmacological basis of therapeutics, ed. 5, New York, 1975, The Macmillan Co.

Goth, A.: Medical pharmacology, ed. 9, St. Louis, 1978, The C. V. Mosby Co.

Hawken, M., and Ozuna, J.: Special points that must be considered in caring for patients receiving anticonvulsant medications, Am. J. Nurs. **79**(6):1062, 1979.

Hussar, D. A.: New drugs '78 '79, Nursing 79 **9**(5):35, 1979.

Kastrup, E. K., and Boyd, J. R.: Facts and comparisons, St. Louis, 1979, Facts and Comparisons, Inc.

Levine, R.: Pharmacology: drug actions and reactions, ed. 2, Boston, 1978, Little, Brown, & Co.

Meyers, F. J., Jawetz, E., and Goldfien, A.: Review of medical pharmacology, ed. 6, Los Altos, Calif., 1978, Lange Medical Publications.

Modell, W., editor: Drugs of choice, 1978-1979, St. Louis, 1978, The C. V. Mosby Co.

Physicians' desk reference, ed. 34, Oradell, N.J., 1980, Medical Economics Co.

Rodman, M. J.: The year's new drugs: cefamandole, bretylium, butorphanol, R.N. **42**(1):33-40, 1979.

Ryan, S. A., and Clayton, B. D.: Handbook of practical pharmacology, ed. 2, St. Louis, 1980, The C. V. Mosby Co.

Silman, J.: The management of pain, Am. J. Nurs. **79**(1):74-78, 1979.

Spruck, M.: Gold therapy for rheumatoid arthritis, Am. J. Nurs. **79**(7):1246-1248, 1979.

Unlisted drugs, various monthly publications, New York, 1979, Special Libraries Association.

U.S. pharmacopeia, ed. 20, Easton, Pa., 1980, The Mack Publishing Co.

Chapter 11

American Hospital Formulary Service, Washington, D.C., 1979, American Society of Hospital Pharmacists.

American Pharmaceutical Association: Handbook of nonprescription drugs, ed. 6, Washington, D.C., 1979, American Pharmaceutical Association.

American Medical Association: Drug evaluations, eds. 4 and 5, Acton, Mass., 1978, 1979, Publishing Sciences Group, Inc.

Bergersen, B. S.: Pharmacology in nursing, ed. 14, St. Louis, 1979, The C. V. Mosby CO.

Falconer, M. W., and others: The drug, the nurse, the patient, ed. 6, Philadelphia, 1978, W. B. Saunders Co.

Goodman, L. S., and Gilman, A., editors: The pharmacological basis of therapeutics, ed. 5, New York, 1975, The Macmillan Co.

Goth, A.: Medical pharmacology, ed. 9, St. Louis, 1978, The C. V. Mosby Co.

Kastrup, E. K., and Boyd, J. R.: Facts and comparisons, St. Louis, 1979, Facts and Comparisons, Inc.

Lalli, S.: The complete Swan-Ganz, R.N. **41**(9):66-67, 1978.

Lewis, A. J., editor: Modern drug encyclopedia, ed. 14, New York, 1977, Dun-Donnelley Publishing Corp.

Littman, A., and Pine, B. H.: Antacids and anticholinergic drugs, Ann. Intern. Med. **82:**(544), 1975.

Meyers, F. J., Jawetz, E., and Goldfien, A.: Review of medical pharmacology, ed. 6, Los Altos, Calif., 1978, Lange Medical Publications.

Modell, W., editor: Drugs of choice, 1978-1979, St. Louis, 1978, The C. V. Mosby Co.

Physicians' desk reference, ed. 34, Oradell, N.J., 1980, Medical Economics Co.

Purin-Parkinson, C.: Sorting out the adrenergic/cholinergic drugs, R.N. **42**(7):52-54, 1979.

Rodman, M. J.: Adrenergic drugs and adrenergic blockers, R.N. **37:**55, 1974.

Ryan, S. A., and Clayton, B. D.: Handbook of practical pharmacology, ed. 2, St. Louis, 1980, The C. V. Mosby Co.

Up-data: Inderal: drug found to inhibit migraine, Am. J. Nurs. **79**(7):1301, 1979.

U.S. pharmacopeia, ed. 20, Easton, Pa., 1980, The Mack Publishing Co.

Woods, S.: Monitoring pulmonary artery pressures, Am. J. Nurs. **76**(11):1765-1771, 1976.

Chapter 12

Bergersen, B. S.: Pharmacology in nursing, ed. 14, St. Louis, 1979, The C. V. Mosby Co.

Dell, D. D., and Snyder, J. A.: Marijuana: pro and con, Am. J. Nurs. **77:**630, 1977.

Ellinwood, E., and Kilbey, M., editors: Cocaine and other stimulants, New York, 1977, Plenum Press.

Goodman, L. S., and Gilman, A., editors: The pharmacological basis of therapeutics, ed. 5, New York, 1975, The Macmillan Co.

Goth, A.: Medical pharmacology, ed. 9, St. Louis, 1978, The C. V. Mosby Co.

Methadone maintenance, Med. Letter Drugs Ther. **16**(26), 1974.

Meyers, F. J., Jawetz, E., and Goldfien, A.: Review of medical pharmacology, ed. 6, Los Altos, Calif., 1978, Lange Medical Publications.

Nahas, G.: The fight against marijuana, Guideposts **35**(8):21-24, 1980.

Pradhan, S. N., and Dutta, S. N., editors: Drug abuse: clinical and basic aspects, St. Louis, 1977, The C. V. Mosby Co.

Ray, O. S.: Drugs, society and human behavior, ed. 2, St. Louis, 1978, The C. V. Mosby Co.

U.S. Government Printing Office References, Public Documents Department, Washington, D.C. 20402.

Latest revisions of following references, documents, pamphlets:

Amphetamines, report by the Select Committee on Crime, Catalog No. 91-2:H. rp. 1807.

Before your kid tries drugs, Catalog No. FS 2.22:D 84/10.

Community mental health approach to drug addiction, Catalog No. FS 17.2:D 84.

Community program guide, drug abuse prevention, Catalog No. J 24.8:D 84/2.

Drugs and you, Catalog No. D 2.14:FS-51.

Drugs of abuse, Catalog No. J 24-2:D 84.

Federal source book: Answers to the most frequently asked questions about drug abuse, Catalog No. PrEx 13.2: An 8.

Guidelines for drug abuse prevention education, Catalog No. J 24.8:D 84/4.

Handbook of federal narcotic and dangerous drug laws, Catalog No. J 24.8:N 16.

Hashish, pot, acid, speed, barbiturates, LSD; will they turn you on or will they turn on you, Catalog No. HE 20.2421: W 66.

Heroin and heroin paraphernalia, report by the Select Committee on Crime, Catalog No. 91-2:H. rp. 1808.

LSD: some questions and answers, Catalog No. HE 20.2402:L99/971.

LSD-25, a factual account, layman's guide to pharmacology, physiology, psychology, and sociology of LSD, Catalog No. J 24.8:L 99/rep.

Marihuana, some questions and answers, Catalog No. HE 20.2402:M33/2/970.

Marijuana fables and facts, Catalog No. HE 20.2402:M 33.

Narcotic drug addiction, Catalog No. FS 2.22/31:2.

Narcotics, some questions and answers, Catalog No. HE 20.2402:N16/2/971.

Recent research on narcotics, LSD, marihuana, and other dangerous drugs, Catalog No. HE 20.2402:N 16/4.

Resource book for drug abuse education, Catalog No. FS 2.22:D 84/12.

Sedatives, some questions and answers, Catalog No. HE 20.2402:SE 2.

Students and drug abuse, Catalog No. HE 20.2402:D 84/2.

Terms and symptoms of drug abuse, Catalog No. J 24.2:D 84/3.

Wild hemp (marijuana), how to control it, Catalog No. A 1.68:969.

Youthful drug use, Catalog No. HE 17.2:D 84/2.

Wiley, L., editor: Managing a hospitalized drug addict, Nursing '77 **7**(6):46, 1977.

Yowell, S., and Brose, C.: Working with drug abuse patients in the ER, Am. J. Nurs. **77:**82, 1977.

Chapter 13

American Hospital Formulary Service, Washington, D.C., 1979, American Society of Hospital Pharmacists.

Goodman, L. S., and Gilman, A., editors: The pharmacological basis of therapeutics, ed. 5, New York, 1975, The Macmillan Co.

Goth, A.: Medical pharmacology, ed. 9, St. Louis, 1978, The C. V. Mosby Co.

Lichtiger, M., and Moya, F., editors: Introduction to the practice of anesthesia, ed. 2, New York, 1978, Harper and Row, Publishers, Inc.

Wade, A.: Martindale—the extra pharmacopoeia, ed. 27, London, 1977, The Pharmaceutical Press.

Willson, J. R., Beecham, C. T., and Carrington, E. R.: Obstetrics and gynecology, ed. 5, St Louis, 1975, The C. V. Mosby Co.

Chapter 14

American Hospital Formulary Service, Washington, D.C., 1979, American Society of Hospital Pharmacists.

American Pharmaceutical Association: Evaluations of drug interactions, ed. 2, Washington, D.C., 1976, American Pharmaceutical Association.

Goodman, L. S., and Gilman, A., editors: The pharmacological basis of therapeutics, ed. 5, New York, 1975, The Macmillan Co.

Goth, A.: Medical pharmacology, ed. 9, St. Louis, 1978, The C. V. Mosby Co.

Kastrup, E. K., and Boyd, J. R.: Facts and comparisons, St. Louis, 1979, Facts and Comparisons, Inc.

Lichtiger, M., and Moya, F., editors: Introduction to the practice of anesthesia, ed. 2, New York, 1978, Harper and Row Publishers, Inc.

Modell, W., editor: Drugs of choice, 1978-1979, St. Louis, 1978, The C. V. Mosby Co.

Physician's desk reference, ed. 34, Oradell, N.J., 1980, Medical Economics Co.

Webber-Jones, J., and Bryant, M.: Over-the-counter bronchodilators: what are the risks of ''relief in seconds''?, Nursing 80 **10**(1):34-39, 1980.

Webb-Johnson, D., and Andrews, J. L., Jr.: Drug therapy: bronchodilator therapy, N. Engl. J. Med. **297:**758, 1977.

Chapter 15

American Hospital Formulary Service, Washington, D.C., 1979, American Society of Hospital Pharmacists.

American Medical Association: Drug evaluations, eds. 4 and 5, Acton, Mass., 1978, 1979, Publishing Sciences Group, Inc.

Bergersen, B. S.: Pharmacology in nursing, ed. 14, St. Louis, 1979, The C. V. Mosby Co.

Drug Data: Motrin, Am. J. Nurs. **75**(4):651, 1975.

Drug Data: Sinemet, Am. J. Nurs. **75**(12):2211, 1975.

Falconer, M. W., and others: The drug, the nurse, the patient, ed. 6, Philadelphia, 1978, W. B. Saunders Co.

Goodman, L. S., and Gilman, A., editors: The pharmacological basis of therapeutics, ed. 5, New York, 1975, The Macmillan Co.

Goth, A.: Medical pharmacology, ed. 9, St. Louis, 1978, The C. V. Mosby Co.

Kastrup, E. K., and Boyd, J. R.: Facts and comparisons, St. Louis, 1979, Facts and Comparisons, Inc.

Levine, R.: Pharmacology: drug actions and reactions, ed. 2, 1978, Little, Brown, & Co.

Lewis, A. J., editor: Modern drug encyclopedia, ed. 14, New York, 1977, Dun-Donnelley Publishing Corp.

Lichtiger, M., and Moya, F., editors: Introduction to the practice of anesthesia, ed. 2, New York, 1978, Harper and Row, Publishers, Inc.

Meyers, F. J., Jawetz, E., and Goldfien, A.: Review of medical pharmacology, ed. 6, Los Altos, Calif., 1978, Lange Medical Publications.

Modell, W., editor: Drugs of choice, 1978-1979, St. Louis, 1978, The C. V. Mosby Co.

Physician's desk reference, ed. 34, Oradell, N.J., 1980, Medical Economics Co.

Chapter 16

American Hospital Formulary Service, Washington, D.C., 1979, American Society of Hospital Pharmacists.

American Medical Association: Drug evaluations, eds. 4 and 5, Acton, Mass., 1978, 1979, Publishing Sciences Group, Inc.

Bergersen, B. S.: Pharmacology in nursing, ed. 14, St. Louis, 1979, The C. V. Mosby Co.

Collinsworth, K. A., and others: The clinical pharmacology of lidocaine as an antiarrhythmic drug, Circulation **50:**1217, 1974.

Deberry, P., and others: Teaching cardiac patients to manage medications, Am. J. Nurs. **75:**2191, 1975.

DiPalma, J. R.: Basic pharmacology in medicine, New York, 1976, McGraw-Hill Book Co.

Gifford, R. W., Jr.: Managing hypertension, Postgrad. Med. **61:**153, 1977.

Goodman, L. S., and Gilman, A., editors: The pharmacological basis of therapeutics, ed. 5, New York, 1975, The Macmillan Co.

Goth, A.: Medical pharmacology: principles and concepts, ed. 9, St. Louis, 1978, The C. V. Mosby Co.

Govani, L. E., and Hayes, J. E.: Drugs and nursing implications, ed. 3, New York, 1978, Appleton-Century-Crofts.

Gringauz, A.: Drugs: how they act and why, St. Louis, 1978, The C. V. Mosby Co.

Hand, J.: Keeping anticoagulants under control: how anticoagulants prevent blood clots, R.N. **42**(4):25-29, 1979.

Harrison, D. C.: Practical guidelines for the use of lidocaine, J.A.M.A. **233:**1202, 1975.

Kastrup, E. K., and Boyd, J. R.: Facts and comparisons, St. Louis, 1979, Facts and Comparisons, Inc.

Kosman, M. E.: Evaluation of a new antihypertensive agent: prazosin hydrochloride (Minipress), J.A.M.A. **238:**157, 1977.

Levine, R.: Pharmacology: drug actions and reactions, ed. 2, 1978, Little, Brown, & Co.

Lewis, A. J., editor: Modern drug encyclopedia, ed. 14, New York, 1977, Dun-Donnelley Publishing Corp.

Mason, D. T.: Digitalis pharmacology and therapeutics: recent advances, Ann. Intern. Med. **80:**520, 1974.

Meyers, F. H., Jawetz, E., and Goldfien, A.: Review of medical pharmacology, ed. 6, Los Altos, Calif., 1978, Lange Medical Publications.

Modell, W., editor: Drugs of choice 1978-1979, St. Louis, 1978, The C. V. Mosby Co.

Nies, A. S., and Shand, D. G.: Clinical pharmacology of propranolol, Circulation **52:**6, 1975.

Physician's desk reference, ed. 34, Oradell, N.J., 1980, Medical Economics Co.

Rodman, M. J.: The year's new drugs, R.N. **42**(1);33-40, 1979.

Rodman, M. J.: Drug therapy today: how to cope with those new antihypertensive drugs, R.N. **42**(10):109-116, 1979.

Ryan, S. A., and Clayton, B. D.: Handbook of practical pharmacology, ed. 2, St. Louis, 1980, The C. V. Mosby Co.

Wade, A.: Martindale—the extra pharmacopoeia, ed. 27, London, 1977, The Pharmaceutical Press.

Walton, C., and Hammond, B.: Angina: teaching your patient to prevent recurring attacks, Nursing 78 **8**(2):32, 1978.

White, S. J., and Williamson, K.: What to watch for when you give digitalis: the digitalis glycosides, R.N. **42**(10):61-63, 1979.

Chapter 17

American Hospital Formulary Service, Washington, D.C., 1979, American Society of Hospital Pharmacists.

American Medical Association: Drug evaluations, eds. 4 and 5, Acton, Mass. 1978, 1979, Publishing Sciences Group, Inc.

Bergersen, B. S.: Pharmacology in nursing, ed. 14, St. Louis, 1979, The C. V. Mosby Co.

Davies, D., and Wilson, G.: Diuretics: mechanism of action and clinical application, Drugs **9**:178, 1975.

Falconer, M. W., and others: The drug, the nurse, the patient, ed. 6, Philadelphia, 1978, W. B. Saunders Co.

Goodman, L. S., and Gilman, A., editors: The pharmacological basis of therapeutics, ed. 5, New York, 1975, The Macmillan Co.

Goth, A.: Medical pharmacology: principles and concepts, ed. 9, St. Louis, 1978, The C. V. Mosby Co.

Greenblatt, D., and others: Chronic toxicity of furosemide in hospitalized patients, Am. Heart J. **94**:6, 1977.

Gringauz, A.: Drugs: how they act and why, St. Louis, 1978, The C. V. Mosby Co.

Jacobson, H., and Kokko, J.: Diuretics: sites and mechanisms of action, Annu. Rev. Pharmacol. Toxicol. **16**:201, 1976.

Jamison, R., and Maffly, R.: The urinary concentrating mechanism, N. Engl. J. Med. **295**:1059, 1976.

Kastrup, E. K., and Boyd, J. R.: Facts and comprisons, St. Louis, 1979, Facts and Comparisons, Inc.

Koda-Kimble, M. A., Katcher, B., and Young, L.: Applied therapeutics for clinical pharmacists, ed. 2, San Francisco, 1978, Applied Therapeutics, Inc.

Levine, R.: Pharmacology: drug actions and reactions, ed. 2, 1978, Little, Brown, & Co.

Meyers, F. H., Jawetz, E., and Goldfien, A.: Review of medical pharmacology, ed. 6, Los Altos, Calif., 1978, Lange Medical Publications.

Modell, W.: editor: Drugs of choice 1978-1979, St. Louis, 1978, The C. V. Mosby Co.

Newmark, S., and Dluhy, R.: Hyperkalemia and hypokalemia, J.A.M.A. **231**:631, 1975.

Physicians' desk reference, ed. 34, Oradell, N.J., 1980, Medical Economics Co.

Rodman, M. J.: Fighting the second most frequent infections (the use of drugs to eradicate or curb urinary tract infections), R.N. **38**:11, 1975.

Ryan, S. A., and Clayton, B. D.: Handbook of practical pharmacology, ed. 2, St. Louis, 1980, The C. V. Mosby Co.

Wade, A.: Martindale—the extra pharmacopoeia, ed. 27, London, 1977, The Pharmaceutical Press.

Chapter 18

American Hospital Formulary Service, Washington, D.C., 1979, American Society of Hospital Pharmacists.

American Medical Association: Drug evaluations, eds. 4 and 5, Acton, Mass., 1978, 1979, Publishing Sciences Group, Inc.

American Pharmaceutical Association: Handbook of nonprescription drugs, ed. 6, Washington, D.C., 1979, American Pharmaceutical Association.

Bergersen, B. S.: Pharmacology in nursing, ed. 14, St. Louis, 1979, The C. V. Mosby Co.

Binder, H.: Pharmacology of laxatives, Annu. Rev. Pharmacol. Toxicol. **17**:355, 1977.

Bodemarg, G., and Wallan, A.: Cimetidine in the treatment of active duodenal and prepyloric ulcers, Lancet **2**:161-164, 1976.

Brown, M.: Over-the-counter gastrointestinal drugs, part 1, antacids, Nurse Practitioner **1**(5):15, 1976.

Brown, M.: Over-the-counter gastrointestinal drugs, part 3, antidiarrheal drugs, Nurse Practitioner **2**(1):23, 1976.

Brunner, L.: What to do (and what to teach your patient) about peptic ulcer, Nursing 76 **6**(11):27, 1976.

Drug Data: Fluorigard, Am. J. Nurs. **75**(5):865, 1975.

Falconer, M. W., and others: The drug, the nurse, the patient, ed. 6, Philadelphia, 1978, W. B. Saunders Co.

Galambos, J., and others: Loperamide: a new antidiarrheal agent in the treatment of chronic diarrhea, Gastroenterology **70**:1026-1029, 1976.

Goodman, L., and Gilman, A., editors: The pharmacological basis of therapeutics, ed. 5, New York, 1975, The Macmillan Co.

Goth, A.: Medical pharmacology, ed. 9, St. Louis, 1978, The C. V. Mosby Co.

Gringauz, A.: Drugs: how they act and why, St. Louis, 1978, The C. V. Mosby Co.

Hansten, P. D.: Drug interactions, ed. 4, Philadelphia, 1979, Lea & Febiger.

Isenberg, J.: Therapy of peptic ulcer, J.A.M.A. **233**:540, 1975.

Kastrup, E. K., and Boyd, J. R.: Facts and comparisons, St. Louis, 1979, Facts and Comparisons, Inc.

Levine, R.: Pharmacology: drug actions and reactions, ed. 2, 1978, Little, Brown, & Co.

Littman, A., and Pine, B.: Antacids and anticholinergic drugs, Ann. Intern. Med. **82**:544, 1975.

Meyers, F. H., Jawetz, E., and Goldfien, A.: Review of medical pharmacology, ed. 6, Los Altos, Calif., 1978, Lange Medical Publications.

Modell, W.: editor: Drugs of choice 1978-1979, St. Louis, 1978, The C. V. Mosby Co.

Physicians' desk reference, ed. 34, Oradell, N.J., 1980, Medical Economics Co.

Ryan, S. A., and Clayton, B. D.: Handbook of practical pharmacology, ed. 2, St. Louis, 1980, The C. V. Mosby Co.

Wade, A.: Martindale—the extra pharmacopoeia, ed. 27, London, 1977, The Pharmaceutical Press.

Chapter 19

American Hospital Formulary Service, Washington, D.C., 1979, American Society of Hospital Pharmacists.

American Medical Association: Drug evaluations, eds. 4 and

5, Acton, Mass., 1978, 1979, Publishing Sciences Group, Inc.

American Pharmaceutical Association: Handbook of nonprescription drugs, ed. 6, Washington, D.C., 1979, American Pharmaceutical Association.

Bergersen, B. S.: Pharmacology in nursing, ed. 14, St. Louis, 1979, The C. V. Mosby Co.

Bodemarg, G., and Wallan, A.: Cimetidine in treatment of active duodenal and prepyloric ulcers, Lancet **2:**161-164, 1976.

Danilevicius, Z.: A new star: how brightly will it shine? J.A.M.A. **237:**2224, 1977.

Falconer, M. W., and others: The drug, the nurse, the patient, ed. 6, Philadelphia, 1978, W. B. Saunders Co.

Fleischer, D., and Samloff, I.: Cimetidine therapy in a patient with a metiamide-induced agranulocytosis, N. Engl. J. Med. **296:**342, 1977.

Goodman, L. S., and Gilman, A., editors: The pharmacological basis of therapeutics, ed. 5, New York, 1975, The Macmillan Co.

Goth, A.: Medical pharmacology, ed. 9, St. Louis, 1978, The C. V. Mosby Co.

Kastrup, E. K., and Boyd, J. R.: Facts and comparisons, St. Louis, 1979, Facts and Comparisons, Inc.

Levine, R.: Pharmacology: drug actions and reactions, ed. 2, 1978, Little, Brown, & Co.

Lewis, A., editor: Modern drug encyclopedia, ed. 14, New York, 1977, Dun-Donnelley Publishing Corp.

Meyers, F. H., Jawetz, E., and Goldfien, A.: Review of medical pharmacology, ed. 6, Los Altos, Calif., 1978, Lange Medical Publications.

Modell, W., editor: Drugs of choice 1978-1979, St. Louis, 1978, The C. V. Mosby Co.

Physicians' desk reference, ed. 34, Oradell, N.J., 1980, Medical Economics Co.

Ryan, S. A., and Clayton, B. D.: Handbook of practical pharmacology, ed. 2, St. Louis, 1980, The C. V. Mosby Co.

Wade, A.: Martindale—the extra pharmacopoeia, ed. 27, London, 1977, The Pharmaceutical Press.

Chapter 20

American Hospital Formulary Service, Washington, D.C., 1979, American Society of Hospital Pharmacists.

American Medical Association: Drug evaluations, eds. 4 and 5, Acton, Mass., 1978, 1979, Publishing Sciences Group, Inc.

Benson, R. C.: Handbook of obstetrics and gynecology, ed. 5, Los Altos, Calif., 1974, Lange Medical Publications.

Bergersen, B. S.: Pharmacology in nursing, ed. 14, St. Louis, 1979, The C. V. Mosby Co.

Brown, M. S.: Syphilis and gonorrhea: an update for nurses, Nursing 76 **6:**171, 1976.

Chan, L., and O'Malley, B.: Mechanism of action of the sex steroid hormones, N. Engl. J. Med. **294:**1322, 1976.

Chung, H.: Arresting premature labor, Am. J. Nurs. **76:**810, 1976.

Cowart, M., and Newton, D.: Oral contraceptives: how best to explain their effects to patients, Nursing 76 **6**(6):44, 1976.

Falconer, M. W., and others: The drug, the nurse, the patient, ed. 6, Philadelphia, 1978, W. B. Saunders Co.

Goldfien, A.: Estrogen replacement therapy in postmenopausal women, Ration. Drug Ther. **11**(1):1, 1977.

Goodman, L. S., and Gilman, A., editors: The pharmacological basis of therapeutics, ed. 5, New York, 1975, The Macmillan Co.

Goth, A.: Medical pharmacology, ed. 9, St. Louis, 1978, The C. V. Mosby Co.

Graber, E., and Barber, H.: The case for and against estrogen therapy, Am. J. Nurs. **75:**10:1766, 1975.

Harvey, S.: New relief for menstrual discomfort, R.N. **42**(9):116, 1979.

Hoover, R., and others: Menopausal estrogens and breast cancer, N. Engl. J. Med. **295:**401, 1976.

Kastrup, E. K., and Boyd, J. R.: Facts and comparisons, St. Louis, 1979, Facts and Comparisons, Inc.

Levine, R.: Pharmacology: drug actions and reactions, ed. 2, 1978, Little, Brown, & Co.

Lewis, A., editor: Modern drug encyclopedia, ed. 14, New York, 1977, Dun-Donnelley Publishing Corp.

Marx, J.: Estrogen drugs: do they increase the risk of cancer? Science **191:**838, 1976.

Meyers, F. H., Jawetz, E., and Goldfien, A.: Review of medical pharmacology, ed. 6, Los Altos, Calif., 1978, Lange Medical Publications.

Modell, W.: editor: Drugs of choice 1978-1979, St. Louis, 1978, The C. V. Mosby Co.

Physicians' desk reference, ed. 34, Oradell, N. J., 1980, Medical Economics Co.

Rodman, M.: Drug therapy today: What we know now about oral contraceptives, R.N. **42**(9):133-146, 1979.

Romney, S. L., and others: Gynecology and obstetrics: the health care of women, New York, 1975, McGraw-Hill Book Co.

Ryan, S. A., and Clayton, B. D.: Handbook of practical pharmacology, ed. 2, St. Louis, 1980, The C. V. Mosby Co.

Swerdloff, R., and others: Complications of oral contraceptive agents—a symposium, West. J. Med. **122:**20, 1975.

Timby, B.: Ovulation method of birth control, Am. J. Nurs. **76:**928, 1976.

Vessey, M. P., and others: Oral contraceptives, and breast cancer: progress report of an epidemiological study, Lancet **1:**941, 1975.

Willson, J. R., Beecham, C. T., and Carrington, E. R.: Obstetrics and gynecology, ed. 5, St. Louis, 1979, The C. V. Mosby Co.

Chapter 21

American Hospital Formulary Service, Washington, D.C., 1979, American Society of Hospital Pharmacists.

American Medical Association: Drug evaluations, ed. 3, Littleton, Mass., 1977, Publishing Science Group, Inc.

Avioli, L.: The therapeutic approach to hypoparathyroidism, Am. J. Med. **54:**34, 1974.

Bergersen, B. S.: Pharmacology in nursing, ed. 14, St. Louis, 1979, The C. V. Mosby Co.

Conn, H., editor: Current therapy 1977, Philadelphia, 1977, W. B. Saunders Co.

DeLuca, H.: Vitamin D endocrinology, Ann. Inter. Med. **85:** 366, 1976.

Falconer, and others: The drug, the nurse, the patient, ed. 6, Philadelphia, 1978, W. B. Saunders Co.

Goodman, L. S., and Gilman, A., editors: The pharmacological basis of therapeutics, ed. 5, New York, 1975, The Macmillan Co.

Goth, A.: Medical pharmacology, ed. 9, St. Louis, 1978, The C. V. Mosby Co.

Hallal, J.: Thyroid disorders, Am. J. Nurs. **77**(3):418, 1977.

Kastrup, E. K., and Boyd, J. R.: Facts and comparisons, St. Louis, 1979, Facts and Comparisons, Inc.

Larsen, P.: Hyperthyroidism, D. M. **22:**10, 1976.

Levine, R.: Pharmacology: drug actions and reactions, ed. 2, 1978, Little, Brown, & Co.

Lewis, A., editor: Modern drug encyclopedia, ed. 14, New York, 1977, Dun-Donnelley Publishing Corp.

Meyers, F. H., Jawetz, E., and Goldfien, A.: Review of medical pharmacology, ed. 6, Los Altos, Calif., 1978, Lange Medical Publications.

Modell, W., editor: Drugs of choice 1978-1979, St. Louis, 1978, The C. V. Mosby Co.

Newton, D., and others: You can minimize the hazards of corticosteroids, Nursing 77 **7**(6):26, 1977.

Physicians' desk reference, ed. 34, Oradell, N.J., 1980, Medical Economics Co.

Ryan, S. A., and Clayton, B. D.: Handbook of practical pharmacology, ed. 2, St. Louis, 1980, The C. V. Mosby Co.

Strobele, B.: How to counsel patients on cortisone, R.N. **38**(7): 57, 1975.

Wade, A.: Martindale—the extra pharmacopoeia, ed. 27, London, 1977, The Pharmaceutical Press.

Walton, J., and Ney, R.: Current concepts of corticosteroids, uses and abuses, Chicago, 1975, Year Book Medical Publishers, Inc.

Willson, J. R., Beecham, C. T., and Carrington, E. R.: Obstetrics and gynecology, ed. 5, St. Louis, 1975, The C. V. Mosby Co.

Chapter 22

American Pharmaceutical Association: Handbook of nonprescription drugs, ed. 6, Washington, D.C., 1979, American Pharmaceutical Association.

Bergersen, B. S.: Pharmacology in nursing, ed. 14, St. Louis, 1979, The C. V. Mosby Co.

Boyd-Monk, H., consultant: Screening for glaucoma, Nursing 79 **9**(8):43-45, 1979.

Conn, H., editor: Current therapy 1977, Philadelphia, 1977, W. B. Saunders Co.

Falconer, M. W., and others: The drug, the nurse, the patient, ed. 6, Philadelphia, 1978, W. B. Saunders Co.

Fernsebner, W.: Early diagnosis of acute-angle-closure glaucoma, Am. J. Nurs. **75**:7:1154, 1975.

Goth, A.: Medical pharmacology, ed. 9, St. Louis, 1978, The C. V. Mosby Co.

Havener, W., and others: Nursing care in eye, ear, nose, and throat disorders, St. Louis, 1974, The C. V. Mosby Co.

Hussar, D.: New drugs '78, '79, Nursing 79 **9**(5):38, 1979.

Kastrup, E. K., and Boyd, J. R.: Facts and comparisons, St. Louis, 1979, Facts and Comparisons, Inc.

Loebl, S., Spratto, G., and Wit, A.: The nurse's drug handbook, New York, 1977, John Wiley & Sons, Inc.

Meyers, F. H., Jawetz, E., and Goldfien, A.: Review of medical pharmacology, ed. 6, Los Altos, Calif., 1978, Lange Medical Publications.

Newell, F. W.: Ophthalmology, principles and concepts, ed. 2, St. Louis, 1969, The C. V. Mosby Co.

Physician's desk reference, 34, Oradell, N.J., 1980, Medical Economics Co.

Chapter 23

American Hospital Formulary Service, Washington, D.C., 1979, American Society of Hospital Pharmacists.

Bergersen, B. S.: Pharmacology in nursing, ed. 14, St. Louis, 1979, The C. V. Mosby Co.

Drug data: What's new in drugs: cefaclor (Ceclor) R.N. **42**(8): 88, 1979.

Drug data: what's new in drugs: a new antibiotic: cyclacillin (Cyclapen), R.N. **43**(1):109, 1980.

Drug data: Mandol (cefamandole nafate), Am. J. Nurs. **79**(9): 1615, 1979.

Goodman, L. S., and Gilman, A., editors: The pharmacological basis of therapeutics, ed. 5, New York, 1975, The Macmillan Co.

Kastrup, E. K., and Boyd, J. R.: Facts and comparisons, St. Louis, 1979, Facts and Comparisons, Inc.

Physician's desk reference, 34, Oradell, N.J., 1980, Medical Economics Co.

Rodman, M. J., and Smith, D. W.: Clinical pharmacology in nursing, Philadelphia, 1974, J. B. Lippincott Co.

Ryan, S. A., and Clayton, B. D.: Handbook of practical pharmacology, ed. 2, St. Louis, 1980, The C. V. Mosby Co.

White, S., and Williamson, K.: What to watch for when you give penicillin: the penicillins, R.N. **42**(6):21-23, 1979.

White, S., and Williamson, K.: What to watch for when you give tetracyclines: the tetracyclines, R.N. **42**(7):31-33, 1979.

White, S., and Williamson, K.: What to watch for when you give a cephalosporin: the cephalosporins, R.N. **42**(8):30-32, 1979.

White, S., and Williamson, K.: What to watch for when you give aminoglycosides: the aminoglycosides, R.N. **42**(9):75-77, 1979.

Chapter 24

American Hospital Formulary Service, Washington, D.C., 1979, American Society of Hospital Pharmacists.

American Pharmaceutical Association: Handbook of nonprescription drugs, ed. 6, Washington, D.C., 1979, American Pharmaceutical Association.

Goodman, L. S., and Gilman, A., editors: The pharmacological basis of therapeutics, ed. 5, New York, 1975, The Macmillan Co.

Kastrup, E. K., and Boyd, J. R.: Facts and comparisons, St. Louis, 1979, Facts and Comparisons, Inc.

Chapter 25

Bergersen, B. S.: Pharmacology in nursing, ed. 14, St. Louis, 1979, The C. V. Mosby Co.

Block, S. S., editor: Disinfection, sterilization and preservation, ed. 2, Philadelphia, 1977, Lea & Febiger.

Goth, A.: Medical pharmacology, ed. 9, St. Louis, 1978, The C. V. Mosby Co.

Kastrup, E. K., and Boyd, J. R.: Facts and comparisons, St. Louis, 1979, Facts and Comparisons, Inc.

Wade, A.: Martindale—the extra pharmacopoeia, ed. 27, London, 1977, The Pharmaceutical Press.

Chapter 26

American Medical Association: Drug evaluations, ed. 3, Littleton, Mass., 1977, Publishing Sciences Group, Inc.

Bergersen, B. S.: Pharmacology in nursing, ed. 14, St. Louis, 1979, The C. V. Mosby Co.

Goodman, L., and Gilman, A., editors: The pharmacological basis of therapeutics, ed. 5, New York, 1975, The Macmillan Co.

Hawkins, K.: Wet dressings: putting the damper on dermatitis, Nursing 78 **8**(2):64, 1978.

Jacoby, F.: Nursing care of the patient with burns, ed. 2, St. Louis, 1976, The C. V. Mosby Co.

Kastrup, E. K., and Boyd, J. R.: Facts and comparisons, St. Louis, 1979, Facts and Comparisons, Inc.

Medication tips: clotrimazole, antifungal agent, R.N. **42**(5):143, 1979.

Meyers, F., Jawetz, E., and Goldfien, A.: Review of medical pharmacology, ed. 6, Los Altos, Calif., 1978, Lange Medical Publications.

Modell, W., editor: Drugs of choice 1978-1979, St. Louis, 1978, The C. V. Mosby Co.

Physicians' desk reference, ed. 34, Oradell, N.J., 1980, Medical Economics Co.

Schumann, L,. and Gaston, S.: Commonsense guide to topical burn therapy, Nursing 79 **9**(3):34-39, 1979.

Chapter 27

Bergersen, B. S.: Pharmacology in nursing, ed. 14, St. Louis, 1979, The C. V. Mosby Co.

Bochow, A.: Cancer immunotherapy; what promise does it hold? Nursing 76 **6**(10):50, 1976.

Burns, N.: Cancer chemotherapy: a systemic approach, Nursing 78 **8**(2):57, 1978.

Chabner, B., and others: The clinical pharmacology of antineoplastic agents, N. Engl. J. Med. **292**:1159, 1975.

Desotell, S.: A brighter future for leukemia patients, Nursing 77 **7**(1):18, 1977.

Falconer, M. W., and others: The drug, the nurse, the patient, ed. 6, Philadelphia, 1978, W. B. Saunders Co.

Goodman, L. S., and Gilman, A., editors: The pharmacological basis of therapeutics, ed. 5, New York, 1975, The Macmillan Co.

Goth, A.: Medical pharmacology: principles and concepts, ed. 9, St. Louis, 1978, The C. V. Mosby Co.

Hoover, R., and others: Menopausal estrogens and breast cancer, N. Engl. J. Med. **295**:401, 1976.

Kastrup, E. K., and Boyd, J. R.: Facts and comparisons, St. Louis, 1979, Facts and Comparisons, Inc.

Keaveny, M., and Wiley, L.: Hodgkin's disease, the curable cancer, Nursing 75 **5**:(3):48, 1975.

Meyers, F., Jawetz, E., and Goldfien, A.: Review of medical pharmacology, ed. 6, Los Altos, Calif., 1978, Lange Medical Publications.

Miller, S. A.: Oncology nurse and chemotherapy, Am. J. Nurs. **77**:989, 1977.

Oswalt, C., and Cruz, A.: Cancer chemotherapeutic agents, Tex. Med. **73**:57, 1977.

Ryan, S. A., and Clayton, B. D.: Handbook of practical pharmacology, ed. 2, St. Louis, 1980, The C. V. Mosby Co.

Scogna, D., and Smalley, R.: Chemotherapy-induced nausea and vomiting, Am. J. Nurs. **79**(9):1512-1514, 1979.

Wackenhut, J. S., and Barnwell, R. A.: Burkitt's lymphoma, Am. J. Nurs. **79**(10):1766-1770, 1979.

Wade, A.: Martindale—the extra pharmacopoeia, ed. 27, London, 1977, The Pharmaceutical Press.

Chapter 28

American Hospital Formulary Service, Washington, D.C., 1979, American Society of Hospital Pharmacists.

American Medical Association: Drug evaluations, ed. 3, Littleton, Mass., 1977, Publishing Sciences Group, Inc.

Bergersen, B. A.: Pharmacology in nursing, ed. 14, St. Louis, 1979, The C. V. Mosby Co.

Brown, M. S.: What you should know about communicable diseases and their immunizations, part 1, Nursing 75 **5**(9):70, 1975.

Brown, M. S.: What you should know about communicable diseases and their immunizations, part 2, Nursing 75 **5**(10):56, 1975.

Brown, M. S.: What you should know about communicable diseases and their immunizations, part 3, Nursing 75 **5**(11):55, 1975.

Falconer, M. W., and others: The drug, the nurse, the patient, ed. 6, Philadelphia, 1978, W. B. Saunders Co.

Goldstein, J., and others: Smallpox vaccination reactions, prophylaxis and therapy of complications, Pediatrics **55**:342, 1975.

Goodman, L. S., and Gilman, A., editors: The pharmacological basis of therapeutics, ed. 5, New York, 1975, The Macmillan Co.

Jackson, G., and Stanley, E.: Prevention and control of influenza by chemoprophylaxis and chemotherapy, J.A.M.A. **235**:2739, 1976.

Kastrup, E. K., and Boyd, J. R.: Facts and comparisons, St. Louis, 1979, Facts and Comparisons, Inc.

Krugman, S., and Katz, S.: Rubella immunization: a five-year progress report, N. Engl. J. Med. **290**:1375, 1974.

Modell, W., editor: Drugs of choice 1978-1979, St. Louis, 1978, The C. V. Mosby Co.

O'Grady, R., and Dolan, T.: Whooping cough in infancy, Am. J. Nurs. **76**:114, 1976.

Physician's desk reference, 34, Oradell, N.J., 1980, Medical Economics Co.

Ryan, S. A., and Clayton, B. D.: Handbook of practical pharmacology, ed. 2, St. Louis, 1980, The C. V. Mosby Co.

Chapter 29

American Hospital Formulary Service, Washington, D.C., 1979, American Society of Hospital Pharmacists.

Goodman, L. S., and Gilman, A., editors: The pharmacological basis of therapeutics, ed. 5, New York, 1975, The Macmillan Co.

Goth, A.: Medical pharmacology, ed. 9, St. Louis, 1978, The C. V. Mosby Co.

Kastrup, E. K., and Boyd, J. R.: Facts and comparisons, St. Louis, 1979, Facts and Comparisons, Inc.

Modell, W., editor: Drugs of choice 1978-1979, St. Louis, 1978, The C. V. Mosby Co.

Physician's desk reference, 34, Oradell, N.J., 1980, Medical Economics Co.

Index

ANSWER BOOK FOR
Basic pharmacology for nurses

JESSIE E. SQUIRE, R.N., B.A., M.Ed.

Professor Emeritus, De Anza College School of Nursing,
Cupertino, California, Foothill Junior College District;
formerly Instructor, Foothill College School of Vocational Nursing,
Los Altos Hills, California, Foothill Junior College District;
formerly Instructor, Hayward-Fairmont School of Vocational Nursing,
Hayward Adult and Technical School, Hayward Unified School District,
Hayward, California

BRUCE D. CLAYTON, B.S., Pharm.D.

Associate Professor and Vice-Chairman,
Department of Pharmacy Practice,
College of Pharmacy,
University of Nebraska Medical Center,
Omaha, Nebraska

SEVENTH EDITION

Copyright © 1981 by The C. V. Mosby Company

ST. LOUIS • TORONTO • LONDON

Printed in the United States of America

Chapter 5

1. a. XVII
   b. LXV
   c. XCIX
   d. C
   e. LXXV
   f. XLV
   g. XXXVIII
   h. LIX
2. a. 110
   b. 60
   c. 45
   d. 30
   e. 48
   f. 4
   g. 25
   h. 90
3. a. 2
   b. 6 1/3
   c. 1
   d. 9 3/5
   e. 8
   f. 5 3/7
   g. 11 1/8
   h. 25
4. a. 23/24
   b. 8 13/30
   c. 1 13/40
   d. 1 73/90
5. a. 0.679
   b. 1.565
   c. 1.4278
6. a. 346.739
   b. 126.492
   c. 2097.29
7. a. 1/2
   b. 1 7/8
   c. 1
   d. 7 3/4
8. a. 7.3
   b. 165.26
   c. 8
   d. 183.71
9. a. 1/8
   b. 27
   c. 32
   d. 13
10. a. 526.89
    b. 51
    c. 728.192
    d. 26.52
11. a. 25/28
    b. 2 2/3
    c. 4/25
12. a. 3.65
    b. 6.3
    c. 34.86
13. a. 1/2
    b. 3/4
    c. 1/150
    d. 1/50

14. a. 0.75
    b. 0.9
    c. 1.5
    d. 4.25
15. a. 50%
    b. 7%
    c. 0.09%
    d. 33%
16. a. 1.6
    b. 10
    c. 0.64
    d. 5
17. a. one
    b. one-tenth
    c. one-tenth
    d. one
    e. five
18. a. 1:8
    b. 1:50
    c. 1:250
    d. 1:125
19. a. 540
    b. 2
    c. 9000
    d. 10
    e. 2
    f. 0.5
    g. 30
    h. 5

Chapter 6

8. 1 lb
9. 16
10. 480 gr, 1 oz
13. 1 f℥
14. 1 f℥
16. 1 pt
17. 1 qt
18. 1 gal
37. a. 225 gr
    b. 450 gr
    c. 15 gr
38. a. .06 g
    b. .325 g
    c. .650 g
    d. 1.0 g
39. a. 1 ml
    b. 4 ml
    c. 500 mg
40. a. 250 mg
    b. 125 mg
    c. 0.6 mg
    d. 500 mg
41. a. 0.5 g
    b. 0.1 g
    c. .0001 g
    d. 0.05 g
    e. 0.2 g
    f. .0006 g

43. a. 1 pt
    b. 2 pt
    c. 20 pt
44. a. 10 qt
    b. 3 qt
    c. 4 qt
45. a. 2 gal
    b. 3 gal
    c. 1 gal

Chapter 8

14. a. 0.2 ml
    b. 0.01 ml
    c. 0.5 ml
    d. 0.1 ml
    e. 0.5 ml
    f. add 2 ampules to 1000 ml D5/W
    g. 0.3 ml
    h. add two 20-mg vials to 250 ml D5/W; set rate at 31 ml/min
    i. 68.1 mg
    j. 100 cc
    k. 1 ml
    l. 12 ml
    m. 0.25 ml
    n. 1 g/20 ml sterile water to 80 cc D5/W; set rate at 100 cc/30 min
    o. 4 ml
    p. add 6 ml penicillin G to 1000 cc D5/W; set rate at 250 cc/hr
    q. dilute powder with 5 ml sterile water; add 5 ml solution to 1000 cc D5W/0.45% NaCl solution
15. 8 minims or 0.5 cc (ml)
16. 12 minims or 0.8 cc (ml)
17. 3 minims or 0.2 cc (ml)
18. 100/2 cc (ml); administer 1.5 cc (ml)
19. 100/2 cc (ml); administer 0.5 cc (ml)
20. 100/1 cc (ml); administer 0.2 cc (ml)
21. 0.5 cc (ml)
23. 0.75 cc (ml)

Chapter 10

90. 1/2 tablet
91. 2 tablets
92. 1 tablet

Chapter 11

31. 3 tablets
32. 1 tablet

Chapter 13

23. Nembutal
    Sodium: 50 mg or
    1 cc (ml), or
    half the dose on hand

    Demerol: 20/50 or
    2/5 of total dose
    of 1 cc (ml) or
    0.4 cc (ml)

    Scopolamine: 0.3/0.5
    or 3/5 x 1 cc (ml)
    or 0.6 cc (ml)

Chapter 14

32. 2 tablets

Chapter 15

15. 1 tablet
16. 1/2 tablet

Chapter 16

62. 3 tablets
63. 1/2 tablet
64. 1 tablet

Chapter 17

25. 1 tablet
26. 1 tablet

Chapter 19

10. 2 tablets

Chapter 20

33. 2 tablets
34. 2 tablets

Chapter 21

21. 2 tablets

Chapter 22

42. 2 tablets

Chapter 23

20. 0.5 g
21. 2 capsules

Chapter 29

9. 2 tablets
10. .5 g (0.5 g)